Medical Terminology

An Illustrated Guide

SIXTH EDITION

Barbara Janson Cohen, MEd

 Wolters Kluwer | Lippincott Williams & Wilkins
Health

Philadelphia • Baltimore • New York • London
Buenos Aires • Hong Kong • Sydney • Tokyo

Senior Publisher: Julie K. Stegman
Product Director: Eric Branger
Associate Product Manager: Erin Cosyn
Marketing Manager: Allison Powell
Design Manager: Stephen Druding
Compositor: Aptara, Inc.
Printer: C&C Offset Printing

351 West Camden Street   530 Walnut St.
Baltimore, MD 21201   Philadelphia, PA 19106

Library of Congress Cataloging-in-Publication Data

Cohen, Barbara J.
  Medical terminology : an illustrated guide / Barbara Janson Cohen. –
6th ed.
     p. ; cm.
  Includes bibliographical references and index.
  ISBN 978-1-60547-604-9 (alk. paper)
  1. Medicine–Terminology. I. Title.
  [DNLM: 1. Terminology as Topic. W 15 C678m 2011]
  R123.C56 2011
  610.1'4–dc22
                                                                    2009048269

DISCLAIMER

Care has been taken to confirm the accuracy of the information present and to describe generally accepted practices. However, the authors, editors, and publisher are not responsible for errors or omissions or for any consequences from application of the information in this book and make no warranty, expressed or implied, with respect to the currency, completeness, or accuracy of the contents of the publication. Application of this information in a particular situation remains the professional responsibility of the practitioner; the clinical treatments described and recommended may not be considered absolute and universal recommendations.

The authors, editors, and publishers have exerted every effort to ensure that drug selection and dosage set forth in this text are in accordance with current recommendations and practice at the time of publication. However, in view of ongoing research, changes in government regulations, and the constant flow of information relating to drug therapy and drug reactions, the reader is urged to check the package insert for each drug for any change in indications and dosage and for added warnings and precautions. This is particularly important when the recommended agent is a new or infrequently employed drug.

Some drugs and medical devices presented in this publication have Food and Drug Administration (FDA) clearance for limited use in restricted research settings. It is the responsibility of the health care provider to ascertain the FDA status of each drug or device planned for use in their clinical practice.

To purchase additional copies of this book, call our customer service department at **(800) 638-3030** or fax orders to **(301) 824-7390**. For other book services, including chapter reprints and large quantity sales, ask for the Special Sales department.

For all other calls originating outside of the United States, please call **(301) 714-2324**.

Visit Stedman's on the Internet: http://www.stedmans.com. Lippincott Williams & Wilkins customer service representatives are available from 8:30 a.m. to 4:30 p.m., EST, Monday through Friday, for telephone access.

Preface

Every career in health care begins with learning the vast and challenging language of medical terminology. Without adequate learning and teaching resources, it can be an overwhelming challenge for students and faculty. This sixth edition of *Medical Terminology: An Illustrated Guide* meets that challenge with clear organization, many full-color illustrations with a strong clinical focus, a wide array of effective pedagogical features, a variety of activities, and useful ancillaries to make teaching and learning more effective. Because the content is so accessible and logically organized, the text can be used as part of classroom instruction, for independent study, or for distance learning.

Organization and Approach

Medical Terminology: An Illustrated Guide, 6th Edition, takes a stepwise approach to learning the language of medical terminology. Part I describes how medical terms are built from separate word parts and gives an overview of body structure. Part II introduces concepts of disease and treatment. Students should study these chapters before proceeding to Part III, which describes each of the body systems. While using the systems approach common to anatomy and physiology texts, this book alters the typical sequence to present systems of the most general medical importance first, the cardiovascular and respiratory systems, for example, followed by chapters on the more focused medical specialties. Individual chapters build on knowledge in stages. The Key Terms sections list the terms most commonly used; more specialized terms are included in a later section entitled "Supplementary Terms." Students may study the latter terms according to the time available and their needs.

Each chapter opens with an indexed chapter outline, a list of student objectives—goals to be accomplished by the completion of the chapter—and a chapter pretest, testing a student's previous knowledge to measure progress. In Part III, the chapters begin with an overview of the normal structure and function of the system under study, followed by a list of key terms with definitions and mention of some roots. Word parts related to each topic are then presented and illustrated, along with exercises on the new material. Next, there is an overview of clinical information pertaining to the system, also followed by a list of key terms with definitions. Most chapters contain reference boxes that unify and simplify material on specific topics. There are also special interest boxes on health care professions, clinical topics, and word derivations and usage.

Pedagogical Features

Features of *Medical Terminology: An Illustrated Guide*, 6th Edition, have been designed to bring the content alive and to aid in understanding and retention (also see the User's Guide).

- **Illustrations**—Detailed, full-color drawings and photographs illuminate the chapters. These include clinical photographs and tissue micrographs. The many figures amplify and clarify the text and are particularly helpful for visual learners.

- **Pronunciations**—This text places great emphasis on pronunciation, and phonetic pronunciations are included with all new terms. It is important to practice saying these words and to be able to recognize them when they are heard.

- **Pretests**—Short quizzes to test previous knowledge begin each chapter. Students should take each quiz before starting the chapter and again after completing the chapter in order to measure progress.

- **Exercises**—Exercises accompany the introduction of all material, and review exercises conclude each chapter. Many of the illustrations have corresponding labeling exercises accompanied by helpful alphabetical word lists. All answers are included in the Answer Key at the end of the book. Students are actively involved in the learning process by answering questions on new material, checking answers with the answer keys, correcting mistakes, and keeping track of progress with review exercises.

- **Use of Dictionaries**—Word exercises that may require dictionary use are included in chapter review exercises. Some information on medical dictionaries is given in Chapter 1. Appendix 9 provides a sample page from a medical dictionary with information on how it is used.

- **Case Studies**—Case studies that present terminology in the context of a medical report are included in all chapters, followed by related questions. Professionals in a variety of health occupations figure in these scenarios to represent the diverse work settings students may encounter. Because they may include information learned in a previous chapter, the case studies also serve as an excellent review. Understanding these cases, especially those in the early parts of the book, may seem challenging for students, but much of the information needed to answer the questions is given in the histories, and students should make their best efforts to figure out the answers. These can be verified with the Answer Key.

- **Glossaries of Word Parts**—In working through the exercises, students can refer to complementary lists at the end of the text. Appendix 3 lists word parts and their meanings, and Appendix 4 lists meanings with corresponding word parts. Appendices 5 through 7 have lists of roots, suffixes, and prefixes alone. The remaining appendices include symbols, abbreviations, and units of the metric system.

- **Flashcards**—Because flashcards offer an excellent way to learn this new vocabulary, a section with more than 100 flashcards is included at the back of the text. Flashcard content is presented in chapter order so that the cards can be removed in sequence as students progress through the book. Students can make additional cards to match the cards in the book by cutting 3 × 5 cards in half. The Student Resources website provides printable flashcards and the capacity to make unlimited additional cards.

Students are also encouraged to create their own learning aids, such as devising a practice test by covering lists of words and testing themselves on the definitions, or by covering definitions and testing themselves on the words. The same can be done with the charts on word parts and their definitions. It is also helpful for students to keep a personal list of words that they find difficult to spell or pronounce.

PASSport to Success® for Students

  Look for this icon throughout the book for pertinent supplementary material on the companion website.

The PASSport to Success® is a practical system that lets students learn faster, remember more, and achieve success. Students discover their unique learning style—visual, auditory, or kinesthetic—with a simple online assessment; they choose from a wealth of resources for each learning style including animations, 16 different types of online learning activities, an audio glossary, an online dictionary application (including audio pronunciations of terms), a flashcard application (including a flashcard generator, which allows you to build your own unique set of flashcards), and other supplemental materials. Throughout the textbook, the graphic icon shown above alerts students to pertinent supplementary material.

The PASSport to Success® is available from the book's companion website at http://thePoint.lww.com/CohenMedTerm6e. See the inside cover of this text for the passcode you will need to gain access to the website, and refer to the User's Guide for all details about the PASSport to Success® and a complete listing of student resources.

Instructor Ancillary Package

A strong package of ancillary materials is available to instructors with this edition. All resources are available to approved adopting instructors online at http://thePoint.lww.com/CohenMedTerm6e. These resources include the following:

- **PowerPoint slides** for each chapter organized by learning objectives
- **Lesson plans** for each chapter, organized around the learning objectives, and include lecture notes and in-class activities and assignments
- **Word search activities**
- **Fill-in-the-blank tables**
- **Image bank** of all images from the text
- **Instructor's Test Generator** with more than 500 questions in different formats (multiple choice, true–false, fill-in-the-blank, and matching)
- **WebCT and Blackboard-ready Cartridge**, which allows you to integrate the ancillary materials, by exercise type, into learning management systems

Summary

An understanding of medical terminology provides an essential foundation for any career in health care. *Medical Terminology: An Illustrated Guide*, 6th Edition, both the textbook and its ancillaries, makes learning and teaching medical terminology a rewarding and exciting process.

Acknowledgments

In preparing this 6th edition of *Medical Terminology: An Illustrated Guide*, my thanks go, once again, to the talented and dedicated staff at Lippincott Williams & Wilkins. Senior Publisher, Julie Stegman, and Product Director, Eric Branger, were at the helm of this project. Erin Cosyn, Associate Product Manager, Amy Rowland, Editorial Assistant, and Heather Rybacki, Senior Production Manager, handled the innumerable daily tasks required for publication of a textbook. Production Manager, Richard Rosenberg, took charge of the electronic ancillaries and their placement on *thePoint*. Allison Noplock was in charge of marketing.

Thanks once more to my able contributor, Jason James Taylor, who wrote many of the special interest boxes that appear in the text and also created all of the original student and instructor resource materials.

I truly appreciate the efforts of the many reviewers who have evaluated past editions of the book as well as this new edition. Their suggestions have greatly improved this text over the years.

For perennially needed advice and assistance, I thank my husband, Matthew, an instructor of anatomy and physiology.

Barbara Janson Cohen

Reviewers

We gratefully acknowledge the generous contributions of the manuscript reviewers whose names appear in the list that follows:

Mary Elizabeth W. Browder, MEd, CMA(AAMA)
Assistant Professor, Medical Assisting
Raymond Walters College
    University of Cincinnati
Cincinnati, Ohio

Schvon Bussey, MSN
Nursing Instructor
Practical Nursing Department
Albany Technical College
Albany, Georgia

Mindy Carr, MEd, BSN, RN
Clinical Director, Paramedic Technology
Adjunct Faculty, Health Science
Pennsylvania College of Technology, Pennsylvania State
    University Affiliate
Williamsport, Pennsylvania

Ursula Dyer, MS, BSRT, (R)(CT)
Program Director
Radiologic Science Program
Kilgore College
Kilgore, Texas

Steven Goldschmidt, DC
Instructor
HCM
Inverhills Community College
Inver Grove Heights, Minnesota

Jennifer Lamé, MPH, RHIT
Coding Certificate Program Coordinator
Health and Human Services Department
Southwest Wisconsin Technical College
Fennimore, Wisconsin

Barbareta A. Welch McGill, RN, MSN, DRS
Clinical Assistant Professor
Nursing
North Carolina Central University
Durham, North Carolina

Elizabeth Pagenkopf, RN, MA
Adjunct Faculty, RN
Health Careers
Harper College
Palatine, Illinois

Shawn Marie Russell
Allied Health Program Coordinator
Assistant Professor of Allied Health
College of Rural and Community Development
    Health Programs
University of Alaska Fairbanks
Fairbanks, Alaska

Beryl Stetson, RNBC, MSN
Assistant Professor—Nursing
Raritan Valley Community College
Somerville, New Jersey
Nursing Education Specialist
Robert Wood Johnson University Hospital
New Brunswick, New Jersey

User's Guide

Medical Terminology: An Illustrated Guide, 6th Edition, was created and developed to help you master the language of medicine. The tools and features in the text will help you work through the material presented. Please take a few moments to look through this User's Guide, which will introduce you to the features that will enhance your learning experience.

Chapter Contents, Objectives, and Pretests

Chapter Contents and Objectives help you identify learning goals and familiarize yourself with the materials covered in the chapter. **Chapter Pretests** quiz students on previous knowledge at the beginning of each chapter. Students should take each Chapter Pretest before starting the chapter and again after completing the chapter in order to measure progress.

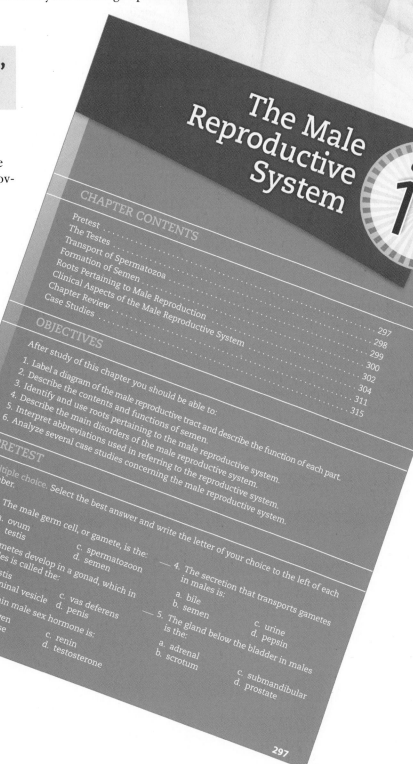

The Male Reproductive System

CHAPTER 14

CHAPTER CONTENTS

OBJECTIVES

After study of this chapter you should be able to:

1. Label a diagram of the male reproductive tract and describe the function of each part.
2. Describe the contents and functions of semen.
3. Identify and use roots pertaining to the male reproductive system.
4. Describe the main disorders of the male reproductive system.
5. Interpret abbreviations used in referring to the reproductive system.
6. Analyze several case studies concerning the male reproductive system.

PRETEST

Multiple choice. Select the best answer and write the letter of your choice to the left of each number.

_____ 1. The male germ cell, or gamete, is the:
   a. ovum
   b. testis
   c. spermatozoon
   d. semen

_____ 2. Gametes develop in a gonad, which in males is called the:
   a. testis
   b. seminal vesicle
   c. vas deferens
   d. penis

_____ 3. The main male sex hormone is:
   a. estrogen
   b. amylase
   c. renin
   d. testosterone

_____ 4. The secretion that transports gametes in males is:
   a. bile
   b. semen
   c. urine
   d. pepsin

_____ 5. The gland below the bladder in males is the:
   a. adrenal
   b. scrotum
   c. submandibular
   d. prostate

297

Detailed Illustrations

Illustrations: Detailed, full-color drawings and photographs illuminate the chapters. These include clinical photographs and tissue micrographs. The many figures amplify and clarify the text and are particularly helpful for visual learners.

Figure 15-12 Ovulation and fertilization. Arrows show the pathway of spermatozoa and ovum. Fertilization occurs in the oviduct, after which the zygote implants in the uterine lining.

Figure 12-4   Intestinal villi. (*A*) Microscopic view of the small intestine's lining showing villi and glands that secrete mucus and digestive juices. The lumen is the central opening. (*B*) An intestinal villus. Each villus has blood vessels and a lacteal (lymphatic capillary) for nutrient absorption.

Figure 4-4   The stages in cell division (mitosis). When it is not undergoing mitosis, the cell is in interphase. The cell shown is for illustration only. It is not a human cell, which has 46 chromosomes.

Figure 18-2   The ear. Structures in the outer, middle, and inner divisions are shown.

Case Studies and Case Study Questions

Case Studies and Case Study Questions in every chapter present terminology in the context of a medical report. These are an excellent review tool as they test your cumulative knowledge of medical terminology, and put terminology into a real-world context.

Case Studies

Case Study 18-1: Medical Records

An electrical fire in the physicians' dictation room left a charred mass of burned and water-damaged medical records. Discharge charts had been stacked awaiting physician sign-off before they could be returned to Medical Records for storage. Several medical transcriptionists spent 3 days sorting through the remains to reassemble the charts, all of which were from the patients of the large otorhinolaryngology practice. In addition to patient identification information, the transcriptionists matched word cues to create piles of similar documents. Patients treated for middle and inner ear problems were identified with words such as stapedectomy, tympanoplasty, myringotomy, cochlear, cholesteatoma, otosclerosis, labyrinth, otitis media, and acoustic neuroma. Patients treated for external ear conditions were grouped using terms such as otoplasty, pinna, postauricular, and otitis externa. Mastoid, laryngeal, and nasal surgery patients were grouped separately. Restoring the charts was an impossible task, and the records were determined to be either incomplete or a total loss. The only document to survive the fire was an audiology report.

Case Study 18-2: Audiology Report

S.R., a 55-year-old man sensitivity in his l to heari

uled procedure. Before transfer to the operating room, she spoke with her ophthalmologist and reviewed the surgical plan. Her right eye was identified as the operative eye and it was marked with a "yes" and the surgeon's initials on the lid. She was given anesthetic drops in the right eye and an intravenous bolus of 2.0 mg of midazolam (Versed).

In the OR, W.S. and her operative eye were again identified by the surgeon, anesthetist, and nurses. After anesthesia and akinesia were achieved, the eye area was prepped and draped in sterile sheets. An operating microscope with video system was positioned over her eye. A 5-0 silk suture was placed through the superior rectus muscle to retract the eye. A lid speculum was placed to open the eye. A minimal conjunctival peritomy was performed, and hemostasis was achieved with wet-field cautery. The anterior chamber was entered at the 10:30 o'clock position. A capsulotomy was performed after Healon was placed in the anterior chamber. Phacoemulsification was carried out without difficulty. The remaining cortex was removed by irrigation and aspiration.

An intraocular lens (IOL) was placed into the posterior chamber. Miochol was injected to achieve papillary miosis, and the wound was closed with one 10-0 suture. Subconjunctival Celestone and Garamycin were injected. The lid speculum and retraction suture were removed. After application of Eserine and Bacitracin ointments, the eye was patched and a shield was applied. W.S. left the OR in good condition and was discharged to home 4 hours later.

CASE STUDY QUESTIONS

Multiple choice. Select the best answer and write the letter of your choice to the left of each number:

_____ 1. The medical specialty of otorhinolaryngology is most often referred to as:
 a. ENT, or ear, nose, and throat
 b. optometry
 c. PERLA
 d. oral surgery
 e. EENT/dental

The surgery to remove one of the microscopic bones of the middle ear is a(n):
 a. stapedectomy
 b. mastoidectomy
 c. myringotomy
 d. tympanoplasty
 e. otoplasty

procedure in question 2 may require con-
tion of a new eardrum, a procedure called

 plasty
 ngotomy
 transfer
 noplasty
 e

(continued)

Case Studies (continued)

_____ 4. Mastoid surgery incisions are made postauricularly, which is:
 a. anterior to the ear drum
 b. over the left ear
 c. behind the ear
 d. inferior to the tympanic membrane
 e. between the ears

_____ 5. The study of hearing is termed:
 a. acousticology
 b. radio frequency
 c. light spectrum
 d. otology
 e. audiology

_____ 6. Sensorineural hearing loss may result from:
 a. damage to the second cranial nerve
 b. otitis media
 c. otosclerosis
 d. damage to the eighth cranial nerve
 e. stapedectomy

_____ 7. Ultrasound destruction and aspiration of the lens is called:
 a. catarectomy
 b. phacoemulsification
 c. stapedectomy
 d. radial keratotomy
 e. refraction

_____ 8. The term akinesia means:
 a. movement
 b. lack of sensation
 c. washing
 d. lack of movement
 e. incision

_____ 9. The term that means "on the same side" is:
 a. contralateral
 b. bilateral
 c. distal
 d. ventral
 e. ipsilateral

_____ 10. Another name for an acoustic neuroma is:
 a. macular degeneration
 b. acoustic neurilemoma
 c. auditory otosclerosis
 d. 8th cranial labyrinthitis
 e. acoustic glaucoma

Write terms from the case studies with the following meanings:

11. record obtained by tympanometry
_____

12. pertaining to or perceived by the ear
_____

13. inflammation of the middle ear
_____

14. inflammation of the external ear
_____

15. physician who specializes in conditions of the eye
_____

16. within the eye
_____

17. abnormal contraction of the pupil
_____

18. generic drug name for Versed
_____

Abbreviations. Define the following abbreviations:

19. Hz

20. BAEP

21. OD

22. IOL

Flashcard Starter Set

More than 100 flashcards are included at the back of the text. Add to this collection with your own cards as you work through the text (please be sure to see the Student Resources section for information on creating your own set of flashcards using the Flashcard Generator).

Student Resources and the PASSport to Success®

Different people learn in different ways. Some students learn by reading. Others take in new information by listening to their instructors. You may prefer to write down notes. A simple self-assessment can tell you whether you are a visual, auditory, or kinesthetic learner. When you understand the way that you process information most effectively, you can choose resources that fit your learning style. The PASSport to Success® is a practical system that lets you learn faster, remember more, and achieve success.

Getting started with the Student Resources and the PASSport to Success®

Your journey begins with your textbook, *Medical Terminology: An Illustrated Guide*, 6th Edition. The textbook is filled with icons that guide you to resources and activities that are designed for your personal learning style.

 Go to the pronunciation glossary on the Student Resources to hear these words pronounced.

Inside the front cover of your textbook, you will find your personal access code. Use it to log on to *the Point*—the companion website for this textbook. On the website, you can search and sort learning activities by learning style and choose the ones that will help you understand the material quickly and efficiently.

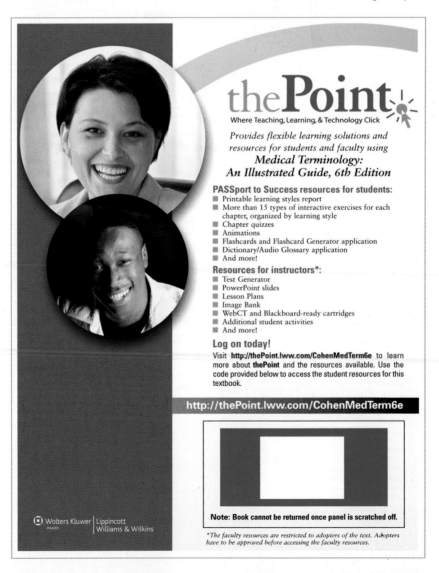

thePoint
Where Teaching, Learning, & Technology Click

Provides flexible learning solutions and resources for students and faculty using
Medical Terminology: An Illustrated Guide, 6th Edition

PASSport to Success resources for students:
- Printable learning styles report
- More than 15 types of interactive exercises for each chapter, organized by learning style
- Chapter quizzes
- Animations
- Flashcards and Flashcard Generator application
- Dictionary/Audio Glossary application
- And more!

Resources for instructors*:
- Test Generator
- PowerPoint slides
- Lesson Plans
- Image Bank
- WebCT and Blackboard-ready cartridges
- Additional student activities
- And more!

Log on today!
Visit **http://thePoint.lww.com/CohenMedTerm6e** to learn more about **thePoint** and the resources available. Use the code provided below to access the student resources for this textbook.

http://thePoint.lww.com/CohenMedTerm6e

Note: Book cannot be returned once panel is scratched off.

Wolters Kluwer | Lippincott Williams & Wilkins
Health

The faculty resources are restricted to adopters of the text. Adopters have to be approved before accessing the faculty resources.

Discover your learning style!

If you like to study animations, illustrations, and diagrams, you may be a visual learner. If you like to sound out new words or discuss material with other students, you may be an auditory (hearing) learner. If you take a lot of notes during class and benefit from hands-on learning activities, you are probably a kinesthetic (touch) learner.

Most people have both a primary and a secondary learning style—and the PASSport to Success® helps you identify both! Once you know *how* you learn best, you can choose learning activities that will help you master new material more efficiently.

Discovering your learning style is easy—and fun! Here's how to begin:

1. Use your web browser to navigate to http://lww.mypowerlearning.com/login.isf.

2. If this is the first time you are visiting the MyPowerLearning website, enter your scratch-off access code from the inside cover of this book into the "Access Code" box and click "Begin!"

3. MyPowerLearning will send you an email with your username and password you will use to log in to MyPowerLearning and complete your Learning Style Assessment (*Don't worry—There are no wrong answers!*).

4. Print and read your own personal learning styles report to better understand how to study most effectively and efficiently.

Once you know your own personal learning style, access thePoint.lww.com/CohenMedterm6e on *thePoint*—the companion website for *Medical Terminology: An Illustrated Guide*, 6th Edition, which will allow you to search and sort PASSport to Success® activities by learning style to choose the most effective way for you to learn the material. Resources and activities available to students include the following:

- Multiple choice, true–false, and fill-in-the blank questions
- Categories
- Listen & Label and Look and Label
- Word Building
- Zooming In
- Pronounce It
- Spell It
- Sound It
- Hangman
- Crossword Puzzles
- Quiz Show

- Concentration
- Case Studies and Case Study Questions
- Dictionary and Audio Glossary application
- Flashcards and Flashcard Generator applications
- Animations
- Audio Drills (which allow for chapter audio files to be downloaded as MP3 files)
- Chapter Quizzes

Contents

Expanded Contents

Concepts of Medical Terminology

CHAPTER CONTENTS

OBJECTIVES

After study of this chapter you should be able to:

1. Explain the purpose of medical terminology.
2. Define the terms *root*, *suffix*, and *prefix*.
3. Explain what combining forms are and why they are used.
4. Name the languages from which most medical word parts are derived.
5. Pronounce words according to the pronunciation guide used in this text.
6. List some features of medical dictionaries.
7. Analyze some concepts of medical terminology in a case study.

PRETEST

Multiple choice. Select the best answer and write the letter of your choice to the left of each number.

___ 1. The main part of a word is called the:

    a. origin   c. root
    b. prefix   d. extension

___ 2. A word part at the beginning of a word is a(n):

    a. prefix   c. preview
    b. combining form   d. root

___ 3. A word part at the end of a word is the:

    a. vowel   c. insertion
    b. adjective   d. suffix

___ 4. Most medical words are derived from the languages:

    a. French and Italian
    b. Greek and Latin
    c. English and German
    d. Greek and Arabic

___ 5. The adjective form of *cervix*, meaning "neck," is:

    a. cervical   c. cervous
    b. cervixal   d. cerviral

___ 6. The *ch* in the word *chemistry* is pronounced like the letter:

    a. s   c. k
    b. h   d. f

___ 7. The *ps* in the word *psychology* is pronounced like the letter:

    a. p   c. j
    b. s   d. k

___ 8. The *pn* in the word *pneumonia* is pronounced like the letter:

    a. p   c. m
    b. u   d. n

___ 9. The symbol ® means

    a. right   c. redirect
    b. review   d. register

Medical terminology is a special vocabulary used by health care professionals for effective and accurate communication. Every health-related field requires an understanding of medical terminology, and this book will highlight selected health care occupations in special boxes (see Box 1-1). Because it is based mainly on Greek and Latin words, medical terminology is consistent and uniform throughout the world. It is also efficient; although some of the terms are long, they often reduce an entire phrase to a single word. The one word *gastroduodenostomy*, for example, stands for "a communication between the stomach and the first part of the small intestine" (Fig. 1-1). The part *gastr* means stomach; *duoden* stands for the duodenum, the first part of the small intestine; *ostomy* means a communication.

The medical vocabulary is vast, and learning it may seem like learning the entire vocabulary of a foreign language. Moreover, like the jargon that arises in all changing fields, it is always expanding. Think of the terms that have been added to our vocabulary with the development of computers, such as software, search engine, e-mail,

chat room, and blog. The task may seem overwhelming, but there are methods to aid in learning and remembering words and even help to make informed guesses about unfamiliar words. Most medical terms can be divided into component parts—roots, prefixes, and suffixes—that maintain the same meaning whenever they appear. By learning these meanings, you can analyze and remember many words.

Word Parts

Word components fall into three categories:

1. The **root** is the fundamental unit of each medical word. It establishes the basic meaning of the word and is the part to which modifying **prefixes** and suffixes are added.

2. A **suffix** is a short word part or series of parts added at the end of a root to modify its meaning. This book indicates suffixes by a dash before the suffix, such as *-itis* (inflammation).

Box 1-1 Health Professions

Health Information Technicians

Every time a patient receives medical treatment, information is added to the patient's medical record, which includes data about symptoms, medical history, test results, diagnoses, and treatment. Health information technicians organize and manage these records, working closely with physicians, nurses, and other health professionals to ensure that they provide a complete and accurate basis for quality patient care.

Accurate medical records are essential for administrative purposes. Health information technicians assign a code to each diagnosis and procedure a patient receives, and this information is used for accurate patient billing. In addition, health information technicians analyze medical records to

reveal trends in health and disease. This research can be used to improve patient care, manage costs, and help establish new medical treatments.

To read and interpret medical records, health information technicians need a thorough background in medical terminology. Most of these technicians work in hospitals and long-term care facilities. Others may work in medical clinics, government agencies, insurance companies, and consulting firms. Because of the growing need for medical care, health information technology is projected to be one of the fastest growing careers in the United States. For more information about this profession, contact the American Health Information Management Association at www.ahima.org.

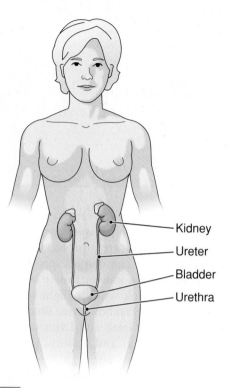

Figure 1-1 **Gastroduodenostomy.** A communication (-stomy) between the stomach (gastr) and the first part of the small intestine, or duodenum (duoden).

3. A prefix is a short word part added before a root to modify its meaning. This book indicates prefixes by a dash after the prefix, such as *pre-* (before).

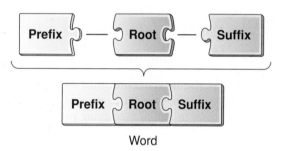

Words are formed from roots, suffixes, and prefixes.

The simple word *learn* can be used as a root to illustrate. If we add the suffix *-er* to form *learner*, we have "one who learns." If we add the prefix *re-* to form *relearn*, we have "to learn again."

Not all roots are complete words. In fact, most medical roots are derived from other languages and are meant to be used in combinations. The Greek word *kardia*, for example, meaning "heart," gives us the root *cardi*. The Latin word *pulmo*, meaning "lung," gives us the root *pulm*. In a few instances, both the Greek and Latin roots are used for the same structure. We find both the Greek root *nephr* and the Latin root *ren* used in words pertaining to the kidney (Fig. 1-2).

Note that the same root may have different meanings in different fields of study, just as the words *spam*, *menu*, *browser*, *surfing*, and *cookie* have different meanings in common vocabulary than in "computerese." The root *myel* means "marrow" and may apply to either the bone marrow or the spinal cord. The root *scler* means "hard" but may also apply to the white of the eye. *Cyst* means "a filled sac or pouch" but also refers specifically to the urinary bladder. You will sometimes have to consider the context of a word before assigning its meaning.

Compound words contain more than one root. The words *eyeball*, *bedpan*, *frostbite*, and *wheelchair* are

Figure 1-2 **Medical terminology uses both the Greek root** *nephr* **and the Latin root** *ren* **to refer to the kidney, an organ of the urinary system.**

examples. Some examples of compound medical words are *cardiovascular* (pertaining to the heart and blood vessels), *urogenital* (pertaining to the urinary and reproductive systems), and *lymphocyte* (a white blood cell found in the lymphatic system).

Combining Forms

When a suffix or another root beginning with a consonant is added to a root, a vowel is inserted between the root and the next word part to aid in pronunciation. This combining vowel is usually an *o*, as seen in the previous example of gastroduodenostomy, but may occasionally be *a*, *e*, or *i*.

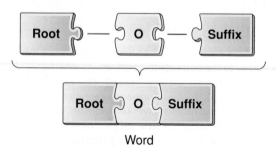

A combining vowel may be added between a root and the word part that follows.

Thus, when the suffix *-logy*, meaning "study of," is added to the root *neur*, meaning "nerve or nervous system," a combining vowel is added:

neur + o + logy = neurology
(study of the nervous system)

Roots shown with a combining vowel are called **combining forms.**

Root — **O**

Root **O**

Combining form

A root with a combining vowel is called a combining form.

This text gives roots with their most common combining vowels added after a slash and refers to them simply as roots, as in *neur/o.*

A combining vowel usually is not used if the ending begins with a vowel. For example, the root *neur* is combined with the suffix *-itis,* meaning "inflammation of," in this way:

neur + itis = neuritis (inflammation of a nerve)

This rule has some exceptions, particularly when they affect pronunciation or meaning, but you will observe these as you work.

Word Derivations

As mentioned, most medical word parts come from Greek (G.) and Latin (L.). The original words and their meanings are included in this text only occasionally. They are interesting, however, and may aid in learning. For example, *muscle* comes from a Latin word that means "mouse" because the movement of a muscle under the skin was thought to resemble the scampering of a mouse.

The coccyx, the tail end of the spine, is named for the cuckoo because it was thought to resemble the cuckoo's bill (Fig. 1-3). For those interested in the derivations of medical words, a good medical dictionary will provide this information.

Words Ending in x

When you add a suffix to a word ending in *x,* the *x* is changed to a *g* or a *c.* If there is a consonant before the *x,* such as *yx* or *nx,* the *x* is changed to a *g.* For example, *pharynx* (throat) becomes *pharyng*eal (*fa-RIN-jē-al*), to mean "pertaining to the throat"; *coccyx* (terminal portion of the spine) becomes *coccyg*eal (*kok-SIJ-ē-al*), to mean "pertaining to the coccyx."

If a vowel comes before the *x,* such as *ax* or *ix,* you change the *x* to a *c.* Thus, *thorax* (chest) becomes *thoracic* (*thō-RAS-ik*) to mean "pertaining to the chest" and *cervix* (neck) becomes *cervic*al (*SER-vi-kal*) to mean "pertaining to a neck."

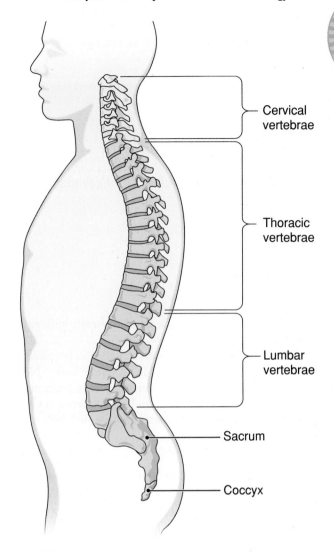

Cervical vertebrae

Thoracic vertebrae

Lumbar vertebrae

Sacrum

Coccyx

Figure 1-3 **The coccyx of the spine looks like the bill of a cuckoo.**

Suffixes Beginning with *rh*

When you add a suffix beginning with *rh* to a root, the *r* is doubled. For example:

hem/o (blood) + -rhage (bursting forth) = hemorrhage (a bursting forth of blood)

men/o (menses) + -rhea (flow, discharge) = menorrhea (menstrual flow)

Pronunciation

This text provides phonetic pronunciations at every opportunity, even in the answer keys. The student resources CD at the back of this book and the student Web resource, *thePoint,* have a large auditory pronunciation dictionary. Take advantage of these aids. Repeat each word aloud as you learn to recognize it in print or hear it on the student resources. The following pronunciation guidelines apply throughout the text.

A vowel (a, e, i, o, u) gets a short pronunciation if it has no pronunciation mark over it, such as

a as in hat

e as in met

i as in bin

o as in not

u as in run

A short line over the vowel gives it a long pronunciation:

ā as in say

ē as in tea

ī as in lie

ō as in hose

ū as in sue

The accented syllable in each word is shown with capital letters, as in *AK-sent*.

Be aware that word parts may change in pronunciation when they are combined in different ways. Note also that accepted pronunciations may vary from place to place. Only one pronunciation for each word is given here, but be prepared for differences (see Box 1-2).

Soft and Hard *c* and *g*

- A soft *c*, as in *racer*, will be written in pronunciations as *s* (*RĀ-ser*).
- A hard *c*, as in *candy*, will be written as *k* (*KAN-dē*).
- A soft *g*, as in *page*, will be written as *j* (*pāj*).
- A hard *g*, as in *grow*, will be written as *g* (*grō*).

Silent Letters and Unusual Pronunciations

A silent letter or unusual pronunciation can be a problem, especially if it appears at the start of a word that you are trying to look up in the dictionary. See Box 1-3 for some examples.

The combinations in Box 1-3 may be pronounced differently when they appear within a word, as in diagnosis (*dī-ag-NŌ-sis*), meaning determination of the cause of disease, in which the *g* is pronounced; apnea (*AP-nē-a*), meaning cessation of breathing, in which the *p* is pronounced; nephroptosis (*nef-rop-TŌ-sis*), meaning dropping of the kidney, in which the *p* is pronounced.

Learning Styles

The term "learning styles" describes how people differ in the senses they most depend on to learn. Visual learners want to see a word in print. They like diagrams, charts, and pictures. Auditory learners need to hear words pronounced. They like to talk over what they have learned and profit from listening again to recorded lessons. Tactile learners use touch, such as writing out answers or retyping notes. They like to follow demonstrations to learn a new skill. You can evaluate your own learning style with an inventory on the student resources CD or *thePoint*. Exercises in these resources are coded as to the learning styles they support.

Of course, we use all of our senses to some degree in learning, and the more channels we use, the more likely it is that we will absorb and remember new information. This text, in combination with the student resources, calls on multiple senses to aid learning: seeing new words in print, writing out answers, using flash cards,

---

Box 1-2 Focus on Words

Pronunciations

When pronunciations are included in a text, it is sometimes difficult for authors to know which pronunciation of a term to use. Pronunciations may vary from country to country and even in different regions of the same country. Think how easy it is to distinguish a southern accent and one from the Midwest or Northeast United States. The general rule is to use the most common pronunciation or to list that pronunciation first if more than one is given.

The word *gynecology* is usually pronounced with a hard g in the United States, but in many areas a soft g is used, as in *jin-e-KOL-ō-jē*. Words pertaining to the cerebrum (largest part of the brain) may have an accent on different syllables. The

adjective is usually pronounced with the accent on the second syllable (*se-RE-bral*), but in cerebrum (*SER-e-brum*) and cerebrospinal (*ser-e-brō-SPĪ-nal*), the accented syllable differs.

The name for the first part of the small intestine (duodenum) is often pronounced *dū-ō-DĒ-num*, although the pronunciation *dū-O-de-num* is also acceptable. And the scientific term for the navel, umbilicus, is usually pronounced with the accent on the second syllable as *um-BIL-i-kus*, but *um-bi-LĪ-kus* is also used. When extreme, some alternative pronunciations can sound like a foreign language. The word we pronounce as *SKEL-e-tal* is pronounced in some other English-speaking countries as *ske-LE-tal*.

Box 1-3 For Your Reference

Silent Letters and Unusual Pronunciations

LETTER(S)	PRONUNCIATION	EXAMPLE	DEFINITION OF EXAMPLE
ch	k	**chemical** *KEM-i-kal*	pertaining to the elements and their interactions (root *chem/o* means "chemical")
dys	dis	**dysfunction** *dis-FUNK-shun*	difficult or abnormal (dys-) function
eu	u	**euphoria** *ū-FOR-ē-a*	exaggerated feeling of well-being (*eu-* means "true" or "good")
gn	n	**gnathic** *NATH-ik*	pertaining to the jaw (gnath/o)
ph	f	**phantom** *FAN-tom*	illusion or imaginary image
pn	n	**pneumonitis** *nū-mō-NĪ-tis*	inflammation of the lungs (pneumon/o)
ps	s	**pseudonym** *SŪ-dō-nim*	false name (-nym)
pt	t	**ptosis** *TŌ-sis*	dropping, downward displacement
rh	r	**rhinoplasty** *RĪ-nō-plas-tē*	plastic repair of the nose (rhin/o)
x	z	**xiphoid** *ZIF-oyd*	pertaining to cartilage attached to the sternum (from Greek *xiphos,* meaning "sword")

listening to pronunciations, and completing exercises on the computer. Unlike the fashion magazines that use perfumed ads to sell products, the olfactory sense has not yet been incorporated into textbooks. Perhaps someday student resources will have a smell feature!

Abbreviations

Shortened words or initials can save time in writing medical reports and case histories. We commonly use TV for television, Jr. for junior, F for Fahrenheit temperature readings, UV for ultraviolet, and Dr. for doctor. A few of the many medical abbreviations are mL for the metric measurement milliliter, dB for decibels, units of sound intensity, CA for cancer, hgb for hemoglobin, and ECG for electrocardiogram.

Phrase Abbreviations

An **acronym** is an abbreviation formed from the first letter of each word in a phrase. Some everyday acronyms are ASAP (as soon as possible), ATM (automated teller machine), and a computer's RAM (random access memory). Acronyms have become popular for

saving time and space in naming objects, organizations, and procedures. They abound in the names of government agencies: FDA (Food and Drug Administration), USDA (United States Department of Agriculture), NIH (National Institutes of Health). Some medical acronyms are BP for blood pressure, MRI for magnetic resonance imaging, AIDS for acquired immunodeficiency syndrome, CNS for the central nervous system, and RN for registered nurse.

Symbols

Symbols are commonly used as shorthand in case histories. Some examples are Ⓛ and Ⓡ for left and right; ↑ and ↓ for increase and decrease. A list of common symbols appears in Chapter 7 and in Appendix 1.

Symbols and abbreviations can save time, but they can also cause confusion if they are not universally understood. Usage varies in different institutions, and the same abbreviation may have different meanings in different fields. Only the most commonly used symbols and abbreviations are given here. These are listed at the end of each chapter, but a more complete alphabetical list appears in Appendix 2. An abbreviation dictionary also is helpful.

Medical Dictionaries

With few exceptions, you can do all the exercises in this book without the aid of a dictionary, but medical dictionaries are valuable references for everyone in health-related fields. These include not only complete, unabridged versions, but also easy-to-carry short versions and dictionaries of medical acronyms and abbreviations. Many of these dictionaries are also available on CD. Dictionaries give information on meanings, pronunciation, synonyms, derivations, and related terms. Those intended for nursing and allied health professions include more complete clinical information, with notes on patient care.

Dictionaries vary in organization; in some, almost all terms are entered as nouns, such as disease, syndrome, procedure, or test. Those with a more clinical approach enter some terms according to their first word, which may be an adjective or proper name, for example, biomedical engineering, Cushing disease, windchill factor. This format makes it easier to look up some terms. All dictionaries have directions on how to use the book and interpret the entries, as shown in Appendix 9, taken from *Stedman's Medical Dictionary*, 28th ed.

In addition to information on individual terms and phrases, medical dictionaries have useful appendices on measurements, clinical tests, drugs, diagnosis, body structure, information resources, and other topics.

Terminology   Key Terms

acronym AK-rō-nim	An abbreviation formed from the first letter of each word in a phrase
combining form kom-BĪ-ning	A word root combined with a vowel that links the root with another word part, such as a suffix or another root. Combining forms are shown with a slash between the root and the vowel, as in *neur/o*
compound word KOM-pownd	A word that contains more than one root
prefix PRĒ-fix	A word part added before a root to modify its meaning
root rūt	The fundamental unit of a word
suffix SU-fix	A word part added to the end of a root to modify its meaning

PASSport to Success®   Go to the student resources to hear these words pronounced.

Chapter Review

Fill in the blanks:

1. A word part that always comes after a root is a(n) _____.

2. A root with a vowel added to aid in pronunciation is called a(n) _____.

3. Combine the word parts *dia-*, meaning "through," and *-rhea*, meaning "flow," to form a word meaning "passage of fluid stool" _____.

4. Combine the root *cardi*, meaning "heart," with the suffix *-logy*, meaning "study of," to form a word meaning "study of the heart" _____.

Chapter Review (continued)

Multiple Choice > Select the best answer and write the letter of your choice to the left of each number:

_____ 5. Which of the following is a compound word?

    a. intestinal

    b. pharmacy

    c. urogenital

    d. muscular

_____ 6. The adjective for *larynx* is

    a. larynxic

    b. laryngeal

    c. larynal

    d. largeal

_____ 7. The combining form for *thorax* (chest)

    a. thorax/o

    b. thor/o

    c. thorac/o

    d. thori/o

_____ 8. An acronym is formed from

    a. a proper name

    b. Latin or Greek

    c. two or more roots

    d. the first letter of each word in a phrase

Pronounce the following words:

  9. dyslexia

10. rheumatism

11. pneumatic

12. chemist

13. pharmacy

Pronounce the following phonetic forms and write the words they represent:

14. *KAR-dē-ak* _____

15. *HĪ-drō-jen* _____

16. *OK-ū-lar* _____

17. *IN-ter-fās* _____

18. *rū-MAT-ik* _____

Chapter Review *(continued)*

Word Building > Write words for the following definitions using the word parts provided. A combining vowel is included. Each word part can be used more than once.

-itis   -logy   -ptosis   nephr   -o-   gastr   cardi   neur

19. Inflammation of the stomach   _____

20. Study of the nervous system   _____

21. Dropping of the kidney   _____

22. Study of the kidney   _____

23. Inflammation of a nerve   _____

24. Downward displacement of the heart   _____

Word Analysis > Define each of the following words and give the meaning of the word parts in each. Use a dictionary if necessary.

25. dysmenorrhea *(dis-men-ō-RĒ-a)* _____.

   a. dys _____

   b. men/o _____

   c. -rhea _____

26. cardiologist *(kar-dē-OL-ō-jist)* _____

   a. cardi/o _____

   b. -log/o _____

   c. -ist _____

27. nephritis *(nef-RĪ-tis)* _____

   a. nephr/o _____

   b. -itis _____

28. renogastric *(rē-nō-GAS-trik)* _____

   a. ren/o _____

   b. gastr/o _____

   c. -ic _____

 PASSport to Success® See Chapter 1 in the student resources for additional review exercises.

Case Study

> ## Case Study 1-1: Multiple Health Problems Secondary to Injury

D.S., a 28-year-old woman, was treated for injuries sustained in a train-derailment accident. During the course of her treatment, she was seen by several specialists. For pain in her knee and hip joints, she was referred to an orthopedist. For migraine headaches and blurry vision, she consulted a neurologist. For pain on urination, occasional bloody urine, and possible nephritis, she saw a urologist. Later, for a persistent dry cough, pharyngitis, and problems resulting from a fractured nose, she was referred to an otorhinolaryngologist.

During D.S.'s initial course of treatment, she had a CT scan of her abdomen and brain and an MRI of her hip and knee. Her many visits also included respiratory endoscopic studies, pulmonary x-rays, and periodic blood tests in the hematology lab.

CASE STUDY QUESTIONS

Multiple choice. Select the best answer and write the letter of your choice to the left of each number:

_____ 1. The *de-* in the word *derailment* is a:
   a. suffix
   b. root
   c. prefix
   d. combining form

_____ 2. The *-ist* in the word *orthopedist* is a:
   a. root
   b. prefix
   c. derivation
   d. suffix

_____ 3. *MRI* stands for magnetic resonance imaging. This term represents a(n):
   a. combining form
   b. acronym
   c. prefix
   d. suffix

_____ 4. The root *nephr/o* in *nephritis* means:
   a. lung
   b. nerve
   c. joint
   d. kidney

_____ 5. The *rh* in the root *rhin/o* is pronounced as:
   a. r
   b. h
   c. er
   d. ro

Fill in the blanks:

6. Use Appendix 4 to find root**s that mean** blood.

_____

7. Use the index to find the chapter that contains information on imaging techniques.

_____

8. Use the flash cards at the back of this book to find the meaning of the prefix *endo-*.

_____

9. Use Appendix 4 to find another word part with the same meaning as *endo-*.

_____

10. Use Appendix 5 to look up the meaning of the roots in *otorhinolaryngology*.

   ot/o _____

   rhin/o _____

   laryng/o _____

11. When the word pharynx has a suffix added, the x is changed to a

_____

12. Appendix 2 tells you that the abbreviation CT in CT scan means

_____

CHAPTER 2

Suffixes

CHAPTER CONTENTS

OBJECTIVES

After study of this chapter you should be able to:

1. Define a suffix.
2. Give examples of how suffixes are used.
3. Recognize and apply some general noun, adjective, and plural suffixes used in medical terminology.
4. Analyze the suffixes used in a case study.

PRETEST

Multiple choice. Select the best answer and write the letter of your choice to the left of each number.

___ 1. The suffix in the word *learning* is:

    a. learn   c. ing
    b. ng   d. earn

___ 2. The suffixes *-ism*, *-ia*, and *-ist* are found in:

    a. verbs   c. adverbs
    b. adjectives   d. nouns

___ 3. The suffixes *-ic*, *-al*, *-ous*, and *-oid* are found in:

    a. adjectives   c. verbs
    b. nouns   d. roots

___ 4. The suffix *-form* means:

    a. excess   c. resembling
    b. origin   d. paired

___ 5. The suffix *-logy* means:

    a. placement   c. vocabulary
    b. study of   d. size

___ 6. The plural of *fungus* is:

    a. fungi   c. fungae
    b. fungal   d. funga

___ 7. The plural of *protozoon* is:

    a. protozoi   c. protozoas
    b. protozoae   d. protozoa

___ 8. The singular of *ova* (eggs) is:

    a. ovi   c. ovum
    b. ovae   d. ovas

___ 9. The singular of *phenomena* is:

    a. phenomenon   c. phenomenas
    b. phenomenae   d. phenomeni

A suffix is a word ending that modifies a root. A suffix may indicate that the word is a noun or an adjective and often determines how the definition of the word will begin (Box 2-1). For example, using the root *myel/o*, meaning "bone marrow," the adjective ending *-oid* forms the word *myeloid*, which means "like or pertaining to bone marrow." The ending *-oma* produces *myeloma*, which is a tumor of the bone marrow. Adding another root, *gen*, which represents genesis or origin, and the adjective ending *-ous* forms the word *myelogenous*, meaning "originating in bone marrow."

The suffixes given in this chapter are general ones that are used throughout medical terminology. They include endings that form:

- Nouns: a person, place, or thing
- Adjectives: words that modify nouns
- Plurals: endings that convert single nouns to multiples

Additional suffixes will be presented in later chapters, as they pertain to disease states, medical treatment, or specific body systems.

Noun Suffixes

The following general suffixes convert roots into nouns. Table 2-1 has suffixes that represent different conditions. Note that the ending *-sis*, may appear with different combining vowels as *-osis*, *-iasis*, *-esis*, or *-asis*. The first two of these denote an abnormal condition.

Box 2-1   Focus on Words

Meaningful Suffixes

Suffixes sometimes take on a color of their own as they are added to different words. The suffix *-thon* is taken from the name of the Greek town Marathon, from which news of a battle victory was carried by a long-distance runner. It has been attached to various words to mean a contest of great endurance. We have bike-athons, dance-athons, telethons, and even major charity fund-raisers called thon-a-thons.

    The adjective ending *-ish*, as in Scottish, can be added to imply that something is not right on target, as in largish, softish, oldish.

In science and medicine, the ending *-tech* is used to imply high technology, and *-pure* may be added to inspire confidence, as in the company name Genentech and the Multi-Pure water filter. The ending *-mate* suggests helping, as in *helpmate*, defined in the dictionary as a helpful companion, more specifically, a wife, or sometimes, a husband. The medical device HeartMate is a pump used to assist a damaged heart.

Table 2-1   Suffixes That Mean "Condition of"

Suffix	Example	Definition of Example
-ia	dementia *dē-MEN-shē-a*	loss of (de-) intellectual function (from L. *mentis*: mind)
-ism	racism *RĀ-sizm*	discrimination based on race
-sis	thrombosis *throm-BŌ-sis*	having a blood clot (thrombus) in a vessel (see Fig. 2-1)
-y	atony *AT-ō-nē*	lack (a-) of muscle tone

Figure 2-1 Thrombosis (having a blood clot, or thrombus, in a vessel). The word *thrombosis* has the noun suffix *-sis*, meaning "condition of."

Table 2-2 has endings that convert roots into medical specialties or specialists. The suffix *-logy* applies to many fields other than medicine. It contains the root *log/o* taken from the Greek word *logos*, which means "word," and generally means a field of study, as in *biology, archeology, terminology,* and *technology* (Box 2-2). Terms with this ending are also used to identify an institutional department or a specialty, as in cardiology, dermatology, radiology, and others.

The two endings *-iatrics* and *-iatry* contain the root *-iatr/o,* based on a Greek word for healing and meaning "physician" or "medical treatment."

EXERCISE 2-1

Write the suffix that means "condition of" in the following words:

1. phobia (unfounded fear; from L. *phobos*: fear)
   FŌ-bē-a   -ia

2. psoriasis (skin disease)
   sō-RĪ-a-sis   _____

3. egotism (exaggerated self-importance; from *ego*: self)
   Ē-gō-tizm   _____

4. dystrophy (changes due to lack of nourishment; root: troph/o)
   DIS-trō-fē   _____

5. anesthesia (loss of sensation; root: esthesi/o) (Fig. 2-2)
   an-es-THĒ-zē-a   _____

6. parasitism (infection with parasites or behaving as a parasite)
   PAR-a-sit-izm   _____

7. stenosis (narrowing of a canal)
   ste-NŌ-sis   _____

8. tetany (sustained muscle contraction)
   TET-a-nē   _____

9. diuresis (increased urination; root: ur/o)
   dī-ū-RĒ-sis   _____

Table 2-2   Suffixes for Medical Specialties

Suffix	Meaning	Example	Definition of Example
-ian	specialist in a field of study	physician *fi-ZISH-un*	practitioner of medicine (from root *physi/o*, meaning "nature")
-iatrics	medical specialty	pediatrics *pē-dē-AT-riks*	care and treatment of children (ped/o) (Fig. 2-3)
-iatry	medical specialty	psychiatry *sī-KĪ-a-trē*	study and treatment of mental (psych/o) disorders
-ics	medical specialty	orthopedics *or-thō-PĒ-diks*	study and treatment of the skeleton and joints (from root *ped/o*, meaning "child," and prefix *ortho*, meaning "straight")
-ist	specialist in a field of study	podiatrist *pō-DĪ-a-trist*	one who studies and treats the foot (pod/o)
-logy	study of	physiology *fiz-ē-OL-ō-jē*	study of function in a living organism (from root *physi/o*, meaning "nature"

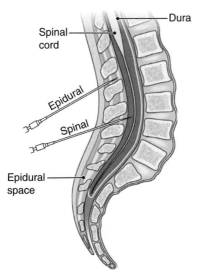

Figure 2-2 **Injection sites for anesthesia.** The word *anesthesia* uses the noun suffix *-ia*, meaning "condition of." The dura is a layer of the meninges, the membranes that cover the brain and spinal cord. One who administers anesthesia is an anesthetist or anesthesiologist.

Figure 2-3 **A practitioner of pediatrics, the care and treatment of children.** The ending *-ics* indicates a medical specialty. This pediatrician, one who practices pediatrics, is testing an infant's reflexes.

Box 2-2 **Health Professions**

Medical Technology

The field of medical technology includes a wide range of clinical laboratory sciences. Medical technologists test blood for abnormalities or infections and cross match it for transfusions. They analyze body fluids, looking for abnormal levels of various substances, such as cholesterol and glucose. They identify and test infectious agents and examine cells for signs of cancer and other diseases. A medical technologist working in a small lab may have to do tests in all these areas; those working in larger labs or hospitals usually specialize in one. Their work requires them to use microscopes, computers, and other complex instruments and equipment.

Most medical technologists have a bachelor's degree, which includes courses in mathematics and life sciences. Programs may also include on-the-job training. Advancement to supervisory positions requires advanced degrees. There are several accrediting agencies for medical technologists, and states vary in their licensing or registration policies. Medical technicians perform similar tasks in the laboratory but generally are required to have a minimum of an associate (2-year) degree and to work under closer supervision. For information on careers in medical technology, contact the American Society for Clinical Laboratory Science at http://www.ascls.org.

EXERCISE 2-2

Write the suffix in the following words that means "study of," "medical specialty," or "specialist in a field of study":

1. cardiologist (specialist in the study and treatment of the heart; root: cardi/o)
kar-dē-OL-ō-jist
_____-ist_____

2. neurology (the study of the nervous system; root: neur/o)
nū-ROL-ō-jē
_____

3. geriatrics (study and treatment of the aged; root: ger/e) (Fig. 2-4)
jer-ē-AT-riks
_____

4. dermatology (study and treatment of the skin, or derma)
der-ma-TOL-ō-jē
_____

5. optician (one who makes and fits corrective lenses
   for the eyes; root: opt/o)
   op-TISH-an
   _____

6. anesthetist (one who administers anesthesia) (see Fig. 2-2)
   a-NES-the-tist
   _____

Write a word for a specialist in the following fields:

7. anatomy (study of body structure)
   a-NAT-ō-mē
   _____

8. pediatrics (care and treatment of children; root: ped/o)
   pē-dē-AT-riks
   _____

9. radiology (use of radiation in diagnosis and treatment)
   rā-dē-OL-ō-jē
   _____

10. psychology (study of the mind; root: psych/o)
    sī-KOL-ō-jē
    _____

11. technology (practical application of science)
    tek-NOL-ō-jē
    _____

12. obstetrics (medical specialty concerning pregnancy and birth)
    ob-STET-riks
    _____

Figure 2-4 **Geriatrics is the care and treatment of the aged.**
A specialist in this field, a geriatrician, is shown.

Adjective Suffixes

The suffixes below are all adjective endings that mean "pertaining to," "like," or "resembling" (Table 2-3). There are no rules for which ending to use for a given noun. Familiarity comes with practice. When necessary, tips on proper usage are given in the text.

Note that for words ending with the suffix *-sis*, the first *s* is changed to a *t* before adding *-ic* to form the adjective, as in genetic, pertaining to genesis (origin); psychotic, pertaining to psychosis (a mental disorder); or diuretic, pertaining to diuresis (increased urination).

Table 2-3	Suffixes That Mean "Pertaining to," "Like," or "Resembling"	
Suffix	**Example**	**Definition of Example**
-ac	cardiac *KAR-dē-ak*	pertaining to the heart
-al	vocal *VŌ-kal*	pertaining to the voice
-ar	nuclear *NŪ-klē-ar*	pertaining to a nucleus
-ary	salivary *SAL-i-var-ē*	pertaining to saliva
-form	muciform *MŪ-si-form*	like or resembling mucus

Table 2-3	Continued	
Suffix	Example	Definition of Example
-ic	anatomic *an-a-TOM-ik*	pertaining to anatomy (see Fig. 2-5)
-ical (ic + al)	electrical *ē-LEK-tri-kal*	pertaining to electricity
-ile	virile *VIR-il*	pertaining to the male; masculine
-oid	lymphoid *LIM-foyd*	pertaining to the lymphatic system
-ory	circulatory *SIR-kū-la-tor-ē*	pertaining to circulation
-ous	cutaneous *kū-TĀ-nē-us*	pertaining to the skin (from L. *cutis*: skin)

EXERCISE 2-3

Identify the suffix meaning "pertaining to," "like," or "resembling" in the following words:

1. dietary (pertaining to the diet)   _____-ary_____
   DĪ-e-tar-ē

2. neuronal (pertaining to a nerve cell, or neuron) (Fig. 2-6)   _____
   NŪ-rō-nal

3. metric (pertaining to a meter or measurement; root metr/o
   means "measure")   _____
   ME-trik

4. venous (pertaining to a vein; root: ven/o)   _____
   VĒ-nus

5. epileptiform (like or resembling epilepsy)   _____
   ep-i-LEP-ti-form

6. toxoid (like or resembling a toxin, or poison)   _____
   TOK-soyd

7. topical (pertaining to a surface)   _____
   TOP-i-kal

8. febrile (pertaining to fever)   _____
   FEB-rīl

9. neurotic (pertaining to neurosis, a mental disorder)   _____
   nū-ROT-ik

10. surgical (pertaining to surgery)   _____
    SUR-ji-kal

11. muscular (pertaining to a muscle)   _____
    MUS-kū-lar

12. urinary (pertaining to urine; root: ur/o)   _____
    Ū-ri-nar-ē

13. respiratory (pertaining to respiration)   _____
    RES-pi-ra-tor-ē

14. pelvic (pertaining to the pelvis) (Fig. 2-7)   _____
    PEL-vik

Figure 2-5 **The anatomic position is standard in the study of anatomy.** A person in this position is facing forward with arms at the side and palms forward (anterior). The adjective suffix *-ic* means "pertaining to."

— Neuron

Figure 2-6 **A neuron is a nerve cell.** The adjective form of *neuron* is *neuronal*.

Figure 2-7 **The pelvis is the bony hip girdle.** The adjective form of *pelvis* is *pelvic*.

Forming Plurals

Many medical words have special plural forms based on the ending of the word. Table 2-4 gives some general rules for the formation of plurals along with examples. The plural endings listed in column 2 are substituted for the word endings in column 1. Note that both singular endings *-on* and *-um* change to *-a* for the plural. You have to learn which singular ending to use for specific words when converting a plural word ending in *-a* to the singular.

Some Exceptions to the Rules

There are exceptions to the rules given for forming plurals, some of which will appear in later chapters. For example, the plural of *sinus* (space) is *sinuses*; the plural of *virus* is *viruses*; and *serums* (thin fluids) is sometimes used instead of *sera*. An *-es* ending may be added to words ending in *-ex* or *-ix* to form a plural, as in *appendixes*, *apexes*, and *indexes*.

Table 2-4	Plural Endings		
Word Ending	**Plural Ending**	**Singular Example**	**Plural Example**
a	ae	vertebra (bone of the spine) VER-*te-bra*	vertebrae (Fig. 2-8) VER-*te-brē*
en	ina	lumen (central opening) LŪ-*men*	lumina (Fig. 2-9) LŪ-*min-a*
ex, ix, yx	ices	matrix (background substance; mold) MĀ-*triks*	matrices MĀ-*tri-sēz*
is	es	diagnosis (determination of a disease or defect) *dī-ag-*NŌ-*sis*	diagnoses *dī-ag-*NŌ-*sēz*
ma	mata	stigma (mark or scar) STIG-*ma*	stigmata *stig-*MAT-*a*
nx (anx, inx, ynx)	nges	phalanx (bone of finger or toe) *fa-*LANKS	phalanges (Fig. 2-10) *fa-*LAN-*jēz*
on	a	ganglion (mass of nervous tissue) GANG-*lē-on*	ganglia GANG-*lē-a*
um	a	serum (thin fluid) SĒ-*rum*	sera SĒ-*ra*
us	i	thrombus (see Fig. 2-1) THROM-*bus*	thrombi THROM-*bī*

2

A

B

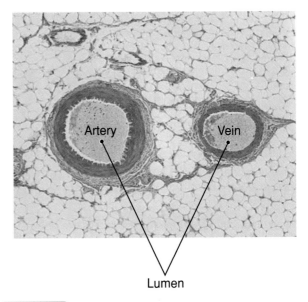

Artery   Vein

Lumen

Figure 2-8 Each bone of the spine is a vertebra (*A*). The spinal column is made of 26 vertebrae (*B*).

Figure 2-9 A lumen is the central opening of an organ or vessel. Two blood vessels are shown, an artery and a vein. The plural of *lumen* is *lumina*.

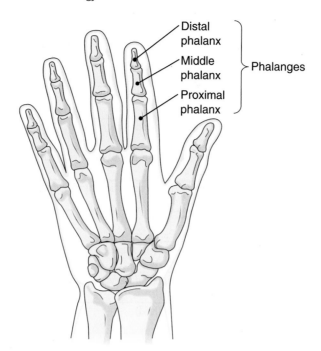

Figure 2-10 **Bones of the right hand, anterior view.** Each bone of a finger or toe is a phalanx. Each hand has 15 phalanges.

Some incorrect plural forms are in common usage, for example, *stigmas* instead of *stigmata*, *referendums* instead of *referenda*, *stadiums* instead of *stadia*. Often people use *phalange* instead of *phalanx* as the singular of *phalanges*. Words ending in *-oma*, meaning "tumor," should be changed to *-omata*, but most people just add an *s* to form the plural. For example, the plural of *carcinoma* (a type of cancer) should be *carcinomata*, but *carcinomas* is commonly used.

EXERCISE 2-4

Write the plural form of the following words. The word ending is underlined in each:

1. patella (kneecap) _____ patellae _____
    pa-TEL-a

2. phenomenon (occurrence or perception) _____
    fe-NOM-e-non

3. omentum (abdominal membrane) _____
    ō-MEN-tum

4. prognosis (prediction of disease outcome) _____
    prog-NŌ-sis

5. apex (tip or peak) _____
    Ā-peks

6. ovum (female reproductive cell; egg) _____
    Ō-vum

7. spermatozoon (male reproductive cell; sperm cell) _____
    sper-ma-tō-ZŌ-on

8. meninx (membrane around the brain and spinal cord) _____
    ME-ninks

9. embolus (circulating blood clot) _____
    EM-bō-lus

Write the singular form of the following words. The word ending is underlined in each.

10. protozo<u>a</u> (single-celled animals)
prō-tō-ZŌ-a

_____

11. append<u>ices</u> (things added)
a-PEN-di-sēz

_____

12. adeno<u>mata</u> (tumors of glands)
ad-e-NŌ-ma-ta

_____

13. fung<u>i</u> (simple, nongreen plants)
FUN-jī

_____

14. pelv<u>es</u>
PEL-vēz

_____

15. foram<u>ina</u> (openings, passageways)
fō-RAM-i-na

_____

16. curricul<u>a</u> (series of courses)
kur-RIK-ū-la

_____

17. ind<u>ices</u> (directories, lists)
IN-di-sēz

_____

18. alveol<u>i</u> (small sacs)
al-VĒ-ō-lī

_____

2

Chapter Review

Identify the suffix that means "condition of" in the following words:

1. alcoholism (AL-kō-hol-izm) (alcohol dependence) _____

2. insomnia (in-SOM-nē-a) (inability to sleep; root: somn/o) _____

3. acidosis (as-i-DŌ-sis) (acid body condition) _____

4. dysentery (DIS-en-ter-ē) (intestinal disorder; root: enter/o) _____

5. psychosis (sī-KŌ-sis) (disorder of the mind) _____

6. anemia (a-NĒ-mē-a) (lack of blood or hemoglobin; root: hem/o) _____

Give the suffix in the following words that means "specialty" or "specialist":

7. psychiatry (sī-KĪ-a-trē) _____

8. orthopedics (or-thō-PĒ-diks) _____

9. anesthesiologist (an-es-thē-zē-OL-ō-jist) _____

10. technician (tek-NISH-un) _____

11. anatomist (a-NAT-ō-mist) _____

12. obstetrician (ob-ste-TRISH-un) _____

Give the name of a specialist in the following fields:

13. pediatrics (pē-dē-A-triks) _____

14. dermatology (der-ma-TOL-ō-jē) _____

15. physiology *(fiz-ē-OL-ō-jē)* _____

16. gynecology *(gī-ne-KOL-ō-jē)* _____

Identify the adjective suffix in the following words that means "pertaining to," "like," or "resembling":

17. pelvic *(PEL-vik)* _____

18. arterial *(ar-TĒ-rē-al)* _____

19. anxious *(ANG-shus)* _____

20. fibroid *(FĪ-broyd)* _____

21. oral *(OR-al)* _____

22. basic *(Bā-sik)* _____

23. binary *(BĪ-nar-ē)* _____

24. skeletal *(SKEL-e-tal)* _____

25. rheumatoid *(RŪ-ma-toyd)* _____

26. febrile *(FEB-rīl)* _____

27. surgical *(SUR-ji-kal)* _____

28. circular *(SIR-ku-lar)* _____

29. exploratory *(ek-SPLOR-a-tor-ē)* _____

Write the plural for the following words. Each word ending is underlined:

30. gingiva (gums) _____
     JIN-ji-va

31. diagnosis (identification of disease) _____
     dī-ag-NŌ-sis

32. ganglion (mass of nervous tissue) _____
     GANG-lē-on

33. lumen (central opening) _____
     LŪ-men

34. focus (center) _____
     FŌ-kus

35. criterion (standard) _____
     kri-TIR-ē-on

36. larynx (voicebox) _____
     LAR-inks

37. vertebra (bone of the spine) _____
     VER-te-bra

38. nucleus (center; core) _____
     NŪ-klē-us

Write the singular form for the following words. Each word ending is underlined:

39. loci (places) _____
     LŌ-sī

Chapter Review *(continued)*

40. alveoli (air sacs) _____
al-VĒ-ō-lī

41. bacteria (type of microorganism) _____
bak-TĒ-rē-a

42. apices (high points, tips) _____
A-pi-sēz

43. foramina (openings) _____
fō-RAM-i-na

44. testes (male reproductive organs) _____
TES-tēz

45. carcinomata (cancers) _____
kar-si-NŌ-ma-ta

Word Building > Write a word for the following definitions using the word parts provided. Each may be used more than once.

-ist   -ic   parasit   -ism   -y   log   -o-

46. pertaining to parasites   _____

47. one who studies parasites   _____

48. a condition of having parasites   _____

49. study of parasites   _____

Word Analysis > Define each of the following words and give the meaning of the word parts in each. Use a dictionary if necessary.

50. geriatrician *(jer-ē-a-TRI-shun)* _____

    a. ger/e _____

    b. iatr/o _____

    c. -ic _____

    d. -ian _____

51. asymmetric _____

    a. a- _____

    b. sym- _____

    c. metr/o _____

    d. -ic _____

52. anesthesia _____

    a. an- _____

    b. esthesi/o _____

    c. -ia _____

PASSport to Success®   See the Student Resources for additional review exercises.

Case Study

➤ Case Study 2-1: Health Problems on Return from the Rain Forest

E.G., a 39-year-old archeologist, returned from a 6-month expedition in the rain forest of South America suffering from a combination of physical symptoms and conditions that would not subside on their own. He was fatigued, yet unable to sleep through the night. He also had a mild fever, night sweats, occasional dizziness, double vision, and mild abdominal pain accompanied by intermittent diarrhea. In addition, he had a nonhealing wound on his ankle from an insect bite. He made an appointment with his family doctor, an internist.

On examination, E.G. was febrile (feverish) with a temperature of 101°F. His heart and lungs were normal, with a slightly elevated heart rate. His abdomen was tender, and his bowel sounds were active and gurgling. His skin was dry and warm. He had symmetrical areas of edema (swelling) around both knees and tenderness over both patellae (kneecaps). The ulceration on his left lateral ankle had a ring of necrosis (tissue death) surrounding an area of granulation tissue. There was a small amount of purulent (pus-containing) drainage.

E.G.'s doctor ordered a series of hematology lab studies and stool cultures for ova and parasites. The doctor suspected a viral disease, possibly carried by mosquitoes, native to tropical rain forests. He also suspected a form of dysentery typically caused by protozoa. E.G. was also possibly anemic, dehydrated, and septic (infected). The doctor was confident that after definitive diagnosis and treatment, E.G. would gain relief from his insomnia, diplopia (double vision), and dizziness.

CASE STUDY QUESTIONS

Multiple choice. Select the best answer and write the letter of your choice to the left of each number:

_____ 1. Diplopia, the condition of having double vision, has the suffix:

    a. -lopia   c. -ia
    b. -pia   d. -plopia

_____ 2. The adjective *septic* is formed from the noun:

    a. septosis   c. septery
    b. septemia   d. sepsis

_____ 3. E.G. was suspected to have anemia (diminished hemoglobin). The adjective form of the noun *anemia* is _____, and the field of health science devoted to the study of blood is called _____.

    a. anemic; hematology
    b. hematosis; hematism
    c. dehemia; hematomegaly
    d. anemic; parasitology

Write the suffix that means "condition of" in the following words:

4. necrosis

_____

5. dysentery

_____

6. insomnia

_____

Write the adjective ending of the following words:

7. febrile

_____

8. symmetrical

_____

9. anemic

_____

Write the singular form of the following words:

10. patellae

_____

11. ova

_____

12. protozoa

_____

Write a word from the case study that means each of the following:

13. The word *virus* used as an adjective

_____

14. The noun form of the adjective *necrotic*

_____

15. Expert in the field of archeology

_____

16. Expert in the field of internal medicine

_____

17. The noun *abdomen* used as an adjective

_____

Prefixes

CHAPTER

3

CHAPTER CONTENTS

OBJECTIVES

After study of this chapter you should be able to:

1. Define a prefix and explain how prefixes are used.
2. Identify and define some of the prefixes used in medical terminology.
3. Use prefixes to form words used in medical terminology.

PRETEST

Multiple choice. Select the best answer and write the letter of your choice to the left of each number.

___ 1. A word prefix appears:

    a. in the middle of the word
    b. after a suffix
    c. at the end of the word
    d. at the beginning of the word

___ 2. The prefix in the words *prefix* and *pretest* means:

    a. before   c. fixed
    b. final   d. superior

___ 3. The prefix in the word *microscopic* is:

    a. mic-   c. micro-
    b. scop-   d. pic-

___ 4. The suffix in the word *microscopic* is:

    a. -ic   c. -micro
    b. -scop   d. -ros

___ 5. The prefixes *mono-*, *tri-*, and *multi-* all refer to:

    a. size   c. location
    b. number   d. shape

___ 6. The prefixes *leuk/o-*, *melan/o-, and erythr/o-* all refer to:

    a. dimensions   c. abnormalities
    b. area   d. color

___ 7. The opposite of hyperglycemia (high blood sugar) is:

    a. hyperglucemia   c. hypoalcemia
    b. hypoglycemia   d. hyperglycemic

___ 8. The opposite of postnatal (after birth) is:

    a. perinatal   c. prenatal
    b. prenatural   d. postpartum

A prefix is a short word part added before a word or word root to modify its meaning. For example, the word *lateral* means "side." Adding the prefix uni-, meaning "one," forms *unilateral*, which means "affecting or involving one side." Adding the prefix *contra-*, meaning "against or opposite," forms *contralateral*, which refers to an opposite side. The term *equilateral* means "having equal sides." Prefixes in this book will be followed by a hyphen to show that word parts will be added to the prefix to form a word.

This chapter introduces most of the prefixes used in medical terminology in Tables 3-1 to 3-8. Although the list is long, almost all of the prefixes you will need to work through this book are presented here. There is just one short additional table of prefixes related to position in Chapter 5 on body structure. The meanings of many of these prefixes will be familiar to you from words that are already in your vocabulary (see Box 3-1). You may not know all the words in the exercises, but make your best guess. The words in the tables are given as examples of usage. Almost all of them will reappear in later chapters. If you forget a prefix as you work, you may refer to this chapter or to the alphabetical lists of word parts and their meanings in Appendices 3 and 4. Appendix 7 lists prefixes only.

All medical personnel are familiar with these prefixes. To learn about one popular field, nursing, see Box 3-2.

Box 3-1 Focus on Words

Prefix Shorthand

Many prefixes catch on rapidly as a form of shorthand. In everyday life, the prefix e- for electronic has spread to words such as e-mail, e-commerce, e-Bay, e-zine, and others. X- for extreme appears in X-games and other X-sports.

The prefix endo- in the names of many surgical instruments signifies new endoscopic instruments that are longer and thinner and have smaller working tips to be used in areas where there is minimal access. Some examples are endoscissors, endosuture, endocautery, endograsper, and endosnare.

Health care products designed for specific age groups are also encoded by prefixes. Geri-, pertaining to old age, as in geriatrics, appears in geri-chair, geri-pads, geri-jacket, and the patent medicine Geritol, among others. Pedi- or pedia-, meaning "child," is found in the names pedi-cath, pedi-dose, pedi-set (instruments), and Pedialyte, a product used for children to replace fluid and electrolytes.

Box 3-2 Health Professions

Registered Nurse

Careers in nursing are the most diverse of all health care occupations and have the greatest number of practitioners. About 60% of nursing jobs are in hospitals, but other sites include offices, clinics, hospices, homes, and private companies. Within these settings, nurses may concentrate on particular specialties, such as emergency or critical care, surgery, psychiatry, and pediatric (child) or geriatric (elderly) care. Registered nurses (RNs) usually engage in direct patient contact, but they also educate patients and their families about medical conditions, give advice and emotional support, keep patient records, help with diagnostic testing, and provide follow-up and rehabilitative care. On a wider scale, they may work in public health, run health screening or immunization centers, or manage blood drives.

The three possible educational pathways that lead to a nursing career are a 4-year bachelor's degree (BSN), a 2- to 3-year associate degree (ADN) from a community or junior college, or a 2- to 3-year diploma from a hospital nursing program. Courses include liberal arts, sciences, behavioral sciences, and nursing. All programs include supervised clinical training in a health care facility. All graduates must pass a national examination, the NCLEX-RN, to obtain a license to practice.

Many people start their career as practical nurses or nurse's aides and then return to school for an RN degree. Others may begin with an associate degree or diploma and then enroll in a bachelor's degree program while working and receiving tuition reimbursement from an employer. There are also accelerated programs for those with a degree in another field who wish to switch into nursing.

RNs who want to advance further in their careers and work more independently can train as nurse anesthetists, nurse midwives, clinical nurse specialists, or nurse practitioners (who can provide primary care and, in some states, prescribe medications). Careers as nursing educators and administrators also require advanced training. The job outlook for nursing is extremely good, especially in medically underserved areas and in home health care. Sources of information on nursing careers include the National League for Nursing at www.nln.org, the American Association of Colleges of Nursing at www.aacn.nche.edu, and the American Nurses Association at http://nursingworld.org.

Common Prefixes

Table 3-1	Prefixes for Numbers*		
Prefix	**Meaning**	**Example**	**Definition of Example**
prim/i-	first	primary *PRĬ-mar-ē*	first
mon/o-	one	monocular *mon-OK-ū-lar*	having one eyepiece or affecting one eye
uni-	one	unite *ū-NĪT*	form into one part
hemi-	half; one side	hemisphere *HEM-i-sfēr*	one half of a rounded structure (Fig. 3-1)
semi-	half; partial	semipermeable *sem-ē-PER-mē-a-bl*	partially permeable (capable of being penetrated)
bi-	two, twice	binary *BĬ-nar-ē*	made up of two parts
di-	two, twice	diatomic *dī-a-TOM-ik*	having two atoms
dipl/o-	double	diplococci *dip-lō-KOK-sī*	round bacteria (cocci) that grow in groups of two
tri-	three	tricuspid *trĬ-KUS-pid*	having three points or cusps (Fig. 3-2)
quadr/i-	four	quadruplet *kwa-DRŬP-let*	one of four babies born together
tetra-	four	tetralogy *tet-RAL-ō-jē*	a group of four
multi-	many	multicellular *mul-tĬ-SEL-ū-lar*	consisting of many cells (Fig. 3-3)
poly-	many, much	polymorphous *pol-ē-MOR-fus*	having many forms (morph/o)

*Prefixes pertaining to the metric system are in Appendix 1.

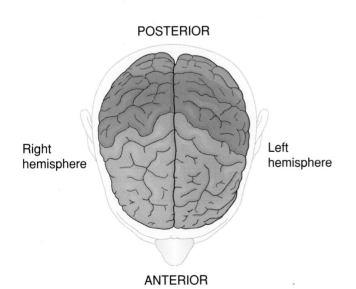

Figure 3-1 **Brain hemispheres.** Each half of the brain is a hemisphere. The prefix *hemi-* means half or one side.

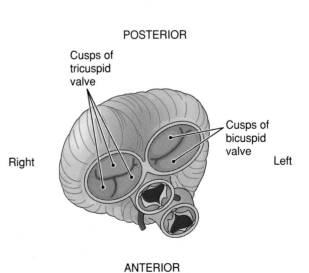

Figure 3-2 **Heart valves.** The valve on the heart's right side, the tricuspid, has three cusps (flaps); the valve on the heart's left side, the bicuspid, has two cusps. The prefixes *bi-* and *tri-* indicate number.

Figure 3-3   **A multicellular organism has more than one cell.** This fungus is a simple multicellular organism.

EXERCISE 3-1

Fill in the blanks:

1. Place the following prefixes in order of increasing numbers:

   a. tri-   **b.** uni-   **c.** tetra-   **d.** bi-

2. A binocular (*bī-NOK-ū-lar*) microscope has _____ eyepieces.

3. A quadruped (*KWAD-rū-ped*) animal walks on _____ feet (ped/o).

4. The term unilateral (*ū-ni-LAT-e-ral*) refers to _____ side (later/o).

5. The term semilunar (*sem-ē-LŪ-nar*) means shaped like a _____ moon.

6. A diploid (*DIP-loyd*) organism has _____ sets of chromosomes (-ploid).

7. A tetrad (*TET-rad*) has _____ components.

8. A tripod (*TRĪ-pod*) has _____ legs.

9. Monophonic sound has _____ channel.

Give a prefix that is similar in meaning to each of the following:

10. di- _____

11. poly- _____

12. hemi- _____

13. mon/o- _____

Table 3-2	Prefixes for Colors		
Prefix	**Meaning**	**Example**	**Definition of Example**
cyan/o-	blue	cyanosis sī-a-NŌ-sis	bluish discoloration of the skin due to lack of oxygen (Fig. 3-4)
erythr/o-	red	erythrocyte e-RITH-rō-sīt	red blood cell (-cyte)
leuk/o-	white, colorless	leukemia lū-KĒ-mē-a	cancer of white blood cells
melan/o-	black, dark	melanin MEL-a-nin	the dark pigment that colors the hair and skin
xanth/o-	yellow	xanthoma zan-THŌ-ma	yellow growth (-oma) on the skin

Figure 3-4 **Cyanosis, a bluish discoloration.** This abnormal coloration is seen in the toenails and toes, as compared to the normal coloration of the fingertips. The prefix *cyan/o-* means "blue."

3

EXERCISE 3-2

Match the following terms and write the appropriate letter to the left of each number:

_____ **1.** melanocyte (*MEL-a-nō-sīt*)

_____ **2.** xanthoderma (*zan-thō-DER-ma*)

_____ **3.** cyanotic (*sī-a-NOT-ik*)

_____ **4.** erythema (*e-ri-THĒ-ma*)

_____ **5.** leukocyte (*LŪ-kō-sīt*)

a. pertaining to bluish discoloration

b. redness of the skin

c. yellow coloration of the skin

d. cell that produces dark pigment

e. white blood cell

Table 3-3   Negative Prefixes

Prefix	Meaning	Example	Definition of Example
a-, an-	not, without, lack of, absence	anhydrous *an-HĪ-drus*	lacking water (hydr/o)
anti-	against	antiseptic *an-ti-SEP-tik*	agent used to prevent infection (sepsis)
contra-	against, opposite	contraindicated *kon-tra-IN-di-kā-ted*	against recommendations; not advisable
de-	down, without, removal, loss	decalcify *dē-KAL-si-fī*	remove calcium (calc/i) from
dis-	absence, removal, separation	dissect *di-SEKT*	to separate tissues for anatomical study
in-*, im- (used before b, m, p)	not	incontinent *in-KON-ti-nent*	not able to contain or control discharge of excretions
non-	not	noncontributory *non-kon-TRIB-ŭ-tor-ē*	not significant; not adding information to a medical diagnosis
un-	not	uncoordinated *un-kō-OR-di-nā-ted*	not working together; not coordinated

*May also mean "in" or "into" as in inject, inhale.

EXERCISE **3-3**

Identify and define the prefix in the following words:

	Prefix	**Meaning of Prefix**
1. aseptic	a-	not, without, lack of, absence
2. antidote	___	___
3. amnesia	___	___
4. disintegrate	___	___
5. contraception	___	___
6. inadequate	___	___
7. depilatory	___	___
8. nonconductor	___	___

Add a prefix to form the negative of the following words:

9. conscious	unconscious
10. significant	___
11. infect	___
12. usual	___
13. specific	___
14. congestant	___
15. compatible	___

Table 3-4	**Prefixes for Direction**

Prefix	Meaning	Example	Definition of Example
ab-	away from	abduct *ab-DUKT*	to move away from the midline (Fig. 3-5)
ad-	toward; near	adduct *ad-DUKT*	to move toward the midline (see Fig. 3-5)
dia-	through	diarrhea *dī-a-RĒ-a*	frequent discharge of fluid fecal matter
per-	through	percutaneous *per-kū-TĀ-nē-us*	through the skin
trans-	through	transfusion *trans-FŪ-zhun*	introduction of blood or blood components into the bloodstream

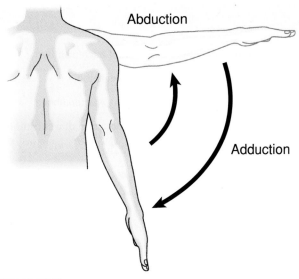

Figure 3-5 **Abduction and adduction.** The prefix *ab-* means "away from"; the arm is moved away from the body in abduction. The prefix *ad-* means "toward"; the arm is moved toward the body in adduction.

EXERCISE 3-4

Identify and define the prefix in the following words:

	Prefix	Meaning of Prefix
1. dialysis	dia-	through
2. percolate	_____	_____
3. adjacent	_____	_____
4. absent	_____	_____
5. diameter	_____	_____
6. transaction	_____	_____

Table 3-5   Prefixes for Degree

Prefix	Meaning	Example	Definition of Example
hyper-	over, excess, abnormally high, increased	hyperglycemia *hī -per-glī-SĒ-mē-a*	high blood sugar (glyc/o)
hypo-*	under, below, abnormally low, decreased	hypotension *hī-pō-TEN-shun*	low blood pressure
olig/o-	few, scanty	oligospermia *ol-i-gō-SPER-mē-a*	abnormally low number of sperm cells in semen
pan-	all	pandemic *pan-DEM-ik*	disease affecting an entire population
super-*	above, excess	supernumerary *su-per-NŪ-mer-ar-ē*	in excess number

*May also show position, as in hypodermic, superficial.

EXERCISE 3-5

Match the following terms and write the appropriate letter to the left of each number:

_____ **1.** hyposecretion (hi-pō-sē-KRĒ-shun)   **a.** excess breathing

_____ **2.** oligodontia (ol-i-gō-DON-shē-a)   **b.** something written above

_____ **3.** panplegia (pan-PLĒ-jē-a)   **c.** underproduction of a substance

_____ **4.** superscript (SŪ-per-skript)   **d.** total paralysis

_____ **5.** hyperventilation (hī-per-ven-ti-LĀ-shun)   **e.** less than the normal number of teeth

Table 3-6   Prefixes for Size and Comparison

Prefix	Meaning	Example	Definition of Example
equi-	equal, same	equilibrium ē-kwi-LIB-rē-um	a state of balance; state in which conditions remain the same
eu-	true, good, easy, normal	euthanasia ū-tha-NĀ-zē-a	easy or painless death (thanat/o)
hetero-	other, different, unequal	heterogeneous het-er-ō-JĒ-nē-us	composed of different materials; not uniform
homo-, homeo-	same, unchanging	homograft HŌ-mō-graft	tissue transplanted to another of the same species
iso-	equal, same	isocellular ī-sō-SEL-ū-lar	composed of similar cells
macro-	large, abnormally large	macroscopic mak-rō-SKOP-ik	large enough to be seen without a microscope
mega-*, megalo-	large, abnormally large	megacolon meg-a-KŌ-lon	enlargement of the colon
micro-*	small	microcyte MĪ-krō-sīt	very small cell (-cyte)
neo-	new	neonate NĒ-ō-nāt	a newborn infant (Fig. 3-6)
normo-	normal	normovolemia nor-mō-vol-Ē-mē-a	normal blood volume
ortho-	straight, correct, upright	orthodontics or-thō-DON-tiks	branch of dentistry concerned with correction and straightening of the teeth (odont/o)
poikilo-	varied, irregular	poikilothermic poy-ki-lō-THER-mik	having variable body temperature (therm/o)
pseudo-	false	pseudoplegia sū-dō-PLĒ-jē-a	false paralysis (-plegia)
re-	again, back	reflux RĒ-flux	backward flow

*Mega- also means 1 million, as in megahertz. Micro- also means 1 millionth, as in microsecond.

Figure 3-6 **A neonate, or newborn.** The prefix *neo-* means "new."

3

EXERCISE 3-6

Match the following terms and write the appropriate letter to the left of each number:

_____ **1.** isograft (*Ī-sō-graft*)

_____ **2.** orthotic (*or-THOT-ik*)

_____ **3.** pseudoreaction (*sū-dō-rē-AK-shun*)

_____ **4.** poikiloderma (*poy-kil-ō-DER-ma*)

_____ **5.** homothermic (*hō-mō-THER-mik*)

a. having a constant body temperature

b. irregular, mottled condition of the skin

c. false response

d. tissue transplanted between identical individuals

e. straightening or correcting deformity

Identify and define the prefix in the following words:

	Prefix	Meaning of Prefix
6. homeostasis	homeo-	same, unchanging
7. equivalent	_____	_____
8. orthopedics	_____	_____
9. regurgitation	_____	_____
10. euthyroidism	_____	_____
11. neocortex	_____	_____
12. megabladder	_____	_____
13. isometric	_____	_____
14. normothermic	_____	_____

Write the opposite of the following words:

15. homogeneous (of uniform composition)
      hō-mō-JĒ-nē-us   _____

16. macroscopic (large enough to see with the naked eye)
      ma-krō-SKOP-ik   _____

Table 3-7	Prefixes for Time and/or Position		
Prefix	**Meaning**	**Example**	**Definition of Example**
ante-	before	antenatal *an-te-NĀ-tal*	before birth (nat/i)
pre-	before, in front of	premature *prĕ-ma-CHUR*	occurring before the proper time
pro-	before, in front of	prodrome *PRŌ-drōm*	symptom that precedes a disease
post-	after, behind	postnasal *pōst-NĀ-sal*	behind the nose (nas/o)

EXERCISE 3-7

Match the following terms and write the appropriate letter to the left of each number:

_____ **1.** postmortem (*pōst-MOR-tem*)

_____ **2.** antedate (*AN-te-dāt*)

_____ **3.** progenitor (*prō-JEN-i-tor*)

_____ **4.** prepartum (*prĕ-PAR-tum*)

_____ **5.** projectile (*prō-JEK-tīl*)

a. to occur before another event

b. ancestor; one who comes before

c. before birth (parturition)

d. throwing or extending forward

e. occurring after death

Identify and define the prefix in the following words:

	Prefix	**Meaning of Prefix**
6. prediction (*prĕ-DIK-shun*)	pre-	before, in front of
7. postmenopausal (*pōst-men-ō-PAW-zal*)	_____	
8. procedure (*prō-SĒD-ūr*)	_____	
9. predisposing (*prĕ-dis-PŌ-zing*)	_____	
10. antepartum (*an-ti-PAR-tum*)	_____	

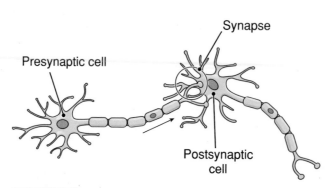

Synapse

Presynaptic cell

Postsynaptic cell

Figure 3-7 **A synapse.** Nerve cells come together at a synapse, as shown by the prefix *syn-*. The presynaptic cell is located before (prefix *pre-*) the synapse; the postsynaptic cell is located after (prefix *post-*) the synapse.

Table 3-8	Prefixes for Position		
Prefix	**Meaning**	**Example**	**Definition of Example**
dextr/o-	right	dextrogastria *deks-trō-GAS-trē-a*	displacement of the stomach (gastr/o) to the right
sinistr/o-	left	sinistromanual *sin-is-trō-MAN-ū-al*	left handed
ec-, ecto-	out, outside	ectopic *ek-TOP-ik*	out of normal position
ex/o-	away from, outside	excise *ek-SĪZ*	to cut out
end/o-	in, within	endoderm *EN-dō-derm*	inner layer of a developing embryo
mes/o-	middle	mesencephalon *mes-en-SEF-a-lon*	middle portion of the brain (encephalon); midbrain
syn-, sym- (used before b, m, p)	together	synapse *SIN-aps*	a junction between two nerve cells (Fig. 3-7)
tel/e-, tel/o-	end	telophase *TEL-ō-fāz*	the last stage of cell division (mitosis)

3

EXERCISE 3-8

Match the following terms and write the appropriate letter to the left of each number:

_____ **1.** mesoderm (*MES-ō-derm*)

_____ **2.** symbiosis (*sim-bī-Ō-sis*)

_____ **3.** sinistrocardia (*sin-is-trō-KAR-dē-a*)

_____ **4.** endoscope (*EN-dō-skōp*)

_____ **5.** telencephalon (*tel-en-SEF-a-lon*)

a. displacement of the heart to the left

b. device for viewing the inside of a structure

c. two organisms living together

d. endbrain

e. middle layer of a developing embryo

Identify and define the prefix in the following words:

	Prefix	**Meaning of Prefix**
6. sympathetic (*sim-pa-THET-ik*)	sym-	together
7. extract (*EKS-tract*)	_____	_____
8. ectoparasite (*ek-tō-PAR-a-sīt*)	_____	_____
9. syndrome (*SIN-drōm*)	_____	_____
10. endotoxin (*en-dō-TOX-in*)	_____	_____

Write the opposite of the following words:

11. exogenous (outside the organism)

eks-OJ-e-nus _____

12. dextromanual (right handed)

deks-trō-MAN-ū-al _____

13. ectoderm (outermost layer of the embryo)

EK-tō-derm _____

Chapter Review

Match the following terms and write the appropriate letter to the left of each number:

_____ **1.** primitive
_____ **2.** biceps
_____ **3.** unify
_____ **4.** dimorphous
_____ **5.** hemithorax

a. one half or one side of the chest
b. having two forms
c. a muscle with two parts
d. combine into one part
e. occurring first in time

_____ **6.** erythroderma
_____ **7.** melanoma
_____ **8.** xanthocyte
_____ **9.** cyanotic
_____ **10.** leukocyte

a. cell with yellow color
b. having a bluish discoloration
c. darkly pigmented tumor
d. redness of the skin
e. white blood cell

_____ **11.** telophase
_____ **12.** mesoderm
_____ **13.** panplegia
_____ **14.** prophase
_____ **15.** diplopia

a. total paralysis
b. first stage of cell division
c. double vision
d. middle layer of tissue
e. final stage of cell division

Match each of the following prefixes with its meaning:

_____ **16.** poikilo-
_____ **17.** eu-
_____ **18.** ortho-
_____ **19.** pseudo-
_____ **20.** oligo-

a. good, true, easy
b. straight, correct
c. false
d. few, scanty
e. varied, irregular

Fill in the blanks:

21. A monocle has _____ lens(es).

22. A triplet is one of _____ babies born together.

23. Sinistrad means toward the _____.

24. A disaccharide is a sugar composed of _____ subunits.

25. A contralateral structure is located on the side _____ to a given point.

26. A tetralogy is composed of _____ part(s).

Identify and define the prefix in the following words:

	Prefix	Meaning of Prefix
27. hyperactive	_____	_____
28. transfer	_____	_____
29. distant	_____	_____
30. posttraumatic	_____	_____
31. regurgitate	_____	_____
32. exhale	_____	_____
33. adhere	_____	_____

Chapter Review *(continued)*

	Prefix	Meaning of Prefix
34. unusual	_____	_____
35. ectoderm	_____	_____
36. detoxify	_____	_____
37. semisolid	_____	_____
38. premenstrual	_____	_____
39. perforate	_____	_____
40. dialysis (*dī-AL-i-sis*)	_____	_____
41. antibody	_____	_____
42. microsurgery	_____	_____
43. disease	_____	_____
44. endoparasite	_____	_____
45. symbiotic (*sim-bī-OT-ik*)	_____	_____
46. prognosis (*prog-NŌ-sis*)	_____	_____
47. insignificant	_____	_____

True–False > Examine the following statements. If the statement is true, write T in the first blank. If the statement is false, write F in the first blank and correct the statement by replacing the underlined word in the second blank.

48. Immune cells are primed by their <u>first</u> exposure to a disease organism.   T   _____

49. A unicellular organism is composed of <u>ten</u> cells.   F   one   _____

50. To bisect is to cut into <u>two</u> parts.   _____   _____

51. A tetrad has <u>five</u> parts.   _____   _____

52. In Latin, the oculus dexter (OD) is the <u>left</u> eye.   _____   _____

53. A triceps muscle has <u>six</u> parts.   _____   _____

54. A polygraph measures <u>many</u> physiologic responses.   _____   _____

55. Quadriplegia is paralysis of <u>four</u> limbs.   _____   _____

Opposites > Write a word that means the opposite of each of the following:

56. humidify   _____

57. abduct   _____

58. permeable   _____

59. heterogeneous   _____

60. exotoxin   _____

61. microscopic   _____

62. hyperventilation   _____

63. postsynaptic   _____

64. septic   _____

Chapter Review *(continued)*

Synonyms > Write a word that means the same as each of the following:

65. supersensitivity   _____

66. megalocyte (extremely
large red blood cell)   _____

67. antenatal   _____

68. isolateral (having equal sides)   _____

Word Building > Write words for the following definitions using the word parts provided. Each may be used more than once.

mon/o   -al   dextr/o   end/o   cardi   cyt   -ic   ecto   micro   -ia

69. Pertaining to a very small cell   _____

70. A condition in which the heart is
outside its normal position   _____

71. Pertaining to a cell with a single nucleus   _____

72. Condition in which the heart is displaced
to the right   _____

73. Pertaining to the innermost layer of
the heart   _____

74. Pertaining to a very large cell   _____

75. Condition in which the heart is
extremely small   _____

Word Analysis > Define each of the following words and give the meaning of the word parts in each. Use a dictionary if necessary.

76. Isometric _____

   a. iso- _____

   b. metr/o _____

   c. -ic _____

77. symbiosis _____

   a. sym- _____

   b. bio _____

   c. -sis _____

78. monoclonal _____

   a. mon/o_____

   b. clon(e)_____

   c. al _____

PASSport
to **Success**®

Go to the Student Resources for additional
review exercises.

Case Studies

> ## Case Study 3-1: Displaced Fracture of the Femoral Neck

While walking home from the train station, M.A., a 72-year-old woman with preexisting osteoporosis, tripped over a broken curb and fell. In the emergency department, she was assessed for severe pain in and swelling and bruising of her right thigh. A radiograph showed a fracture at the neck of the right femur (thigh bone) (Fig. 3-8). M.A. was prepared for surgery and given a preoperative injection of an analgesic to relieve her pain. During surgery, she was given spinal anesthesia and positioned on an operating room table, with her right hip elevated on a small pillow. Intravenous antibiotics were given before the incision was made. Her right hip was repaired with a bipolar hemiarthroplasty (joint reconstruction). Postoperative care included maintaining the right hip in abduction, fluid replacement, physical therapy, and attention to signs of tissue degeneration and possible dislocation.

> ## Case Study 3-2: Sleep Study

The patient is a 58-year-old male 5′10′′, weighing 240 lb, with a history of hypertension and previously treated for thymoma (thymus tumor) and melanoma. He reports excessive daytime sleepiness, snoring, and episodes of apnea (cessation of breathing). A full overnight polysomnography (sleep study) was arranged to evaluate for obstructive sleep apnea syndrome and upper airway resistance syndrome. The studies included electrical tracings of brain, heart, and muscle activity, along with measurement of eye movements and blood oxygen levels. Respiratory effort and airflow were also monitored.

Results showed multiple periods of wakefulness related to sleep-disordered breathing accompanied by recurrent and severe blood oxygen desaturation. Use of

Head
Neck

Anterior view

Figure 3-8 **The right femur (thigh bone).** The femoral neck is the fracture site in Case Study 3-1.

a mask to provide continuous positive airway pressure eliminated the respiratory distress, brought measurements to within normal limits, and eliminated snoring. Continued therapy was recommended, and the patient was also advised to lose weight. Assuming the patient complies with use of the mask, no further treatment or surgery should be necessary.

CASE STUDY QUESTIONS

Identify and define the prefixes in the following words:

	Prefix	Meaning of Prefix
1. preexisting	_____	_____
2. analgesic, anesthesia	_____	_____
3. dislocation, disordered	_____	_____
4. recurrent, replacement	_____	_____
5. bipolar	_____	_____
6. hemiarthroplasty	_____	_____
7. degeneration, desaturation	_____	_____
8. hypertension	_____	_____
9. apnea	_____	_____
10. polysomnography	_____	_____
11. syndrome	_____	_____

(continued)

Case Studies *(continued)*

Fill in the blanks:

12. The suffixes in the words osteoporosis and anesthesia mean _____.

13. The suffixes in the words intravenous, femoral, and analgesic mean _____.

Find a word in the case histories that describes:

14. The time period before surgery _____

15. The time period after surgery _____

16. A position away from the midline of the body _____

17. A darkly pigmented tumor _____

Cells, Tissues, and Organs

CHAPTER

4

CHAPTER CONTENTS

OBJECTIVES

After study of this chapter you should be able to:

1. List the simplest to the most complex levels of a living organism.
2. Describe the main parts of a cell.
3. Label a diagram of a typical cell.
4. Name and give the functions of the four basic types of tissues in the body.
5. Define basic terms pertaining to the structure and function of body tissues.
6. Recognize and use roots and suffixes pertaining to cells, tissues, and organs.
7. Analyze case studies pertaining to cells and tissues.

PRETEST

Multiple choice. Select the best answer and write the letter of your choice to the left of each number.

___ 1. The root that means "cell" is:

    a. spher   c. fibr
    b. cyt   d. gen

___ 2. The root that means "tissue" is:

    a. hist   c. cyst
    b. cellul   d. hem

___ 3. The control center of the cell is the:

    a. membrane   c. virus
    b. ribosome   d. nucleus

___ 4. The process of body cell division is called:

    a. separation   c. mitosis
    b. segregation   d. gestation

___ 5. A compound that speeds the rate of a metabolic reaction is a(n):

    a. gene   c. enzyme
    b. salt   d. mineral

___ 6. The substance that makes up the cell's genetic material is:

    a. DNA   c. acid
    b. protein   d. base

___ 7. Chemicals: cells: tissues: _____: systems: organism. What belongs in the blank?

    a. organs   c. enzymes
    b. genes   d. nuclei

___ 8. The root *morph/o* means:

    a. reproduction   c. form
    b. fat   d. balance

Body Organization

All organisms are built from simple to more complex levels (Fig. 4-1). Chemicals form the materials that make up cells, which are the body's structural and functional units. Groups of cells working together make up **tissues**, which in turn make up the **organs** with specialized functions. Organs become components of the various systems, which together comprise the whole organism. This chapter discusses the terminology related to cells, tissues, and organs, leading to the study of all the organ systems in Part 3.

The Cell

The **cell** is the basic unit of living organisms (Fig. 4-2). Cells accomplish all the activities and produce all the components of the body. They carry out **metabolism**, the sum of all the body's physical and chemical activities. They provide the energy for metabolic reactions in the form of the chemical **ATP** (adenosine triphosphate), commonly described as the energy compound of the cell. The main categories of organic compounds contained in cells are:

- **Proteins**, which include the **enzymes**, some hormones, and structural materials.

- **Carbohydrates**, which include sugars and starches. The main carbohydrate is the sugar **glucose**, which circulates in the blood to provide energy for the cells.

- **Lipids**, which include fats. Some hormones are derived from lipids, and adipose (fat) tissue is designed to store lipids.

Within the **cytoplasm** that fills the cell are subunits called **organelles**, each with a specific function (see Fig. 4-2). The main cell structures are named and described in Box 4-1. Diseases may affect specific parts of cells. Cystic fibrosis and diabetes, for example, involve the plasma membrane. Other disorders originate with mitochondria, ER, lysosomes, or peroxisomes (Box 4-2).

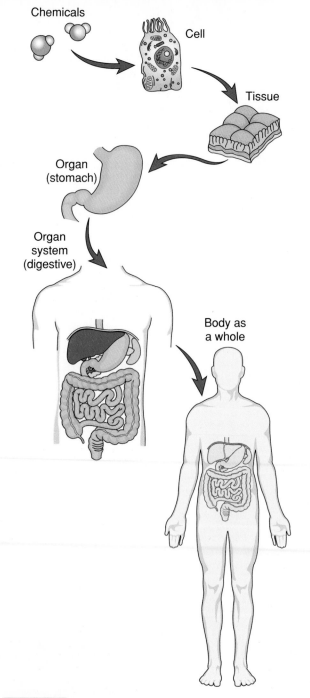

Chemicals

Cell

Tissue

Organ (stomach)

Organ system (digestive)

Body as a whole

Figure 4-1 **Levels of organization.** The organ shown is the stomach, which is part of the digestive system.

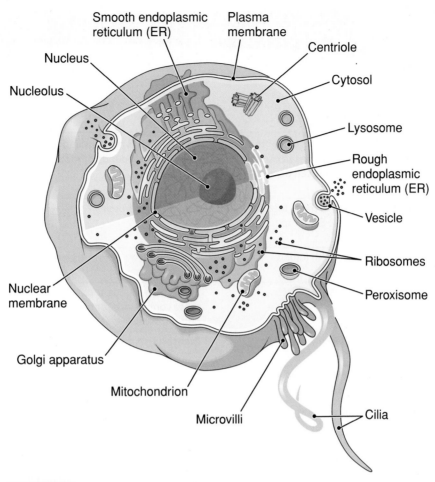

Smooth endoplasmic reticulum (ER)
Plasma membrane
Centriole
Cytosol
Lysosome
Rough endoplasmic reticulum (ER)
Vesicle
Ribosomes
Peroxisome
Cilia
Microvilli
Mitochondrion
Golgi apparatus
Nuclear membrane
Nucleolus
Nucleus

Figure 4-2 **Generalized animal cell, sectional view.** The main organelles are shown.

Box 4-1	For Your Reference

Cell Structures

NAME	DESCRIPTION	FUNCTION
Plasma membrane (*PLAZ-ma*)	Outer layer of the cell; composed mainly of lipids and proteins	Encloses the cell contents; regulates what enters and leaves the cell; participates in many activities, such as growth, reproduction, and interactions between cells
Microvilli (*mī-krō-VIL-ī*)	Short extensions of the cell membrane	Absorb materials into the cell
Nucleus (*NŪ-klē-us*)	Large, dark-staining organelle near the center of the cell, composed of DNA and proteins	Contains the chromosomes, the hereditary units that direct all cellular activities
Nucleolus (*nū-KLĒ-ō-lus*)	Small body in the nucleus; composed of RNA, DNA, and protein	Makes ribosomes
Cytoplasm (*SĪ-tō-plazm*)	Colloidal suspension that fills the cell from the nuclear membrane to the plasma membrane	Site of many cellular activities. Consists of cytosol and organelles
Cytosol (*SĪ-tō-sol*)	The fluid portion of the cytoplasm	Surrounds the organelles

Box 4-1 For Your Reference *(Continued)*

Cell Structures

NAME	DESCRIPTION	FUNCTION
Endoplasmic reticulum (ER) (*en-dō-PLAZ-mik re-TIK-ū-lum*)	Network of membranes within the cytoplasm. Rough ER has ribosomes attached to it; smooth ER does not have ribosomes	Rough ER sorts proteins and forms them into more complex compounds. Smooth ER is involved with lipid synthesis
Ribosomes (*RĪ-bō-sōmz*)	Small bodies free in the cytoplasm or attached to the ER; composed of RNA and protein	Manufacture proteins
Mitochondria (*mī-tō-KON-drē-a*)	Large organelles with folded membranes inside	Convert energy from nutrients into ATP
Golgi apparatus (*GŌL-jē*)	Layers of membranes	Makes compounds containing proteins; sorts and prepares these compounds for transport to other parts of the cell or out of the cell
Lysosomes (*LĪ-sō-sōmz*)	Small sacs of digestive enzymes	Digest substances within the cell
Peroxisomes (*per-OKS-i-sōmz*)	Membrane-enclosed organelles containing enzymes	Break down harmful substances
Vesicles (*VES-i-klz*)	Small membrane-bound sacs in the cytoplasm	Store materials and move materials into or out of the cell in bulk
Centrioles (*SEN-trē-ōlz*)	Rod-shaped bodies (usually two) near the nucleus	Help separate the chromosomes during cell division
Surface projections	Structures that extend from the cell	Move the cell or the fluids around the cell
Cilia (*SIL-ē-a*)	Short, hairlike projections from the cell	Move the fluids around the cell
Flagellum (*fla-JEL-um*)	Long, whiplike extension from the cell	Moves the cell

Box 4-2 Clinical Perspectives

Cell Organelles and Disease

Two organelles that play a vital role in cellular disposal and recycling may also be involved in disease. **Lysosomes** contain enzymes that break down carbohydrates, lipids, proteins, and nucleic acids to safely recycle cellular structures. Lysosomes may also digest the cell itself as a normal part of development. Cells that are no longer needed "self-destruct" by releasing lysosomal enzymes into their own cytoplasm. In Tay–Sachs disease, the lysosomes in nerve cells lack an enzyme that breaks down certain kinds of lipids. These lipids build up inside the cells, causing malfunction that leads to brain injury, blindness, and death.

Peroxisomes resemble lysosomes but contain different kinds of enzymes. They break down toxic substances that enter the cell, such as drugs and alcohol, as well as harmful byproducts of normal metabolism. Disease may result if lysosomes or peroxisomes destroy cells in error. This may occur in cases of autoimmune diseases, in which the body develops an immune response to its own cells. The joint disease rheumatoid arthritis is one such example.

Mitochondria, because they may have been separate organisms early in evolution, have their own DNA. Mutations (changes) in their DNA or in the nuclear DNA that controls their activity can disrupt ATP production and damage organs throughout the body. These mitochondrial disorders are difficult to diagnose because they cause a variety of symptoms and have been confused with epilepsy, cerebral palsy, and multiple sclerosis.

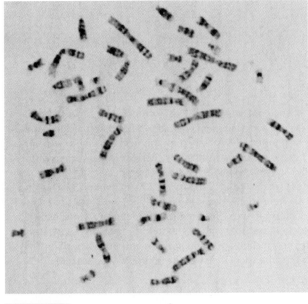

Figure 4-3 **Human chromosomes.** There are 46 chromosomes in each human cell, except the sex cells (egg and sperm).

The **nucleus** is the control region of the cell. It contains the **chromosomes**, which carry genetic information (Fig. 4-3). Each human cell, aside from the reproductive (sex) cells, contains 46 chromosomes. These threadlike structures are composed of a complex organic substance, **DNA (deoxyribonucleic acid)**, which is organized into separate units called **genes**. Genes control the formation of proteins, most particularly enzymes, the catalysts needed to speed the rate of metabolic reactions. To help manufacture proteins, the cells use a compound called **RNA (ribonucleic acid)**, which is chemically related to DNA. Changes (mutations) in the genes or chromosomes are the source of hereditary diseases, as described in Chapter 15.

When a body cell divides by the process of **mitosis**, the chromosomes are doubled and then equally distributed to the two daughter cells. The stages in mitosis are shown in Figure 4-4. When a cell is not dividing, it remains in a stage called *interphase*. In cancer, cells multiply without control causing cellular overgrowth and tumors. Reproductive cells (egg and sperm) divide by a related process, meiosis, that halves the chromosomes in preparation for fertilization. The role of meiosis in reproduction is further explained in Chapter 14.

The study of cells is **cytology** (*sī-TOL-ō-jē*), based on the root *cyt/o*, meaning "cell." Box 4-3 has career information in the field of cytology.

Tissues

Cells are organized into four basic types of tissues that perform specific functions:

- Epithelial (*ep-i-THĒ-lē-al*) tissue covers and protects body structures and lines organs, vessels, and

Figure 4-4 **The stages in cell division (mitosis).** When it is not undergoing mitosis, the cell is in interphase. The cell shown is for illustration only. It is not a human cell, which has 46 chromosomes.

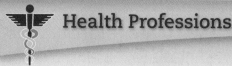

Box 4-3   Health Professions

Cytotechnologist

Cytotechnology is the laboratory study of cells. Cytotechnologists work with pathologists to diagnose cancer, infections, and other diseases based on cellular changes. This profession developed initially for the study of Pap smears, used in the diagnosis of cervical cancer, but has since expanded to include analysis of specimens from many other body sites, such as glands, lymph nodes, organs, and body cavities. In addition to direct microscopic study, the work of cytotechnologists also now includes molecular analysis and immunologic chemistry, often involving complex automated and computerized instruments.

Someone interested in a cytotechnology career should be meticulous and independent and should possess a high degree of responsibility. Preparation for this field requires a bachelor's degree with courses in anatomy, chemistry, microbiology, histology, and mathematics plus specialized laboratory training. Those interested in a supervisory, management, or teaching position need an advanced degree and 3 to 5 years of professional experience. The American Society for Cytotechnology develops practice standards, monitors regulatory issues, evaluates new technologies, and provides educational opportunities for the profession. Their website is http://www.asct.com.

cavities (Fig. 4-5). Simple epithelium, composed of cells in a single layer, functions to absorb substances from one system to another, as in the respiratory and digestive tracts. Stratified epithelium, with cells in multiple layers, protects deeper tissues, as in the mouth and vagina. Most of the active cells in glands are epithelial cells. Glands are described in more detail in Chapter 16.

- Connective tissue supports and binds body structures (Fig. 4-6). It contains fibers and other nonliving material between the cells. Included are adipose (fat) tissue, cartilage, bone (Chapter 19), and blood (Chapter 10).

- Muscle tissue (root: *my/o*) contracts to produce movement (Fig. 4-7). There are three types of muscle tissue:

  - Skeletal muscle moves the skeleton. It has visible cross-bands, or striations, that are involved in contraction. Because it is under conscious control, it is also called voluntary muscle. Skeletal muscle is discussed in greater detail in Chapter 20.

  - Cardiac muscle forms the heart. It functions without conscious control and is described as involuntary. Chapter 9 describes the heart and its actions.

  - Smooth, or visceral, muscle forms the walls of the abdominal organs; it is also involuntary. Many organs described in later chapters on the systems have walls made of smooth muscle. The walls of ducts and blood vessels also are composed mainly of smooth muscle.

- Nervous tissue (root: *neur/o*) makes up the brain, spinal cord, and nerves (Fig. 4-8). It coordinates and controls body responses by the transmission of electrical impulses. The basic cell in nervous tissue is the neuron, or nerve cell. The nervous system and senses are discussed in Chapters 17 and 18.

Figure 4-5 **Epithelial tissue.** The cells in simple epithelium (*A*) are in a single layer and absorb materials from one system to another. The cells in stratified epithelium (*B*) are in multiple layers and protect deeper tissues.

Membranes

The simplest tissues are membranes. Mucous membranes secrete **mucus**, a thick fluid that lubricates surfaces and

Figure 4-6 **Connective tissue.** Examples of connective tissue are adipose tissue (*A*), which stores fat; cartilage (*B*), which is used for protection and reinforcement; and bone (*C*), which makes up the skeleton.

Figure 4-7 **Muscle tissue.** Skeletal muscle (*A*) moves the skeleton. It has visible bands (striations) that produce contraction. Cardiac muscle (*B*) makes up the wall of the heart. Smooth muscle (*C*) makes up the walls of hollow organs, ducts, and vessels.

Figure 4-8 **Nervous tissue.** The functional cell of the nervous system is the neuron (*A*). Neuron fibers join to form nerves (*B*). Nervous tissue also makes up the spinal cord and brain (*C*), where it is divided into gray matter and white matter.

Box 4-4   **Clinical Perspectives**

Laboratory Study of Tissues

Biopsy is the removal and examination of living tissue to determine a diagnosis. The term is also applied to the specimen itself. *Biopsy* comes from the Greek word *bios*, meaning "life," plus *opsis*, meaning "vision." Together they mean the visualization of living tissue.

Some other terms that apply to cells and tissues come from Latin. *In vivo* means "in the living body," as contrasted with *in vitro*, which literally means "in glass," and refers to procedures and experiments done in the laboratory, as compared with studies done in living organisms. *In situ* means "in its original place" and is used to refer to tumors that have not spread.

In toto means "whole" or "completely," as in referring to a structure or organ removed totally from the body. *Postmortem* literally means "after death," as in referring to an autopsy performed to determine the cause of death.

---

protects underlying tissue, as in the lining of the digestive tract and respiratory passages. Serous membranes, which secrete a thin, watery fluid, line body cavities and cover organs. These include the membranes around the heart and lungs. Fibrous membranes cover and support organs, as found around the bones, the brain, and spinal cord.

The study of tissues is **histology** (*his-TOL-ō-jē*), based on the root *hist/o*, meaning "tissue." Box 4-4 describes some terms used in histology.

Organs and Organ Systems

Tissues are arranged into organs, which serve specific functions, and organs, in turn, are grouped into systems. Figure 4-9 shows the organs of the digestive system as an example. Grouped according to functions, the body systems are:

- Circulation:
  - Cardiovascular system, consisting of the heart and blood vessels.
  - Lymphatic system, organs and vessels that aid circulation and help protect the body from foreign materials.

- Nutrition and fluid balance:
  - Respiratory system, which obtains the oxygen needed for metabolism and eliminates carbon dioxide, a byproduct of metabolism.
  - Digestive system, which takes in, breaks down, and absorbs nutrients and eliminates undigested waste.
  - Urinary system, which eliminates soluble waste and balances the volume and composition of body fluids.

- Production of offspring:
  - The male and female reproductive systems.

- Coordination and control:
  - Nervous system, consisting of the brain, spinal cord, and nerves, and including the sensory system. This system receives and processes stimuli and directs responses.

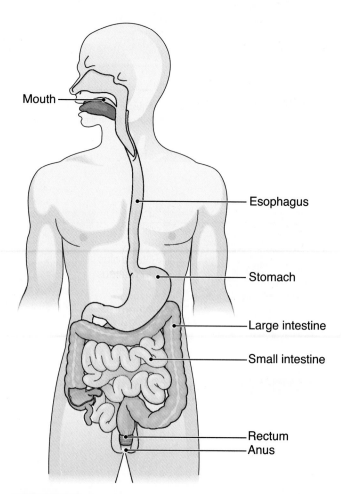

Figure 4-9 **Organs of the digestive tract.** Other organs and glands contribute to digestion, as described in Chapter 12.

- Endocrine system, individual glands that produce hormones.
- Body structure and movement:
  - Skeletal system, the bones and joints.
  - Muscular system, which moves the skeleton and makes up organs. The muscular system and skeleton protect vital organs.
- Body covering:

- The skin, or integumentary system, which functions in protection and also helps to regulate body temperature.

Each of the body systems is discussed in Part 3. Bear in mind, however, that the body functions as a whole—no system is independent of the others. They work together to maintain the body's state of internal stability, termed **homeostasis**.

Terminology — Key Terms

Term	Definition
ATP	The energy compound of the cell that stores energy needed for cell activities. ATP stands for adenosine triphosphate (*a-DEN-ō-sēn trī-FOS-fāt*)
carbohydrate *kar-bō-HĪ-drāt*	The category of organic compounds that includes sugars and starches
cell *sel*	The basic structural and functional unit of the living organism; a microscopic unit that combines with other cells to form tissues (root: *cyt/o*)
chromosome *KRŌ-mō-sōm*	A threadlike body in a cell's nucleus that contains genetic information
cytology *sī-TOL-ō-jē*	Study of cells
cytoplasm *SĪ-tō-plazm*	The fluid that fills a cell and holds the organelles
DNA	The genetic compound of the cell; makes up the genes. DNA stands for deoxyribonucleic (*dē-ok-sē-rī-bō-nū-KLĒ-ik*) acid
enzyme *EN-zīm*	An organic substance that speeds the rate of a metabolic reaction
gene *jēn*	A hereditary unit composed of DNA and combined with other genes to form the chromosomes
glucose *GLŪ-kōs*	A simple sugar that circulates in the blood; the main energy source for metabolism (roots: *gluc/o, glyc/o*)
histology *his-TOL-ō-jē*	Study of tissues
homeostasis *hō-mē-ō-STĀ-sis*	A steady state; a condition of internal stability and constancy
lipid *LIP-id*	A category of organic compounds that includes fats (root: *lip/o*)
metabolism *me-TA-bō-lizm*	The sum of all the physical and chemical reactions that occur within an organism
mitosis *mī-TŌ-sis*	Cell division
mucus *MŪ-kus*	A thick fluid secreted by cells in membranes and glands that lubricates and protects tissues (roots: *muc/o, myx/o*); the adjective is *mucous*
nucleus *NŪ-klē-us*	The cell's control center; directs all cellular activities based on the information contained in its chromosomes (roots: *nucle/o, kary/o*)
organ *OR-gan*	A part of the body with a specific function. A component of a body system

(continued)

Terminology	Key Terms (continued)
organelle OR-ga-nel	A specialized structure in the cytoplasm of a cell
protein PRŌ-tēn	A category of organic compounds that includes structural materials, enzymes, and some hormones
RNA	An organic compound involved in the manufacture of proteins within cells. RNA stands for ribonucleic (rī-bō-nū-KLĒ-ik) acid
tissue TISH-ū	A group of cells that acts together for a specific purpose (roots: hist/o, histi/o)

PASSport to Success® Go to the pronunciation glossary on the Student Resources to hear these words pronounced.

Word Parts Pertaining to Cells, Tissues, and Organs

See Tables 4-1 to 4-3

Table 4-1	Roots for Cells and Tissues

Root	Meaning	Example	Definition of Example
morph/o	form	polymorphous pol-ē-MOR-fus	having many forms
cyt/o, -cyte	cell	cytologist sī-TOL-ō-jist	one who studies cells
nucle/o	nucleus	nuclear NŪ-klē-ar	pertaining to a nucleus
kary/o	nucleus	karyotype KAR-ē-ō-tīp	picture of a cell's chromosomes organized according to size (Fig. 4-10)
hist/o, histi/o	tissue	histocompatibility his-tō-kom-pat-i-BIL-i-tē	tissue similarity that permits transplantation
fibr/o	fiber	fibrosis fī-BRŌ-sis	abnormal formation of fibrous tissue
reticul/o	network	reticulum re-TIK-ū-lum	a network
aden/o	gland	adenoma ad-e-NO-ma	tumor (-oma) of a gland
papill/o	nipple	papilla pa-PIL-a	projection that resembles a nipple
myx/o	mucus	myxadenitis miks-ad-e-NĪ-tis	inflammation (-itis) of a mucus-secreting gland
muc/o	mucus, mucous membrane	mucorrhea mū-kō-RĒ-a	increased flow (-rhea) of mucus
somat/o, -some	body, small body	chromosome KRŌ-mō-sōm	small body that takes up color (dye) (chrom/o)

Figure 4-10 **Human karyotype.** The 46 chromosomes are in 23 pairs arranged according to size. The XY sex chromosomes, the 23rd pair at the lower right, indicate that the cell is from a male; a female cell has XX sex chromosomes.

EXERCISE **4-1**

4

Fill in the blanks:

1. Cytogenesis is the formation (genesis) of _____.

2. A fibril (FĪ-bril) is a small _____.

3. A histologist (his-TOL-ō-jist) studies _____.

4. A dimorphic (dī-MOR-fik) organism has two _____.

5. Karyomegaly (kar-ē-ō-MEG-a-lē) is enlargement (-megaly) of the _____.

6. Nucleoplasm is the substance that fills the _____.

7. Adenitis (ad-e-NĪ-tis) is inflammation (-itis) of a(n) _____.

8. A papillary (PAP-i-lar-ē) structure resembles a(n) _____.

9. A myxoma (mik-SŌ-ma) is a tumor of tissue that secretes _____.

10. A reticulocyte (re-TIK-ū-lō-sīt) is a cell that contains a(n) _____.

11. The term *mucosa* (mu-KŌ-sa) is used to describe a membrane that secretes _____.

12. Somatotropin (sō-ma-tō-TRŌ-pin), also called growth hormone, has a general stimulating effect on the
_____.

Use the suffix -logy to build a word with each of the following meanings:

13. The study of form _____

14. The study of cells _____

15. The study of tissues _____

Table 4-2	Roots for Cell Activity		

Root	Meaning	Example	Definition of Example
blast/o, -blast	immature cell, productive cell, embryonic cell	histioblast *HIS-tē-ō-blast*	a tissue-forming cell
gen	origin, formation	karyogenesis *kar-ē-ō-JEN-e-sis*	formation of a nucleus
phag/o	eat, ingest	autophagy *aw-TOF-a-jē*	self (auto) destruction of a cell's organelles
phil	attract, absorb	basophilic *bā-sō-FIL-ik*	attracting basic stain
plas	formation, molding, development	hyperplasia *hī-per-PLĀ-zē-a*	overdevelopment of an organ or tissue
trop	act on, affect	chronotropic *kron-o-TROP-ik*	affecting rate or timing (chron/o)
troph/o	feeding, growth, nourishment	atrophy *A-trō-fē*	tissue wasting

The roots in Table 4-2 are often combined with a simple noun suffix (*-in*, *-y*, or *-ia*) or an adjective suffix (*-ic*) and used as word endings. Such combined forms that routinely appear as word endings will simply be described and used as suffixes in this book. Examples from the above list are *-trophy*, *-plasia*, *-tropin*, *-philic*, and *-genic*.

EXERCISE 4-2

Match the following terms and write the appropriate letter to the left of each number:

_____ **1.** phagocyte (FAG-ō-sīt)   **a.** overdevelopment of tissue

_____ **2.** histogenesis (his-tō-JEN-e-sis)   **b.** study of heredity

_____ **3.** leukoblast (LŪ-kō-blast)   **c.** formation of tissue

_____ **4.** genetics (je-NET-iks)   **d.** cell that ingests waste

_____ **5.** hypertrophy (hī-PER-trō-fē)   **e.** immature white blood cell

_____ **6.** neoplasia (nē-ō-PLĀ-jē-a)   **a.** attracting color

_____ **7.** gonadotropin (gon-a-dō-TRŌ-pin) **b.** pertaining to the body

_____ **8.** aplasia (a-PLĀ-jē-a)   **c.** substance that acts on the sex glands

_____ **9.** somatic (sō-MAT-ik)   **d.** new formation of tissue

_____ **10.** chromophilic (krō-mō-FIL-ik)   **e.** lack of development

Identify and define the root in the following words:

	Root	Meaning of Root
11. genesis (JEN-e-sis)	_____	_____
12. esophagus (e-SOF-a-gus)	_____	_____
13. normoblast (NOR-mō-blast)	_____	_____
14. aplastic (a-PLAS-tik)	_____	_____
15. dystrophy (DIS-trō-fē)	_____	_____

Table 4-3	Suffixes and Roots for Body Chemistry

Word Part	Meaning	Example	Definition of Example
Suffixes			
-ase	enzyme	lipase *LĪ-pās*	enzyme that digests fat (lipid)
-ose	sugar	lactose *LAK-tōs*	milk sugar
Roots			
hydr/o	water, fluid	hydration *hī-DRĀ-shun*	addition of water; relative amount of water present
gluc/o	glucose	glucogenesis *glū-kō-JEN-e-sis*	production of glucose
glyc/o	sugar, glucose	normoglycemia *nor-mō-glī-SĒ-mē-a*	normal blood sugar level
sacchar/o	sugar	polysaccharide *pol-ē-SAK-a-rīd*	compound containing many simple sugars
amyl/o	starch	amyloid *AM-i-loyd*	resembling starch
lip/o	lipid, fat	lipophilic *lip-ō-FIL-ik*	attracting or absorbing lipid
adip/o	fat	adiposuria *ad-i-pō-SŪR-ē-a*	presence of fat in the urine (ur/o)
steat/o	fatty	steatorrhea *stē-a-tō-RĒ-a*	discharge (-rhea) of fatty stools
prote/o	protein	protease *PRŌ-tē-ās*	enzyme that digests protein

4

EXERCISE 4-3

Fill in the blanks:

1. A disaccharide (*dī-SAK-a-rīd*) is a compound that contains two _____.

2. The ending *-ose* indicates that fructose is a(n) _____.

3. Hydrophobia (*hī-drō-FŌ-bē-a*) is an aversion (-phobia) to _____.

4. Amylase (*AM-i-lās*) is an enzyme that digests _____.

5. Liposuction (*LIP-ō-suk-shun*) is the surgical removal of _____.

6. A glucocorticoid (*glū-kō-KOR-ti-koyd*) is a hormone that controls the metabolism of _____.

7. An adipocyte (*AD-i-pō-sīt*) is a cell that stores _____.

Identify and define the root in the following words:

		Root	Meaning of Root
8.	asteatosis (*as-tē-a-TŌ-sis*)	_____	_____
9.	lipoma (*lī-PŌ-ma*)	_____	_____
10.	hyperglycemia (*hī-per-glī-SĒ-mē-a*)	_____	_____
11.	glucolytic (*glū-kō-LIT-ik*)	_____	_____

Terminology   Supplementary Terms

amino acids *a-MĒ-nō*	The nitrogen-containing compounds that make up proteins
anabolism *a-NAB-ō-lizm*	The type of metabolism in which body substances are made; the building phase of metabolism
catabolism *ka-TAB-ō-lizm*	The type of metabolism in which substances are broken down for energy and simple compounds
collagen *KOL-a-jen*	A fibrous protein found in connective tissue
cortex *KOR-tex*	The outer region of an organ
glycogen *GLĪ-kō-jen*	A complex sugar compound stored in liver and muscles and broken down into glucose when needed for energy
interstitial *in-ter-STISH-al*	Between parts, such as the spaces between cells in a tissue
medulla *me-DUL-la*	The inner region of an organ; marrow (root: *medull/o*)
parenchyma *par-EN-ki-ma*	The functional tissue of an organ
parietal *pa-RĪ-e-tal*	Pertaining to a wall; describes a membrane that lines a body cavity
soma *SŌ-ma*	The body
stem cell	An immature cell that has the capacity to develop into any of a variety of different cell types. A precursor cell
visceral *VIS-er-al*	Pertaining to the internal organs, describes a membrane on the surface of an organ

 PASSport to Success®   Go to the pronunciation glossary on the Student Resources to hear these words pronounced.

Chapter Review

LABELING EXERCISE

Diagram of a Typical Animal Cell > Write the name of each numbered part on the corresponding line of the answer sheet.

Centriole
Cilia
Cytosol
Golgi apparatus
Lysosome
Microvilli
Mitochondrion
Nuclear membrane

Nucleolus
Nucleus
Peroxisome
Plasma membrane
Ribosomes
Rough ER
Smooth ER
Vesicle

1. _____
2. _____
3. _____
4. _____
5. _____
6. _____
7. _____
8. _____
9. _____
10. _____
11. _____
12. _____
13. _____
14. _____
15. _____
16. _____

TERMINOLOGY

Matching > Match the following terms and write the appropriate letter to the left of each number:

_____ **1.** cytoplasm
_____ **2.** DNA
_____ **3.** nucleoplasm
_____ **4.** homeostasis
_____ **5.** ATP

a. state of internal stability
b. material that holds the cellular organelles
c. energy compound of the cells
d. genetic material
e. material that fills the nucleus

_____ **6.** mitosis
_____ **7.** ribosomes
_____ **8.** mitochondria
_____ **9.** blastocyte
_____ **10.** liposomes

a. immature cell
b. organelles that produce ATP
c. organelles that contain RNA
d. small bodies that store fat
e. cell division

Chapter Review *(continued)*

_____ **11.** reticular
_____ **12.** adenoid
_____ **13.** fibroma
_____ **14.** megakaryocyte
_____ **15.** chromosome

a. resembling a gland
b. fibrous tumor
c. cell with a very large nucleus
d. pertaining to a network
e. structure that contains genes

_____ **16.** autotroph
_____ **17.** papilliform
_____ **18.** cytogenesis
_____ **19.** atrophy
_____ **20.** somatic

a. resembling a nipple
b. wasting of tissue
c. formation of cells
d. pertaining to the body
e. organism that can manufacture its own food

_____ **21.** fibroplasia
_____ **22.** hypoplasia
_____ **23.** dysphagia
_____ **24.** amorphous
_____ **25.** lipolysis

a. difficulty in eating
b. dissolving of fat
c. underdevelopment of an organ or tissue
d. formation of fibrous tissue
e. having no specific form

_____ **26.** glucosuria
_____ **27.** proteolytic
_____ **28.** adiposuria
_____ **29.** polysaccharide
_____ **30.** hydrotherapy

a. presence of fat in the urine
b. presence of glucose in the urine
c. treatment using water
d. compound composed of many simple sugars
e. destroying or dissolving protein

Supplementary Terms

_____ **31.** amino acid
_____ **32.** collagen
_____ **33.** glycogen
_____ **34.** cortex
_____ **35.** catabolism

a. outer region of an organ
b. building block of protein
c. fibrous protein in connective tissue
d. complex sugar stored in liver and muscles
e. breakdown phase of metabolism

Fill in the blanks:

36. All the activity of a cell makes up its _____.

37. The four basic tissue types are _____.

38. The study of tissues is called _____.

39. The simple sugar that is the main energy source for metabolism is _____.

40. The control center of the cell is the _____.

41. An organic compound that speeds the rate of metabolic reactions is a(n) _____.

42. A cytotoxic substance is poisonous or damaging to _____.

43. The term *dehydration* refers to a loss or deficiency of _____.

44. The study of form and structure is called _____.

45. A myxocyte is found in tissue that secretes _____.

Chapter Review *(continued)*

True–False > Examine the following statements. If the statement is true, write T in the first blank. If the statement is false, write F in the first blank, and correct the statement by replacing the underlined word in the second blank.

46. An adipocyte is a cell that stores <u>proteins</u>.   _____   _____

47. Hydrophobia is an aversion to <u>fats</u>.   _____   _____

48. A megakaryocyte is a cell with a large <u>nucleus</u>.   _____   _____

49. There are <u>46</u> chromosomes in each human cell, aside from the reproductive cells.   _____   _____

50. A whiplike extension of a cell is a <u>flagellum</u>.   _____   _____

Word Building > Write a word for each of the following definitions using the word parts provided. Each may be used more than once.

-oid   amyl/o   muc/o   aden/o   -ase   lip/o   leuk/o   histi/o   blast

51. Like or resembling a gland   _____

52. Immature white blood cell   _____

53. Enzyme that digests fat   _____

54. Resembling mucus   _____

55. Cell that gives rise to tissue   _____

56. Enzyme that digests starch   _____

57. Resembling starch   _____

Word Analysis > Define each of the following words and give the meaning of the word parts in each. Use a dictionary if necessary.

58. somatotropic (sō-ma-tō-TROP-ik) _____

    a. somat/o _____

    b. trop/o _____

    c. -ic _____

59. autophagy (aw-TOF-a-jē) _____

    a. auto _____

    b. phag/o _____

    c. -y _____

60. asteatosis (as-tē-a-TŌ-sis) _____

    a. a- _____

    b. steat/o _____

    c. -sis _____

PASSport to Success®   Go to Student Resources for additional review exercises.

Case Studies

➤ Case Study 4-1: Hematology Laboratory Studies

J.E. had a blood test as required for preoperative anesthesia assessment in preparation for scheduled plastic surgery on her breasts. The report read as follows:

Complete blood count (CBC) and differential
Red blood cell (RBC) count—4.5 million/μL
Hemoglobin (Hgb)—12.6 g/dL
Hematocrit (Hct)—38%
White blood cell (WBC) count—8500/μL
Neutrophils—58%
Lymphocytes—34%
Monocytes—6%
Eosinophils—1.5%
Basophils—0.5%
Platelet count—200,000/μL
Prothrombin time (PT)—11.5 seconds
Partial thromboplastin time (PTT)—65 seconds
Blood glucose—84 mg/dL

The surgeon reviewed these results and concluded that they were within normal limits (WNL).

➤ Case Study 4-2: Pathology Laboratory Tests

R.C., the manager of the clinical and pathology laboratory, received several surgical specimens taken from a 26-year-old female patient with a 4-week history of nonspecific pelvic pain. The specimens included several small containers of pink-tinged cloudy fluid labeled *pelvic lavage* (washing) *for cytology*, which R.C. took to the cytology laboratory to be placed on slides and checked microscopically for abnormal cells. R.C. also received a tissue specimen labeled *uterine myoma*, a wedge biopsy of a right ovarian neoplasm, and four jars, each labeled *pelvic lymph nodes*. She took all of the tissue specimens to the pathology laboratory for gross and microscopic evaluation. A test tube half filled with a cloudy gel and a cotton-tipped applicator labeled *swab of pelvic fluid for culture and sensitivity and Gram stain* was taken to the microbiology laboratory to be streaked on a culture plate and incubated to look for growth. Any organisms that grew out would be gram stained and tested for sensitivity to antibiotics that might be used in treatment.

The laboratory form was accompanied by a surgeon's note stating that the patient's preoperative diagnosis was cervical dysplasia with atypical cells and a positive urine leukocyte esterase, indicating a urinary tract infection. R.C. placed a copy of the laboratory forms and surgeon's note on the desk of the pathologist who was doing a research project on carcinogenesis (causes of cancer).

CASE STUDY QUESTIONS

Multiple choice. Select the best answer and write the letter of your choice to the left of each number:

_____ 1. J.E.'s blood test results were within normal limits. She could be described as being in a state of:
  a. normosmosis
  b. dysplasia
  c. homeostasis
  d. hematophilia
  e. myogenesis

_____ 2. The suffix in *glucose* indicates that this compound is a(n):
  a. cervix
  b. enzyme
  c. protein
  d. sugar
  e. fat

_____ 3. The suffix in *esterase* indicates that this compound is a(n):
  a. sugar
  b. carbohydrate
  c. cell
  d. enzyme
  e. lipid

_____ 4. The root *gen* in carcinogenesis refers to a cancer's:
  a. origin
  b. treatment
  c. location
  d. laboratory results
  e. severity

Identify and give the meaning of the prefixes in the following words:

	Prefix	Meaning of Prefix
5. monocytes	_____	_____
6. prothrombin	_____	_____
7. neoplasm	_____	_____
8. atypical	_____	_____
9. leukocyte	_____	_____

Find words in the case studies for the following:

10. Three words that contain a root that means *attract, absorb*: _____

11. Three words with a root that means *formation, molding, development*: _____

12. Four words with a root that means *cell*: _____

- right and left iliac (*IL-ē-ak*) regions, named for the upper bone of the hip, the ilium. These regions are also called the inguinal (*ING-gwi-nal*) regions, with reference to the groin.

More simply, but less precisely, the abdomen can be divided into four sections by a single vertical line and a single horizontal line that intersect at the umbilicus (navel) (Fig. 5-5). The sections are the right upper quadrant (RUQ), left upper quadrant (LUQ), right lower quadrant (RLQ), and left lower quadrant (LLQ).

Additional terms for body regions are shown in Figures 5-6 and 5-7. You may need to refer to these illustrations as you work through the book.

Positions

In addition to the anatomic position, there are other standard positions in which the body is placed for special purposes, such as examination, tests, surgery, or fluid drainage. The most common of these positions and some of their uses are described in Box 5-4.

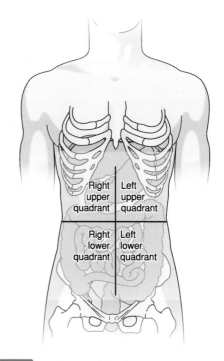

Figure 5-5 **Quadrants of the abdomen.** Some organs within the quadrants are indicated.

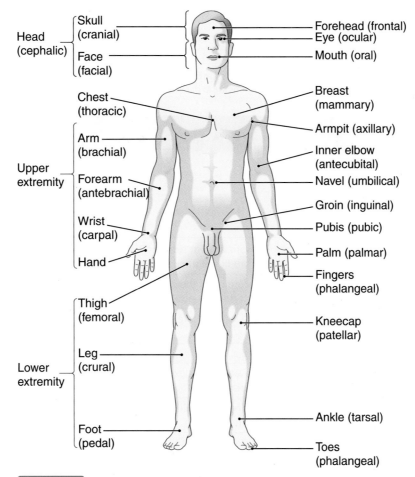

Figure 5-6 **Common terms for body regions, anterior view.** Anatomic adjectives for regions are in parentheses.

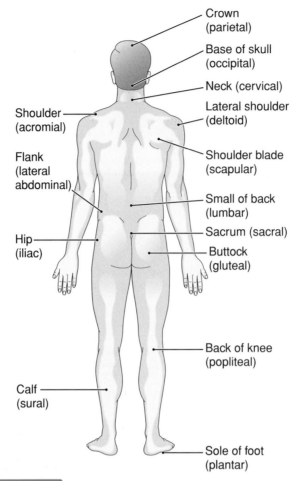

Figure 5-7 **Common terms for body regions, posterior view.**
Anatomic adjectives for regions are in parentheses.

Box 5-4 For Your Reference

Body Positions

POSITION	DESCRIPTION
anatomic position *an-a-TOM-ik*	standing erect, facing forward, arms at sides, palms forward, legs parallel, toes pointed forward; used for descriptions and studies of the body
decubitus position *dē-KŪ-bi-tus*	lying down, specifically according to the part of the body resting on a flat surface, as in left or right lateral decubitus, or dorsal or ventral decubitus
dorsal recumbent position *rē-KUM-bent*	on back, with legs bent and separated, feet flat; used for obstetrics and gynecology
Fowler position	on back, head of bed raised about 18 in., knees elevated; used to ease breathing and for drainage
jackknife position *JAK-nīf*	on back with shoulders elevated, legs flexed and thighs at right angles to the abdomen; used to introduce a tube into the urethra
knee–chest position	on knees, head and upper chest on table, arms crossed above head; used in gynecology and obstetrics and for flushing the intestine
lateral recumbent position	on the side with one leg flexed; arm position may vary
lithotomy position *li-THOT-ō-mē*	on back, legs flexed on abdomen, thighs apart; used for gynecologic and urologic surgery

| Box 5-4 | For Your Reference (Continued) |

Body Positions

POSITION	DESCRIPTION
prone	lying face down
Sims position	on left side, right leg drawn up high and forward, left arm along back, chest forward resting on bed; used for kidney and uterine surgery, colon examination, and enemas
supine* SŪ-pīn	lying face up
Trendelenburg position tren-DEL-en-berg	on back with head lowered by tilting bed back at 45° angle; used for pelvic and abdominal surgery, treatment of shock

*To remember the difference between prone and supine, look for the word *up* in supine.

Terminology Key Terms

abdominal cavity ab-DOM-i-nal	The large ventral cavity below the diaphragm and above the pelvic cavity
abdominopelvic cavity ab-dom-i-nō-PEL-vik	The large ventral cavity between the diaphragm and pelvis that includes the abdominal and pelvic cavities
anatomic position an-a-TOM-ik	Standard position for anatomic studies, in which the body is erect and facing forward, the arms are at the sides with palms forward, and the feet are parallel
cranial cavity KRĀ-nē-al	The dorsal cavity that contains the brain
diaphragm DĪ-a-fram	The muscle that separates the thoracic from the abdominal cavity
frontal (coronal) plane ko-RŌN-al	Plane of section that separates the body into anterior (front) and posterior (back) portions
pelvic cavity PEL-vik	The ventral cavity that is below the abdominal cavity
peritoneum per-i-tō-NĒ-um	The large serous membrane that lines the abdominopelvic cavity and covers the organs within it
sagittal plane SAJ-i-tal	Plane that divides the body into right and left portions
spinal cavity (canal) SPĪ-nal	Dorsal cavity that contains the spinal cord
thoracic cavity thō-RAS-ik	The ventral cavity above the diaphragm; the chest cavity
transverse (horizontal) plane trans-VERS	Plane that divides the body into superior (upper) and inferior (lower) portions

PASSport to Success® Go to the pronunciation glossary on the Student Resources to hear these words pronounced.

Word Parts Pertaining to Body Structure

See Tables 5-1 to 5-3.

Table 5-1	Roots for Regions of the Head and Trunk		
Root	**Meaning**	**Example**	**Definition of Example**
cephal/o	head	megacephaly *meg-a-SEF-a-lē*	abnormal largeness of the head
cervic/o	neck	cervicofacial *ser-vi-kō-FĀ-shal*	pertaining to the neck and face
thorac/o	chest, thorax	thoracotomy *thō-ra-KOT-Ō-mē*	incision (-tomy) into the chest
abdomin/o	abdomen	intra-abdominal *in-tra-ab-DOM-i-nal*	within the abdomen
celi/o	abdomen	celiocentesis *sē-lē-ō-sen-TĒ-sis*	surgical puncture (centesis) of the abdomen
lapar/o	abdominal wall	laparoscope *LAP-a-rō-skōp*	instrument (-scope) for viewing the peritoneal cavity through the abdominal wall
lumb/o	lumbar region, lower back	thoracolumbar *thō-rak-ō-LUM-bar*	pertaining to the chest and lumbar region
periton, peritone/o	peritoneum	peritoneal *per-i-tō-NĒ-al*	pertaining to the peritoneum

EXERCISE 5-1

Write the adjective for each of the following definitions. The correct suffix is given in parentheses:

1. Pertaining to (-al) the abdomen _____abdominal_____

2. Pertaining to (-ic) the head _____

3. Pertaining to (-al) the neck _____

4. Pertaining to the chest (-ic) _____

5. Pertaining to (-ar) the lower back _____

Fill in the blanks:

6. Peritonitis (*per-i-tō-NĪ-tis*) is inflammation (-itis) of the _____.

7. The adjective celiac (*SĒ-lē-ak*) pertains to the _____.

8. Mesocephalic refers to an average size of the _____.

9. A laparotomy (*lap-a-ROT-ō-mē*) is an incision through the _____.

| Table 5-2 | Roots for the Extremities | | |

Root	Meaning	Example	Definition of Example
acro	extremity, end	acrocyanosis *ak-rō-sī-a-NŌ-sis*	bluish discoloration of the extremities
brachi/o	arm	antebrachium *an-tē-BRĀ-kē-um*	forearm
dactyl/o	finger, toe	polydactyly *pol-ē-DAK-til-ē*	having more than the normal number of fingers or toes
ped/o	foot	pedometer *pe-DOM-e-ter*	instrument that measures footsteps
pod/o	foot	podiatric *pō-dē-AT-rik*	pertaining to study and treatment of the foot

EXERCISE 5-2

Fill in the blanks:

1. Acrokinesia (*ak-rō-kī-NĒ-sē-a*) is excess motion (-kinesia) of the _____.

2. Animals that brachiate (*BRĀ-kē-āt*), such as monkeys, swing from place to place using their _____.

3. A dactylospasm (*DAK-til-ō-spazm*) is spasm (cramp) of a(n) _____.

4. The term brachiocephalic (*brā-kē-ō-se-FAL-ik*) refers to the _____.

5. Sinistropedal (*si-nis-trō-PĒ-dal*) refers to the use of the left _____.

5

| Table 5-3 | Prefixes for Position and Direction | | |

Prefix	Meaning	Example	Definition of Example
circum-	around	circumoral *ser-kum-OR-al*	around the mouth
peri-	around	periorbital *per-ē-OR-bit-al*	around the orbit (eye socket)
intra-	in, within	intravascular *in-tra-VAS-kū-lar*	within a vessel (vascul/o)
epi-	on, over	epithelial *ep-i-THĒ-lē-al*	referring to epithelium, tissue that covers surfaces
extra-	outside	extrathoracic *eks-tra-thō-RAS-ik*	outside the thorax
infra-*	below	infrascapular *in-fra-SKAP-ū-lar*	below the scapula (shoulder blade)
sub-*	below, under	sublingual *sub-LING-gwal*	under the tongue (lingu/o)
inter-	between	intercostal *in-ter-KOS-tal*	between the ribs (cost/o)

(continued)

| Table 5-3 | **Continued** | | |

Prefix	Meaning	Example	Definition of Example
juxta-	near, beside	juxtaposition *juks-ta-pō-ZI-shun*	a location near or beside another structure
para-	near, beside	parasagittal *par-a-SAJ-i-tal*	near or beside a sagittal plane
retro-	behind, backward	retrouterine *re-trō-Ū-ter-in*	behind the uterus
supra-	above	suprapatellar *su-pra-pa-TEL-ar*	above the patella (kneecap)

*Also indicates degree.

EXERCISE 5-3

Synonyms. Write a word that means the same as each of the following:

1. perioral   circumoral _____

2. subscapular   _____

3. perivascular   _____

4. infracostal   _____

5. circumorbital   _____

Opposites. Write a word that means the opposite of each of the following:

6. infrapatellar   suprapatellar _____

7. intracellular   _____

8. subscapular   _____

9. extrathoracic   _____

Define the following words:

10. paranasal (*par-a-NĀ-zal*) _____

11. retroperitoneal (*re-trō-per-i-tō-NĒ-al*) _____

12. supra-abdominal (*sū-pra-ab-DOM-i-nal*) _____

13. intrauterine (*in-tra-Ū-ter-in*) _____

Refer to Figures 5-6 and 5-7 to define the following terms:

14. periumbilical (*per-ē-um-BIL-i-kal*) _____

15. intergluteal (*in-ter-GLŪ-tē-al*) _____

16. epitarsal (*ep-i-TAR-sal*) _____

17. intraocular (*in-tra-OK-ū-lar*) _____

18. parasacral (*par-a-SĀ-kral*) _____

Terminology — Supplementary Terms

Term	Definition
digit *DIJ-it*	A finger or toe (adjective: digital)
epigastrium *ep-i-GAS-trē-um*	The epigastric region
fundus *FUN-dus*	The base or body of a hollow organ; the area of an organ farthest from its opening
hypochondrium *hī-pō-KON-drē-um*	The hypochondriac region (left or right)
lumen *LŪ-men*	The central opening within a tube or hollow organ
meatus *mē-Ā-tus*	A passage or opening
orifice *OR-i-fis*	The opening of a cavity
os	Mouth; any body opening
septum *SEP-tum*	A wall dividing two cavities
sinus *SĬ-nus*	A cavity, as within a bone
sphincter *SFINK-ter*	A circular muscle that regulates an opening

 Go to the pronunciation glossary on the Student Resources to hear these words pronounced.

Terminology — Abbreviations

LLQ	Left lower quadrant
LUQ	Left upper quadrant
RLQ	Right lower quadrant
RUQ	Right upper quadrant

Chapter Review

LABELING EXERCISE

Directional Terms > Write the name of each numbered part on the corresponding line of the answer sheet.

Anterior (ventral)   Medial
Distal   Posterior (dorsal)
Inferior (caudal)   Proximal
Lateral   Superior (cranial)

1. _____
2. _____
3. _____
4. _____
5. _____
6. _____
7. _____
8. _____

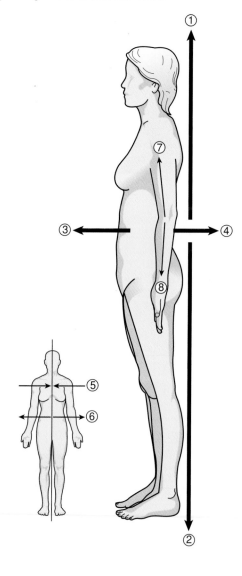

Planes of Division > Write the name of each numbered part on the corresponding line of the answer sheet.

Frontal (coronal) plane   Transverse (horizontal) plane
Sagittal plane

1. _____

2. _____

3. _____

Body Cavities, Lateral View > Write the name of each numbered part on the corresponding line of the answer sheet.

Abdominal cavity   Pelvic cavity
Abdominopelvic cavity   Spinal cavity (canal)
Cranial cavity   Thoracic cavity
Dorsal cavity   Ventral cavity
Diaphragm

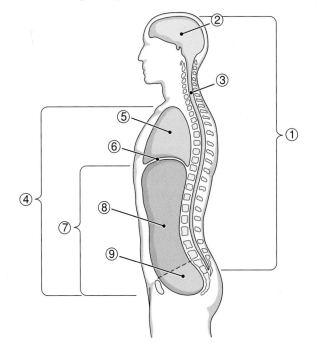

1. _____

2. _____

3. _____

4. _____

5. _____

6. _____

7. _____

8. _____

9. _____

5

The Nine Regions of the Abdomen > Write the name of each numbered part on the corresponding line of the answer sheet.

Epigastric region   Right hypochondriac region
Hypogastric region   Right iliac (inguinal) region
Left hypochondriac region   Right lumbar region
Left iliac (inguinal) region   Umbilical region
Left lumbar region

1. _____

2. _____

3. _____

4. _____

5. _____

6. _____

7. _____

8. _____

9. _____

TERMINOLOGY

Matching > Match the following terms and write the appropriate letter to the left of each number:

_____ **1.** cephalad   **a.** surgical puncture of the chest
_____ **2.** acrodermatitis   **b.** skin inflammation of the extremities
_____ **3.** laparoscopy   **c.** pertaining to the right foot
_____ **4.** dextropedal   **d.** examination through the abdominal wall
_____ **5.** thoracentesis   **e.** toward the head

_____ **6.** microcephaly   **a.** circular cut
_____ **7.** celiotomy   **b.** excessive size of the feet
_____ **8.** macropodia   **c.** outer layer of the skin
_____ **9.** epidermis   **d.** abnormal smallness of the head
_____ **10.** circumcision   **e.** incision of the abdomen

Supplementary Terms

_____ **11.** septum   **a.** central opening of a tube
_____ **12.** fundus   **b.** circular muscle that regulates an opening
_____ **13.** lumen   **c.** dividing wall
_____ **14.** sphincter   **d.** cavity, as in a bone
_____ **15.** sinus   **e.** base of a hollow organ

Chapter Review (continued)

True–False > Examine each of the following statements. If the statement is true, write T in the first blank. If the statement is false, write F in the first blank and correct the statement by replacing the underlined word in the second blank.

16. The cranial and spinal cavities are the <u>ventral</u> body cavities.   __F__   _____dorsal_____

17. A <u>midsagittal plane</u> divides the body into equal right and left parts.   _____   _____

18. The wrist is <u>distal</u> to the elbow.   _____   _____

19. A <u>transverse plane</u> divides the body into anterior and posterior parts.   _____   _____

20. The abdominal cavity is <u>inferior</u> to the thoracic cavity.   _____   _____

21. The hypogastric region is <u>superior</u> to the umbilical region.   _____   _____

22. In the <u>supine</u> position, a person is lying face-down.   _____   _____

23. The left hypochondriac region is in the <u>LUQ</u>.   _____   _____

Adjectives > Name the part of the body referred to in the following adjectives:

24. lumbar   _____

25. carpal   _____

26. popliteal   _____

27. occipital   _____

28. phalangeal   _____

29. cervical   _____

30. celiac   _____

31. brachial   _____

Define the following words:

32. perioral   _____

33. suprapubic   _____

34. infraumbilical   _____

35. intercostal   _____

36. sublingual   _____

37. retroperitoneal   _____

38. bipedal   _____

Synonyms > Write a word that means the same as each of the following:

39. posterior   _____

40. circumocular   _____

41. submammary   _____

42. ventral   _____

Opposites > Write a word that means the opposite of each of the following:

43. megacephaly _____

44. deep _____

45. proximal _____

46. subscapular _____

47. extracellular _____

48. superior _____

Eliminations > In each of the sets below, underline the word that does not fit in with the rest and explain the reason for your choice:

49. thoracic cavity — spinal cavity — pelvic cavity — abdominal cavity — abdominopelvic cavity

_____

50. umbilical region — hypochondriac region — epigastric region — cervical region — iliac region

_____

51. jackknife — supine — sagittal — decubitus — prone

_____

52. lumb/o — dactyl/o — brachi/o — acro — pod/o

_____

Word Building > Write a word for each of the following definitions using the word parts provided.

spasm   cephal   -o-   dactyl   extra-   -ic   infra-   syn-   thorac   a-   intra-   -y   poly-

53. within the head _____

54. below the chest _____

55. outside the chest _____

56. condition of having extra fingers or toes _____

57. fusion of the fingers or toes _____

58. pertaining to the head and chest _____

59. absence of a finger or toe _____

60. cramp of a finger or toe _____

61. absence of a head _____

Word Analysis > Define each of the words below and give the meaning of the word parts in each. Use a dictionary if necessary.

62. megacephaly (*meg-a-SEF-a-lē*) _____

   a. mega- _____

   b. cephal/o _____

   c. -y _____

63. acrocyanosis (*ak-rō-sī-a-NŌ-sis*) _____

    a. acro _____

    b. cyan/o _____

    c. -sis _____

64. antebrachial (*an-tē-BRĀ-kē-al*) _____

    a. ante- _____

    b. brachi/o _____

    c. -al _____

65. epigastric (*ep-i-GAS-trik*) _____

    a. epi- _____

    b. gastr/o _____

    c. -ic _____

PASSport to Success® Go to the Student Resources for additional review exercises.

Case Study

➤ Case Study 5-1: Emergency Care

During a triathlon, paramedics responded to a scene with multiple patients involved in a serious bicycle accident. B.R., a 20-year-old woman, lost control of her bike while descending a hill at approximately 40 mph. As she fell, two other cyclists collided with her, sending all three crashing to the ground.

At the scene, B.R. reported pain in her head, back, chest, and leg. She also had numbness and tingling in her legs and feet. Other injuries included a cut on her face and on her right arm and an obvious deformity to both her shoulder and knee. She had slight difficulty breathing.

The paramedic did a rapid cephalocaudal assessment and immobilized B.R.'s neck in a cervical collar. She was secured on a backboard and given oxygen. After her bleeding was controlled and her injured extremities were immobilized, she was transported to the nearest emergency department.

During transport, the paramedic in charge radioed ahead to provide a prehospital report to the charge nurse. His report included the following information: occipital and frontal head pain; laceration to right temple, superior and anterior to right ear; lumbar pain; bilateral thoracic pain on inspiration at midclavicular line on the right and midaxillary line on the left; dull aching pain of the posterior proximal right thigh; bilateral paresthesia (numbness and tingling) of distal lower legs circumferentially; varus (knock-knee) adduction deformity of left knee; and posterior displacement deformity of left shoulder.

At the hospital, the emergency department physician ordered radiographs for B.R. Before the procedure, the radiology technologist positioned a lead gonadal shield centered on the midsagittal line above B.R.'s symphysis pubis to protect her ovaries from unnecessary irradiation by the primary beam. The technologist knew that gonadal shielding is important for female patients undergoing imaging of the lumbar spine, sacroiliac joints, acetabula, pelvis, and kidneys. Shields should not be used for any examination in which an acute abdominal condition is suspected.

(continued)

Case Study *(continued)*

CASE STUDY QUESTIONS

Multiple choice. Select the best answer and write the letter of your choice to the left of each number:

_____ 1. The term for the time span between injury and admission to the emergency department is:
   a. preoperative
   b. prehospital
   c. pre-emergency
   d. pretrauma
   e. intrainjury

_____ 2. A cephalocaudal assessment goes from _____.
   a. stem to stern
   b. front to back
   c. head to toe
   d. side to side
   e. skin to bone

_____ 3. The victim's injured extremities were immobilized before transport. Immobilized means:
   a. abducted as far as possible
   b. internally rotated and flexed
   c. adducted so that the limbs are crossed
   d. rotated externally
   e. held in place to prevent movement

_____ 4. A cervical collar was placed on the victim to stabilize and immobilize the _____.
   a. uterus
   b. shoulders
   c. chin
   d. neck
   e. pelvis

_____ 5. The singular form of acetabula is:
   a. acetyl
   b. acetabulum
   c. acetabia
   d. acetab
   e. acetabulae

Draw or shade the appropriate area(s) on one or both diagrams for each question:

6. Draw dots over the areas of the victim's occipital and frontal head pain.

7. Draw a dash (—) over the area of the right temporal laceration—superior and anterior to the right ear.

8. Cross-hatch the area of lumbar pain.

9. Place an X over the area of thoracic pain at the anterior left midaxillary line.

10. Draw a star at the area of the pain on the right proximal posterior thigh.

11. Shade the area of the bilateral paresthesia of the distal lower legs, circumferentially.

12. Draw an arrow to show the direction of the varus adduction of the left knee.

13. Draw an arrow to show the direction of the posterior displacement of the left shoulder.

14. Draw a fig leaf to show the gonadal shield on the midsagittal line above the symphysis pubis.

15. Draw a circle around the area of the sacroiliac joints.

CHAPTER

6

Disease

CHAPTER CONTENTS

OBJECTIVES

After study of this chapter you should be able to:

1. List the major categories of diseases.
2. Compare the common types of infectious organisms, and list some diseases caused by each.
3. Describe the common responses to disease.
4. Define and give examples of neoplasia.
5. Identify and use word parts pertaining to diseases.
6. Define the major terms describing types of diseases.
7. List and define the major manifestations of diseases.
8. Analyze the disease terminology in several case studies.

PRETEST

Multiple choice. Select the best answer and write the letter of your choice to the left of each number.

___ 1. Any organism so small that it can only be seen with a microscope is a:

    a. miniorganism   c. microcell
    b. macroorganism d. microorganism

___ 2. A disease that has a sudden and severe onset is described as:

    a. chronic   c. acute
    b. mild   d. infectious

___ 3. Abnormal and uncontrolled growth of tissue is termed:

    a. anemia   c. parasitism
    b. neoplasia   d. toxicity

___ 4. Round bacteria are called:

    a. cocci   c. fungi
    b. yeasts   d. bacilli

___ 5. Single-celled animals, as a group, are called:

    a. algae   c. protozoa
    b. molds   d. vibrios

___ 6. Heat, pain, redness, and swelling are the characteristics signs of:

    a. immunity   c. inflammation
    b. fever   d. healing

___ 7. White blood cells engulf foreign organisms by the process of:

    a. phagocytosis   c. ejection
    b. egestion   d. dysphagia

___ 8. The sum of all body defenses against infectious disease is termed:

    a. pyosis   c. secretion
    b. complementation   d. immunity

A disease is any disorder of normal body function. Diseases can be grouped into a number of different but often overlapping categories.

Types of Diseases

- Infectious diseases—caused by certain harmful microorganisms and other **parasites** that live at the expense of another organism. Any disease-causing organism is described as a **pathogen**.

- Degenerative diseases—resulting from wear and tear, aging, or **trauma** (injury) that can result in a **lesion** (wound) and perhaps **necrosis** (death of tissue). Common examples include arthritis, cardiovascular problems, and certain respiratory disorders such as emphysema. Structural malformations such as congenital malformations, **prolapse** (dropping), or **hernia** (rupture) may also result in degenerative changes.

- Neoplasia—abnormal and uncontrolled growth of tissue.

- Immune disorders—This category includes failures of the immune system, allergies, and autoimmune diseases, in which the body makes antibodies to its own tissues. (Immune disorders receive more detailed discussion in Chapter 10.)

- Metabolic disorders—resulting from lack of enzymes or other factors needed for cellular functions. Many hereditary disorders fall into this category. Malnutrition caused by inadequate intake of nutrients or inability of the body to absorb and use nutrients also upsets metabolism. (Metabolic disorders are discussed in more detail in Chapter 12, and hereditary disorders are discussed in Chapter 15.)

- Hormonal disorders—caused by underproduction or overproduction of hormones or by inability of the hormones to function properly. One example is diabetes mellitus. (Chapter 16 has more detail on hormonal disorders.)

- Mental and emotional disorders—disorders that affect the mind and adaptation of an individual to his or her environment. (Chapter 17 has further discussion on behavioral disorders.)

Some methods for naming diseases are described in Box 6-1.

Box 6-1   Focus on Words

Name That Disease

Diseases get their names in a variety of ways. Some are named for the places where they were first found, such as Lyme disease for Lyme, Connecticut; West Nile disease and Rift Valley fever for places in Africa; and hantavirus fever for a river in Korea. Others are named for the people who first described them, such as Cooley anemia; Crohn disease, an inflammatory bowel disease; and Hodgkin disease of the lymphatic system.

Many diseases are named on the basis of the symptoms they cause. Tuberculosis causes small lesions known as tubercles in the lungs and other tissues. Skin anthrax produces lesions that turn black, and its name comes from the same root as anthracite coal. In sickle cell anemia, red blood cells become distorted into a crescent shape when they give up oxygen. Having lost their smooth, round form, the cells jumble together, blocking small blood vessels and depriving tissues of oxygen.

Bubonic plague causes painful and enlarged lymph nodes called buboes. Lupus erythematosus, a systemic autoimmune disorder, is named for the Latin term for wolf, because the red rash that may form on the face of people with this disease gives them a wolflike appearance. Yellow fever, scarlet fever, and rubella (German measles) are named for colors associated with the pathology of these diseases.

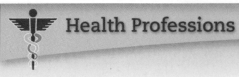

Box 6-2   Health Professions

Emergency Medical Technicians

Emergency medical technicians (EMTs) are the first health professionals to arrive at the scene of an automobile accident, heart attack, or other emergency situation. EMTs must assess and respond rapidly to a medical crisis, taking a medical history, performing a physical examination, stabilizing the patient, and, if necessary, transporting the patient to the nearest medical facility.

To perform their lifesaving duties, EMTs need extensive training, including a thorough understanding of anatomy and physiology. EMTs must know how to use specialized equipment, such as backboards to immobilize injuries, electrocardiographs to monitor heart activity, and defibrillators to treat cardiac arrest; they must also be proficient at giving intravenous fluids, oxygen, and certain lifesaving medications. At medical facilities, EMTs work closely with physicians and nurses, reporting on histories, physical examinations, and measures taken to stabilize the patient. Most EMTs receive their training from a college or technical school and must be certified in the state where they are employed.

As the American population ages and becomes concentrated in urban centers, the rate of accidents and other emergencies is expected to rise. Thus, the need for EMTs remains high. For more information about this career, contact the National Association of Emergency Medical Technicians at http://www.naemt.org.

The cause of a disease is its **etiology** (ē-tē-OL-ō-jē), although many diseases have multiple interacting causes. An **acute** disease is sudden and severe and of short duration.

A **chronic** disease is of long duration and progresses slowly. One health profession that deals with the immediate effects of acute disease is the Emergency Medical Technician (EMT) (Box 6-2).

A Diplococci

B Streptococci

Infectious Diseases

Infectious diseases are caused by viruses, bacteria, fungi (yeasts and molds), protozoa (single-celled animals), and worms (Box 6-3). Infecting organisms can enter the body through several routes, or portals of entry, including damaged skin, the respiratory tract, digestive system, and the urinary and reproductive tracts. An infected person's bodily discharges may contain organisms that spread infection through the air, food, water, or direct contact. Microorganisms often produce disease by means of the **toxins** (poisons) they release. The presence of harmful microorganisms or their toxins in the body is termed **sepsis**.

C Staphylococci

D Streptococci, photomicrograph

Figure 6-1   Cocci, round bacteria, Gram stained. (*A*) Cells growing in pairs, diplococci. (*B*) Cells in chains, streptococci. (*C*) Cells in clusters, staphylococci. (*D*) Streptococci viewed under a microscope in a photomicrograph. Gram-positive cells are purple; gram-negative cells are red.

Bacteria

In shape, bacteria are:

- Round, or cocci, shown in Figure 6-1
- Rod-shaped, or bacilli, shown in Figure 6-2
- Curved, including vibrios and spirochetes, shown in Figure 6-3

Box 6-3   For Your Reference

Common Infectious Organisms

TYPE OF ORGANISM	DESCRIPTION	EXAMPLES OF DISEASES CAUSED
bacteria *bak-TĒ-rē-a*	simple microscopic organisms that are widespread throughout the world; some can produce disease; singular: bacterium (*bak-TĒ-rē-um*)	
cocci *KOK-sī*	round bacteria; may be in clusters (staphylococci), chains (streptococci), and other formations; singular, coccus (*KOK-us*)	pneumonia, rheumatic fever, food poisoning, septicemia, urinary tract infections, gonorrhea
bacilli *ba-SIL-ī*	rod-shaped bacteria; singular, bacillus (*ba-SIL-us*)	typhoid, dysentery, salmonellosis, tuberculosis, botulism, tetanus
vibrios *VIB-rē-ōz*	short curved rods	cholera, gastroenteritis
spirochetes *SPĪ-rō-kētz*	corkscrew-shaped bacteria that move with a twisting motion	Lyme disease, syphilis, Vincent disease
chlamydia *kla-MID-ē-a*	extremely small bacteria that, like viruses, grow in living cells, but are susceptible to antibiotics	conjunctivitis, trachoma, pelvic inflammatory disease (PID), and other sexually transmitted infections (STIs)
rickettsia *ri-KET-sē-a*	extremely small bacteria that grow in living cells but are susceptible to antibiotics	typhus, Rocky Mountain spotted fever
viruses *VĪ-rus-es*	submicroscopic infectious agents that can live and reproduce only within living cells	colds, herpes, hepatitis, measles, varicella (chickenpox), influenza, AIDS
fungi *FUN-jī*	simple, nongreen plants, some of which are parasitic; includes yeasts and molds; singular, fungus (*FUN-gus*)	candidiasis, skin infections (tinea, ringworm), valley fever
protozoa *prō-tō-ZŌ-a*	single-celled animals; singular, protozoon (*prō-tō-ZŌ-on*)	dysentery, *Trichomonas* infection, malaria
helminths *HEL-minths*	worms	trichinosis; infestations with roundworms, pinworms, hookworms

A Bacilli

B Bacilli, photomicrograph

Figure 6-2 **Bacilli, rod-shaped bacteria.** (*A*) Drawing of bacilli. (*B*) Photomicrograph of bacilli.

Bacteria may be named according to their shape and also by the arrangements they form (see Fig. 6-1). They are also described according to the dyes they take up when stained in the laboratory. The most common laboratory bacterial stain is the **Gram stain,** with which gram-positive organisms stain purple and gram-negative organisms stain red (see Fig. 6-1).

Chlamydia and rickettsia are two bacterial groups that are smaller than typical bacteria and can grow only within living host cells (see Box 6-3).

A Vibrios

B Spirochetes

C Spirochetes, photomicrograph

Figure 6-3 **Curved bacteria.** (*A*) Vibrios are short curved rods. (*B*) Spirochetes are spiral shaped. (*C*) Spirochetes shown in a photomicrograph.

A

B

Figure 6-4 **Edema.** (*A*) A normal foot showing veins, tendons, and bones. (*B*) Edema (swelling) obscures surface features.

Responses to Disease

Inflammation

A common response to infection and to other forms of disease is **inflammation**. When cells are injured, they release chemicals that allow blood cells and fluids to move into the tissues. This inflow of blood results in the four signs of inflammation:

- heat
- pain
- redness
- swelling

The suffix *-itis* indicates inflammation, as in appendicitis (inflammation of the appendix) and tonsillitis (inflammation of the tonsils).

Inflammation is one possible cause of **edema**, a swelling or accumulation of fluid in the tissues (Fig. 6-4).

Other causes of edema include fluid blockage, heart failure, and imbalance in body fluid composition, as described in later chapters.

PASSport to Success®   Go to the Student Resources to view an animation on inflammation.

Phagocytosis

The body uses **phagocytosis** to get rid of invading microorganisms, damaged cells, and other types of harmful debris. Certain white blood cells are capable of engulfing these materials and destroying them internally (Fig. 6-5). Phagocytic cells are found circulating in the blood, in the tissues, and in the lymphatic system (see Chapters 9

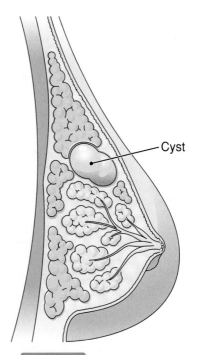

Figure 6-5 **Phagocytosis.** (*A*) A phagocytic white blood cell squeezes through a capillary wall to engulf a bacterium. (*B*) Lysosomal enzymes destroy the bacterium, and the waste products are eliminated.

and 10). The remains of phagocytosis consist of fluid and white blood cells; this mixture is called **pus**.

Immunity

Immunity refers to all our defenses against infectious disease. Inflammation and phagocytosis are examples of inborn or innate protective mechanisms, which are based on a person's genetic makeup and do not require any previous exposure to a disease organism. Other defenses that fall into this category are mechanical barriers, such as intact skin and mucous membranes, as well as body secretions, such as stomach acid and enzymes in saliva and tears.

Immunity that we acquire during life from exposure to disease organisms is termed *adaptive immunity*. This type of immunity is specific for particular diseases encountered by natural exposure or by the administration of vaccines (see Chapter 10). The system responsible for adaptive immunity consists of cells in the blood, lymphatic system, and other tissues. These cells recognize different foreign invaders and get rid of them by direct attack and by production of circulating antibodies that immobilize and help to destroy them. The immune system also monitors the body continuously for abnormal and malfunctioning cells, such as cancer cells. The immune system may overreact to produce allergies and may react to one's own tissues to cause autoimmune diseases.

Neoplasia

As noted earlier, a **neoplasm** is an abnormal and uncontrolled growth of tissue—a tumor or growth. A **benign** neoplasm does not spread, that is, undergo **metastasis** to other tissues, although it may cause damage at the site where it grows. An invasive neoplasm that can metastasize to other tissues is termed **malignant**, and is commonly called *cancer*. A malignant tumor that involves epithelial tissue is a **carcinoma**. If the tumor arises in glandular epithelium, it is an adenocarcinoma (the root *aden/o* means "gland"); a cancer of pigmented epithelial cells (melanocytes) is a melanoma. A neoplasm that involves connective tissue or muscle is a **sarcoma**. Cancers of the blood, lymphatic system, and nervous system are classified according to the cell types involved and other clinical features. Further descriptions of these cancers appear in Chapters 10 and 17.

Often mistaken for a malignancy is a **cyst**, a sac or pouch filled with fluid or semisolid material that is abnormal but not cancerous (Fig. 6-6). Common sites for cyst formation are the breasts, the skin's sebaceous glands, and the ovaries. Causes of cyst formation include infection or blockage of a duct.

Figure 6-6 **Cyst in the breast.**

Terminology | Key Terms

acute *a*-KŪT	Sudden, severe; having a short course
benign *bē*-NĪN	Not recurrent or malignant; favorable for recovery; describing a tumor that does not spread (metastasize) to other tissues
carcinoma *kar-si*-NŌ-*ma*	A malignant neoplasm composed of epithelial cells (from Greek root *carcino*, meaning "crab") (adjective: carcinomatous)
chronic KRON-*ĭk*	Of long duration; progressing slowly
cyst *sist*	An abnormal filled sac or pouch (see Fig. 6-6). Used as a root meaning a normal bladder or sac, such as the urinary bladder or gallbladder (root: cyst/o)
edema *e*-DĒ-*ma*	Accumulation of fluid in the tissues; swelling. Adjective edematous (*e*-DĒ-*ma-tus*) (see Fig. 6-4)
etiology *ē-tē*-OL-*ō-jē*	The cause of a disease
Gram stain	A laboratory staining procedure that divides bacteria into two groups: gram-positive, which stain purple, and gram-negative, which stain red (see Fig. 6-1)
hernia HER-*nē-a*	Protrusion of an organ through an abnormal opening; a rupture (Fig. 6-7)
inflammation *in-fla*-MĀ-*shun*	A localized response to tissue injury characterized by heat, pain, redness, and swelling
lesion LĒ-*zhun*	A distinct area of damaged tissue; an injury or wound
malignant *ma*-LIG-*nant*	Growing worse; harmful; tending to cause death; describing an invasive tumor that can spread (metastasize) to other tissues
metastasis *me*-TAS-*ta-sis*	Spread from one part of the body to another; characteristic of cancer. Verb is metastasize (*me*-TAS-*ta-sīz*); adjective: metastatic (*met-a*-STAT-*ĭk*)
necrosis *ne*-KRŌ-*sis*	Death of tissue (root *necr/o* means "death"); adjective: necrotic (*ne*-KROT-*ĭk*)
neoplasm NĒ-*ō-plazm*	An abnormal and uncontrolled growth of tissue, namely, a tumor; may be benign or malignant. From prefix *neo-* meaning "new" and root *plasm* meaning "formation." The root *onc/o* and the suffix *-oma* refer to neoplasms
parasite PAR-*a-sīt*	An organism that grows on or in another organism (the host), causing damage to it
pathogen PATH-*ō-jen*	An organism capable of causing disease (root *path/o* means "disease")
phagocytosis *fag-ō-sī*-TŌ-*sis*	The ingestion of organisms, such as invading bacteria or small particles of waste material by a cell (root *phag/o* means "to eat"). The phagocytic cell, or phagocyte, then destroys the ingested material (see Fig. 6-5)
prolapse PRŌ-*laps*	A dropping or downward displacement of an organ or part; ptosis
pus	A product of inflammation consisting of fluid and white blood cells (root: py/o)
sarcoma *sar*-KŌ-*ma*	A malignant neoplasm arising from connective tissue (from Greek root *sarco*, meaning "flesh") (adjective: sarcomatous)

(continued)

Terminology   **Key Terms** (continued)

sepsis SEP-sis	The presence of harmful microorganisms or their toxins in the blood or other tissues (adjective: septic)
toxin TOKS-in	A poison (adjective: toxic) (roots: tox/o, toxic/o)
trauma TRAW-ma	A physical or psychological wound or injury

See also Box 6-3 on infectious organisms.

PASSport to Success®   Go to the pronunciation glossary on the Student Resources to hear these words pronounced.

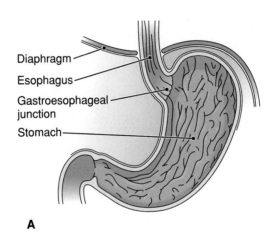

Diaphragm

Esophagus

Gastroesophageal junction

Stomach

A

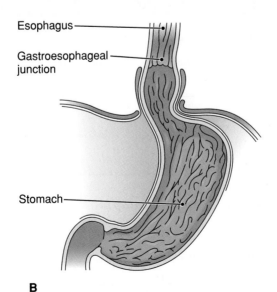

Esophagus

Gastroesophageal junction

Stomach

B

Figure 6-7   **Hernia (A) A normal stomach. (B) Hiatal hernia.**
The stomach protrudes through the diaphragm into the thoracic cavity, raising the level of the junction between the esophagus and the stomach.

6

Word Parts Pertaining to Disease

See Tables 6-1 to 6-5.

Table 6-1	Roots for Disease		
Root	Meaning	Example	Definition of Example
alg/o, algi/o, algesi/o	pain	algesia *al-JĒ-zē-a*	condition of having pain
carcin/o	cancer, carcinoma	carcinoid *KAR-si-noyd*	resembling a carcinoma
cyst/o	filled sac or pouch, cyst, bladder	cystic *SIS-tik*	pertaining to or having cysts
lith	calculus, stone	lithiasis *lith-Ī-a-sis*	stone formation
onc/o	tumor	oncogenic *on-kō-JEN-ik*	causing a tumor
path/o	disease	pathogen *PATH-ō-jen*	organism that produces disease
py/o	pus	pyocyst *PĪ-ō-sist*	cyst filled with pus
pyr/o, pyret/o	fever, fire	pyrexia *pī-REK-sē-a*	fever
scler/o	hard	sclerosis *skle-RŌ-sis*	hardening of tissue
tox/o, toxic/o	poison	endotoxin *en-dō-TOK-sin*	toxin within bacterial cells

EXERCISE 6-1

Identify and define the root in each of the following words:

	Root	Meaning of Root
1. antipyretic *an-tē-pī-RET-ik*	_____	_____
2. pathology *pa-THOL-ō-jē*	_____	_____
3. empyema *em-pī-Ē-ma*	_____	_____
4. intoxicate *in-TOK-si-kāt*	_____	_____

Fill in the blanks:

5. A carcinogen (*kar-SIN-ō-jen*) is a substance that causes _____.

6. Pyoderma (*pī-ō-DER-ma*) is a skin disease associated with _____.

7. A pyrogenic (*pī-rō-JEN-ik*) agent induces _____.

8. The term *pathogenic* (*path-ō-JEN-ik*) means producing _____.

9. A urolith (Ŭ-rō-lith) is a(n) _____ in the urinary tract (ur/o).

10. An exotoxin (ek-sō-TOK-sin) is a(n) _____ secreted by bacterial cells.

11. Arteriosclerosis (ar-tē-rē-ō-skle-RŌ-sis) is a(n) _____ of the arteries.

12. An algesimeter (al-je-SIM-e-ter) is used to measure sensitivity to _____.

13. An oncogene (ON-kō-jĕn) is a gene that causes a(n) _____.

Table 6-2	Prefixes for Disease		
Prefix	**Meaning**	**Example**	**Definition of Example**
brady-	slow	bradypnea brad-ip-NĒ-a	slow breathing (-pnea) rate
dys-	abnormal, painful, difficult	dysplasia dis-PLĀ-jē-a	abnormal development (plas) of tissue
mal-	bad, poor	malabsorption mal-ab-SŌRP-shun	poor absorption of nutrients
pachy-	thick	pachycephaly pak-i-SEF-a-lē	abnormal thickness of the skull
tachy-	rapid	tachycardia tak-i-KAR-dē-a	rapid heart (cardiac) rate
xero-	dry	xeroderma zē-rō-DER-ma	dryness of the skin

EXERCISE 6-2

Match the following terms and write the appropriate letter to the left of each number:

_____ **1.** dystrophy (DIS-trō-fē)

_____ **2.** pachydactyly (pak-ē-DAK-til-ē)

_____ **3.** tachypnea (tak-IP-nē-a)

_____ **4.** bradycardia (brad-i-KAR-dē-a)

_____ **5.** dysphagia (dis-FĀ-jē-a)

a. abnormal thickness of the fingers

b. abnormal nourishment of tissue

c. difficulty in swallowing

d. rapid breathing

e. slow heart rate

Identify and define the prefix in each of the following words:

	Prefix	Meaning of Prefix
6. xerosis (zē-RŌ-sis)	_____	_____
7. dysentery (DIS-en-ter-ē)	_____	_____
8. maladjustment (mal-ad-JUST-ment)	_____	_____

6

Table 6-3	Suffixes for Disease		
Suffix	**Meaning**	**Example**	**Definition of Example**
-algia, -algesia	pain	neuralgia nū-RAL-jē-a	pain in a nerve (neur/o)
-cele	hernia, localized dilation	gastrocele GAS-trō-sēl	hernia of the stomach (gastr/o)
-clasis, -clasia	breaking	karyoclasis kar-ē-OK-la-sis	breaking of a nucleus (kary/o)
-itis	inflammation	cystitis sis-TĪ-tis	inflammation of the urinary bladder (cyst/o)
-megaly	enlargement	hepatomegaly hep-a-tō-MEG-a-lē	enlargement of the liver (hepat/o)
-odynia	pain	urodynia ū-rō-DIN-ē-a	pain on urination (ur/o)
-oma*	tumor	lipoma lī-PŌ-ma	tumor of fat cells
-pathy	any disease of	nephropathy nef-ROP-a-thē	any disease of the kidney (nephr/o)
-rhage†, -rhagia†	bursting forth, profuse flow, hemorrhage	hemorrhage HEM-or-ij	profuse flow of blood
-rhea†	flow, discharge	pyorrhea pī-ō-RĒ-a	discharge of pus
-rhexis†	rupture	amniorrhexis am-nē-ō-REK-sis	rupture of the amniotic sac (bag of waters)
-schisis	fissure, splitting	retinoschisis ret-i-NOS-ki-sis	splitting of the retina of the eye

*Plurals: -omas, -omata.
†Remember to double the r when adding this suffix to a root.

EXERCISE 6-3

Match the following terms and write the appropriate letter to the left of each number:

_____ **1.** adipocele (AD-i-pō-sēl)   **a.** tumor of immature cells

_____ **2.** blastoma (blas-TŌ-ma)   **b.** fissure of the chest

_____ **3.** thoracoschisis (thō-ra-KOS-ki-sis)   **c.** breaking of a bone

_____ **4.** melanoma (mel-a-NŌ-ma)   **d.** hernia containing fat

_____ **5.** osteoclasis (os-tē-OK-la-sis)   **e.** tumor of pigmented cells

_____ **6.** analgesia (an-al-JĒ-zē-a)   **a.** local dilatation containing fluid

_____ **7.** hydrocele (HĪ-drō-sēl)   **b.** pain in a gland

_____ **8.** menorrhagia (men-ō-RĀ-jē-a)   **c.** absence of pain

_____ **9.** adenodynia (ad-e-nō-DIN-ē-a)   **d.** profuse menstrual flow

_____ **10.** hepatorrhexis (hep-a-tō-REK-sis)   **e.** rupture of the liver

The root *my/o* means "muscle." Define the following terms:

11. myalgia (mī-AL-jē-a)_____ pain in a muscle_____

12. myopathy (mī-OP-a-thē) _____

13. myorrhexis (mī-ō-REK-sis) _____

14. myodynia (mī-ō-DIN-ē-a) _____

15. myoma (mī-Ō-ma) _____

Some words pertaining to disease are used as suffixes in compound words (see Table 6-4). As previously noted, the term *suffix* is used in this book to mean any word part that consistently appears at the end of words. This may be a simple suffix (such as -y, -ia, -ic), a word, or a root–suffix combination, such as -megaly, -rhagia, -pathy.

Table 6-4 Words for Disease Used as Suffixes

Word	Meaning	Example	Definition of Example
dilation*, dilatation*	expansion, widening	vasodilation *vas-ō-dī-LĀ-shun*	widening of blood vessels (vas/o)
ectasia, ectasis	dilation, dilatation, distension	gastrectasia *gas-trek-TĀ-sē-a*	dilatation of the stomach (gastr/o)
edema	accumulation of fluid, swelling	cephaledema *sef-al-e-DĔ-ma*	swelling of the head
lysis*	separation, loosening, dissolving, destruction	dialysis *dī-AL-i-sis*	separation of substances by passage through (dia-) a membrane
malacia	softening	craniomalacia *krā-nē-ō-ma-LĀ-shē-a*	softening of the skull (crani/o)
necrosis	death of tissue	osteonecrosis *os-tē-ō-ne-KRŌ-sis*	death of bone (oste/o) tissue
ptosis	dropping, downward displacement, prolapse	blepharoptosis *blef-e-rop-TŌ-sis*	drooping of the eyelid (blephar/o; Fig. 6-8)
sclerosis	hardening	phlebosclerosis *fleb-ō-skle-RŌ-sis*	hardening of veins (phleb/o)
spasm	sudden contraction, cramp	arteriospasm *ar-TĒR-ē-ō-spazm*	spasm of an artery
stasis*	suppression, stoppage	menostasis *men-OS-ta-sis*	suppression of menstrual (men/o) flow
stenosis	narrowing, constriction	bronchostenosis *brong-kō-ste-NŌ-sis*	narrowing of a bronchus (air passageway)
toxin	poison	nephrotoxin *nef-rō-TOK-sin*	substance poisonous or harmful for the kidneys

*May also refer to treatment.

6

EXERCISE **6-4**

Match the following terms and write the appropriate letter to the left of each number:

_____ **1.** myolysis (*mī-OL-i-sis*)

_____ **2.** osteomalacia (*os-tē-ō-ma-LĀ-shē-a*)

_____ **3.** cardionecrosis (*kar-dē-ō-ne-KRŌ-sis*)

_____ **4.** hemolysis (*hē-MOL-i-sis*)

_____ **5.** hemostasis (*hē-mō-STĀ-sis*)

a. destruction of blood cells

b. death of heart tissue

c. stoppage of blood flow

d. softening of a bone

e. dissolving of muscle

The root *splen/o* means "spleen." Define the following words:

6. splenomalacia (*splē-nō-ma-LĀ-shē-a*) _____

7. splenoptosis (*splē-nop-TŌ-sis*) _____

8. splenotoxin (*splē-nō-TOK-sin*) _____

Table 6-5	Prefixes and Roots for Infectious Diseases		
Word Part	**Meaning**	**Example**	**Definition of Example**
Prefixes			
staphyl/o	grapelike cluster	staphylococcus *staf-i-lō-KOK-us*	a round bacterium that forms clusters
strept/o	twisted chain	streptobacillus *strep-tō-ba-SIL-us*	a rod-shaped bacterium that forms chains
Roots			
bacill/i, bacill/o	bacillus	bacilluria *bas-i-LŪ-rē-a*	bacilli in the urine (-uria)
bacteri/o	bacterium	bacteriostatic *bak-tēr-ē-ō-STAT-ik*	stopping (stasis) the growth of bacteria
myc/o	fungus, mold	mycotic *mī-KOT-ik*	pertaining to a fungus
vir/o	virus	viremia *vī-RĒ-mē-a*	presence of viruses in the blood (-emia)

Normal lid   Drooping lid

Figure 6-8 **Blepharoptosis (drooping of the eyelid).** Ptosis means a downward displacement.

EXERCISE **6-5**

Fill in the blanks:

1. A bactericidal (*bak-tēr-i-SĪ-dal*) agent kills _____.

2. A mycosis (*mī-KŌ-sis*) is any disease caused by a(n) _____.

3. The term bacillary (*BAS-il-a-rē*) means pertaining to _____.

4. The prefix *staphyl/o-* means _____.

5. The prefix *strept/o-* means _____.

Use the suffix *-logy* to write a word that means the same as each of the following:

6. Study of fungi _____

7. Study of viruses _____

8. Study of bacteria _____

Terminology Supplementary Terms

acid-fast stain	A laboratory staining procedure used mainly to identify the tuberculosis (TB) organism
communicable *ko-MŪN-i-ka-bl*	Capable of passing from one person to another, such as an infectious disease
endemic *en-DEM-ik*	Occurring at a low level but continuously in a given region, such as the common cold
epidemic *ep-i-DEM-ik*	Affecting many people in a given region at the same time; a disease that breaks out in a large proportion of a population at a given time
exacerbation *eks-zas-er-BĀ-shun*	Worsening of disease; increase in severity of a disease or its symptoms
iatrogenic *i-at-rō-JEN-ik*	Caused by the effects of treatment (from Greek root *iatro-*, meaning "physician")
idiopathic *id-ē-ō-PATH-ik*	Having no known cause (root *idio* means "self-originating")
in situ *in SĪ-tū*	Localized, noninvasive (literally "in position"); said of tumors that do not spread, such as carcinoma in situ (CIS)
normal flora *FLŌ-ra*	The microorganisms that normally live on or in the body. These organisms are generally harmless, and are often beneficial, but they can cause disease under special circumstances, such as injury or failure of the immune system
nosocomial *nos-ō-KŌ-mē-al*	Describing an infection acquired in a hospital (root *nos/o* means "disease," and *comial* refers to a hospital). Such infections can be a serious problem, especially if they are resistant to antibiotics; for example, there are now strains of methicillin-resistant *Staphylococcus aureus* (MRSA) and vancomycin-resistant *S. aureus* (VRSA), which cause dangerous infections in hospital settings
opportunistic *op-por-tū-NIS-tik*	Describing an infection that occurs because of a host's poor or altered condition
pandemic *pan-DEM-ik*	Describing a disease that is prevalent throughout an entire region or the world. AIDS is now pandemic in certain regions of the world

(continued)

Terminology   Supplementary Terms (continued)

remission rē-MISH-un	A lessening of disease symptoms; the period during which such lessening occurs
septicemia sep-ti-SĒ-mē-a	Presence of pathogenic bacteria in the blood; blood poisoning
systemic sis-TEM-ik	Pertaining to the whole body

Manifestations of Disease

abscess AB-ses	A localized collection of pus
adhesion ad-HĒ-zhun	A uniting of two surfaces or parts that may normally be separated
anaplasia a-na-PLĀ-jē-a	Lack of normal differentiation, as shown by cancer cells
ascites a-SĪ-tēz	Accumulation of fluid in the peritoneal cavity
cellulitis sel-ū-LĪ-tis	A spreading inflammation of tissue
effusion e-FŪ-zhun	Escape of fluid into a cavity or other body part
exudate EKS-ū-dāt	Material that escapes from blood vessels as a result of tissue injury
fissure FISH-ur	A groove or split
fistula FIS-tū-la	An abnormal passage between two organs or from an organ to the surface of the body
gangrene GANG-grēn	Death of tissue, usually caused by lack of blood supply; may be associated with bacterial infection and decomposition
hyperplasia hī-per-PLĀ-jē-a	Excessive growth of normal cells in normal arrangement
hypertrophy hī-PER-trō-fē	An increase in size of an organ without increase in the number of cells; may result from an increase in activity, as in muscles
induration in-dū-RĀ-shun	Hardening; an abnormally hard spot or place
metaplasia met-a-PLĀ-jē-a	Conversion of cells to a form that is not normal for that tissue (prefix *meta-* means "change")
polyp POL-ip	A tumor attached by a thin stalk
purulent PUR-ū-lent	Forming or containing pus
suppuration sup-ū-RĀ-shun	Pus formation

 Go to the pronunciation glossary on the Student Resources to hear these words pronounced.

Terminology   Abbreviations

AF	Acid fast		Gm⁻	Gram-negative
CA	Cancer		MRSA	Methicillin-resistant *Staphylococcus aureus*
CIS	Carcinoma in situ		staph	Staphylococcus
FUO	Fever of unknown origin		strep	Streptococcus
Gm+	Gram-positive		VRSA	Vancomycin-resistant *Staphylococcus aureus*

Chapter Review

Terminology > Match the following terms and write the appropriate letter to the left of each number:

_____ **1.** adenocarcinoma   **a.** pertaining to profuse flow of blood
_____ **2.** neuroma   **b.** cancer of glandular tissue
_____ **3.** gastromegaly   **c.** tumor of a nerve
_____ **4.** encephalitis   **d.** enlargement of the stomach
_____ **5.** hemorrhagic   **e.** inflammation of the brain

_____ **6.** sclerotic   **a.** stone formation
_____ **7.** oncolysis   **b.** dry
_____ **8.** analgesia   **c.** destruction of a tumor
_____ **9.** xerotic   **d.** absence of pain
_____ **10.** lithiasis   **e.** hardened

_____ **11.** dactyledema   **a.** swelling of the fingers or toes
_____ **12.** apyrexia   **b.** thickness of the skin
_____ **13.** pachyderma   **c.** discharge of pus
_____ **14.** dysphagia   **d.** difficulty in swallowing
_____ **15.** pyorrhea   **e.** absence of fever

_____ **16.** nephroptosis   **a.** local wound or injury
_____ **17.** hemostasis   **b.** stoppage of blood flow
_____ **18.** carcinoid   **c.** dilatation
_____ **19.** lesion   **d.** resembling cancer
_____ **20.** ectasia   **e.** dropping of the kidney

_____ **21.** spasm   **a.** any disease of a gland
_____ **22.** cardiorrhexis   **b.** hardening of a vein
_____ **23.** venosclerosis   **c.** like a poison
_____ **24.** toxoid   **d.** sudden contraction or cramp
_____ **25.** adenopathy   **e.** rupture of the heart

6

Chapter Review (continued)

Supplementary Terms

_____ **26.** abscess
_____ **27.** adhesion
_____ **28.** fistula
_____ **29.** polyp
_____ **30.** effusion

a. abnormal passageway
b. escape of fluid into a cavity
c. tumor attached by a thin stalk
d. localized collection of pus
e. union of two surfaces or parts

_____ **31.** idiopathic
_____ **32.** purulent
_____ **33.** ascites
_____ **34.** nosocomial
_____ **35.** exacerbation

a. worsening
b. having no known cause
c. acquired in a hospital
d. forming or containing pus
e. fluid in the abdominal cavity

Fill in the blanks:

36. Heat, pain, redness, and swelling are the four major signs of _____.

37. Any abnormal and uncontrolled growth of tissue, whether benign or malignant, is called a(n) _____.

38. The spreading of cancer to other parts of the body is the process of_____.

39. Protrusion of an organ through an abnormal opening is a(n) _____.

40. Toxicology is the study of _____.

41. Death of tissue is called _____.

42. An oncoprotein is a protein associated with a(n)_____.

Use the suffix *-genesis* to write words with the following meanings:

43. Formation of cancer _____ carcinogenesis _____

44. Formation of pus _____

45. Origin of any disease _____

46. Formation of a tumor _____

The root *bronch/o* pertains to a bronchus, an air passageway in the lungs. Add a suffix to this root to form words with the following meanings:

47. Sudden contraction of a bronchus _____

48. Inflammation of a bronchus _____

49. Narrowing of a bronchus _____

50. Excessive flow or discharge from a bronchus _____

Use the root *oste/o*, meaning "bone," to form words with the following meanings:

51. Death of bone tissue _____

52. Softening of a bone _____

53. Breaking of a bone _____

54. Tumor of a bone _____

55. Destruction of bone tissue _____

Chapter Review (continued)

True–False > Examine the following statements. If the statement is true, write T in the first blank. If the statement is false, write F in the first blank and correct the statement by replacing the underlined word in the second blank.

56. A mycosis is an infection with a <u>fungus</u>.   _____   _____

57. Round bacteria in chains are <u>staphylococci</u>.   _____   _____

58. A sudden disease of short duration is <u>chronic</u>.   _____   _____

59. A tumor that does not metastasize is termed <u>benign</u>.   _____   _____

60. A slower than normal heart rate is <u>tachycardia</u>.   _____   _____

61. A tumor of connective tissue is classified as a <u>sarcoma</u>.   _____   _____

Eliminations > In each of the sets below, underline the word that does not fit in with the rest and explain the reason for your choice:

62. cocci — helminths — chlamydia — bacilli — vibrios

_____

63. neoplasm — tumor — carcinoma — pathogen — oncology

_____

64. septicemic — endemic — metastatic — opportunistic — epidemic

_____

Word Building > Use the word parts given to build words for the following definitions.

tox   pyr   gen   o   py   oma   tox   y   path   nephr   logy   ic

65. poisonous for the kidney   _____

66. producing pus   _____

67. tumor of the kidney   _____

68. study of disease   _____

69. producing fever   _____

70. study of the kidney   _____

71. producing disease   _____

72. any disease of the kidney   _____

73. producing kidney tissue   _____

Define the following words and give the meaning of the word parts in each. Use a dictionary if necessary.

74. antipyretic (*an-tē-pī-RET-ik*) _____

    a. anti- _____

    b. pyret/o _____

    c. -ic _____

6

Chapter Review (continued)

75. arteriosclerosis (*ar-tē-rē-ō-skle-RŌ-sis*) _____

   a. arterio/o _____

   b. scler/o _____

   c. -sis _____

76. homeostasis (*hō-mē-ō-STĀ-sis*) _____

   a. homeo- _____

   b. stasis _____

PASSport to Success®

Go to the Student Resources for additional review exercises.

Case Studies

▶ Case Study 6-1: Esophageal Spasm

B.R., a 53-year-old woman, consulted with her primary physician because of occasional episodes of dysphagia with moderate to severe tight, gripping pain in her midthorax. She reported that the onset was sudden after ingestion of certain foods or beverages, beginning retrosternally and radiating to the cervical and dorsal regions. The pain was not relieved by assuming a supine position or holding her breath. B.R. also stated that she felt like her heart was racing and that she might be having a heart attack. She denied any dyspepsia, vomiting, or dyspnea. Her doctor suspected acute esophageal spasm or possibly a paraesophageal hiatal hernia and referred B.R. to a gastroenterologist for a gastroscopy and esophageal manometry study (pressure measurement). She also underwent a barium swallow study under fluoroscopic imaging.

▶ Case Study 6-2: HIV Infection and Tuberculosis

T.H., a 48-year-old man, was an admitted intravenous (IV) drug user and occasionally abused alcohol. Over 4 weeks, he had experienced fever, night sweats, malaise, a cough, and a 10-lb weight loss. He was also concerned about several discolored lesions that had erupted weeks before on his arms and legs.

T.H. made an appointment with a physician assistant (PA) at the neighborhood clinic. On exami-

nation, the PA noted bilateral anterior cervical and axillary lymphadenopathy and pyrexia. T.H.'s temperature was 39°C. The PA sent T.H. to the hospital for further studies.

T.H.'s chest radiograph (x-ray image) showed paratracheal adenopathy and bilateral interstitial infiltrates, suspicious of tuberculosis (TB). His blood study results were positive for human immunodeficiency virus (HIV) and showed a low lymphocyte count. Sputum and bronchoscopic lavage (washing) fluid were positive for an acid-fast bacillus (AFB); a PPD (purified protein derivative) skin test result was also positive. Based on these findings, T.H. was diagnosed with HIV, TB, and Kaposi sarcoma related to past IV drug abuse.

▶ Case Study 6-3: Endocarditis

D.A., a 37-year-old man, sought treatment after experiencing several days of high fever and generalized weakness on return from his vacation. D.A.'s family doctor suspected cardiac involvement because of D.A.'s history of rheumatic fever. The doctor was concerned because D.A.'s brother had died of acute malignant hyperpyrexia during surgery at the age of 12. D.A. was referred to a cardiologist, who scheduled an electrocardiogram (ECG) and a transesophageal echocardiogram (TEE).

D.A. was admitted to the hospital with subacute bacterial endocarditis (SBE) and placed on high-dose IV antibiotics and bed rest. He had also developed a heart murmur, which was diagnosed as idiopathic hypertrophic subaortic stenosis (IHSS).

(continued)

Case Studies (continued)

CASE STUDY QUESTIONS

Multiple choice. Select the best answer and write the letter of your choice to the left of each number:

_____ 1. The cervical region is the region of the:
- a. heart
- b. uterus
- c. neck
- d. leg
- e. head

_____ 2. A word that has the same meaning as dorsal is:
- a. anterior
- b. posterior
- c. caudal
- d. inferior
- e. superior

_____ 3. In referring to tissues, the term *interstitial* means:
- a. around cells
- b. under cells
- c. between cells
- d. through cells
- e. within cells

_____ 4. The term *axillary* refers to the:
- a. bladder
- b. abdomen
- c. wrist
- d. armpit
- e. groin

_____ 5. The term *pyrexia* refers to a:
- a. fever
- b. stone
- c. tumor
- d. spasm
- e. poison

_____ 6. Dyspepsia refers to indigestion. Dysphagia and dyspnea refer to difficulty with:
- a. breathing and coughing
- b. swallowing and urinating
- c. walking and chewing gum
- d. swallowing and breathing
- e. sleeping and breathing

_____ 7. Paraesophageal and paratracheal refer to a position _____ the esophagus and trachea.
- a. under
- b. superior to
- c. near
- d. in between
- e. within

_____ 8. The endocardium is the tissue lining the heart's chambers. Endocarditis refers to a(n) _____ of this lining.
- a. narrowing
- b. inflammation
- c. overgrowth of tissue
- d. cancerous growth
- e. thinning

_____ 9. D.A.'s heart murmur was caused by a stenosis, or _____ of the heart's aortic valve.
- a. narrowing
- b. inflammation
- c. overgrowth
- d. cancer
- e. thinning

_____ 10. The term for a condition or disease of unknown etiology is:
- a. stenosis
- b. hypertrophic
- c. chronic
- d. acute
- e. idiopathic

Fill in the blanks:

11. The word in the case studies that means "protrusion of an organ through an abnormal body opening" is _____.

12. Adenopathy is any disease of a(n) _____.

13. Tuberculosis is caused by a bacterium that is rod shaped, thus described as a(n) _____.

14. A malignant neoplasm arising from muscle or connective tissue is a(n) _____.

15. A potentially fatal disease condition characterized by a very high fever is called _____.

Give the meaning of the following abbreviations:

16. HIV _____

17. PPD _____

18. ECG _____

19. AFB _____

6

Diagnosis and Treatment; Surgery

OBJECTIVES

After study of this chapter you should be able to:

1. List the main components of a patient history.
2. Describe the main methods used in patient examination.
3. Name and describe nine imaging techniques.
4. Name possible forms of treatment.
5. Describe theories of alternative and complementary medicine and some healing practices used in these fields.
6. Describe staging and grading as they apply to cancer.
7. Define basic terms pertaining to medical examination, diagnosis, and treatment.
8. Identify and use the roots and suffixes pertaining to diagnosis and surgery.
9. Interpret symbols and abbreviations used in diagnosis and treatment.
10. Interpret a case history containing terms related to diagnosis and treatment.

PRETEST

Multiple choice. Select the best answer and write the letter of your choice to the left of each number.

___ 1. Determination of a disease's nature and cause is called:

    a. prognosis   c. titration
    b. diagnosis   d. admission

___ 2. Measurements of the basic functions needed to maintain life, such as breathing and pulse, together are called:

    a. respiration   c. vital signs
    b. health signs   d. etiology

____ 3. The two phases recorded when measuring blood pressure are:

    a. systolic and sinoatrial
    b. diastolic and symbiotic
    c. superior and inferior
    d. systolic and diastolic

____ 4. A simple device for listening to sounds within the body is a:

    a. cystoscope   c. barometer
    b. speculum   d. stethoscope

____ 5. Removal of tissue for microscopic study is a(n):

    a. biopsy   c. endoscopy
    b. aeration   d. CT scan

____ 6. Prediction of a disease's outcome is a(n):

    a. evidence   c. history
    b. prognosis   d. therapy

____ 7. A process used to evaluate the severity of cancer is:

    a. radiation   c. laparoscopy
    b. staging   d. endoscopy

____ 8. An appendectomy is:

    a. therapy of the appendix
    b. measurement of the appendix
    c. imaging of the appendix
    d. surgical removal of the appendix

____ 9. A tracheotomy is:

    a. surgical incision of the trachea
    b. placement of a tracheal tube
    c. removal of a tracheal tube
    d. removal of the trachea

Medical care begins with assessing a disorder using information gathered from the patient and a variety of testing and examination methods. Based on these results, a course of treatment is recommended, which may include surgery.

Diagnosis

Medical **diagnosis**, the determination of the nature and cause of an illness, begins with a patient history. This includes a history of the present illness with a description of **symptoms** (evidence of disease), a past medical history, and a family and a social history.

A physical examination, which includes a review of all systems and observation of any **signs** of illness, follows the history taking. Practitioners use the following techniques in performing physicals:

- **Inspection**: visual examination.
- **Palpation**: touching the surface of the body with the hands or fingers (Fig. 7-1).
- **Percussion**: tapping the body to evaluate tissue according to the sounds produced (Fig. 7-2).
- **Auscultation**: listening to body sounds with a **stethoscope** (Fig. 7-3).

Vital signs (VS) are also recorded for comparison with normal ranges. VS are measurements that reflect basic functions necessary to maintain life and include:

- Temperature (T).

- Pulse rate, measured in beats per minute (bpm) (Fig. 7-4). Pulse rate normally corresponds to the heart rate (HR), the number of times the heart beats per minute.

- Respiration rate (R), measured in breaths per minute.

- Blood pressure (BP), measured in millimeters of mercury (mm Hg) and recorded when the heart is contracting (systolic pressure) and relaxing (diastolic

Figure 7-1 **Palpation.** The practitioner touches the body surface with the hands or fingers.

99

Figure 7-2 **Percussion.** The practitioner taps the body to evaluate tissues.

Figure 7-4 **Pulse rate.** The practitioner palpates an artery to measure pulse rate in beats per minute.

pressure) (Fig. 7-5). An examiner typically uses a stethoscope and a blood pressure cuff, or **sphygmo-manometer** (*sfig-mō-ma-NOM-e-ter*), to measure blood pressure. Newer devices that read blood pressure directly and give a digital reading are also in use. Chapter 9 has more information on blood pressure.

Additional tools used in physical examinations include the **ophthalmoscope** (Fig. 7-6A), for examination of the eyes; the **otoscope** (see Fig. 7-6B), for examination of the ears; and hammers, for testing reflexes.

The skin, hair, and nails provide easily observable indications of a person's state of health. Skin features such as color, texture, thickness, and presence of lesions (local injuries) are noted throughout the course of the physical examination. Chapter 21 contains a discussion of the skin and skin diseases.

Diagnosis is further aided by laboratory test results. These may include tests on blood, urine, and other body fluids, and the identification of infectious organisms. Additional tests may include study of the electrical activity of tissues such as the brain and heart, examination of body cavities by means of an **endoscope** (Fig. 7-7), and imaging techniques. **Biopsy** is the removal of tissue for microscopic examination. Biopsy specimens can be obtained by:

- needle withdrawal (aspiration) of fluid, as from the chest or from a cyst

- a small punch, as of the skin

- endoscopy, as from the respiratory or digestive tract

- surgical removal, as of a tumor or node

When new tests appear, as in all other areas of health sciences, new terminology is added to the medical vocabulary (see Box 7-1).

Figure 7-3 **Auscultation.** The practitioner uses a stethoscope to listen to body sounds.

Figure 7-5 **Blood pressure.** The practitioner uses a blood pressure cuff (sphygmomanometer) and a stethoscope to measure systolic and diastolic pressures.

A

B

Figure 7-6 **Examination tools.** (*A*) Ophthalmoscope for eye examination. (*B*) Otoscope for ear examination.

Bronchoscope

Lungs

Figure 7-7 **Endoscope.** A bronchoscope is a type of endoscope used to examine the respiratory bronchi.

Imaging Techniques

Imaging techniques employ various types of energy to produce visual images of the body. The most fundamental imaging method is **radiography** (Fig. 7-8), which uses x-rays to produce an image (radiograph) on film or to produce a digital image that can be viewed on a monitor. Radiography is the preferred method for imaging dense tissues, such as bone. Some soft tissue structures can be demonstrated as well, but a contrast medium, such as a barium mixture, may be needed to enhance visualization. Other forms of energy used to produce diagnostic images include sound waves, radioactive isotopes, radio

waves, and magnetic fields. See Box 7-2 for a description of the most commonly used imaging methods and Reference Box 7-3 for a summary of these and other imaging techniques in use.

Treatment

If diagnosis so indicates, treatment, also termed **therapy**, is begun. This may consist of counseling, drugs, surgery, radiation, physical therapy, occupational therapy, psychiatric treatment, or some combination of these. See Chapter 8 for a discussion of drugs and their actions. **Palliative** therapy is treatment that provides relief but is not intended as a cure. Terminally ill patients, for example, may receive treatment that eases pain and provides comfort but is not expected to change the outcome of their disease. During diagnosis and throughout the course of treatment, a patient is evaluated to establish a **prognosis**—that is, a prediction of the disease's outcome.

Box 7-1 Focus on Words

Terminology Evolves with Medical Science

The science of medicine never stands still, nor does its terminology. One can never say that his or her work in learning medical terminology is complete because vocabulary is constantly being added as new diagnoses, treatments, and technologies are discovered or developed.

A generation ago, gene therapy, genetic engineering, in vitro fertilization, cloning, and stem cell research were unknown to the public. PET scans, MRI, DNA fingerprinting, radioimmunoassay, bone density scans for identifying osteoporosis, and other diagnostic techniques were not in use.

Some of the new categories of drugs, such as statins for reducing cholesterol, antiviral agents, histamine antagonists for treating ulcers, ACE inhibitors for treating hypertension, and breast cancer preventives were undiscovered. The genes associated with certain forms of cancer and with certain hereditary abnormalities had yet to be isolated.

Each of these advances brings new terminology into use. Anyone who wants to keep current with medical terminology has a lifetime of learning ahead.

7

Figure 7-8 **Radiography.** The action of x-rays on sensitized film produced this image (radiograph) of a normal right hand.

Surgery

Surgery is a method for treating disease or injury by manual operations. Surgery may be done through an existing body opening, but usually it involves cutting or puncturing tissue with a sharp instrument in the process of **incision**. See Reference Box 7-4 for descriptions of surgical instruments and Figure 7-11 for pictures of surgical instruments. Surgery usually requires some form of **anesthesia** to dull or eliminate pain. After surgery, incisions must be closed for proper healing. Traditionally, surgeons have used stitches or **sutures** to close wounds, but today they also use adhesive strips, staples, and skin glue.

Many types of operations are now performed with a **laser**, an intense beam of light. Some procedures require destruction of tissue by a harmful agent, such as by heat or a chemical, in the process of **cautery** or cauterization.

Some of the purposes of surgery include:

- Treatment: For **excision** (cutting out) of diseased or abnormal tissue, such as a tumor or an inflamed appendix. Surgical methods are also used to repair wounds or injuries, as in skin grafting for burns or for realigning broken bones. Surgical methods are used to correct circulatory problems and to return structures to their normal position, as in raising a prolapsed organ, such as the bladder, in a surgical **fixation** procedure.

- Diagnosis: To remove tissue for laboratory study in a biopsy, as described above. Exploratory surgery to investigate the cause of symptoms is performed less frequently now because of advances in noninvasive diagnostic and imaging techniques.

Box 7-2 **Clinical Perspectives**

Medical Imaging

Three imaging techniques that have revolutionized medicine are radiography, computed tomography (CT), and magnetic resonance imaging (MRI). With them, physicians today can "see" inside the body without making a single cut.

The oldest technique is radiography (rā-dē-OG-ra-fē), in which a machine beams x-rays (a form of radiation) through the body onto a piece of film. The resulting image is called a radiograph. Dark areas indicate where the beam passed through the body and exposed the film, whereas light areas show where the beam did not pass through. Dense tissues (bone, teeth) absorb most of the x-rays, preventing them from exposing the film. For this reason, radiography is commonly used to visualize bone fractures and tooth decay as well as abnormally dense tissues like tumors. Radiography does not provide clear images of soft tissues because most of the beam passes through and exposes the film, but contrast media can help make structures like blood vessels and hollow organs more visible. For example, barium sulfate (which absorbs x-rays) coats the digestive tract when ingested.

During a CT scan, a machine revolves around the patient, beaming x-rays through the body onto a detector. The detector takes numerous images of the beam and a computer assembles them into transverse sections, or "slices." Unlike conventional radiography, CT produces clear images of soft structures such as the brain, liver, and lungs. It is commonly used to visualize brain injuries and tumors, and even blood vessels when used with contrast media.

MRI uses a strong magnetic field and radio waves. The patient undergoing MRI lies inside a chamber within a very powerful magnet. The molecules in the patient's soft tissues align with the magnetic field inside the chamber. When radio waves hit the soft tissue, the aligned molecules emit energy that the MRI machine detects, and a computer converts these signals into an image. MRI produces even clearer images of soft tissue than does CT and can create detailed views of blood vessels without contrast media. MRI can visualize brain injuries and tumors that might be missed using CT.

Box 7-3 For Your Reference

Imaging Techniques

METHOD	DESCRIPTION
cineradiography sin-e-rā-dē-OG-ra-fē	making of a motion picture of successive images appearing on a fluoroscopic screen
computed tomography (CT, CT scan) tō-MOG-ra-fē	use of a computer to generate an image from a large number of x-rays passed at different angles through the body; a three-dimensional image of a cross section of the body is obtained; reveals more about soft tissues than does simple radiography (Fig. 7-9A)
fluoroscopy flū-ROS-kō-pē	use of x-rays to examine deep structures; the shadows cast by x-rays passed through the body are observed on a fluorescent screen; the device used is called a fluoroscope
magnetic resonance imaging (MRI)	production of images through the use of a magnetic field and radio waves; the characteristics of soft tissue are revealed by differences in molecular properties; eliminates the need for x-rays and contrast media (see Fig. 7-9B)
positron emission tomography (PET)	production of sectional body images by administration of a natural substance, such as glucose, labeled with a positron-emitting isotope; the rays subsequently emitted are interpreted by computer to show the internal distribution of the substance administered; PET has been used to follow blood flow through an organ and to measure metabolic activity within an organ, such as the brain, under different conditions
radiography rā-dē-OG-ra-fē	use of x-rays passed through the body to make a visual record (radiograph) of internal structures on specially sensitized film. Also called roentgenography (rent-ge-NOG-ra-fē) after the developer of the technique
scintigraphy sin-TIG-ra-fē	imaging the radioactivity distribution in tissues after internal administration of a radioactive substance (radionuclide); the images are obtained with a scintillation camera; the record produced is a scintiscan (SIN-ti-skan) and usually specifies the part examined or the isotope used for the test, as in bone scan, gallium scan
single-photon emission computed tomography (SPECT)	scintigraphic technique that permits visualization of a radioisotope's cross-sectional distribution
ultrasonography ul-tra-son-OG-ra-fē	generation of a visual image from the echoes of high-frequency sound waves traveling back from different tissues; also called sonography (so-NOG-ra-fē) and echography (ek-OG-ra-fē) (Fig. 7-10)

- Restoration: Surgery may compensate for lost function, as when a section of the intestine is redirected in a colostomy; a tube is inserted to allow breathing in a tracheostomy; a feeding tube is inserted; or an organ is transplanted. Surgeons may perform plastic or reconstructive surgery to accommodate a prosthesis (substitute part), to restore proper appearance, or for cosmetic reasons.

- Relief: Palliative surgery relieves pain or discomfort, as by cutting the nerve supply to an organ or reducing the size of a tumor to relieve pressure.

Surgery may be done in an emergency or urgent situation under conditions of acute danger, as in traumatic injury or severe blockage. Other procedures, such as cataract removal from the eye, may be planned when convenient. Elective or optional surgery would not cause serious consequences if delayed or not done.

Over time, surgery has extended beyond the classic operating room of a hospital to other hospital areas and to private surgical facilities where people can be treated within 1 day as outpatients. Preoperative care is given before surgery and includes examination, obtaining the patient's informed consent for the procedure, and preadmission testing. Postoperative care includes recovery from anesthesia, follow-up evaluations, and instructions for home care.

Box 7-5 describes some aspects of careers in surgical technology.

Box 7-4 For Your Reference

Surgical Instruments

INSTRUMENT	DESCRIPTION
bougie *BOO-zhē*	slender, flexible instrument for exploring and dilating tubes
cannula *KAN-ū-la*	tube enclosing a trocar (see below) that allows escape of fluid or air after removal of the trocar
clamp	instrument used to compress tissue
curet (curette) *KŪ-ret*	spoon-shaped instrument for removing material from the wall of a cavity or other surface (see Fig. 7-11)
elevator *EL-e-vā-tor*	instrument for lifting tissue or bone
forceps *FOR-seps*	instrument for holding or extracting (see Fig. 7-11)
Gigli saw *JĒL-yēz*	flexible wire saw
hemostat *HĒ-mō-stat*	small clamp for stopping blood flow from a vessel (see Fig. 7-11)
rasp	surgical file
retractor *rē-TRAK-tor*	instrument used to maintain exposure by separating a wound and holding back organs or tissues (see Fig. 7-11)
rongeur *ron-ZHUR*	gouge forceps
scalpel *SKAL-pel*	surgical knife with a sharp blade (see Fig. 7-11)
scissors *SIZ-ors*	a cutting instrument with two opposing blades
sound *sownd*	instrument for exploring a cavity or canal (see Fig. 7-11)
trocar *TRŌ-kar*	sharp pointed instrument contained in a cannula used to puncture a cavity

Box 7-5 Health Professions

Surgical Technology

Surgical technologists, also known as operating room technicians, prepare for and assist with surgical procedures under the supervision of surgeons and nurses. They prepare the operating room, surgical instruments, and equipment. They help the surgical team to scrub and put on gowns, gloves, and masks. They also prepare patients for surgery, helping to position them on the table and draping them with sterile linens. During an operation, surgical technologists hand instruments and other materials to the surgeon, maintain supplies, and operate special equipment. Finally, they help count materials to be sure that all have been removed from the patient at the conclusion of surgery, and they assist in suturing. They also take responsibility for specimens removed for laboratory testing. The job requires stamina, manual dexterity, and quick reaction time.

A career in surgical technology requires training in a surgical technology program and certification. Preparation for this training should include courses in basic sciences, math, and computer applications. The Association of Surgical Technologists at www.ast.org has additional information on this career.

Right portal vein
(to liver)

Diaphragm

Contrast medium in stomach

Main portal vein (to liver)

Inferior vena cava (vein)

Aorta

Spleen

Vertebra of spine

Ribs

A

Liver

Left breast

Portal veins (to liver)

Hepatic veins (from liver)

Stomach

Inferior vena cava (vein)

Spleen

Aorta

Vertebra of spine

Spinal cord

B

Figure 7-9 **Imaging techniques.** Shown are cross sections through the liver and spleen. (*A*) Computed tomography (CT). (*B*) Magnetic resonance imaging (MRI).

Figure 7-10 **Ultrasonography.** The practitioner is using ultrasound to monitor pregnancy.

Curette   Forceps   Hemostat

Retractor   Sound   Scalpel

Figure 7-11 Surgical instruments.

Alternative and Complementary Medicine

During the past century, the leading causes of death in industrialized countries have gradually shifted from infectious diseases to chronic diseases of the cardiovascular and respiratory systems and cancer. In addition to advancing age, life habits and the environment greatly influence these conditions. As a result, many people have begun to consider healing practices from other philosophies and cultures as alternatives and complements to conventional Western medicine. Some of these philosophies include **osteopathy, naturopathy,** homeopathy, and **chiropractic.** Techniques of **acupuncture, biofeedback, massage,** and **meditation** may also be used, as well as herbal remedies (see Chapter 8) and nutritional counseling on diet, vitamins, and minerals. Complementary and alternative therapies emphasize maintaining health rather than treating disease and allowing the body the opportunity to heal itself. These ideas fit into the concept of **holistic health care,** which promotes treating an individual as a whole with emotional, social, and spiritual needs in addition to physical needs and encouraging people to be involved in their own health maintenance.

The U.S. government has established the National Center for Complementary and Alternative Medicine (NCCAM) within the National Institutes of Health (NIH) to study these therapies.

Cancer

Methods used in the diagnosis of cancer include physical examination, biopsy, imaging techniques, and laboratory tests for abnormalities, or "markers," associated with specific types of malignancies. Some cancer markers are byproducts, such as enzymes, hormones, and cellular proteins, that are abnormal or are produced in abnormal amounts. Researchers have also linked specific genetic mutations to certain forms of cancer.

Oncologists (cancer specialists) use two methods, **grading** and **staging,** to classify cancers, to select and evaluate therapy, and to estimate disease outcome. Grading is based on histologic (tissue) changes observed in tumor cells when they are examined microscopically. Grades increase from I to IV with increasing cellular abnormality.

Staging is a procedure for establishing the clinical extent of tumor spread, both at the original site and in other parts of the body (metastases). The TNM system is commonly used. These letters stand for primary tumor (T), regional lymph nodes (N), and distant metastases (M). Evaluation in these categories varies for each type of tumor. Based on TNM results, a stage ranging in severity from I to IV is assigned. Cancers of the blood, lymphatic system, and nervous system are evaluated by different standards.

The most widely used methods for treatment of cancer are surgery, radiation therapy, and **chemotherapy** (treatment with chemicals). Newer methods of **immunotherapy** use substances that stimulate the immune system as a whole or vaccines prepared specifically against a tumor. Hormone therapy may also be effective against certain types of tumors. When no active signs of the disease remain, the cancer is said to be in **remission.**

Terminology	Key Terms

anesthesia *an-es-THĒ-zē-a*	Loss of the ability to feel pain, as by administration of a drug
auscultation *aws-kul-TĀ-shun*	Listening for sounds within the body, usually within the chest or abdomen (see Fig. 7-3)
biopsy *BĪ-op-sē*	Removal of a small amount of tissue for microscopic examination
cautery *KAW-ter-ē*	Destruction of tissue by a damaging agent, such as a harmful chemical, heat, or electric current (electrocautery); cauterization
chemotherapy *kē-mō-THER-a-pē*	Use of chemicals to treat disease. The term is often applied specifically to the treatment of cancer with chemicals
diagnosis *dī-ag-NŌ-sis*	The process of determining the cause and nature of an illness
endoscope *EN-dō-skōp*	An instrument for examining the inside of an organ or cavity through a body opening or small incision; most endoscopes use fiberoptics for viewing (see Fig. 7-7)
excision *ek-SIZH-un*	Removal by cutting (suffix: *-ectomy*)
fixation *fik-SĀ-shun*	Holding or fastening a structure in a firm position (suffix: *-pexy*)
grading *GRĀ-ding*	A method for evaluating a tumor based on microscopic examination of the cells
immunotherapy *im-ū-nō-THER-a-pē*	Treatment that involves stimulation or suppression of the immune system, either specifically or nonspecifically
incision *in-SIZH-un*	A cut, as for surgery; also the act of cutting (suffix: *-tomy*)
inspection *in-SPEK-shun*	Visual examination of the body
laser *LĀ-zer*	A device that transforms light into a beam of intense heat and power; used for surgery and diagnosis
ophthalmoscope *of-THAL-mō-skōp*	An instrument for examining the interior of the eye (see Fig. 7-6A)
otoscope *Ō-tō-skōp*	Instrument used to examine the ears (see Fig. 7-6B)
palliative *PAL-ē-a-tiv*	Providing relief but not cure; a treatment that provides such relief
palpation *pal-PĀ-shun*	Examining by placing the hands or fingers on the surface of the body to determine characteristics such as texture, temperature, movement, and consistency (see Fig. 7-1)
percussion *per-KUSH-un*	Tapping the body lightly but sharply to assess the condition of the underlying tissue by the sounds obtained (see Fig. 7-2)
prognosis *prog-NŌ-sis*	Prediction of a disease's course and outcome
radiography *rā-dē-OG-ra-fē*	Use of x-rays passed through the body to make a visual record (radiograph) of internal structures on specially sensitized film; roentgenography (*rent-ge-NOG-ra-fē*)
remission *rē-MISH-un*	Lessening of disease symptoms; the period during which this decrease occurs or the period when no sign of a disease exists
sign *sīn*	Objective evidence of disease that can be observed or tested; examples are fever, rash, high blood pressure, and blood or urine abnormalities; an objective symptom

7

(continued)

Terminology   Key Terms (continued)

sphygmomanometer *sfig-mō-ma-NOM-e-ter*	Blood pressure apparatus or blood pressure cuff; pressure is read in millimeters of mercury (mm Hg) when the heart is contracting (systolic pressure) and when the heart is relaxing (diastolic pressure) and is reported as systolic/diastolic (see Fig. 7-5)
staging *STĀ-jing*	The process of classifying malignant tumors for diagnosis, treatment, and prognosis
stethoscope *STETH-ō-skōp*	An instrument used for listening to sounds produced within the body (from the Greek root *steth/o,* meaning "chest") (see Fig. 7-3)
surgery *SUR-jer-ē*	A method for treating disease or injury by manual operations
suture *SŪ-chur*	To unite parts by stitching them together; also the thread or other material used in that process or the seam formed by surgical stitching (suffix: *-rhaphy*)
symptom *SIM-tum*	Any evidence of disease; sometimes limited to subjective evidence of disease, as experienced by the individual, such as pain, dizziness, and weakness
therapy *THER-a-pē*	Treatment; intervention
vital signs	Measurements that reflect basic functions necessary to maintain life

Alternative and Complementary Medicine

acupuncture *AK-ū-punk-chur*	An ancient Chinese method of inserting thin needles into the body at specific points to relieve pain, induce anesthesia, or promote healing; similar effects can be obtained by using firm finger pressure at the surface of the body in the technique of *acupressure*
biofeedback *bī-ō-FĒD-bak*	A method for learning control of involuntary physiologic responses by using electronic devices to monitor bodily changes and feeding this information back to a person
chiropractic *kī-rō-PRAK-tik*	A science that stresses the condition of the nervous system in diagnosis and treatment of disease; often, the spine is manipulated to correct misalignment. Most patients consult for musculoskeletal pain and headaches (from Greek *cheir,* meaning "hand")
holistic health care *hō-LIS-tik*	Practice of treating a person as a whole entity with physical, emotional, social, and spiritual needs. It stresses comprehensive care, involvement in one's own care, and the maintenance of good health rather than the treatment of disease
homeopathy *hō-mē-OP-a-thē*	A philosophy of treating disease by administering drugs in highly diluted form along with promoting healthy life habits and a healthy environment (from *home/o,* meaning "same," and *path/o,* meaning "disease")
massage *ma-SAHJ*	Manipulation of the body or portion of the body to calm, relieve tension, increase circulation, and stimulate muscles
meditation *med-i-TĀ-shun*	Process of clearing the mind by concentrating on the inner self while controlling breathing and perhaps repeating a word or phrase (mantra)
naturopathy *nā-chur-OP-a-thē*	A therapeutic philosophy of helping people to heal themselves by developing healthy lifestyles; naturopaths may use some of the methods of conventional medicine (from *nature* and *path/o,* meaning "disease")
osteopathy *os-tē-OP-a-thē*	A system of therapy based on the theory that the body can overcome disease when it has normal structure, a favorable environment, and proper nutrition. Osteopaths use standard medical practices for diagnosis and treatment but stress the identification and correction of faulty body structure (from *oste/o,* meaning "bone," and *path/o,* meaning "disease")

PASSport to Success®   Go to the pronunciation glossary in the Student Resources to hear these words pronounced.

Word Parts Pertaining to Diagnosis and Treatment

See Tables 7-1 to 7-3.

Table 7-1	Roots for Physical Forces		
Root	**Meaning**	**Example**	**Definition of Example**
aer/o	air, gas	aerobic *ār-Ō-bik*	pertaining to or requiring air (oxygen)
bar/o	pressure	barometer *ba-ROM-e-ter*	instrument used to measure pressure
chrom/o, chromat/o	color, stain	chromatic *krō-MAT-ik*	having color
chron/o	time	chronologic *kron-ō-LOJ-ik*	arranged according to the time of occurrence
cry/o	cold	cryoprobe *KRĪ-ō-prōb*	instrument used to apply extreme cold
electro/o	electricity	electrolysis *ē-lek-TROL-i-sis*	decomposition of a substance by means of electric current
erg/o	work	synergistic *sin-er-JIS-tik*	working together with increased effect, such as certain drugs in combination
phon/o	sound, voice	phonograph *FŌ-nō-graf*	instrument used to reproduce sound
phot/o	light	photoreaction *fō-tō-rē-AK-shun*	response to light
radi/o	radiation, x-ray	radiology *rā-dē-OL-ō-jē*	study and use of radiation
son/o	sound	Sonogram *SON-ō-gram*	record obtained by use of ultrasound
therm/o	heat, temperature	hypothermia *hī-pō-THER-mē-a*	abnormally low body temperature

EXERCISE 7-1

Match the following terms and write the appropriate letter to the left of each number:

_____ **1.** radioactive (*rā-dē-ō-AK-tiv*)

_____ **2.** chromophilic (*krō-mō-FIL-ik*)

_____ **3.** synchrony (*SIN-krō-nē*)

_____ **4.** hyperthermia (*hī-per-THER-mē-a*)

_____ **5.** hyperbaric (*hī-per-BAR-ik*)

a. attracting color (stain)

b. abnormally high body temperature

c. pertaining to increased pressure

d. occurrence at the same time

e. giving off radiation

Identify and define the root in each of the following words:

	Root	**Meaning of Root**
6. ultrasonic (*ul-tra-SON-ik*)	son/o	sound
7. anaerobic (*an-er-Ō-bik*)		
8. exergonic (*eks-er-GON-ik*)		
9. homeothermic (*hō-mē-ō-THER-mik*)		
10. chronic (*KRON-ik*)		
11. achromatic (*ak-rō-MAT-ik*)		

Fill in the blanks:

12. Barotrauma (*bar-ō-TRAW-ma*) is injury caused by _____.

13. Cryotherapy (*krī-ō-THER-a-pē*) is treatment using _____.

14. A photograph (*FŌ-tō-graf*) is an image produced by means of _____.

15. The term electroconvulsive (*ē-lek-trō-con-VUL-siv*) means causing convulsions by means of _____.

16. Phonetics (*fō-NET-iks*) is the study of _____.

Table 7-2	Suffixes for Diagnosis		
Suffix	**Meaning**	**Example**	**Definition of Example**
-graph	instrument for recording data	polygraph *POL-ē-graf*	instrument used to record many physiologic responses simultaneously; lie detector
-graphy	act of recording data*	echography *ek-OG-ra-fē*	recording data obtained by ultrasound
-gram†	a record of data	electrocardiogram *e-lek-trō-KAR-dē-ō-gram*	record of the heart's electrical activity
-meter	instrument for measuring	calorimeter *kal-ō-RIM-e-ter*	instrument for measuring the caloric energy of food
-metry	measurement of	audiometry *aw-dē-OM-e-trē*	measurement of hearing (audi/o)
-scope	instrument for viewing or examining	bronchoscope *BRONG-kō-skōp*	instrument for examining the bronchi (breathing passages) (see Fig. 7-7)
-scopy	examination of	celioscopy *sē-lē-OS-kō-pē*	examination of the abdominal cavity (celi/o)

*This ending is often used to mean not only the recording of data but also the evaluation and interpretation of the data.
†An image prepared simply using x-rays is called a radiograph. When special techniques are used to image an organ or region with x-rays, the ending -gram is used with the root for that area, as in urogram (urinary tract), angiogram (blood vessels), and mammogram (breast).

EXERCISE 7-2

Match the following terms and write the appropriate letter to the left of each number:

_____ **1.** microscope (*MĪ-krō-skōp*)

a. instrument for examining very small objects

_____ **2.** sonogram (*SON-ō-gram*)

b. instrument for measuring temperature

_____ **3.** thermometer (*ther-MOM-e-ter*)

c. measurement of work done

_____ **4.** laparoscopy (*lap-a-ROS-kō-pē*)

d. a record of sound

_____ **5.** ergometry (*er-GOM-e-trē*)

e. examination of the abdomen

_____ **6.** audiometer (*aw-dē-OM-e-ter*)

a. a record of sound

_____ **7.** phonogram (*FŌ-nō-gram*)

b. instrument for measuring time

_____ **8.** endoscope (*EN-dō-skōp*)

c. instrument for viewing the inside of a cavity or organ

_____ **9.** electroencephalograph (*e-lek-trō-en-SEF-a-lō-graf*)

d. instrument used to measure hearing

_____ **10.** chronometer (*kron-OM-e-ter*)

e. instrument used to record the brain's electrical activity

Table 7-3	Suffixes for Surgery		
Suffix	**Meaning**	**Example**	**Definition of Example**
-centesis	puncture, tap	arthrocentesis *ar-thrō-sen-TĒ-sis*	puncture of a joint (arthr/o)
-desis	binding, fusion	pleurodesis *plū-ROD-e-sis*	binding of the pleura (membranes around the lungs)
-ectomy	excision, surgical removal	hepatectomy *hep-a-TEK-tō-mē*	excision of liver tissue (hepat/o)
-pexy	surgical fixation	hysteropexy *HIS-ter-ō-pek-sē*	surgical fixation of the uterus (hyster/o)
-plasty	plastic repair, plastic surgery, reconstruction	rhinoplasty *RĪ-nō-plas-tē*	plastic surgery of the nose (rhin/o)
-rhaphy	surgical repair, suture	herniorrhaphy *her-nē-OR-a-fē*	surgical repair of a hernia (herni/o)
-stomy	surgical creation of an opening	tracheostomy *trā-kē-OS-tō-mē*	creation of an opening into the trachea (trache/o)
-tome	instrument for incising (cutting)	microtome *MĪ-krō-tōm*	instrument for cutting thin sections of tissue for microscopic study
-tomy	incision, cutting	laparotomy *lap-a-ROT-ō-mē*	surgical incision of the abdomen (lapar/o)
-tripsy	crushing	neurotripsy *nū-rō-TRIP-sē*	crushing of a nerve (neur/o)

EXERCISE 7-3

Match the following terms and write the appropriate letter to the left of each number:

_____ **1.** thoracentesis (*thor-a-sen-TĒ-sis*)

_____ **2.** mammoplasty (*MAM-ō-plas-tē*)

_____ **3.** adenectomy (*ad-e-NEK-tō-mē*)

_____ **4.** lithotripsy (*LITH-ō-trip-sē*)

_____ **5.** celiocentesis (*sē-lē-ō-sen-TĒ-sis*)

a. crushing of a stone

b. puncture of the chest

c. puncture of the abdomen

d. excision of a gland

e. plastic surgery of the breast

The root *cyst/o* means "urinary bladder." Use this root to write a word that means each of the following:

6. Incision into the bladder _____ cystotomy _____

7. Surgical repair of the bladder _____

8. Creation of an opening into the bladder _____

9. Surgical fixation of the bladder _____

10. Plastic repair of the bladder _____

The root *arthr/o* means "joint." Use this root to write a word that means each of the following:

11. Puncture of a joint _____ arthrocentesis _____

12. Instrument for incising a joint _____

13. Fusion of a joint _____

14. Plastic repair of a joint _____

15. Incision of a joint _____

Write a word for each of the following definitions using the roots given:

16. Incision into the trachea (trache/o) _____

17. Surgical fixation of the stomach (gastr/o) _____

18. Creation of an opening into the colon (col/o) _____

| **Terminology** | **Supplementary Terms** |

Symptoms

clubbing KLUB-ing	Enlargement of the ends of the fingers and toes because of soft-tissue growth of the nails; seen in a variety of diseases, especially lung and heart diseases (Fig. 7-12)
colic KOL-ik	Acute abdominal pain associated with smooth-muscle spasms
cyanosis sī-a-NŌ-sis	Bluish discoloration of the skin due to lack of oxygen
diaphoresis dī-a-fō-RĒ-sis	Profuse sweating
malaise ma-LĀZ	A feeling of discomfort or uneasiness, often indicative of infection
nocturnal nok-TUR-nal	Pertaining to or occurring at night (roots noct/i and nyct/o mean "night")
pallor PAL-or	Paleness; lack of color
prodrome PRŌ-drōm	A symptom indicating an approaching disease
sequela se-KWEL-a	A lasting effect of a disease (plural: sequelae)
syncope SIN-kō-pē	A temporary loss of consciousness because of inadequate blood flow to the brain; fainting

Diagnosis

alpha-fetoprotein (AFP) AL-fa fē-tō-PRŌ-tēn	A fetal protein that appears in the blood of adults with certain types of cancer
bruit brwē	A sound, usually abnormal, heard in auscultation
facies FĀ-shē-ēz	The expression or appearance of the face
febrile FEB-ril	Pertaining to fever
nuclear medicine	The branch of medicine concerned with the use of radioactive substances (radionuclides) for diagnosis, therapy, and research
radiology rā-dē-OL-ō-jē	The branch of medicine that uses radiation, such as x-rays, in the diagnosis and treatment of disease; a specialist in this field is a radiologist
radionuclide rā-dē-ō-NŪ-klīd	A substance that gives off radiation; used for diagnosis and treatment; also called radioisotope or radiopharmaceutical
speculum SPEK-ō-lum	An instrument for examining a canal (Fig. 7-13)
syndrome SIN-drōm	A group of signs and symptoms that together characterize a disease condition

(continued)

Terminology Supplementary Terms (continued)

Treatment

catheter KATH-e-ter	A thin tube that can be passed into the body; used to remove fluids from or introduce fluids into a body cavity (Fig. 7-14)
clysis KLĪ-sis	The introduction of fluid into the body, other than orally, as into the rectum or abdominal cavity; also refers to the solution thus used
irrigation ir-i-GĀ-shun	Flushing of a tube, cavity, or area with a fluid (see Fig. 7-14)
lavage la-VAJ	The washing out of a cavity; irrigation
normal saline solution (NSS) SĀ-lēn	A salt (NaCl) solution compatible with living cells; also called physiologic saline solution (PSS)
paracentesis par-a-sen-TĒ-sis	Puncture of a cavity for removal of fluid
prophylaxis prō-fi-LAK-sis	Prevention of disease

Surgery

drain	Device for allowing matter to escape from a wound or cavity; common types include Penrose (cigarette), T-tube, Jackson–Pratt (J–P), and Hemovac
ligature LIG-a-chur	A tie or bandage; the process of binding or tying (also called ligation)
resection rē-SEK-shun	Partial excision of a structure
stapling STĀ-pling	In surgery, the joining of tissue by using wire staples that are pushed through the tissue and then bent
surgeon SUR-jun	One who specializes in surgery

PASSport to Success® Go to the pronunciation glossary in the Student Resources to hear these words pronounced.

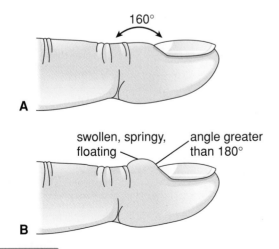

Figure 7-12 **Clubbing.** (*A*) Normal. (*B*) Clubbing; the end of the finger is enlarged because of soft-tissue growth around the nail.

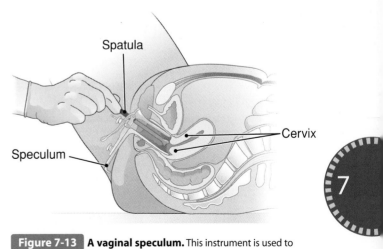

Figure 7-13 **A vaginal speculum.** This instrument is used to examine the vagina and cervix and to obtain a cervical sample for testing.

Fluid in
irrigation bag

Drip chamber

Clamp

Catheter

Bladder

Tubing to
irrigation port

Port for inflation
of catheter balloon

Drainage
bag

Figure 7-14   **Continuous bladder irrigation using a catheter.**

Terminology	Symbols		
1°	primary	>	greater than
2°	secondary (to)	<	less than
Δ	change	∧	above
Ⓛ	left	∨	below
Ⓡ	right	=	equal to
↑	increase(d)	≠	not equal to
↓	decrease(d)	±	doubtful, slight
♂	male	~	approximately
♀	female	×	times
°	degree	#	number, pound

Terminology   Abbreviations

History and Physical Examination

ADL	Activities of daily living
BP	Blood pressure
bpm	Beats per minute
C	Celsius (centigrade)
CC	Chief complaint
c/o	Complains of
EOMI	Extraocular muscles intact
ETOH	Alcohol (ethyl alcohol)
F	Fahrenheit
HEENT	Head, eyes, ears, nose, and throat
HIPAA	Health Insurance Portability and Accountability Act
h/o	History of
H & P	History and physical
HPI	History of present illness
HR	Heart rate
Hx	History
I & O	Intake and output
IPPA	Inspection, palpation, percussion, auscultation
IVDA	Intravenous drug abuse
NAD	No apparent distress
NKDA	No known drug allergies
P	Pulse
PE	Physical examination
PE(R)RLA	Pupils equal (regular) react to light and accommodation
PMH	Past medical history
pt	Patient
R	Respiration
R/O	Rule out
ROS	Review of systems
T	Temperature
TPR	Temperature, pulse, respiration
VS	Vital signs
WD	Well developed
WNL	Within normal limits
w/o	Without

Diagnosis and Treatment

ABC	Aspiration biopsy cytology
AFP	Alpha-fetoprotein
BS	Bowel sounds
bx	Biopsy
CAM	Complementary and alternative medicine
Ci	Curie (unit of radioactivity)
C & S	Culture and (drug) sensitivity (of bacteria)
CT	Computed tomography
D/C, dc	Discontinue, discharge
Dx	Diagnosis
EBL	Estimated blood loss
ICU	Intensive care unit
I & D	Incision and drainage
MET	Metastasis
MRI	Magnetic resonance imaging
NCCAM	National Center for Complementary and Alternative Medicine
NS, N/S	Normal saline
NSS	Normal saline solution
PCA	Patient-controlled analgesia
PET	Positron emission tomography
PICC	Peripherally inserted central catheter
postop	Postoperative
preop	Preoperative
PSS	Physiologic saline solution
RATx	Radiation therapy
Rx	Drug, prescription, therapy
SPECT	Single-photon emission computed tomography
TNM	(Primary) tumor, (regional lymph) nodes, (distant) metastases
UV	Ultraviolet

Views for Radiography

AP	Anteroposterior
LL	Left lateral
PA	Posteroanterior
RL	Right lateral

7

(continued)

Terminology | Abbreviations (continued)

Orders

AMA	Against medical advice		NPO	Nothing by mouth (Latin, *non per os*)
AMB	Ambulatory		OOB	Out of bed
BRP	Bathroom privileges		QNS	Quantity not sufficient
CBR	Complete bed rest		QS	Quantity sufficient
DNR	Do not resuscitate		STAT	Immediately
KVO	Keep vein open		TKO	To keep open

Drug-related abbreviations are located in Chapter 8.

Chapter Review

Match the following terms and write the appropriate letter to the left of each number:

_____	**1.** electrolyte	**a.**	evidence of disease
_____	**2.** staging	**b.**	classification of malignant tumors
_____	**3.** symptom	**c.**	substance that conducts electric current
_____	**4.** syndrome	**d.**	to unite parts by stitching them together
_____	**5.** suture	**e.**	a group of symptoms that characterizes a disease
_____	**6.** cautery	**a.**	removal of tissue for microscopic study
_____	**7.** scintiscan	**b.**	pain caused by cold
_____	**8.** cryalgesia	**c.**	destruction of tissue with a damaging agent
_____	**9.** vasotripsy	**d.**	image obtained with a radionuclide
_____	**10.** biopsy	**e.**	crushing of a vessel
_____	**11.** ergometer	**a.**	instrument used to cut bone
_____	**12.** osteotome	**b.**	organism that produces color
_____	**13.** acupuncture	**c.**	instrument to measure work output
_____	**14.** biofeedback	**d.**	method for controlling involuntary responses
_____	**15.** chromogen	**e.**	treatment by insertion of thin needles

Supplementary Terms

_____	**16.** sequelae	**a.**	enlargement of the ends of the fingers and toes
_____	**17.** prophylaxis	**b.**	lasting effects of disease
_____	**18.** clubbing	**c.**	prevention of disease
_____	**19.** prodrome	**d.**	partial excision
_____	**20.** resection	**e.**	symptom indicating an approaching disease
_____	**21.** catheter	**a.**	thin tube
_____	**22.** colic	**b.**	feeling of discomfort
_____	**23.** diaphoresis	**c.**	acute abdominal pain
_____	**24.** malaise	**d.**	washing out of a cavity
_____	**25.** lavage	**e.**	profuse sweating

Identify and define the root in each of the following words:

	Root	Meaning of Root
26. achromatous	_____	_____
27. ultrasonic	_____	_____
28. radiology	_____	_____
29. thermal	_____	_____
30. allergy	_____	_____
31. chronology	_____	_____
32. anaerobic	_____	_____

Fill in the blanks:

33. Photochromic eyeglass lenses change color in response to _____.

34. Plastic repair of the bladder is called _____.

35. Fusion of a joint is _____.

36. Surgical creation of an opening in the trachea is a(n) _____.

37. Another word for treatment is _____.

Use the root -*hepat*/o, meaning "liver," to write a word for each of the following:

38. Incision of the liver _____

39. Excision of liver tissue _____

40. Surgical fixation of the liver _____

41. Surgical repair of the liver _____

True–False > Examine the following statements. If the statement is true, write T in the first blank. If the statement is false, write F in the first blank and correct the statement by replacing the underlined word in the second blank.

42. Adenectomy is surgical removal of a <u>gland</u>.   _____   _____

43. An image produced by x-rays is a <u>radiogram</u>.   _____   _____

44. An otoscope is used to examine the <u>ear</u>.   _____   _____

45. A baroreceptor is sensitive to <u>temperature</u>.   _____   _____

46. An echogram is produced by <u>ultrasound</u>.   _____   _____

47. An arthroscope is used to examine a <u>joint</u>.   _____   _____

Eliminations > In each of the sets below, underline the word that does not fit in with the rest and explain the reason for your choice:

48. percussion — inspection — palpation — remission — auscultation

_____

49. ophthalmoscope — sphygmomanometer — stethoscope — syncope — endoscope

_____

50. curette — forceps — speculum — scalpel — hemostat

_____

Chapter Review (continued)

51. TNM — MRI — PET — CT — SPECT

_____

Word Building > Write words for the following definitions using the word parts provided.

lith/o   -rhaphy   neur/o   -tripsy   -tome   r   -pexy   -scopy   cyst/o

52. Instrument used to incise a nerve _____

53. Endoscopic examination of the bladder _____

54. Bladder stone _____

55. Surgical repair of a nerve _____

56. Crushing of a stone _____

57. Surgical fixation of the bladder _____

58. Surgical repair of the bladder _____

59. Crushing of a nerve _____

60. Instrument used to incise the bladder _____

Word Analysis > Define each of the following words, and give the meaning of the word parts in each. Use a dictionary if necessary.

61. isochromatophilic (_ī-sō-krō-mat-ō-FIL-ik_) _____

    a. iso- _____

    b. chromat/o _____

    c. phil _____

    d. -ic _____

62. synchronous (_SIN-krō-nus_) _____

    a. syn- _____

    b. chron/o _____

    c. -ous _____

63. phonocardiography (_fō-nō-kar-dē-OG-ra-fē_) _____

    a. phon/o _____

    b. cardi/o _____

    c. -graphy _____

64. chromogenesis (_krō-mō-JEN-e-sis_) _____

    a. chrom/o _____

    b. gen/e _____

    c. -sis _____

PASSport to Success® Go to the word exercises in the Student Resources for additional review exercises.

Case Studies

▶ Case Study 7-1: Comprehensive History and Physical

C.F., a 46-year-old married Asian woman, works as an office manager for an insurance company. This morning, she had a follow-up visit with her oncologist and was sent to the hospital for immediate admission for possible recurrence or sequelae of her ovarian cancer. She is alert, articulate, and a reliable reporter.

CC: C.F. presents with mild, low, aching pelvic pain and low abdominal fullness. She states, "I feel like I have cramps and am bloated. Sometimes I'm so tired I cannot do my work without a short nap."

HPI: C.F. has been in remission for 14 months from aggressively treated ovarian carcinoma. She presents with mild abdominal distention and tenderness on deep palpation of the lower pelvis. C.F. claims a feeling of fullness in the lower abdomen, loss of appetite, and inability to sleep through the night. She is afraid that her cancer was not cured. Sometimes her heart races and she cannot catch her breath, but with two children in college, she cannot afford to miss work.

MEDS: Therapeutic vitamin × 1/day. Valium 5 mg every 6 hours (q6h) as needed (prn) for anxiety. Benadryl 25 mg at bedtime (hs) prn for insomnia. Echinacea tea 3 cups/day to prevent colds or flu. Ginkgo biloba 3 caps/day for energy.

ALLERGIES: NKDA; no food allergies

PMH: C.F. was diagnosed with ovarian CA 4 years ago and treated with surgery, radiation, and chemotherapy. A total abdominal hysterectomy (removal of the uterus) with bilateral removal of the oviducts and ovaries was performed. At the time of surgery, the pelvic lymph nodes tested negative for disease. Chemotherapy and radiation therapy occurred after surgical recovery. C.F. has been well and capable of full ADL until 4 weeks ago. Childhood history is unremarkable, with normal childhood diseases, including measles, mumps, and chicken pox. C.F. was born and raised in this country. She has no other adult diseases, surgery, or injuries.

CURRENT HEALTH Hx: Denies tobacco, ETOH, or recreational drugs or substances. She exercises three to five times per week with aerobic exercise class and treadmill. She is a vegetarian and drinks one to five cups of green tea per day. Immunizations are up to date; unsure of last tetanus booster. Recent negative mammogram and negative TB test (PPD).

FAMILY Hx: Both parents alive and well. Maternal aunt died of "stomach tumor" at age 37.

TPR & BP & PAIN: 37C-96-22 126/72 in no acute distress.

HEENT: WNL. Mesocephalic, fundi benign, PERRLA, uncorrected 20/20 vision, mouth clear, good dental health, neck supple w/o rigidity, thyromegaly, or cervical lymphadenopathy; trachea midline. No carotid bruits (sounds).

LUNGS: All lobes clear to auscultation and percussion.

HEART: Rate 96 bpm, regular; no murmurs, gallops, or rubs.

BREASTS: Symmetrical, w/o masses or discharge.

ABDOMEN: Skin intact with healed suprapubic midline surgical incision and a symmetrical area of discoloration and dermal thickness from radiation therapy. Bowel sounds active and normal. Suprapubic tenderness on palpation. No hepatosplenomegaly. Absence of inguinal lymph nodes on palpation. Kidneys palpable. Rectal exam WNL. Hemoccult test (stool test for blood) result negative.

GU: Unremarkable. Surgical menopause.

MUSCULOSKELETAL: WNL. No weakness, limitation of mobility, joint pain, stiffness, or edema.

NEUROLOGIC: All reflexes intact. No syncope, paralysis, numbness.

DIAGNOSTIC IMPRESSION: Possible recurrence of ovarian CA, ascites.

TREATMENT PLAN: Send blood for CA-125 (genetic marker for ovarian cancer). Schedule abdominal paracentesis and second-look diagnostic laparoscopy with biopsy and tissue staging. D/C all herbal supplements.

▶ Case Study 7-2: Diagnostic Laparoscopy

For a laparoscopy, C.F. was given general anesthesia and her trachea was intubated. She was placed in lithotomy position with arms abducted. Her abdomen was insufflated with carbon dioxide (CO_2) through a thin needle placed below the umbilicus. Three trocar punctures were made to insert the telescope with camera and the cutting and grasping instruments. Biopsies were taken of several pelvic lymph nodes and sent to the pathology laboratory. There were many adhesions from prior surgery, which were lysed to mobilize her organs and enhance visualization. A loop of small bowel, which had adhered to the anterior abdominal wall, had been punctured when the trocar was introduced. The surgeon repaired the defect with an endoscopic stapler and irrigated the abdomen with 3 L of NSS mixed with antibiotic solution.

▶ Case Study 7-3: Postoperative Care

After surgery, C.F. reported numbness and tingling in her right arm and bilateral subscapular discomfort when she stood. The retained CO_2 was eventually absorbed. The subscapular discomfort decreased and was judged to have originated from hyperabduction of the arms during surgery.

Biopsy results were negative, there was no fluid found on paracentesis to explain the abdominal symptoms, and the CA-125 was below 35 U/mL, which is

(continued)

Case Studies (continued)

negative for recurrence. Psychological counseling was recommended to help C.F. verbalize her fears and gain a sense of control. She will call her oncologist to schedule a follow-up visit for reevaluation.

CASE STUDY QUESTIONS

Write the word from the case study that completes each of the following statements:

1. Secondary conditions, complications, or lasting effects of C.F.'s cancer would be called _____.

2. Examination by touching the surface of the body is _____.

3. The size and shape of C.F.'s head was described as _____.

4. A collection of abdominal fluid (ascites) is drained by a cavity puncture and drainage procedure called a(n) _____.

5. Removal of tissue for microscopic examination is _____.

6. A surgical procedure in which an endoscope is inserted through the abdominal wall to visualize the abdominal cavity and determine the cause of a disorder is a(n) _____.

7. Extreme or overextension of an arm or leg away from the midline of the body is _____.

Multiple choice. Select the best answer and write the letter of your choice to the left of each number:

_____ 8. C.F.'s cancer was in a state of apparent cure with no active signs of disease. This state is called:
   a. exacerbation
   b. syndrome
   c. remission
   d. sequelae
   e. tumor staging

_____ 9. The abbreviation NKDA refers to allergies to:
   a. lactose
   b. wheat
   c. eggs
   d. drugs
   e. dust

_____ 10. C.F. claimed that her heart races and she cannot catch her breath. The terms for these conditions are:
   a. tachypnea and dyspnea
   b. tachycardia and dyspnea
   c. dyspnea and tachycardia
   d. tachycardia and bradypnea
   e. bradycardia and tachypulmono

_____ 11. Syncope is:
   a. fainting
   b. nosebleed
   c. inflammation
   d. palpitations
   e. anxiety

_____ 12. Hepatosplenomegaly means:
   a. removal of the liver and spleen
   b. prolapse of the heart and spleen
   c. hemorrhage of the liver and spleen
   d. enlargement of the liver and spleen
   e. surgical repair of the kidney and liver

_____ 13. C.F.'s abdominal cavity and organs were bound with fibrous tissue bands, which had to be lysed during surgery. These bands are called:
   a. prodromes
   b. sequelae
   c. adhesions
   d. ascites
   e. fibroids

_____ 14. The accidental puncture of the intestine was not an expected outcome of surgery. It was an incident that occurred despite attempts to protect her from harm. The term for this type of disorder is (see Chapter 6):
   a. iatrogenic
   b. nosocomial
   c. idiopathic
   d. etiologic
   e. surgical misadventure

Give the meaning of each of the following abbreviations:

15. HPI _____

16. CA _____

17. TPR _____

18. ADL _____

19. bpm _____

20. WNL _____

21. D/C _____

22. NSS _____

Drugs

CHAPTER CONTENTS

OBJECTIVES

After study of this chapter you should be able to:

1. Explain the difference between over-the-counter and prescription drugs.
2. List some potential adverse side effects of drugs.
3. Explain ways in which drugs can interact.
4. Explain the difference between the generic name and the brand name of a drug.
5. List several drug references.
6. Describe some of the issues involved in the use of herbal medicines.
7. Identify and use word parts pertaining to drugs.
8. Recognize the major categories of drugs and how they act.
9. List some common herbal medicines and how they act.
10. List common routes for drug administration.
11. List standard forms in which liquid and solid drugs are prepared.
12. Define abbreviations related to drugs and their use.
13. Analyze the terminology related to drugs in several case studies.

PRETEST

Multiple choice. Select the best answer and write the letter of your choice to the left of each number.

___ 1. The federal agency that approves drugs for sale is the:

    a. Food and Drug Administration
    b. U.S. Department of Agriculture
    c. Department of Health and Human Services
    d. Occupational Safety and Health Administration

_____ 2. A reason for not using a specific drug is a:

    a. prescription   c. counterpurpose
    b. prognosis   d. contraindication

_____ 3. A manufacturer's registered name for a drug is its:

    a. chemical name
    b. generic name
    c. brand name
    d. over-the-counter name

_____ 4. A written and signed order for a drug is a(n):

    a. license   c. indication
    b. prescription   d. therapy

_____ 5. The word root for drug or medicine is:

    a. pharm   c. log
    b. scop   d. lapar

_____ 6. An analgesic is a drug used for:

    a. fractures   c. coma
    b. water retention d. pain

_____ 7. An antihypertensive drug affects:

    a. blood pressure   c. growth
    b. diet   d. ovulation

_____ 8. The solvent in an aqueous solution is:

    a. acid   c. salt
    b. water   d. base

_____ 9. The abbreviation IV means:

    a. inverted   c. intravenous
    b. introverted   d. inviable

_____ 10. The abbreviation prn means:

    a. as needed   c. each night
    b. once a day   d. before meals

Drugs

A **drug** is a substance that alters body function. Traditionally, drugs have been derived from natural plant, animal, and mineral sources. Today, most are manufactured synthetically by pharmaceutical companies. A few, such as certain hormones and enzymes, have been produced by genetic engineering.

Many drugs, described as over-the-counter (OTC) drugs, are available without a signed order, or **prescription (Rx)**. Others require a health care provider's prescription for use. Responsibility for the safety and **efficacy** of all drugs sold in the United States lies with the Federal Food and Drug Administration (FDA), which must approve all drugs before they are sold.

Adverse Drug Effects

An unintended effect of a drug or other form of treatment is a **side effect**. Most drugs have potential adverse side effects that must be evaluated before they are prescribed. In addition, there may be **contraindications**, or reasons not to use a particular drug for a specific individual based on that person's medical conditions, current medications, sensitivity, or family history. While a patient is under treatment, it is important to be alert for signs of adverse effects such as digestive upset, changes in the blood, or signs of allergy, such as hives or skin rashes. **Anaphylaxis** is an immediate and severe allergic reaction that may be caused by a drug. It can lead to life-threatening respiratory distress and circulatory collapse.

Because drugs given in combination may interact, the prescriber must know of any drugs the patient is taking before prescribing another. In some cases, a combination may result in **synergy** or **potentiation**, meaning that the drugs together have a greater effect than either of the drugs acting alone. In other cases, one drug may act as an **antagonist** of another, interfering with its action. Drugs may also react adversely with certain foods or substances used socially, such as alcohol and tobacco.

Drugs that act on the central nervous system may lead to a psychological or physical **substance dependence**, in which a person has a chronic or compulsive need for a drug regardless of its bad effects. With repeated use, a drug **tolerance** may develop, whereby a constant dose has less effect and the dose must be increased to produce the original response. Cessation of the drug then leads to symptoms of substance **withdrawal**, a state that results from a drug's removal or dose reduction. Certain symptoms are associated with withdrawal from specific drugs.

Drug Names

Drugs may be cited by either their generic or their **brand names**. (Box 8-1 has information on drug naming.) The **generic name** is usually a simple version of the chemical name for the drug and is not capitalized. The brand name (trade name, proprietary name) is a registered trademark of the manufacturer and is written with an initial capital letter. For example, Tylenol is the brand name for the analgesic compound acetaminophen; the antidepressant Prozac is fluoxetine. A brand name is protected by a patent; only the company that holds the patent can produce and sell that drug under its brand name until the patent expires. Reference Box 8-3, which

Box 8-1 Focus on Words

Where Do Drugs Get Their Names?

Drug names are derived in a variety of ways. Some are named for their origin. Adrenaline, for example, is named for its source, the adrenal gland. Even its generic name, epinephrine, informs us that it comes from the gland that is above (epi-) the kidney (nephr/o). Pitocin, a drug used to induce labor, is named for its source, the pituitary gland, combined with the chemical name of the hormone, oxytocin. Botox, currently injected into the skin for cosmetic removal of wrinkles, is the toxin from the organism that causes botulism, a type of food poisoning. Aspirin (an antiinflammatory agent), Taxol (an antitumor agent), digitalis (used to treat heart failure), and atropine (a smooth-muscle relaxant) are all named for the plants they come from. For example, aspirin is named for the blossoms of Spiraea, from which it is derived. Taxol comes from a yew (evergreen) of the genus *Taxus*. Digitalis is from purple foxglove, genus *Digitalis*. Atropine comes from the plant *Atropa belladonna*.

Some names tell about the drug or its actions. The name for Humulin, a form of insulin made by genetic engineering, points out that this is human insulin and not a hormone from animal sources. Lomotil reduces intestinal motility and is used to treat diarrhea. The name *Belladonna* is from Italian and means "fair lady," because this drug dilates the pupils of the eyes, making women appear more beautiful.

---

appears later in this chapter, has many more examples of generic and brand names. Note that the same drug may be marketed by different companies under different brand names. Both Motrin and Advil, for example, are the generic antiinflammatory agent ibuprofen.

Drug Information

In the United States, the standard for drug information is the *United States Pharmacopeia* (USP). This reference is published by a national committee of pharmacologists and other scientists. It contains formulas for drugs sold in the United States; standards for testing the strength, quality, and purity of drugs; and standards for the preparation and dispensing of drugs. The American Society of Health System Pharmacists (ASHP) publishes extensive drug information; The *Physicians' Desk Reference*, published yearly by Thomson Healthcare, contains information supplied by drug manufacturers. An enormous amount of drug information is available online through the Web sites for these publications and others. Another excellent source of up-to-date information on drugs is a community or hospital pharmacist. See Box 8-2 for information on careers in pharmacy.

Box 8-2 Health Professions

Pharmacists and Pharmacy Technicians

Medications are chemicals designed to treat illness and improve quality of life. The role of pharmacists and pharmacy technicians is to ensure that patients receive the correct medications and the education they need to use them effectively and derive their intended health benefits.

As key members of the health care team, pharmacists need a strong clinical background with a thorough understanding of chemistry, anatomy, and physiology. Pharmacists not only dispense prescription medications and monitor patients' responses to them, they also educate patients about their appropriate use. They share their expertise with other health professionals and also participate in clinical research on drugs and their effects.

Pharmacy technicians assist pharmacists with their duties. Their training also requires a thorough background in basic sciences. State rules and regulations vary, but pharmacy technicians may perform many of the tasks related to dispensing medications, such as preparing drugs and packaging them with appropriate labels and instructions for use.

Most pharmacists and pharmacy technicians work in retail pharmacies; others work in hospitals and long-term care facilities. Job prospects are promising because of the growing need for health care. In fact, pharmacy is projected to be one of the fastest-growing careers in the United States. For more information about careers in pharmacy, contact the American Association of Colleges of Pharmacy at www.aacp.org.

Herbal Medicines

For hundreds of years, people have used plants to treat diseases, a practice described as herbal medicine or **phytomedicine**. Many people in industrialized countries are now turning to herbal products as alternatives or complements to conventional medicines. Although plants are the source of many conventional drugs, pharmaceutical companies usually purify, measure, and often modify or synthesize the active ingredients in these plants rather than presenting them in their natural state.

Some issues have arisen with the increased use of herbal medicines, including questions about their purity, safety, concentration, and efficacy. Another issue is drug interactions. Health care providers should ask about the use of herbal remedies when taking a patient's drug history, and patients should report any herbal medicines they take when under treatment. The FDA does not test or regulate herbal medicines, and there are no requirements to report adverse effects. There are, however, restrictions on the health claims that can be made by the manufacturers of herbal medicines. The U.S. government has established the Office of Dietary Supplements (ODS) to support and coordinate research in this field.

Terminology   Key Terms

anaphylaxis an-a fi-LAK-sis	An extreme allergic reaction that can lead to respiratory distress, circulatory collapse, and death
antagonist an-TAG-o-nist	A substance that interferes with or opposes the action of a drug
brand name	The trade or proprietary name of a drug, a registered trademark of the manufacturer; written with an initial capital letter
contraindication kon-tra-in-di-KĀ-shun	A factor that makes the use of a drug undesirable or dangerous
drug	A substance that alters body function
efficacy EF-i-ka-sē	The power to produce a specific result; effectiveness
generic name je-NER-ik	The nonproprietary name of a drug; that is, a name that is not privately owned or trademarked; usually a simplified version of the chemical name; not capitalized
phytomedicine fī-tō-MED-i-sin	Another name for herbal medicine (root *phyt/o* meaning "plant")
potentiation pō-ten-shē-Ā-shun	Increased potency created by two drugs acting together
prescription (Rx) prē-SKRIP-shun	Written and signed order for a drug with directions for its administration
side effect	A result of drug therapy or other therapy that is unrelated to or an extension of its intended effect. The term usually applies to an undesirable effect of treatment
substance dependence	A condition that may result from chronic use of a drug, in which a person has a chronic or compulsive need for a drug regardless of its adverse effects; dependence may be psychological or physical
synergy SIN-er-jē	Combined action of two or more drugs working together to produce an effect greater than any of the drugs could produce when acting alone; also called synergism (SIN-er-jizm); adjective: synergistic (sin-er-JIS-tik)
tolerance	A condition in which chronic use of a drug results in loss of effectiveness and the dose must be increased to produce the original response
withdrawal	A condition that results from cessation or reduction of a drug that has been used regularly

 PASSport to Success® Go to the pronunciation glossary on the Student Resources to hear these words pronounced.

Table 8-1	**Word Parts Pertaining to Drugs**		
	Meaning	Example	Definition of Example
Suffixes			
-lytic (adjective of lysis)	dissolving, reducing, loosening	thrombolytic *throm-bō-LIT-ik*	agent that dissolves a blood clot (thrombus)
-mimetic	mimicking, simulating	sympathomimetic *sim-pa-thō-mi-MET-ik*	mimicking the effects of the sympathetic nervous system
-tropic	acting on	psychotropic *sī-kō-TROP-ik*	acting on the mind (psych/o)
Prefixes			
anti-	against	antiemetic *an-tē-e-MET-ik*	drug that prevents vomiting (emesis)
contra-	against, oppose	contraceptive *kon-tra-SEP-tiv*	preventing conception
counter-	opposite, against	countertransport *kown-ter-TRANS-port*	movement in an opposite direction
Roots			
alg/o, algi/o, algesi/o	pain	algesia *al-JĒ-zē-a*	sense of pain
chem/o	chemical	chemotherapy *kē-mō-THER-a-pē*	treatment with drugs
hypn/o	sleep	hypnosis *hip-NŌ-sis*	induced state of sleep
narc/o	stupor	narcotic *nar-KOT-ik*	agent that induces a state of stupor with decreased sensation
pharm, pharmac/o	drug, medicine	pharmacy *FAR-ma-sē*	the science of preparing and dispensing drugs, or the place where these activities occur
pyr/o, pyret/o	fever	antipyretic *an-ti-pī-RET-ik*	counteracting fever
tox/o, toxic/o	poison, toxin	toxicity *tok-SIS-i-tē*	state of being poisonous
vas/o	vessel	vasodilation *vas-ō-dī-LĀ-shun*	widening of a vessel

EXERCISE 8-1

Identify and define the suffix in each of the following words:

	Suffix	Meaning of Suffix
1. anxiolytic (*ang-zī-ō-LIT-ik*)	_____	_____
2. chronotropic (*kron-ō-TROP-ik*)	_____	_____
3. parasympathomimetic (*par-a-sim-pa-thō-mi-MET-ik*)	_____	_____

Using the prefixes listed in Table 8-1, write the opposite of each of the following words:

4. inflammatory _____

5. indicated _____

6. septic _____

7. act _____

8. toxin _____

9. pyretic _____

Identify and define the root in each of the following words:

	Root	Meaning of Root
10. hypnotic	_____	_____
11. toxicology	_____	_____
12. analgesia	_____	_____
13. chemistry	_____	_____
14. narcosis	_____	_____

Define each of the following words:

15. vasoconstriction _____

16. pharmacology _____

17. mucolytic _____

18. gonadotropic _____

Terminology Abbreviations

Drugs and Drug Formulations

APAP	Acetaminophen
ASA	Acetylsalicylic acid (aspirin)
ASHP	American Society of Health System Pharmacists
cap	Capsule
elix	Elixir
FDA	Food and Drug Administration
INH	Isoniazid (antituberculosis drug)
MED(s)	Medicine(s), medication(s)
NSAID(s)	Nonsteroidal antiinflammatory drug(s)
ODS	Office of Dietary Supplements
OTC	Over-the-counter
PDR	*Physicians' Desk Reference*
Rx	Prescription
supp	Suppository
susp	Suspension
tab	Tablet
tinct	Tincture
ung	Ointment
USP	*United States Pharmacopeia*

Dosages and Directions

ā	Before (Latin, *ante*)
āā	Of each (Greek, *ana*)
ac	Before meals (Latin, *ante cibum*)
ad lib	As desired (Latin, *ad libitum*)
aq	Water (Latin, *aqua*)
bid	Twice a day (Latin, *bis in die*)
c̄	With (Latin, *cum*)
D/C, dc	Discontinue
DS	Double strength
gt(t)	Drop(s) (Latin, *gutta*)
hs	At bedtime (Latin, *hora somni*)
ID	Intradermal(ly)
IM	Intramuscular(ly)
IU	International unit
IV	Intravenous(ly)
LA	Long-acting
mcg	Microgram
mg	Milligram

(continued)

Terminology Abbreviations *(continued)*

Dosages and Directions

mL	Milliliter		s̄	Without (Latin, *sine*)
p	After, post		SA	Sustained action
pc	After meals (Latin, *post cibum*)		SC, SQ, subcu	Subcutaneous(ly)
po	By mouth (Latin, *per os*)		SL	sublingual(ly)
pp	Postprandial (after a meal)		SR	Sustained release
prn	As needed (Latin, *pro re nata*)		s̄s̄	Half (Latin, *semis*)
qam	Every morning (Latin, *quaque ante meridiem*)		tid	Three times per day (Latin, *ter in die*)
qh	Every hour (Latin, *quaque hora*)		U	Unit(s)
q __ h	Every _____ hours		x	Times
qid	Four times a day (Latin, *quater in die*)			

Drug Reference Information

So far, this chapter has been an overview of drugs and the terminology for drugs and drug usage. The next section of the chapter contains informational boxes that you can examine now and refer to again as you work through Part 3 of the text. Box 8-3 outlines the major categories of drugs and cites examples by both generic and brand names. Box 8-4 lists some common herbal medicines and their uses. Boxes 8-5 through 8-7 have information on routes of administration, drug preparations, and injectable drugs.

Box 8-3   For Your Reference

Common Drugs and Their Actions

CATEGORY	ACTIONS; APPLICATIONS	GENERIC NAME	BRAND NAME(S)
Adrenergics *ad-ren-ER-jiks* (sympathomimetics *[sim-pa-thō-mi-MET-iks]*)	Mimic the action of the sympathetic nervous system, which responds to stress; used to treat bronchospasms, allergic reactions, hypotension	epinephrine phenylephrine pseudoephedrine dopamine	Bronkaid Neo-Synephrine Sudafed Intropin
Analgesics *an-al-JĒ-siks*	Alleviate pain		
Narcotics *nar-KO-tiks*	Decreases pain sensation in central nervous system; chronic use may lead to physical dependence	codeine morphine meperidine oxycodone	Demerol Percodan, Percocet
Nonnarcotics *non-nar-KO-tiks*	Acts peripherally to inhibit prostaglandins (local hormones); they may also be antiinflammatory and antipyretic (reduce fever). Cox-2 inhibitors limit an enzyme that causes inflammation without affecting a related enzyme that protects the stomach lining	aspirin (acetylsalicylic acid; ASA) acetaminophen (APAP) ibuprofen celecoxib (Cox-2 inhibitor)	Tylenol Motrin, Advil Celebrex

(continued)

Box 8-3   For Your Reference   *(Continued)*

Common Drugs and Their Actions

CATEGORY	ACTIONS; APPLICATIONS	GENERIC NAME	BRAND NAME(S)
Anesthetics *an-es-THET-iks*	Reduce or eliminate sensation (esthesi/o)	Local: lidocaine bupivacaine General: nitrous oxide midazolam thiopental	Xylocaine Marcaine Versed Pentothal
Anticoagulants *an-ti-kō-AG-ū-lants*	Prevent coagulation and formation of blood clots	heparin warfarin	Coumadin
Anticonvulsants *an-ti-kon-VUL-sants*	Suppress or reduce the number and/or intensity of seizures	phenobarbital phenytoin carbamazepine valproic acid	 Dilantin Tegretol Depakene
Antidiabetics *an-ti-dī-a-BET-iks*	Prevent or alleviate diabetes	insulin glyburide acarbose glipizide	Humulin (injected) Diabeta Precose Glucotrol
Antiemetics *an-tē-e-MET-iks*	Relieve symptoms of nausea and prevent vomiting (emesis)	ondansetron dimenhydrinate prochlorperazine scopolamine promethazine	Zofran Dramamine Compazine TRANSDERM-SCŌP Phenergan
Antihistamines *an-ti-HIS-ta-mēnz*	Prevent responses mediated by histamine: allergic and inflammatory reactions	diphenhydramine fexofenadine loratadine cetirizine	Benadryl Allegra Claritin Zyrtec
Antihypertensives *an-ti-hī-per-TEN-sivs*	Lower blood pressure by reducing cardiac output, dilating vessels, or promoting excretion of water by the kidneys. ACE inhibitors block production of a substance that raises blood pressure. See also calcium-channel blockers and beta-blockers under cardiac drugs; diuretics	amlodipine atenolol clonidine prazosin minoxidil captopril enalapril	Norvasc Tenormin Catapres Minipress Loniten Capoten Vasotec
Antiinflammatory drugs *an-tē-in-FLAM-a-tō-rē*	Counteract inflammation and swelling		
Corticosteroids *kor-ti-kō-STER-oyds*	Hormones from the cortex of the adrenal gland; used for allergy, respiratory, and blood diseases, injury, and malignancy; suppress the immune system	dexamethasone cortisone prednisone hydrocortisone fluticasone	Decadron Cortone Deltasone Hydrocortone, Cortef Flonase
Nonsteroidal antiinflammatory drugs (NSAIDs) *non-ster-OYD-al*	Reduce inflammation and pain by interfering with synthesis of prostaglandins; also antipyretic	aspirin ibuprofen indomethacin naproxen celecoxib	 Motrin, Advil Indocin Naprosyn, Aleve Celebrex
Antiinfective agents	Kill or prevent the growth of infectious organisms		
Antibacterials; *an-ti-bak-TĒ-rē-als*	Effective against bacteria	amoxicillin penicillin V erythromycin	Polymox Pen-Vee K Erythrocin

Box 8-3 For Your Reference *(Continued)*

Common Drugs and Their Actions

CATEGORY	ACTIONS; APPLICATIONS	GENERIC NAME	BRAND NAME(S)
antibiotics *an-ti-bī-OT-iks*		vancomycin gentamicin cephalexin tetracycline ciprofloxacin (for ulcer-causing *H. pylori*) isoniazid (INH) (tuberculosis)	Vancocin Garamycin Keflex Achromycin Cipro Nydrazid
Antifungals *an-ti-FUNG-gals*	Effective against fungi	amphotericin B miconazole nystatin	Fungizone Monistat Nilstat
Antiparasitics *an-ti-par-a-SIT-iks*	Effective against parasites: protozoa, worms	iodoquinol (amebae) quinacrine	Yodoxin Atabrine
Antivirals *an-ti-VI-rals*	Effective against viruses	acyclovir zanamivir (influenza) zidovudine (HIV) indinavir (HIV protease inhibitor)	Zovirax Relenza Retrovir Crixivan
Antineoplastics *an-ti-nē-ō-PLAS-tiks*	Destroy cancer cells; they are toxic for all cells but have greater effect on cells that are actively growing and dividing; hormones and hormone inhibitors also are used to slow tumor growth	cyclophosphamide doxorubicin methotrexate vincristine tamoxifen (estrogen inhibitor)	Cytoxan Adriamycin Folex Oncovin Nolvadex
Cardiac drugs *KAR-dē-ak*	Act on the heart		
Antiarrhythmics *an-tē-a-RITH-miks*	Correct or prevent abnormalities of heart rhythm	quinidine lidocaine digoxin	Quinidex Xylocaine Lanoxin
Beta-adrenergic blockers (beta-blockers) *bā-ta-ad-ren-ER-jik*	Inhibit sympathetic nervous system; reduce rate and force of heart contractions	propranolol metoprolol atenolol	Inderal Toprol-XL Tenormin
Calcium-channel blockers *KAL-sē-um*	Dilate coronary arteries, slow heart rate, reduce contractions	diltiazem nifedipine verapamil	Cardizem Procardia Covera
Hypolipidemics *hī-pō-lip-i-DĒ-miks*	Lower cholesterol in patients with high serum levels that cannot be controlled with diet alone; hypocholesterolemics, statins	lovastatin pravastatin atorvastatin simvastatin	Mevacor Pravachol Lipitor Zocor
Nitrates; *NĪ-trātz* antianginal agents *an-ti-AN-ji-nal*	Dilate coronary arteries and reduce heart's workload by lowering blood pressure and reducing venous return	nitroglycerin isosorbide	Nitrostat Isordil
CNS stimulants	Stimulate the central nervous system	methylphenidate amphetamine (chronic use may lead to drug dependence)	Ritalin Adderall, Dexedrine

(continued)

Box 8-3 For Your Reference *(Continued)*

Common Drugs and Their Actions

CATEGORY	ACTIONS; APPLICATIONS	GENERIC NAME	BRAND NAME(S)
Diuretics dī-ū-RET-iks	Promote excretion of water, sodium, and other electrolytes by the kidneys; used to reduce edema and blood pressure. Loop diuretics act on the kidney tubules (see Chapters 9 and 13)	furosemide ethacrynic acid mannitol hydrochlorothiazide (HCTZ) triamterene + HCTZ	Lasix Edecrin Osmitrol HydroDIURIL Dyazide
Gastrointestinal drugs gas-trō-in-TES-tin-al	Act on the digestive tract		
Antidiarrheals an-ti-di-a-RĒ-als	Treat or prevent diarrhea by reducing intestinal motility or absorbing irritants and soothing the intestinal lining	diphenoxylate loperamide attapulgite atropine	Lomotil Imodium Kaopectate
Histamine H₂ antagonists HIS-ta-mēn	Decrease stomach acid secretion by interfering with the action of histamine at H₂ receptors; used to treat ulcers and other gastrointestinal problems	cimetidine ranitidine	Tagamet Zantac
Laxatives LAK-sa-tivs	Promote elimination from the large intestine; types include: stimulants hyperosmotics (retain water) stool softeners bulk-forming agents	bisacodyl lactulose docusate psyllium	Dulcolax Constilac, Chronulac Colace, Surfak Metamucil
Proton pump inhibitors PRŌ-ton	Reduce stomach acidity by blocking transport of hydrogen ions (protons) into the stomach	esomeprazole lansoprazole omeprazole	Nexium Prevacid Prilosec
Hypnotics hip-NOT-iks	Induce sleep or dull the senses; see antianxiety agents (below, under psychotropics)		
Muscle relaxants rē-LAK-sants	Depress nervous system stimulation of skeletal muscles; used to control muscle spasms and pain	baclofen carisoprodol methocarbamol	Lioresal Soma Robaxin
Psychotropics sī-kō-TROP-iks	Affect the mind, altering mental activity, mental state, or behavior		
Antianxiety agents an-tē-ang-ZĪ-e-tē	Reduce or dispel anxiety; tranquilizers; anxiolytic agents	lorazepam chlordiazepoxide diazepam hydroxyzine alprazolam buspirone	Ativan Librium Valium Atarax Xanax BuSpar
Antidepressants an-ti-dē-PRES-sants	Relieve depression by raising brain levels of neurotransmitters (chemicals active in the nervous system)	amitriptyline imipramine fluoxetine paroxetine sertraline	Elavil Tofranil Prozac Paxil Zoloft
Antipsychotics an-ti-sī-KOT-iks	Act on nervous system to relieve symptoms of psychoses	chlorpromazine haloperidol risperidone olanzapine	Thorazine Haldol Risperdal Zyprexa

Box 8-3 For Your Reference *(Continued)*

Common Drugs and Their Actions

CATEGORY	ACTIONS; APPLICATIONS	GENERIC NAME	BRAND NAME(S)
Respiratory drugs	Act on the respiratory system		
Antitussives *an-ti-TUS-sivs*	Suppress coughing	dextromethorphan	Benylin DM
Asthma maintenance drugs	Used for prevention of asthma attacks and chronic treatment of asthma	fluticasone montelukast	Flovent Singulair
Bronchodilators *brong-kō-dī-LĀ-tors*	Prevent or eliminate spasm of the bronchi (breathing tubes) by relaxing bronchial smooth muscle; used to treat asthma attacks and bronchitis	albuterol epinephrine metaproterenol	Proventil Sus-Phrine Alupent
Expectorants *ek-SPEK-tō-rants*	Induce productive coughing to eliminate respiratory secretions	guaifenesin	Robitussin
Mucolytics *mū-kō-LIT-iks*	Loosen mucus to promote its elimination	acetylcysteine	Mucomyst
Sedatives/hypnotics *SED-a-tivs/hip-NOT-iks*	Induce relaxation and sleep; lower (sedative) doses promote relaxation leading to sleep; higher (hypnotic) doses induce sleep; antianxiety agents also used	phenobarbital zolpidem	Ambien
Tranquilizers *tran-kwi-LĪZ-ers*	Reduce mental tension and anxiety; see Antianxiety agents (above, under Psychotropics)		

Box 8-4 For Your Reference

Therapeutic Uses of Herbal Medicines

NAME	PART USED	THERAPEUTIC USES
Aloe *AL-ō*	Leaf	Treatment of burns and minor skin irritations
Black cohosh *KŌ-hosh*	Root	Reduction of menopausal hot flashes
Chamomile *KAM-ō-mīl*	Flower	Antiinflammatory, gastrointestinal antispasmodic, sedative
Echinacea *e-ki-NĀ-shē-a*	All	May reduce severity and duration of colds; may stimulate the immune system; used topically for wound healing
Evening primrose oil *PRIM-rōz*	Seed	Source of essential fatty acids important for the health of the cardiovascular system; treatment of premenstrual syndrome (PMS), rheumatoid arthritis, skin disorders
Flax	Seed	Source of fatty acids important in maintaining proper lipids (e.g., cholesterol) in the blood
Ginkgo *GING-kō*	Leaf	Improves blood circulation in and function of the brain; improves memory; used to treat dementia; antianxiety agent; protects the nervous system
Ginseng *JIN-seng*	Root	Stress reduction; lowers blood cholesterol and blood sugar

(continued)

Box 8-4   For Your Reference *(Continued)*

Therapeutic Uses of Herbal Medicines

NAME	PART USED	THERAPEUTIC USES
Green tea	Leaf	Antioxidant; acts against cancer of the gastrointestinal tract and skin; oral antimicrobial agent; reduces dental caries
Kava *KA-va*	Root	Antianxiety agent; sedative
Milk thistle *thisl*	Seeds	Protects the liver against toxins; antioxidant
Saw palmetto *pal-MET-ō*	Berries	Used to treat benign prostatic hyperplasia (BPH)
Slippery elm	Bark	As lozenge for throat irritation; for gastrointestinal irritation and upset; protects irritated skin
Soy	Bean	Rich source of nutrients; protective estrogenic effects in menopausal symptoms, osteoporosis, cardiovascular disease, cancer prevention
St. John's wort	Flower	Treatment of anxiety and depression; antibacterial and antiviral properties (Note: this product can interact with a variety of drugs)
Tea tree oil	Leaf	Antimicrobial; used to heal cuts, skin infections, burns
Valerian *va-LĒ-rē-an*	Root	Sedative; sleep aid

Box 8-5   For Your Reference

Routes of Drug Administration

ROUTE	DESCRIPTION
BY ABSORPTION	
Absorption *ab-SORP-shun*	Drug taken into the circulation through the digestive tract or by transfer across another membrane
Inhalation *in-ha-LĀ-shun*	Administration through the respiratory system, as by breathing in an aerosol or nebulizer spray
Instillation *in-stil-LĀ-shun*	Liquid is dropped or poured slowly into a body cavity or on the surface of the body, such as into the ear or onto the conjunctiva of the eye (Fig. 8-1)
Oral *OR-al*	Given by mouth; per os (po)
Rectal *REK-tal*	Administered by rectal suppository or enema
Sublingual (SL) *sub-LING-gwal*	Administered under the tongue
Topical *TOP-i-kal*	Applied to the surface of the skin
Transdermal *trans-DER-mal*	Absorbed through the skin, as from a patch placed on the surface of the skin

Box 8-5   **For Your Reference** *(Continued)*

Routes of Drug Administration

ROUTE	DESCRIPTION
BY INJECTION	
Injection (Fig. 8-2) *in-JEK-shun*	Administered by a needle and syringe (Fig. 8-3); described as parenteral (*pa-REN-ter-al*) routes of administration
Epidural *ep-i-DUR-al*	Injected into the space between the meninges (membranes around the spinal cord) and the spine
Hypodermoclysis *hī-pō-der-MOK-li-sis*	Administration of a solution by subcutaneous infusion. Useful for fluid delivery as an alternative for intravenous infusion
Intradermal (ID) *in-tra-DER-mal*	Injected into the skin
Intramuscular (IM) *in-tra-MUS-kū-lar*	Injected into a muscle
Intravenous (IV) *in-tra-VĒ-nus*	Injected into a vein
Spinal (intrathecal) *in-tra-THĒ-kal*	Injected through the meninges into the spinal fluid
Subcutaneous (SC) *sub-kū-TĀ-nē-us*	Injected beneath the skin; hypodermic

Figure 8-1 **Instillation of a drug.** A practitioner pulls down the lower lid to administer eye drops into the lower conjunctival sac.

Figure 8-2 **Injection.** Comparison of the angles of insertion for intramuscular, subcutaneous, and intradermal injections.

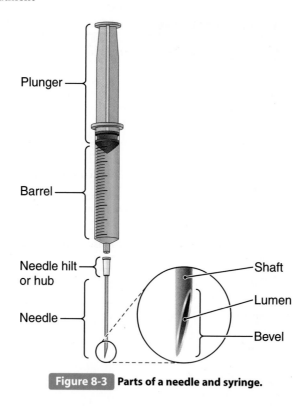

Figure 8-3 Parts of a needle and syringe.

Box 8-6   For Your Reference

Drug Preparations

FORM	DESCRIPTION
LIQUID	
Aerosol *AR-o-sol*	Solution dispersed as a mist to be inhaled
Aqueous solution *AK-wē-us*	Substance dissolved in water
Elixir (elix) *ē-LIK-sar*	A clear, pleasantly flavored and sweetened hydroalcoholic liquid intended for oral use
Emulsion *ē-MUL-shun*	A mixture in which one liquid is dispersed but not dissolved in another liquid
Lotion *LŌ-shun*	Solution prepared for topical use
Suspension (susp) *sus-PEN-shun*	Fine particles dispersed in a liquid; must be shaken before use
Tincture (tinct) *TINK-chur*	Substance dissolved in an alcoholic solution
SEMISOLID	
Cream *krēm*	A semisolid emulsion used topically
Ointment (ung) *OYNT-ment*	Drug in a base that keeps it in contact with the skin

Box 8-6   For Your Reference *(Continued)*

Drug Preparations

FORM	DESCRIPTION
SOLID	
Capsule (cap) KAP-sŭl	Material in a gelatin container that dissolves easily in the stomach
Lozenge LOZ-enj	A pleasant-tasting medicated tablet or disk to be dissolved in the mouth, such as a cough drop
Suppository (supp) su-POZ-i-tor-ē	Substance mixed and molded with a base that melts easily when inserted into a body opening
Tablet (tab) TAB-let	A solid dosage form containing a drug in a pure state or mixed with a nonactive ingredient and prepared by compression or molding; also called a pill

Box 8-7   For Your Reference

Terms Pertaining to Injectable Drugs

TERM	MEANING
Ampule AM-pŭl	A small sealed glass or plastic container used for sterile intravenous solutions (Fig. 8-4)
Bolus BŌ-lus	A concentrated amount of a diagnostic or therapeutic substance given rapidly intravenously
Catheter KATH-e-ter	A thin tube that can be passed into a body cavity, organ, or vessel (Fig. 8-5)
Syringe sir-INJ	An instrument for injecting fluid (see Figs. 8-3 and 8-4)
Vial VĪ-al	A small glass or plastic container (see Fig. 8-4)

Figure 8-4 **Injectable drug containers.** An ampule (*top left*), a vial (*top right*), and a syringe (*bottom*) are shown.

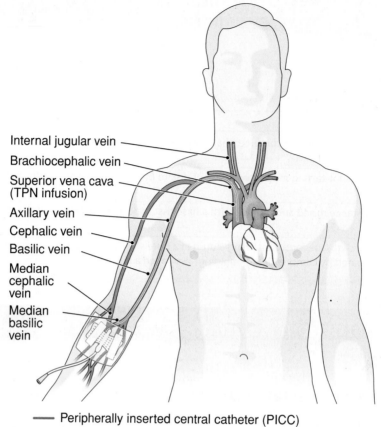

Internal jugular vein
Brachiocephalic vein
Superior vena cava
(TPN infusion)
Axillary vein
Cephalic vein
Basilic vein
Median
cephalic
vein
Median
basilic
vein

—— Peripherally inserted central catheter (PICC)

Figure 8-5 **Catheter.** Shown is placement of a peripherally inserted central catheter (PICC).

Chapter Review

Match the following terms and write the appropriate letter to the left of each number:

_____ **1.** potentiation
_____ **2.** antiemetic
_____ **3.** countercurrent
_____ **4.** hyperpyrexia
_____ **5.** diuretic

a. promoting excretion of water
b. flowing in an opposite direction
c. agent that prevents vomiting
d. combined drug action to greater effect
e. abnormally high body temperature

_____ **6.** efficacy
_____ **7.** adrenergic
_____ **8.** vasomotor
_____ **9.** chronotropic
_____ **10.** anaphylaxis

a. sympathomimetic
b. affecting timing
c. extreme allergic reaction
d. effectiveness
e. pertaining to vessel movement

_____ **11.** po
_____ **12.** ad lib
_____ **13.** aq
_____ **14.** s̄
_____ **15.** tid

a. without
b. as desired
c. by mouth
d. three times a day
e. water

_____ **16.** green tea	**a.** antimicrobial
_____ **17.** aloe	**b.** source of fatty acids
_____ **18.** valerian	**c.** used to treat burns, irritation
_____ **19.** tea tree oil	**d.** antioxidant
_____ **20.** flax seed	**e.** sedative

Multiple Choice > Select the best answer and write the letter of your choice to the left of each number:

_____ **21.** Another term for brand name is:
  a. indicated name
  b. generic name
  c. prescription name
  d. chemical name
  e. trade name

_____ **22.** A drug that is administered topically is:
  a. swallowed
  b. injected
  c. applied to the skin
  d. placed under the tongue
  e. inserted with a catheter

_____ **23.** Drug administration by injection is described as:
  a. partial
  b. instilled
  c. encapsulated
  d. nebulized
  e. parenteral

_____ **24.** An ampule is a(n):
  a. concentrated amount given rapidly
  b. mist to be inhaled
  c. tablet to dissolve in the mouth
  d. small sealed container
  e. alcoholic solution

_____ **25.** A hypolipidemic drug
  a. lowers cholesterol
  b. increases urination
  c. fights infection
  d. reduces inflammation
  e. diminishes sensation

_____ **26.** Another term for *hypodermic* is:
  a. intrathecal
  b. spinal
  c. epidural
  d. subcutaneous
  e. aqueous

_____ **27.** NSAIDs are used to treat:
  a. inflammation
  b. convulsions
  c. nausea
  d. hypertension
  e. diabetes

_____ **28.** Proton pump inhibitors
   a. relieve depression
   b. relax muscle spasms
   c. are used to treat asthma
   d. are used to administer drugs
   e. reduce stomach acidity

Fill in the blanks:

29. An analgesic is used to treat _____.

30. An intravenous injection is given into a(n) _____.

31. When a drug has lost its effect at a constant dose, the patient has developed _____.

32. Phytomedicine is the practice of treating with _____.

33. A transdermal route of administration is through the _____.

34. A toxicologist is one who studies _____.

35. The study of drugs and their actions is called _____.

36. An antipyretic drug counteracts _____.

Eliminations > In each of the sets below, underline the word that does not fit in with the rest and explain the reason for your choice:

37. antitussive — histamine H$_2$ antagonist — expectorant — mucolytic — bronchodilator

_____

38. solution — elixir — tincture — emulsion — tablet

_____

39. antineoplastics — nitrates — antiarrhythmics — calcium-channel blockers — beta-blockers

_____

40. anesthetic — analgesic — narcotic — adrenergic — sedative

_____

Define each of the following words:

41. bronchodilation _____

42. sublingual _____

43. anxiolytic _____

44. psychotropic _____

Opposites > Write a word that means the opposite of each of the following:

45. convulsant _____

46. vasoconstriction _____

47. balance _____

48. toxin _____

49. indicated _____

50. coagulant _____

Chapter Review *(continued)*

Define each of the following abbreviations:

51. prn _____

52. USP _____

53. IU _____

54. Rx _____

55. mg _____

56. NSAIDs _____

57. FDA _____

58. D/C _____

Word Building > Write a word for each of the following definitions using the word parts given.

narc/o   -lytic   thromb/o   muc/o   toxic/o   -sis   anxi/o   hypn/o

59. an induced sleep-like state _____

60. reducing anxiety _____

61. condition caused by poisoning _____

62. dissolving a blood clot _____

63. condition of having a blood clot _____

64. a state of stupor _____

65. dissolving mucus _____

Word Analysis > Define each of the following words, and give the meaning of the word parts in each. Use a dictionary if necessary.

66. hypodermoclysis (*hī-pō-der-MOK-li-sis*) _____

    a. hypo- _____

    b. derm/o _____

    c. clysis _____

67. adrenergic (*ad-ren-ER-jik*) _____

    a. adren/o _____

    b. erg/o _____

    c. -ic _____

68. pharmacokinetic (*far-ma-kō-ki-NET-ik*) _____

    a. pharmac/o _____

    b. kinet/o _____

    c. -ic _____

 PASSport to Success®   Go to the word exercises on the Student Resources for additional review exercises.

Case Studies

➤ Case Study 8-1: Cardiac Disease and Crisis

P.L., who has a 4-year history of heart disease, was brought to the emergency room by ambulance with chest pain that radiated down her arm, dyspnea, and syncope. Her routine meds included Lanoxin to slow and strengthen her heart beat, Inderal to support her heart rhythm, Lipitor to decrease her cholesterol, Catapres to lower her hypertension, nitroglycerin prn for chest pain, HydroDIURIL to eliminate fluid and decrease the workload of her heart, Diabinese for her diabetes, and Coumadin to prevent blood clots. She also took Tagamet for her stomach ulcer and several OTC preparations, including a herbal sleeping potion that she mixed in tea, and Metamucil mixed in orange juice every morning for her bowels. Shortly after admission, P.L.'s heart rate deteriorated into full cardiac arrest. Immediate resuscitation was instituted with cardiopulmonary resuscitation (CPR), defibrillation, and a bolus of IV epinephrine. Between shocks she was given a bolus of lidocaine and a bolus of diltiazem plus repeated doses of epinephrine every 5 minutes. P.L. did not respond to resuscitation. On the death certificate, her primary cause of death was listed as cardiac arrest. Multiple secondary diagnoses were listed, including polypharmacy.

➤ Case Study 8-2: Inflammatory Bowel Disease

A.E., a 19-year-old college student, was diagnosed at the age of 13 with Crohn disease, a chronic inflammatory disease that can affect the entire gastrointestinal tract from mouth to anus. A.E.'s disease is limited to his large bowel. During a 9-month period of disease exacerbation, characterized by severe cramping and bloody stools, he took oral corticosteroids (prednisone) to reduce the inflammatory response. He experienced many of the drug's side effects, but has been in remission for 4 years. Currently, A.E.'s condition is managed on drugs that reduce inflammation by suppressing the immune response. He takes Pentasa (mesalamine) 250 mg 4 caps po bid. Pentasa is of the 5-ASA (acetylsalicylic acid or aspirin) group of antiinflammatory agents, which work topically on the inner surface of the bowel. It has an enteric coating, which dissolves in the bowel environment. He also takes 6-mercaptopurine (Purinethol) 75 mg po daily and a therapeutic vitamin with breakfast. A.E. may take acetaminophen for pain but must avoid NSAIDs, which will irritate the intestinal mucosa (inner lining) and cause a flare-up of the disease.

➤ Case Study 8-3: Asthma

E.N., a 20-year-old woman with asthma, visited the preadmission testing unit 1 week before her cosmetic surgery to meet with the nurse and anesthesiologist. Her current meds included several bronchodilators, which she takes by mouth and by inhalation, and a tranquilizer that she takes when needed for nervousness. She sometimes receives inhalation treatments with Mucomyst, a mucolytic agent. On E.N.'s preoperative note, the nurse wrote:

> Theo-Dur 1 cap tid
> Flovent inhaler 1 spray (50 mcg each nostril bid)
> Ativan (lorazepam) 1 mg po bid
> Albuterol-metered dose inhaler 2 puffs (180 mcg) prn q4–6h for bronchospasm and before exercise

E.N. stated that she has difficulty with her asthma when she is anxious and when she exercises. She also admitted to occasional use of marijuana and ecstasy, a hallucinogen and mood-altering illegal recreational drug. The anesthesiologist wrote an order for lorazepam 4 mg IV 1 hour preop. The plastic surgeon recommended several herbal products to complement her surgery and her recovery. He ordered a high-potency vitamin 3 tabs with breakfast and dinner to support tissue health and healing. He also prescribed Bromelain, an enzyme from pineapple, to decrease inflammation, 1 po qid 3 days before surgery and postoperatively for 2 weeks. Arnica Montana was prescribed to decrease discomfort, swelling, and bruising; 3 tabs sublingual tid the evening after surgery and for the following 10 days.

CASE STUDY QUESTIONS

Multiple choice. Select the best answer and write the letter of your choice to the left of each number:

_____ 1. P.L.'s nitroglycerine is ordered: prn SL. This means:
    a. as needed, under the tongue
    b. at bedtime, under the tongue
    c. as needed, on the skin
    d. by mouth, on the skin
    e. by mouth, under the skin

_____ 2. P.L. took several OTC preparations. OTC means:
    a. on the cutaneous
    b. off the cuff
    c. over the counter
    d. do not need a prescription
    e. c and d

_____ 3. P.L.'s herbal sleeping potion was mixed into tea and taken at bedtime. The dissolved mixture is called a(n) _____ and is taken at _____.
    a. elixir/QAM
    b. emulsion/bid
    c. suspension/hs
    d. aqueous solution/hs
    e. aqueous solution/QAM

_____ 4. During P.L.'s resuscitation, epinephrine was given in an IV bolus. This means it was administered:
    a. intrathecally in a continuous drip
    b. parenterally in a topical solution
    c. intravenously in a continuous drip
    d. intravenously in a rapid concentrated dose
    e. intrathecally in a rapid concentrated dose

(continued)

Case Studies *(continued)*

_____ 5. P.L. had a secondary diagnosis of polypharmacy. This means that she:
   a. used more than one drug store
   b. had polyps
   c. used more prescription than OTC drugs
   d. had a toxic dose
   e. used many different drugs

_____ 6. A.E. takes several drugs to prevent or act against his inflammatory response. These agents are described as
   a. contrainflammatory
   b. counterinflammatory
   c. antiinflammatory
   d. proinflammatory
   e. hypoinflammatory

_____ 7. A.E. presented with several untoward results or risks from the corticosteroid therapy. These sequelae are called:
   a. contraindications
   b. side effects
   c. antagonistic effects
   d. exacerbations
   e. synergy states

_____ 8. A.E. takes four 250-mg capsules of Pentasa po bid. How many capsules does he take in 1 day?
   a. 2000
   b. 1000
   c. 4
   d. 8
   e. 12

_____ 9. A.E. must avoid NSAIDs because, in cases of inflammatory bowel disease, these drugs are
   a. contraindicated
   b. indicated
   c. complementary
   d. synergistic
   e. prescriptive

_____ 10. E.N. used a mucolytic drug when needed. This drug's action is to:
   a. increase secretions
   b. decrease spasm
   c. calm anxiety
   d. decrease mucus secretions
   e. simulate mucus

_____ 11. E.N.'s Flovent inhaler is indicated as 1 spray of 50 mcg in each nostril bid. How many micrograms (mcg) does she get in 1 day?
   a. 100 mcg
   b. 200 mcg
   c. 250 mcg
   d. 500 mcg
   e. 5000 mcg

_____ 12. The Ativan that E.N. takes for nervousness is a(n) _____ drug.
   a. anxiolytic
   b. potentiating
   c. antiemetic
   d. analgesic
   e. bronchodilator

_____ 13. The anesthesiologist ordered lorazepam (Ativan) to be given IV preop to decrease anxiety and to smooth E.N.'s anesthesia induction. The complementary way that lorazepam and anesthesia work together is called:
   a. antagonistic
   b. complementary medicine
   c. parasympathomimetic
   d. tolerance
   e. synergy

_____ 14. Bromelain and Arnica Montana are herbal products that can be described as all of the following except:
   a. phytopharmaceutical
   b. alternative
   c. herbal
   d. complementary
   e. chronotropic

_____ 15. Arnica Montana was prescribed 3 tabs SL tid. How many tabs would E.N. take in 1 day?
   a. 6
   b. 9
   c. 12
   d. 21
   e. 33

_____ 16. Flovent is administered as an inhalant. The form in which the drug is prepared is called a(n):
   a. emulsion
   b. elixir
   c. aerosol
   d. suspension
   e. unguent

PART III

Body Systems

CHAPTER 9

Circulation: The Cardiovascular and Lymphatic Systems

CHAPTER CONTENTS

OBJECTIVES

After study of this chapter you should be able to:

1. Label a diagram of the heart.
2. Trace the path of blood flow through the heart.
3. Trace the path of electrical conduction through the heart.
4. Identify the components of an electrocardiogram.
5. Differentiate among arteries, arterioles, capillaries, venules, and veins.
6. Explain blood pressure and describe how blood pressure is measured.
7. Identify and use the roots pertaining to the cardiovascular and lymphatic systems.
8. Describe the main disorders that affect the cardiovascular and lymphatic systems.
9. Define medical terms pertaining to the cardiovascular and lymphatic systems.
10. List the functions and components of the lymphatic system.
11. Interpret medical abbreviations referring to circulation.
12. Analyze case studies involving circulation.

Multiple choice. Select the best answer and write the letter of your choice to the left of each number.

___ 1. The cardiovascular system includes the heart and:

    a. lungs   c. digestive organs
    b. blood vessels   d. endocrine system

___ 2. The thick, muscular layer of the heart wall is the:

    a. endocardium   c. myocardium
    b. valve   d. apex

___ 3. The lower chambers of the heart are the:

    a. ventricles   c. base
    b. atria   d. systole

___ 4. A vessel that carries blood away from the heart is a(n):

    a. vein   c. lymph node
    b. chamber   d. artery

___ 5. The tonsils, spleen, thymus, and nodes are part of the:

    a. digestive   c. epicardium
       system   d. lymphatic
    b. endocrine   system
       system

___ 6. Study of the heart's electrical activity is:

    a. electrocardiography
    b. electromyography
    c. fluoroscopy
    d. electroencephalography

___ 7. The medical term for a "heart attack" is:

    a. myocardial   c. aneurysm
       infarction   d. pneumonia
    b. cerebrovascular
       accident

___ 8. Any abnormality in the heart's rhythm is called:

    a. monorrhythmia c. arrhythmia
    b. embolism   d. dysphagia

___ 9. The accumulation of fatty deposits in the lining of a vessel is called:

    a. obesity   c. stent
    b. atherosclerosis d. angiogenesis

___ 10. Phlebitis is inflammation of a:

    a. blood cell   c. heart
    b. vein   d. nerve

9

Blood circulates throughout the body in the **cardiovascular system**, which consists of the **heart** and the blood vessels (Fig. 9-1). This system forms a continuous circuit that delivers oxygen and nutrients to all cells and carries away waste products. The **lymphatic system** also functions in circulation. Its **vessels** drain fluid and proteins left in the tissues and return them to the bloodstream. The lymphatic system plays a part in immunity and in the digestive process as well, as explained in Chapters 10 and 12. This chapter discusses the circulatory system in detail, in both its normal and clinical aspects, and then proceeds to study of the lymphatic system.

The Heart

The **heart** is located between the lungs, with its point or **apex** directed toward the inferior and left (Fig. 9-2). The wall of the heart consists of three layers, all named with the root *cardi*, meaning "heart." Moving from the innermost to the outermost layer, these are the:

1. **Endocardium**—a thin membrane that lines the chambers and **valves** (the prefix *endo-* means "within")

2. **Myocardium**—the thick muscle layer that makes up most of the heart wall (the root *my/o* means "muscle")

3. **Epicardium**—a thin membrane that covers the heart (the prefix *epi-* means "on")

A fibrous sac, the **pericardium**, contains the heart and anchors it to surrounding structures, such as the sternum (breastbone) and diaphragm (the prefix *peri-* means "around").

Each of the heart's upper receiving chambers is an **atrium** (plural: atria). Each of the lower pumping chambers is a **ventricle** (plural: ventricles). The chambers of the heart are divided by walls, each of which is called a **septum**. The interventricular septum separates the two ventricles; the interatrial septum divides the two atria. There is also a septum between the atrium and ventricle on each side.

The heart pumps blood through two circuits. The right side pumps blood to the lungs to be oxygenated through the **pulmonary circuit**. The left side pumps to the remainder of the body through the **systemic circuit** (see Fig. 9-1).

PASSport to Success® See the Student Resources for the animation *Blood Circulation.*

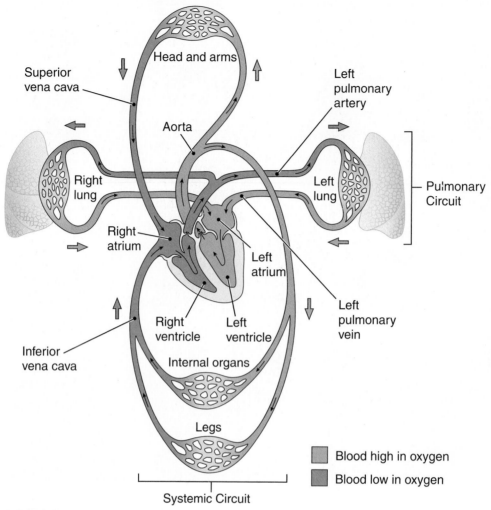

Right lung

Right atrium

Right ventricle

Inferior vena cava

Superior vena cava

Head and arms

Aorta

Left atrium

Left ventricle

Internal organs

Legs

Left pulmonary artery

Left lung

Pulmonary Circuit

Left pulmonary vein

Blood high in oxygen

Blood low in oxygen

Systemic Circuit

Figure 9-1 **The cardiovascular system.** The pulmonary circuit carries blood to and from the lungs; the systemic circuit carries blood to and from all other parts of the body.

Blood Flow through the Heart

The pathway of blood through the heart is shown by the arrows in Figure 9-2. The sequence is as follows:

1. The right atrium receives blood low in oxygen, or deoxygenated, from all body tissues through the **superior vena cava** and the **inferior vena cava.**

2. The blood then enters the right ventricle and is pumped to the lungs through the **pulmonary artery.**

3. Blood returns from the lungs high in oxygen, or oxygenated, and enters the left atrium through the **pulmonary veins.**

4. Blood enters the left ventricle and is forcefully pumped into the **aorta** to be distributed to all tissues.

One-way **valves** in the heart keep blood moving in a forward direction. The valves between the atrium and ventricle on each side are the **atrioventricular (AV) valves** (see Fig. 9-2). The valve between the right atrium and

ventricle is the **right AV valve**, also known as the tricuspid valve because it has three cusps (flaps). The valve between the left atrium and ventricle is the **left AV valve**, which is a bicuspid valve with two cusps; it is often called the **mitral valve** (so named because it resembles a bishop's miter).

The valves leading into the pulmonary artery and the aorta have three cusps. Each cusp is shaped like a half-moon, so these valves are described as *semilunar valves.* The valve at the entrance to the pulmonary artery is specifically named the **pulmonary valve**; the valve at the entrance to the aorta is the **aortic valve.**

See the Student Resources for the animation *Cardiac Cycle.*

Heart sounds are produced as the heart functions. The loudest of these, the familiar lub and dup that can be

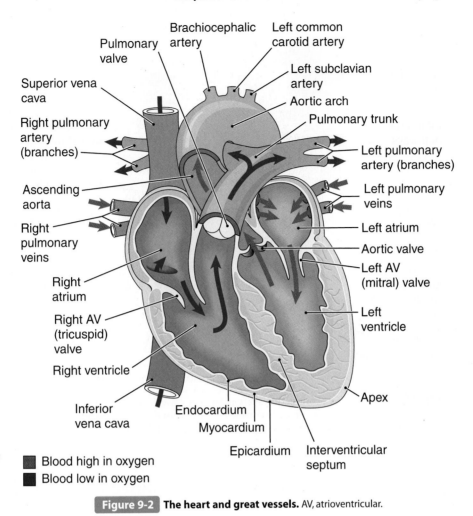

Pulmonary valve
Brachiocephalic artery
Left common carotid artery
Superior vena cava
Left subclavian artery
Aortic arch
Right pulmonary artery (branches)
Pulmonary trunk
Ascending aorta
Left pulmonary artery (branches)
Right pulmonary veins
Left pulmonary veins
Left atrium
Aortic valve
Right atrium
Left AV (mitral) valve
Right AV (tricuspid) valve
Left ventricle
Right ventricle
Apex
Inferior vena cava
Endocardium
Myocardium
Epicardium
Interventricular septum

Blood high in oxygen
Blood low in oxygen

Figure 9-2 **The heart and great vessels.** AV, atrioventricular.

heard through the chest wall, are produced by alternate closing of the valves. The first heart sound (S_1) is heard when the valves between the chambers close. The second heart sound (S_2) is produced when the valves leading into the aorta and pulmonary artery close. Any sound made as the heart functions normally is termed a **functional murmur**. (The word *murmur* used alone with regard to the heart describes an abnormal sound.)

The Heartbeat

Each contraction of the heart, termed **systole** (*SIS-tō-lē*), is followed by a relaxation phase, **diastole** (*dī-AS-tō-lē*), during which the chambers fill. Each time the heart beats, both atria contract and immediately thereafter both ventricles contract. The number of times the heart contracts per minute is the **heart rate**. The wave of increased pressure produced in the vessels each time the ventricles contract is the **pulse**. Pulse rate is usually counted by palpating a peripheral artery, such as the radial artery at the wrist or the carotid artery in the neck (see Fig. 7-4).

Cardiac contractions are stimulated by a built-in system that regularly transmits electrical impulses through the heart. The components of this conduction system are shown in Figure 9-3. In the sequence of action they include the:

1. **Sinoatrial (SA) node**, located in the upper right atrium and called the pacemaker because it sets the rate of the heartbeat.
2. **Atrioventricular (AV) node**, located at the bottom of the right atrium near the ventricle. Internodal fibers between the SA and AV node carry stimulation throughout both atria.
3. **AV bundle** (bundle of His) at the top of the interventricular septum.
4. Left and right **bundle branches**, which travel along the left and right sides of the septum.
5. **Purkinje** (*pur-KIN-jē*) **fibers**, which carry stimulation throughout the walls of the ventricles. (See information on naming in Box 9-1.)

Although the heart itself generates the heartbeat, factors such as nervous system stimulation, hormones, and drugs can influence the rate and the force of contractions.

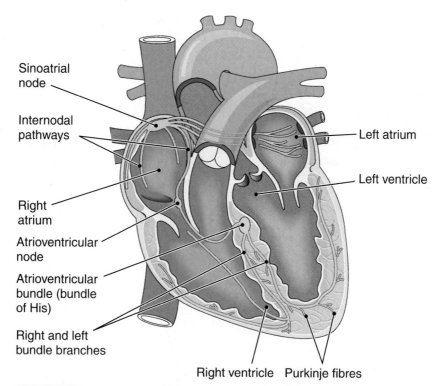

Sinoatrial node

Internodal pathways

Right atrium

Atrioventricular node

Atrioventricular bundle (bundle of His)

Right and left bundle branches

Left atrium

Left ventricle

Right ventricle   Purkinje fibres

Figure 9-3 **The heart's conduction system.** Impulses travel from the sinoatrial (SA) node to the atrioventricular (AV) node, then to the atrioventricular bundle, bundle branches, and Purkinje fibers. Internodal pathways carry impulses throughout the atria.

Box 9-1   Focus on Words

Name That Structure

An eponym (*EP-o-nim*) is a name that is based on the name of a person, usually the one who discovered a particular structure, disease, principle, or procedure. Everyday examples are graham cracker, Ferris wheel, and boycott. In the heart, the bundle of His and Purkinje fibers are part of that organ's conduction system. Korotkoff sounds are heard in the vessels when taking blood pressure. Cardiovascular disorders named for people include the tetralogy of Fallot, a combination of four congenital heart defects; Raynaud disease of small vessels; and the cardiac arrhythmia known as Wolff–Parkinson–White syndrome. In treatment, Doppler echocardiography is named for a physicist of the 19th century. The Holter monitor and the Swan–Ganz catheter give honor to their developers.

In other systems, the islets of Langerhans are cell clusters in the pancreas that secrete insulin. The graafian follicle in the ovary surrounds the developing egg cell. The eustachian tube connects the middle ear to the throat.

Many disease names are eponymic: Parkinson and Alzheimer, which affect the brain; Graves, a disorder of the thyroid; Addison and Cushing, involving the adrenal cortex; and Down syndrome, a hereditary disorder. The genus and species names of microorganisms often are based on the names of their discoverers, *Escherichia*, *Salmonella*, *Pasteurella*, and *Rickettsia* to name a few.

Many reagents, instruments, and procedures are named for their developers. The original name for a radiograph was roentgenograph (*RENT-jen-ō-graf*), named for Wilhelm Roentgen, discoverer of x-rays. A curie is a measure of radiation, derived from the name of Marie Curie, a codiscoverer of radioactivity.

Although eponyms give honor to physicians and scientists of the past, they do not convey any information and may be more difficult to learn. There is a trend to replace these names with more descriptive ones; for example, auditory tube instead of eustachian tube, ovarian follicle for graafian follicle, pancreatic islets for islets of Langerhans, and trisomy 21 for Down syndrome.

B

Electrocardiography (ECG). (*A*) ECG tracing showing a normal sinus rhythm. (*B*) Components of a normal ECG tracing. Shown are the P, QRS, T, and U waves, which represent electrical activity in different parts of the heart. Intervals measure from one wave to the next; segments are smaller components of the tracing.

ELECTROCARDIOGRAPHY

Electrocardiography (ECG) measures the heart's electrical activity as it functions (Fig. 9-4). Electrodes (leads) placed on the body's surface detect the electrical signals, which are then amplified and recorded as a tracing. A normal, or **sinus rhythm**, which originates at the SA node, is shown in Figure 9-4A. Figure 9-4B shows the letters assigned to individual components of one complete cycle:

1. The P wave represents electrical change, or **depolarization**, of the atrial muscles.

2. The QRS component shows depolarization of the ventricles.

3. The T wave shows return, or **repolarization**, of the ventricles to their resting state. Atrial repolarization is hidden by the QRS wave.

4. The small U wave, if present, follows the T wave. It is of uncertain origin.

An *interval* measures the distance from one wave to the next; a *segment* is a smaller component of the tracing. Many heart disorders, some of which are described later in the chapter, appear as abnormalities in ECG components.

The Vascular System

The vascular system consists of:

1. **Arteries** that carry blood away from the heart (Fig. 9-5).

2. **Arterioles**, vessels smaller than arteries that lead into the capillaries.

3. **Capillaries**, the smallest vessels, through which exchanges take place between the blood and the tissues.

4. **Venules**, small vessels that receive blood from the capillaries and drain into the veins.

5. **Veins** that carry blood back to the heart (Fig. 9-6).

All arteries, except the pulmonary artery (and the umbilical artery in the fetus), carry oxygenated blood. They are thick-walled, elastic vessels that carry blood under high pressure. All veins, except the pulmonary vein (and the umbilical vein in the fetus), carry deoxygenated blood. Veins have thinner, less elastic walls and tend to give way under pressure. Like the heart, veins have one-way valves that keep blood flowing forward.

Principal systemic arteries.

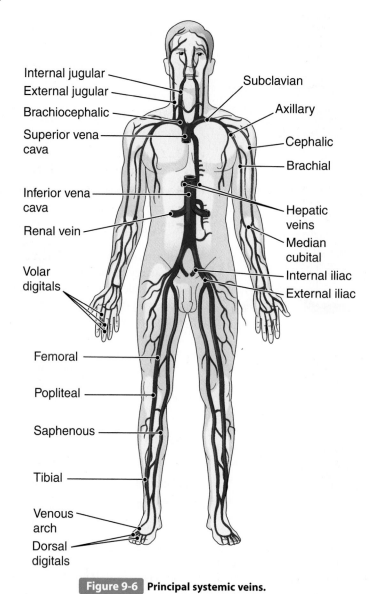

Figure 9-6 **Principal systemic veins.**

Nervous system stimulation can cause the diameter of a vessel to increase (vasodilation) or decrease (vasoconstriction). These changes alter blood flow to the tissues and affect blood pressure.

Blood Pressure

Blood pressure (BP) is the force exerted by blood against the wall of a blood vessel. It falls as the blood travels away from the heart and is influenced by a variety of factors, including cardiac output, vessel diameters, and total blood volume. Vasoconstriction increases blood pressure in a vessel; vasodilation decreases pressure.

Blood pressure is commonly measured in a large artery with an inflatable cuff (Fig. 9-7) known as a blood pressure cuff or blood pressure apparatus, but

Figure 9-7 **Blood pressure cuff (sphygmomanometer).**
Shown are the cuff, the bulb for inflating the cuff, and the manometer for measuring pressure.

Box 9-2   Clinical Perspectives

Cardiac Catheterization: Measuring Blood Pressure from Within

Because arterial blood pressure decreases as blood flows further away from the heart, measurement of blood pressure with a simple inflatable cuff around the arm is only a reflection of the pressure in the heart and pulmonary arteries. Precise measurement of pressure in these parts of the cardiovascular system is useful in diagnosing certain cardiac and pulmonary disorders.

More accurate readings can be obtained using a catheter (thin tube) inserted directly into the heart and large vessels. One type commonly used is the pulmonary artery catheter (also known as the Swan–Ganz catheter), which has an inflatable balloon at the tip. This device is threaded into the right side of the heart through a large vein. Typically, the right internal jugular vein is used because it is the shortest and most direct route to the heart, but the subclavian and femoral veins may also be used. The catheter's position in the heart is confirmed by a chest x-ray and, when appropriately positioned, the atrial and ventricular blood pressures are recorded. As the catheter continues into the pulmonary artery, pressure in this vessel can be read. When the balloon is inflated, the catheter becomes wedged in a branch of the pulmonary artery, blocking blood flow. The reading obtained is called the **pulmonary capillary wedge (PCW) pressure.** It gives information on pressure in the heart's left side and on resistance in the lungs. Combined with other tests, cardiac catheterization can be used to diagnose cardiac and pulmonary disorders such as shock, pericarditis, congenital heart disease, and heart failure.

technically called a **sphygmomanometer.** The examiner inflates the cuff to stop blood flow in a vessel. He or she then uses a stethoscope to listen for blood flow in the vessel as the pressure is slowly released (see Fig. 7-5). The blood pressure reading includes both systolic pressure, measured while the heart is contracting, and diastolic pressure, measured when the heart relaxes. These are reported as systolic then diastolic separated by a slash, such as 120/80. Pressure is expressed as millimeters of mercury (mm Hg)—that is, the height to which the pressure can push a column of mercury in a tube. Blood pressure is a valuable diagnostic measurement that is easily obtained. (See Box 9-2 for more information on blood pressure measurement.)

Terminology   Key Terms

CARDIOVASCULAR SYSTEM

Normal Structure and Function

aorta ā-OR-ta	The largest artery. It receives blood from the left ventricle and branches to all parts of the body (root: *aort/o*)
aortic valve ā-OR-tik	The valve at the entrance to the aorta
apex Ā-peks	The point of a cone-shaped structure (adjective: apical). The apex of the heart is formed by the left ventricle and is pointed toward the inferior and left
artery AR-te-rē	A vessel that carries blood away from the heart. All except the pulmonary and umbilical arteries carry oxygenated blood (roots: *arter, arteri/o*)
arteriole ar-TĒ-rē-ōl	A small vessel that carries blood from the arteries into the capillaries (root: *arteriol/o*)
atrioventricular (AV) node ā-trē-ō-ven-TRIK-ū-lar	A small mass in the lower septum of the right atrium that passes impulses from the sinoatrial (SA) node toward the ventricles
AV bundle	A band of fibers that transmits impulses from the atrioventricular (AV) node to the top of the interventricular septum. It divides into the right and left bundle branches, which descend along the two sides of the septum; the bundle of His
atrioventricular (AV) valve	A valve between the atrium and ventricle on the right and left sides of the heart. The right AV valve is the tricuspid valve; the left is the mitral valve

(continued)

Terminology | Key Terms *(continued)*

atrium Ā-trē-um	An entrance chamber, one of the two upper receiving chambers of the heart (root: *atri/o*)
blood pressure	The force exerted by blood against the wall of a vessel
bundle branches	Branches of the AV bundle that divide to the right and left sides of the interventricular septum
capillary KAP-i-lar-ē	A microscopic blood vessel through which materials are exchanged between the blood and the tissues
cardiovascular system kar-dē-ō-VAS-kū-lar	The part of the circulatory system that consists of the heart and the blood vessels
depolarization dē-pō-lar-i-ZĀ-shun	A change in electrical charge from the resting state in nerves or muscles
diastole dī-AS-tō-lē	The relaxation phase of the heartbeat cycle; adjective: diastolic
electrocardiography (ECG) ē-lek-trō-kar-dē-OG-ra-fē	Study of the electrical activity of the heart as detected by electrodes (leads) placed on the surface of the body. Also abbreviated EKG from the German *electrokardiography*
endocardium en-dō-KAR-dē-um	The thin membrane that lines the chambers of the heart and covers the valves
epicardium ep-i-KAR-dē-um	The thin outermost layer of the heart wall
functional murmur	Any sound produced as the heart functions normally
heart hart	The muscular organ with four chambers that contracts rhythmically to propel blood through vessels to all parts of the body (root: *cardi/o*)
heart rate	The number of times the heart contracts per minute; recorded as beats per minute (bpm)
heart sounds	Sounds produced as the heart functions. The two loudest sounds are produced by alternate closing of the valves and are designated S_1 and S_2
inferior vena cava VĒ-na KĀ-va	The large inferior vein that brings blood back to the right atrium of the heart from the lower body
left AV valve	The valve between the left atrium and the left ventricle; the mitral valve or bicuspid valve
mitral valve MĪ-tral	The valve between the left atrium and the left ventricle; the left AV valve or bicuspid valve
myocardium mī-ō-KAR-dē-um	The thick middle layer of the heart wall composed of cardiac muscle
pericardium per-i-KAR-dē-um	The fibrous sac that surrounds the heart
pulmonary artery PUL-mō-nār-ē	The vessel that carries blood from the right side of the heart to the lungs
pulmonary circuit SER-kit	The system of vessels that carries blood from the right side of the heart to the lungs to be oxygenated and then back to the left side of the heart
pulmonary veins	The vessels that carry blood from the lungs to the left side of the heart
pulmonary valve PUL-mō-nār-ē	The valve at the entrance to the pulmonary artery
pulse puls	The wave of increased pressure produced in the vessels each time the ventricles contract
Purkinje fibers pur-KIN-jē	The terminal fibers of the cardiac conducting system. They carry impulses through the walls of the ventricles
repolarization rē-pō-lar-i-ZĀ-shun	A return of electrical charge to the resting state in nerves or muscles

(continued)

Terminology	Key Terms (continued)	

right AV valve	The valve between the right atrium and right ventricle; the tricuspid valve
septum SEP-tum	A wall dividing two cavities, such as two chambers of the heart
sinus rhythm SĪ-nus	Normal heart rhythm
sinoatrial (SA) node sī-nō-Ā-trē-al	A small mass in the upper part of the right atrium that initiates the impulse for each heartbeat; the pacemaker
sphygmomanometer sfig-mō-man-OM-e-ter	An instrument for determining arterial blood pressure (root *sphygm/o* means "pulse"); blood pressure apparatus or cuff
superior vena cava VĒ-na KĀ-va	The large superior vein that brings deoxygenated blood back to the right atrium from the upper body
systemic circuit sis-TEM-ik SER-kit	The system of vessels that carries oxygenated blood from the left side of the heart to all tissues except the lungs and returns deoxygenated blood to the right side of the heart
systole SIS-tō-lē	The contraction phase of the heartbeat cycle; adjective: systolic
valve valv	A structure that keeps fluid flowing in a forward direction (roots: *valv/o, valvul/o*)
vein vān	A vessel that carries blood back to the heart. All except the pulmonary and umbilical veins carry blood low in oxygen (roots: *ven/o, phleb/o*)
ventricle VEN-trik-l	A small cavity. One of the two lower pumping chambers of the heart (root: *ventricul/o*)
venule VEN-ūl	A small vessel that carries blood from the capillaries to the veins
vessel VES-el	A tube or duct to transport fluid (roots: *angi/o, vas/o, vascul/o*)

PASSport to Success® Go to the pronunciation glossary on the Student Resources to hear these words pronounced.

Roots Pertaining to the Cardiovascular System

See Tables 9-1 and 9-2.

Table 9-1	Roots for the Heart		

Root	Meaning	Example	Definition of Example
cardi/o	heart	cardiomyopathy* kar-dē-ō-mī-OP-a-thē	any disease of the heart muscle
atri/o	atrium	atriotomy ā-trē-OT-ō-mē	surgical incision of an atrium
ventricul/o	cavity, ventricle	supraventricular sū-pra-ven-TRIK-ū-lar	above a ventricle
valv/o, valvul/o	valve	valvulotome VAL-vū-lō-tōm	instrument for incising a valve

*Preferred over myocardiopathy.

EXERCISE 9-1

Fill in the blanks:

1. The word *cardiogenic* (*kar-dē-ō-GEN-ik*) means originating in the _____.

2. Interatrial (*in-ter-Ā-trē-al*) means between the _____.

3. Ventriculotomy (*ven-trik-ū-LOT-ō-mē*) means surgical incision of a(n) _____.

4. A valvuloplasty (*val-vū-lō-PLAS-tē*) is plastic repair of a(n) _____.

Write the adjective for the following definitions. The proper suffix is given for each.

5. Pertaining to the heart (-ac) _____

6. Pertaining to the myocardium (-al; ending differs from adjective ending for the heart) _____

7. Pertaining to an atrium (-al) _____

8. Pertaining to a valve (-ar) _____

9. Pertaining to a ventricle (-ar) _____

10. Pertaining to the pericardium (-al) _____

Following the example, write a word for the following definitions pertaining to the tissues of the heart:

11. Inflammation of the lining of the heart (usually at a valve) _____ endocarditis _____

12. Inflammation of the heart muscle _____

13. Inflammation of the fibrous sac around the heart _____

Write a word for the following definitions:

14. Pertaining to an atrium and a ventricle _____

15. Between (inter-) the ventricles _____

16. Study (-logy) of the heart _____

17. Surgical incision of a valve _____

18. Enlargement (-megaly) of the heart _____

Table 9-2   Roots for the Blood Vessels

Root	Meaning	Example	Definition of Example
angi/o*	vessel	angiography *an-jē-OG-ra-fē*	x-ray imaging of a vessel
vas/o, vascul/o	vessel, duct	vasospasm *vas-ō-spazm*	sudden contraction of a vessel
arter/o, arteri/o	artery	endarterial *end-ar-TĒ-rē-al*	within an artery
arteriol/o	arteriole	arteriolar *ar-tē-rē-Ō-lar*	pertaining to an arteriole
aort/o	aorta	aortoptosis *ā-or-top-TŌ-sis*	downward displacement of the aorta
ven/o, ven/i	vein	venous *VĒ-nus*	pertaining to a vein
phleb/o	vein	phlebotomy *fle-BOT-ō-mē*	incision of a vein to withdraw blood

*The root *angi/o* usually refers to a blood vessel but is used for other types of vessels as well. *Hemangi/o* refers specifically to a blood vessel.

EXERCISE 9-2

Fill in the blanks:

1. Vasoconstriction (vas-ō-kon-STRIK-shun) means narrowing of a(n) _____.

2. Endarterectomy (end-ar-ter-EK-tō-mē) is removal of the inner lining of a(n) _____

_____.

3. Arteriolitis (ar-tē-rē-ō-LĪ-tis) is inflammation of a(n) _____.

4. Angioedema (an-jē-ō-e-DĒ-ma) is localized swelling caused by changes in _____

_____.

5. Aortostenosis (ā-or-tō-ste-NŌ-sis) is narrowing of the _____.

6. Phlebectasia (fleb-ek-TĀ-zē-a) is dilatation of a(n) _____.

7. The term microvascular (mī-krō-VAS-kū-lar) means pertaining to small _____

_____.

Define the following words:

8. cardiovascular (kar-dē-ō-VAS-kū-lar) _____

9. intraaortic (in-tra-ā-OR-tik) _____

10. angiitis (an-jē-Ī-tis) (note spelling); also angitis or vasculitis _____

11. arteriorrhexis (ar-tē-rē-ō-REK-sis) _____

12. phlebitis (fleb-Ī-tis) _____

Use the ending -gram to form a word for a radiograph of the following:

13. vessels (use angi/o) _____

14. aorta _____

15. veins _____

Use the root angi/o to write words with the following meanings:

16. Formation (-genesis) of a vessel _____

17. Dilatation (-ectasis) of a vessel _____

18. Any disease (-pathy) of a vessel _____

19. Plastic repair (-plasty) of a vessel _____

Use the appropriate root to write words with the following meanings:

20. Within (intra-) a vein _____

21. Incision of an artery _____

22. Excision of a vein _____

23. Hardening (-sclerosis) of the aorta _____

Clinical Aspects of the Cardiovascular System

Atherosclerosis

The accumulation of fatty deposits within the lining of an **artery** is termed **atherosclerosis** (Fig. 9-8). This type of deposit, called **plaque** (*plak*), begins to form when a vessel receives tiny injuries, usually at a point of branching. Plaques gradually thicken and harden with fibrous material, cells, and other deposits, restricting the vessel's lumen (opening) and reducing blood flow to the tissues, a condition known as **ischemia** (*is-KĒ-mē-a*). A major risk factor for the development of atherosclerosis is **dyslipidemia**, abnormally high levels or imbalance in **lipoproteins** that are carried in the blood, especially high levels of cholesterol-containing, low-density lipoproteins (LDLs). Other risk factors for atherosclerosis include smoking, high blood pressure, poor diet, inactivity, stress, and a family history of the disorder. Atherosclerosis may involve any arteries, but most of its effects are seen in the coronary vessels of the heart, the aorta, the carotid arteries in the neck, and vessels in the brain. The techniques described later for treating coronary artery disease (CAD) are used for these other vessels as well.

Atherosclerosis is the most common form of a more general condition known as **arteriosclerosis** in which vessel walls harden from any cause. In addition to plaque, calcium salts and scar tissue may contribute to arterial wall thickening, with a narrowing of the lumen and loss of elasticity.

Thrombosis and Embolism

Atherosclerosis predisposes a person to **thrombosis**, the formation of a blood clot within a vessel (see Fig. 9-8). The clot, called a **thrombus**, interrupts blood flow to the tissues supplied by that vessel, resulting in necrosis (tissue death). Blockage of a vessel by a thrombus or other mass carried in the bloodstream is **embolism**, and the mass itself is called an **embolus**. Usually, the mass is a blood clot that breaks loose from a vessel's wall, but it may also be air (as from injection or trauma), fat (as from marrow released after a bone break), bacteria, or other solid materials. Often a venous thrombus will travel through the heart and then lodge in an artery of the lungs, resulting in a life-threatening pulmonary embolism. An embolus from a carotid artery often blocks a cerebral vessel, causing a **cerebrovascular accident** (**CVA**), commonly called **stroke** (see Chapter 17).

Aneurysm

An arterial wall weakened by atherosclerosis, malformation, injury, or other changes may balloon out, forming an **aneurysm**. If an aneurysm ruptures, hemorrhage results. Rupture of a cerebral artery is another cause of stroke. The abdominal aorta and carotid arteries are also common aneurysm sites. In a **dissecting aneurysm** (Fig. 9-9), blood hemorrhages into the arterial wall's thick middle layer, separating the muscle as it spreads and sometimes rupturing the vessel. The aorta is most commonly involved. It may be possible to repair a dissecting aneurysm surgically with a graft.

Hypertension

High blood pressure, or **hypertension** (HTN), is a contributing factor in all of the conditions described above. In simple terms, HTN is defined as a systolic pressure greater than 140 mm Hg or a diastolic pressure greater than 90 mm Hg. HTN causes the left ventricle to enlarge (hypertrophy) as a result of increased work. Some cases of HTN are secondary to other disorders, such as kidney malfunction or endocrine disturbance, but most of the

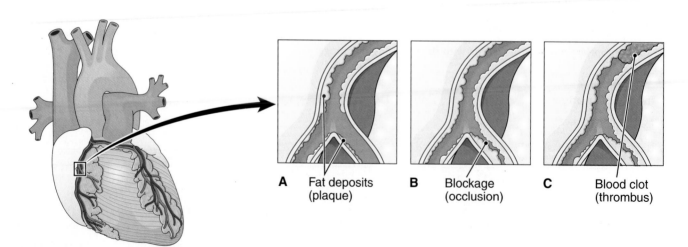

Figure 9-8 **Coronary atherosclerosis.** (*A*) Fat deposits (plaque) narrow an artery, leading to ischemia (lack of blood supply). (*B*) Plaque causes blockage (occlusion) of a vessel. (*C*) Formation of a blood clot (thrombus) in a vessel leads to myocardial infarction (MI).

A Fat deposits (plaque) **B** Blockage (occlusion) **C** Blood clot (thrombus)

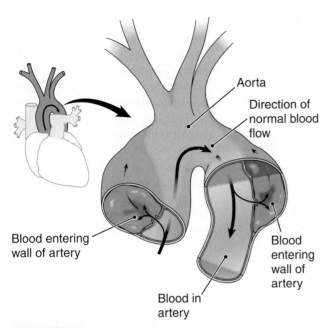

Aorta

Direction of normal blood flow

Blood entering wall of artery

Blood entering wall of artery

Blood in artery

Figure 9-9 **Dissecting aortic aneurysm.** Blood separates the layers of the arterial wall.

time the causes are unknown, a condition described as primary, or essential, HTN.

Changes in diet and life habits are the first line of defense in controlling HTN. Drugs that are used include diuretics to eliminate fluids, vasodilators to relax the blood vessels, and drugs that prevent the formation or action of angiotensin, a substance in the blood that normally acts to increase blood pressure (see Chapter 13).

PASSport to Success® The animation *Hypertension* on the Student Resources illustrates the effects of this disorder.

Heart Disease

CORONARY ARTERY DISEASE
CAD, which results from atherosclerosis in the vessels that supply blood to the heart muscle, is a leading cause of death in industrialized countries (see Fig. 9-8). An early sign of CAD is the type of chest pain known as **angina pectoris**. This is a feeling of constriction around the heart or pain that may radiate to the left arm or shoulder, usually brought on by exertion. Often there is anxiety, **diaphoresis** (profuse sweating), and **dyspnea** (difficulty in breathing). CAD is diagnosed by ECG, **stress tests**, **coronary angiography** (imaging), **echocardiography**, and other tests. Researchers have also found that a substance called **C-reactive protein (CRP)** is associated with poor cardiovascular health. This protein is produced during systemic inflammation, which may contribute to atherosclerosis. CRP levels can indicate cardio-

vascular disease and predict its outcome (prognosis). A more specific test for heart attack risk is the more accurate hs-CRP (high-sensitivity CRP) test.

CAD is treated by control of exercise and administration of nitroglycerin to dilate coronary vessels. Other drugs may be used to regulate the heartbeat, strengthen the force of heart contraction, or prevent blood clot formation.

Patients with severe cases of CAD may be candidates for **angioplasty**, surgical dilatation of the blocked vessel by means of a balloon catheter, a procedure technically called **percutaneous transluminal coronary angioplasty (PTCA)** (Fig. 9-10). Angioplasty may include placement of a **stent**, a small mesh tube, to keep the vessel open (Fig. 9-11). Stents prevent recoil of the vessel, and newer versions release drugs to prevent vascular restenosis.

If further intervention is required, surgeons can bypass the blocked vessel or vessels with a vascular graft (Fig. 9-12). In this procedure, known as a **coronary artery bypass graft (CABG)**, another vessel or a piece of another vessel, usually the left internal mammary artery or part of the leg's saphenous vein, is grafted to carry blood from the aorta to a point past the coronary vessel obstruction.

MYOCARDIAL INFARCTION
Degenerative changes in the arteries predispose a person to thrombosis and sudden coronary artery **occlusion** (obstruction). The resultant area of myocardial necrosis is termed an **infarct** (Fig. 9-13), and the process is known as **myocardial infarction (MI)**, the "heart attack" that may cause sudden death. Symptoms of MI include pain over the heart (precordial pain) or upper part of the abdomen (epigastric pain) that may extend to the jaw or arms, pallor (paleness), diaphoresis, nausea, fatigue, anxiety, and dyspnea. There may be a burning sensation similar to indigestion or heartburn. In women, because degenerative changes more commonly affect multiple small vessels rather than the major coronary pathways, MI symptoms are often more long-term and more subtle and diffuse than the intense chest pain that is more typical in men.

MI is diagnosed by ECG and assays for specific substances in the blood. **Creatine kinase** (CK) is an enzyme normal to muscle cells. It is released in increased amounts when muscle tissue is injured. The form of CK specific to cardiac muscle cells is creatine kinase MB (CK-MB). **Troponin** (Tn) is a protein that regulates contraction in muscle cells. Increased serum levels, particularly the forms TnT and TnI, indicate MI.

Patient outcome is based on the degree of damage and the speed of treatment to dissolve the clot and to reestablish normal blood flow and heart rhythm.

ARRHYTHMIA
Arrhythmia is any irregularity of heart rhythm, such as an altered heart rate, extra beats, or a change in the

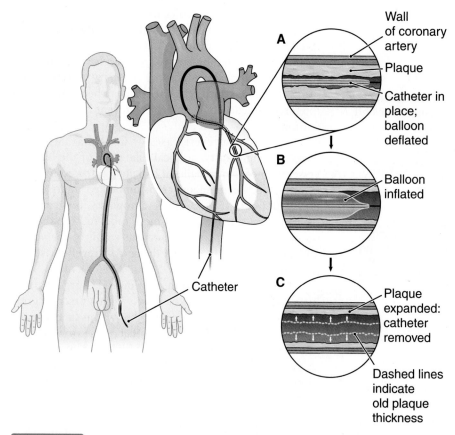

branch is designated as a left or right bundle branch block (BBB).

If, for any reason, the SA node is not generating a normal heartbeat or there is heart block, an **artificial pacemaker** may be implanted to regulate the beat (Fig. 9-15). Usually, the pacemaker is inserted under the skin below the clavicle, and leads are threaded through veins into one or both of the right chambers. Some pacemakers act only when the heart is not functioning on its own, and some adjust to the need for a change in heart rate based on activity.

MI is also a common cause of **fibrillation**, an extremely rapid, ineffective heartbeat, especially dangerous when it affects the ventricles. **Cardioversion** is the general term for restoration of a normal heart rhythm, either by drugs or application of electric current. Hospital personnel use external chest "paddles" for emergency electrical **defibrillation**. In addition to **cardiopulmonary resuscitation** (CPR), automated external defibrillators (AEDs) can help save lives when available for high-risk patients or in public places, such as malls, aircraft, and sports venues. The AED detects fatal arrhythmia and automatically delivers a correct preprogrammed shock. An implantable cardioverter–defibrillator (ICD), applied much like a pacemaker, detects potential fibrillation and automatically shocks the heart to restore normal rhythm.

Figure 9-10 **Coronary angioplasty (PTCA).** (*A*) A guide catheter is threaded into the coronary artery. (*B*) A balloon catheter is inserted through the occlusion. (*C*) The balloon is inflated and deflated until plaque is flattened and the vessel is opened.

pattern of the beat. **Bradycardia** is a slower-than-average rate, and **tachycardia** is a higher-than-average rate.

Damage to cardiac tissue, as by MI, may result in **heart block**, an interruption in the heart's electrical conduction system resulting in arrhythmia (Fig. 9-14). Heart block is classified in order of increasing severity as first-, second-, or third-degree heart block. Block in a bundle

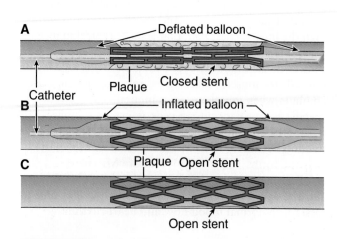

Figure 9-11 **Arterial stent.** (*A*) Stent closed, before balloon inflation. (*B*) Stent open, balloon inflated; stent will remain expanded after balloon is deflated and removed. (*C*) Stent open, balloon removed.

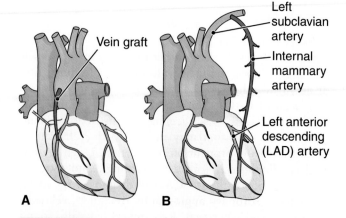

Figure 9-12 **Coronary artery bypass graft (CABG).** (*A*) A segment of the saphenous vein carries blood from the aorta to a part of the right coronary artery that is distal to an occlusion. (*B*) The mammary artery is used to bypass an obstruction in the left anterior descending (LAD) coronary artery.

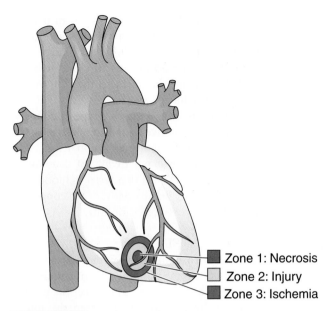

Zone 1: Necrosis
Zone 2: Injury
Zone 3: Ischemia

Figure 9-13 **Myocardial infarction (MI).** A blood clot (thrombus) causes a zone of necrosis (tissue death). Surrounding tissue suffers from lack of blood supply (ischemia).

A newer approach to the treatment of heart rhythm irregularities is **ablation**, or destruction, of that portion of the conduction pathway that is involved in the arrhythmia. Electrode catheter ablation uses high-frequency sound waves, freezing (cryoablation), or electrical energy delivered through an intravascular catheter to ablate a defect in the conduction pathway.

HEART FAILURE

The general term **heart failure** refers to any condition in which the heart fails to empty effectively. The resulting increased pressure in the venous system leads to **edema**, justifying the description *congestive heart failure* (CHF). Left-side failure results in pulmonary edema with breathing difficulties (dyspnea); right-side failure causes periph-

Pacemaker lead enters external jugular vein

Pacemaker

Tip of lead lodged in apex of right ventricle

Pacemaker placed beneath skin in pectoral region

Figure 9-15 **Placement of a pacemaker.** The lead is placed in an atrium or ventricle, usually on the right side. A dual-chamber pacemaker has leads in both chambers.

eral edema with tissue swelling, especially in the legs, along with weight gain from fluid retention. Other symptoms of CHF are **cyanosis** and **syncope** (fainting).

Heart failure is treated with rest, drugs to strengthen heart contractions, diuretics to eliminate fluid, and restriction of salt in the diet.

 PASSport to Success® See the animation *Heart Failure* on the Student Resources.

Heart failure is one cause of **shock**, a severe disturbance in the circulatory system resulting in inadequate blood delivery to the tissues. Shock is classified according to cause as:

- Cardiogenic shock, caused by heart failure
- Hypovolemic shock, caused by loss of blood volume
- Septic shock, caused by bacterial infection
- Anaphylactic shock, caused by severe allergic reaction

CONGENITAL HEART DISEASE

A congenital defect is any defect that is present at birth. The most common type of congenital heart defect is a **septal defect**, a hole in the septum (wall) that separates

Bundle of His

Bundle branches

AV node

Figure 9-14 **Potential sites for heart block in the atrioventricular (AV) portion of the heart's conduction system.**

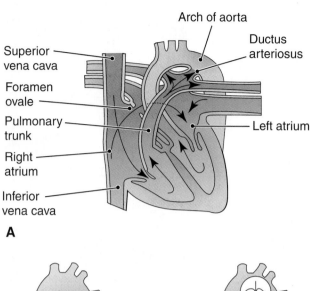

Arch of aorta

Superior vena cava

Foramen ovale

Pulmonary trunk

Right atrium

Inferior vena cava

Ductus arteriosus

Left atrium

A

B

D

C

E

Figure 9-16 **Congenital heart defects.** (*A*) Normal fetal heart showing the foramen ovale and ductus arteriosus. (*B*) Persistence of the foramen ovale results in an atrial septal defect. (*C*) A ventricular septal defect. (*D*) Persistence of the ductus arteriosus (patent ductus arteriosus) forces blood back into the pulmonary artery. (*E*) Coarctation of the aorta restricts outward blood flow in the aorta.

the atria or the septum that separates the ventricles (Fig. 9-16). An atrial septal defect often results from persistence of an opening, the foramen ovale, that allows blood to bypass the lungs in fetal circulation. A septal defect permits blood to shunt from the left to the right side of the heart and return to the lungs instead of flowing out to the body. The heart has to work harder to meet the tissues' oxygen needs. Symptoms of septal defect include cyanosis (leading to the description "blue baby"), syncope, and **clubbing** of the fingers.

Another congenital defect that results from persistence of a fetal modification is **patent ductus arteriosus** (see Fig. 9-16D). In this case, a small bypass between the pulmonary artery and the aorta fails to close at birth. Blood then can flow from the aorta to the pulmonary artery and return to the lungs.

Heart valve malformation is another type of congenital heart defect. Failure of a valve to open or close properly is evidenced by a **murmur**, an abnormal sound heard as the heart cycles. A localized aortic narrowing, or **coarctation of the aorta**, is a congenital defect that restricts blood flow through that vessel (see Fig. 9-16E). Most of the congenital defects described can be corrected surgically.

RHEUMATIC HEART DISEASE

In **rheumatic heart disease**, infection with a specific type of streptococcus sets up an immune reaction that ultimately damages the heart valves. The infection usually begins as a "strep throat," and most often the mitral valve is involved. Scar tissue fuses the valve's leaflets, causing a narrowing or **stenosis** that interferes with proper function. People with rheumatic heart disease are subject to repeated valvular infections and may need to take antibiotics prophylactically (preventively) before invasive medical or dental procedures. Severe cases of rheumatic heart disease may require surgical correction or even valve replacement. The incidence of rheumatic heart disease has declined with the use of antibiotics.

Disorders of the Veins

A breakdown in the valves of the veins in combination with a chronic dilatation of these vessels results in **varicose veins** (Fig. 9-17). These appear twisted and swollen under

Figure 9-17 **Varicose veins.**

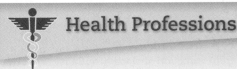

Box 9-3   Health Professions

Vascular Technology

Vascular technologists obtain information about the blood vessels and circulation to help physicians in the diagnosis of vascular disorders. They use a wide range of noninvasive instrumentation, mainly ultrasound, in their studies. Using ultrasound techniques, they obtain two-dimensional images of blood vessels and measure the speed and direction of blood flow (Doppler ultrasound). Using other instruments, they can measure blood pressure, changes in blood volume, and the blood's oxygen saturation. Based on clinical signs, they typically investigate circulation to the brain, extremities, or abdominal organs.

Most vascular technologists work in hospitals, where they prepare patients for tests, take clinical histories, perform physical examinations, carry out appropriate tests, and report results.

They may also work in offices, clinics, or laboratories. Many of their patients are debilitated or critically ill and may need mobile service and/or assistance to undergo testing.

Unlike early workers in this field who often were trained on the job, most vascular technologists today complete a 2- or 4-year educational program accredited by the Commission on Accreditation of Allied Health Education Programs (CAAHEP). Certification specific to vascular technology is available from the American Registry for Diagnostic Medical Sonography at www.ardms.org and from other organizations. Certification requires appropriate education, clinical experience, examination, and continuing education. Additional information on this career is available from the Society for Vascular Ultrasound at www.svunet.org.

---

the skin, most commonly in the legs. Contributing factors include heredity, obesity, prolonged standing, and pregnancy, which increases pressure in the pelvic veins. Varicosities can impede blood flow and lead to edema, thrombosis, hemorrhage, or ulceration. Treatment includes the wearing of elastic stockings and, in some cases, surgical removal of the varicose veins, after which collateral circulation is naturally established. A varicose vein in the rectum or anal canal is referred to as a **hemorrhoid.**

Phlebitis is any inflammation of the veins and may be caused by infection, injury, poor circulation, or dam-

age to valves in the veins. Such inflammation typically initiates blood clot formation, resulting in **thrombophlebitis.** Any veins are subject to thrombophlebitis, but the more serious condition involves the deep veins as opposed to the superficial veins, in the condition termed **deep vein thrombosis** (DVT). The most common sites for DVT are the deep leg veins, causing serious reduction in venous drainage from these areas.

Vascular technologists obtain information on the blood vessels and circulation to aid in diagnosis. See Box 9-3 for information on this career.

Terminology	**Key Terms**

Cardiovascular Disorders

aneurysm AN-ū-rizm	A localized abnormal dilation of a blood vessel, usually an artery, caused by weakness of the vessel wall; may eventually burst
angina pectoris an-JĪ-na PEK-tō-ris	A feeling of constriction around the heart or pain that may radiate to the left arm or shoulder, usually brought on by exertion; caused by insufficient blood supply to the heart
arrhythmia a-RITH-mē-a	Any abnormality in the rate or rhythm of the heartbeat (literally "without rhythm"; note doubled r). Also called *dysrhythmia*
arteriosclerosis ar-tēr-ē-ō-skler-Ō-sis	Hardening (sclerosis) of the arteries, with loss of capacity and loss of elasticity, as from fatty deposits (plaque), deposit of calcium salts, or scar tissue formation
atherosclerosis ath-er-ō-skler-Ō-sis	The development of fatty, fibrous patches (plaques) in the lining of arteries, causing narrowing of the lumen and hardening of the vessel wall. The most common form of arteriosclerosis is hardening of the arteries. The root *ather/o* means "porridge" or "gruel"
bradycardia brad-ē-KAR-dē-a	A slow heart rate, of less than 60 bpm

(continued)

Terminology Key Terms (continued)

cerebrovascular accident (CVA) *ser-e-brō-VAS-kū-lar*	Sudden damage to the brain resulting from reduction of blood flow. Causes include atherosclerosis, embolism, thrombosis, or hemorrhage from a ruptured aneurysm; commonly called stroke
clubbing *KLUB-ing*	Enlargement of the ends of the fingers and toes caused by growth of the soft tissue around the nails (see Fig. 7-12). Seen in a variety of diseases in which there is poor peripheral circulation
coarctation of the aorta *kō-ark-TĀ-shun*	Localized narrowing of the aorta with restriction of blood flow (see Fig. 9-16E)
C-reactive protein (CRP)	Protein produced during systemic inflammation, which may contribute to atherosclerosis; high CRP levels can indicate cardiovascular disease and its prognosis
cyanosis *sī-a-NŌ-sis*	Bluish discoloration of the skin caused by lack of oxygen (see Fig. 3-4)
deep vein thrombosis (DVT)	Thrombophlebitis involving the deep veins
diaphoresis *dī-a-fō-RĒ-sis*	Profuse sweating
dissecting aneurysm	An aneurysm in which blood enters the arterial wall and separates the layers. Usually involves the aorta (see Fig. 9-9)
dyslipidemia *dis-lip-i-DĒ-mē-a*	Disorder in serum lipid levels, which is an important factor in development of atherosclerosis. Includes hyperlipidemia (high lipids), hypercholesterolemia (high cholesterol), and hypertriglyceridemia (high triglycerides)
dyspnea *DYSP-nē-a*	Difficult or labored breathing (-pnea)
edema *e-DĒ-ma*	Swelling of body tissues caused by the presence of excess fluid (see Fig. 6-4). Causes include cardiovascular disturbances, kidney failure, inflammation, and malnutrition
embolism *EM-bō-lizm*	Obstruction of a blood vessel by a blood clot or other matter carried in the circulation
embolus *EM-bō-lus*	A mass carried in the circulation. Usually a blood clot, but also may be air, fat, bacteria, or other solid matter from within or from outside the body
fibrillation *fi-bri-LĀ-shun*	Spontaneous, quivering, and ineffectual contraction of muscle fibers, as in the atria or the ventricles
heart block	An interference in the conduction system of the heart resulting in arrhythmia (see Fig. 9-14)
heart failure	A condition caused by the inability of the heart to maintain adequate blood circulation
hemorrhoid *HEM-ō-royd*	A varicose vein in the rectum
hypertension *hī-per-TEN-shun*	A condition of higher-than-normal blood pressure. Essential (primary, idiopathic) hypertension has no known cause
infarct *in-FARKT*	An area of localized tissue necrosis (death) resulting from a blockage or a narrowing of the artery that supplies the area
ischemia *is-KĒ-mē-a*	Local deficiency of blood supply caused by circulatory obstruction (root: hem/o)
murmur	An abnormal heart sound
myocardial infarction (MI) *mī-ō-KAR-dē-al in-FARK-shun*	Localized necrosis (death) of cardiac muscle tissue resulting from blockage or narrowing of the coronary artery that supplies that area. Myocardial infarction is usually caused by formation of a thrombus (clot) in a vessel (see Fig. 9-13)

Terminology	**Key Terms** *(continued)*

occlusion ō-KLŪ-zhun	A closing off or obstruction, as of a vessel
patent ductus arteriosus PĀ-tent DUK-tus ar-tēr-ē-Ō-sus	Persistence of the ductus arteriosus after birth. The ductus arteriosus is a vessel that connects the pulmonary artery to the descending aorta in the fetus to bypass the lungs (see Fig. 9-16D)
phlebitis fle-BĪ-tis	Inflammation of a vein
plaque plak	A patch. With regard to the cardiovascular system, a deposit of fatty material and other substances on a vessel wall that impedes blood flow and may block the vessel. Atheromatous plaque
rheumatic heart disease rū-MAT-ik	Damage to heart valves after infection with a type of streptococcus (group A hemolytic streptococcus). The antibodies produced in response to the infection produce valvular scarring, usually involving the mitral valve
septal defect SEP-tal	An opening in the septum between the atria or ventricles; a common cause is persistence of the foramen ovale (for-Ā-men ō-VAL-ē), an opening between the atria that bypasses the lungs in fetal circulation (see Fig. 9-16B and C)
shock	Circulatory failure resulting in an inadequate blood supply to the tissues. Cardiogenic shock is caused by heart failure; hypovolemic shock is caused by a loss of blood volume; septic shock is caused by bacterial infection
sinus rhythm SĪ-nus	A normal heart rhythm originating from the sinoatrial (SA) node
stenosis ste-NŌ-sis	Constriction or narrowing of an opening
stroke	See *cerebrovascular accident*
syncope SIN-kō-pē	A temporary loss of consciousness caused by inadequate blood flow to the brain; fainting
tachycardia tak-i-KAR-dē-a	An abnormally rapid heart rate, usually over 100 bpm
thrombophlebitis throm-bō-fle-BĪ-tis	Inflammation of a vein associated with formation of a blood clot
thrombosis throm-BŌ-sis	Development of a blood clot within a vessel
thrombus THROM-bus	A blood clot that forms within a blood vessel (root: *thromb/o*)
varicose vein VAR-i-kōs	A twisted and swollen vein resulting from breakdown of the valves, pooling of blood, and chronic dilatation of the vessel (root: *varic/o*); also called varix (VAR-iks) or varicosity (var-i-KOS-i-tē) (see Fig. 9-17)

Diagnosis and Treatment

angioplasty AN-jē-ō-plas-tē	A procedure that reopens a narrowed vessel and restores blood flow. Commonly accomplished by surgically removing plaque, inflating a balloon within the vessel, or installing a device (stent) to keep the vessel open (see Figs. 9-10 and 9-11)
artificial pacemaker	A battery-operated device that generates electrical impulses to regulate the heartbeat. It may be external or implanted, may be designed to respond to need, and may have the capacity to prevent tachycardia (see Fig. 9-15)
cardiopulmonary resuscitation (CPR) rē-sus-i-TĀ-shun	Restoration of cardiac output and pulmonary ventilation after cardiac arrest using artificial respiration and chest compression or cardiac massage

(continued)

Terminology   Key Terms (continued)

cardioversion KAR-dē-ō-ver-zhun	Correction of an abnormal cardiac rhythm. May be accomplished pharmacologically, with antiarrhythmic drugs, or by application of electric current (see defibrillation)
coronary angiography an-jē-OG-ra-fē	Radiographic study of the coronary arteries after introduction of an opaque dye by means of a catheter
coronary artery bypass graft (CABG)	Surgical creation of a shunt to bypass a blocked coronary artery. The aorta is connected to a point past the obstruction with another vessel or a piece of another vessel, usually the left internal mammary artery or part of the leg's saphenous vein (see Fig. 9-12)
creatine kinase MB (CK-MB) krē-a-tin KĪ-nāz	Enzyme released in increased amounts from cardiac muscle cells following myocardial infarction (MI). Serum assays help diagnose MI and determine the extent of muscle damage
defibrillation dē-fib-ri-LĀ-shun	Use of an electronic device (defibrillator) to stop fibrillation by delivering a brief electric shock to the heart. The shock may be delivered to the surface of the chest, as by an automated external defibrillator (AED), or directly into the heart through wire leads, using an implantable cardioverter defibrillator (ICD)
echocardiography ek-ō-kar-dē-OG-ra-fē	A noninvasive method that uses ultrasound to visualize internal cardiac structures
lipoprotein lip-ō-PRŌ-tēn	A compound of protein with lipid. Lipoproteins are classified according to density as very-low-density (VLDL), low-density (LDL), and high-density (HDL). Relatively higher levels of HDLs have been correlated with cardiovascular health
percutaneous transluminal coronary angioplasty (PTCA)	Dilatation of a sclerotic blood vessel by means of a balloon catheter inserted into the vessel and then inflated to flatten plaque against the arterial wall (see Fig. 9-10)
stent	A small metal device in the shape of a coil or slotted tube that is placed inside an artery to keep the vessel open after balloon angioplasty (see Fig. 9-11)
stress test	Evaluation of physical fitness by continuous ECG monitoring during exercise. In a thallium stress test, a radioactive isotope of thallium is administered to trace blood flow through the heart during exercise
troponin (Tn) trō-PŌ-nin	A protein in muscle cells that regulates contraction. Increased serum levels, primarily in the forms TnT and TnI, indicate recent myocardial infarction (MI)

PASSport to Success®   Go to the pronunciation glossary on the Student Resources to hear these words pronounced.

The Lymphatic System

The lymphatic system is a widely distributed system with multiple functions (Fig. 9-18). Its role in circulation is to return excess fluid and proteins from the tissues to the bloodstream. Blind-ended lymphatic capillaries pick up these materials in the tissues and carry them into larger vessels (Fig. 9-19). The fluid carried in the lymphatic system is called **lymph**. Lymph drains from the lower part of the body and the upper left side into the **thoracic duct** (left lymphatic duct), which travels upward through the chest and empties into the left subclavian vein near the heart (see Fig. 9-18). The **right lymphatic duct** drains the body's upper right side and empties into the right subclavian vein.

Another major function of the lymphatic system is to protect the body from impurities and invading microorganisms (see discussion of immunity in Chapter 10). Along the path of the lymphatic vessels are small masses of lymphoid tissue, the **lymph nodes** (Fig. 9-20). Their function is to filter the lymph as it passes through. They are concentrated in the cervical (neck), axillary

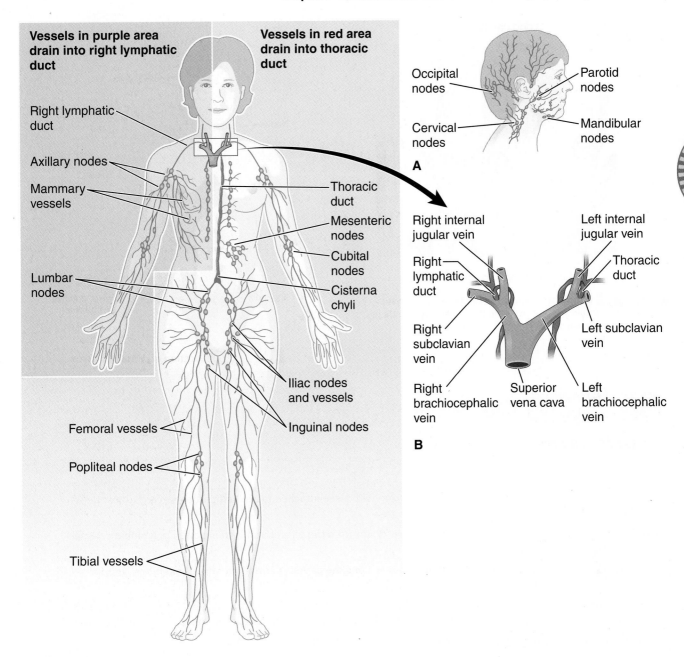

Vessels in purple area drain into right lymphatic duct

Vessels in red area drain into thoracic duct

Right lymphatic duct
Axillary nodes
Mammary vessels
Lumbar nodes
Femoral vessels
Popliteal nodes
Tibial vessels

Thoracic duct
Mesenteric nodes
Cubital nodes
Cisterna chyli
Iliac nodes and vessels
Inguinal nodes

Occipital nodes
Cervical nodes
Parotid nodes
Mandibular nodes

A

Right internal jugular vein
Right lymphatic duct
Right subclavian vein
Right brachiocephalic vein

Left internal jugular vein
Thoracic duct
Left subclavian vein
Superior vena cava
Left brachiocephalic vein

B

9

Figure 9-18 **Lymphatic system.** (A) Lymph nodes and vessels of the head. (B) Drainage of the right lymphatic duct and the thoracic duct into the subclavian veins.

(armpit), mediastinal (chest), and inguinal (groin) regions. Other protective organs and tissues of the lymphatic system include the:

■ **Tonsils,** located in the throat (pharynx). They filter inhaled or swallowed materials and aid in immunity early in life. The tonsils are further discussed in Chapter 11.

■ **Thymus gland** in the chest, above the heart. It processes and stimulates lymphocytes active in immunity.

■ **Spleen** in the upper left region of the abdomen. It filters blood and destroys old red blood cells.

■ **Appendix,** attached to the large intestine. It may aid in the development of immunity.

■ **Peyer patches,** in the lining of the intestine. They help protect against invading microorganisms.

A final function of the lymphatic system is to absorb digested fats from the small intestine (see Chapter 12). These fats are then added to the blood with the lymph that drains from the thoracic duct.

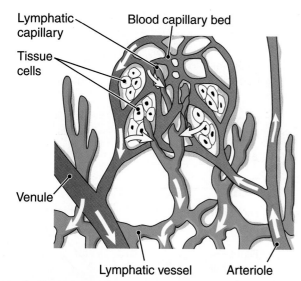

Figure 9-19 **Lymphatic drainage in the tissues.** Lymphatic capillaries pick up fluid and proteins left in the tissues and carry them back to the bloodstream.

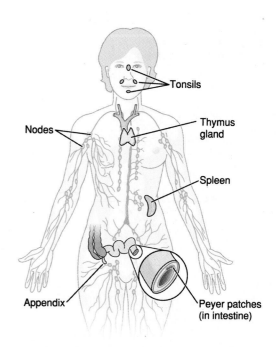

Figure 9-20 **Location of lymphoid tissue.**

Terminology Key Terms

LYMPHATIC SYSTEM

Normal Structure and Function

appendix *a-PEN-diks*	A small, fingerlike mass of lymphoid tissue attached to the first part of the large intestine
lymph *limf*	The thin plasmalike fluid that drains from the tissues and is transported in lymphatic vessels (root: *lymph/o*)
lymph node	A small mass of lymphoid tissue along the path of a lymphatic vessel that filters lymph (root: *lymphaden/o*)
lymphatic system *lim-FAT-ik*	The system that drains fluid and proteins from the tissues and returns them to the bloodstream. This system also participates in immunity and aids in absorption of fats from the digestive tract
Peyer patches *PĪ-er*	Aggregates of lymphoid tissue in the lining of the intestine
right lymphatic duct	The lymphatic duct that drains fluid from the body's upper right side
spleen	A large reddish-brown organ in the upper left region of the abdomen. It filters blood and destroys old red blood cells (root: *splen/o*)
thoracic duct	The lymphatic duct that drains fluid from the upper left side of the body and all of the lower body; left lymphatic duct
thymus gland *THĪ-mus*	A gland in the upper part of the chest beneath the sternum. It functions in immunity (root: *thym/o*)
tonsils *TON-silz*	Small masses of lymphoid tissue located in regions of the throat (pharynx)

 PASSport to Success® Go to the pronunciation glossary on the Student Resources to hear these words pronounced.

Roots Pertaining to the Lymphatic System

See Table 9-3.

Table 9-3	Roots for the Lymphatic System		
Root	**Meaning**	**Example**	**Definition of Example**
lymph/o	lymph, lymphatic system	lymphoid *LIM-foyd*	resembling lymph or lymphatic tissue
lymphaden/o	lymph node	lymphadenitis *lim-fad-e-NĪ-tis*	inflammation of a lymph node
lymphangi/o	lymphatic vessel	lymphangiogram *lim-FAN-jē-ō-gram*	x-ray image of lymphatic vessels
splen/o	spleen	splenalgia *splē-NAL-jē-a*	pain in the spleen
thym/o	thymus gland	athymia *a-THĪ-mē-a*	absence of the thymus gland
tonsill/o	tonsil	tonsillar *TON-sil-ar*	pertaining to a tonsil

EXERCISE 9-3

Fill in the blanks:

1. Lymphedema (*limf-e-DĒ-ma*) means swelling caused by obstruction of the flow of _____ .

2. Lymphadenectomy (*lim-fad-e-NEK-tō-mē*) is surgical removal of a(n) _____.

3. A lymphangioma (*lim-fan-jē-Ō-ma*) is a tumor of _____.

4. The adjective *splenic* (*SPLEN-ik*) means pertaining to the _____.

5. Thymectomy (*thī-MEK-tō-mē*) is surgical removal of the _____.

6. Tonsillopathy (*ton-sil-OP-a-thē*) is any disease of the _____.

Identify and define the root in the following words:

	Root	**Meaning of Root**
7. lymphangial (*lim-FAN-jē-al*)	lymphangi/o	lymphatic vessel
8. perisplenitis (*per-i-splē-NĪ-tis*)	_____	_____
9. lymphadenography (*lim-fad-e-NOG-ra-fē*)	_____	_____
10. tonsillectomy (*ton-sil-EK-tō-mē*)	_____	_____
11. hypothymism (*hī-pō-THĪ-mizm*)	_____	_____

Use the appropriate root to write words with the following meanings:

12. Inflammation of lymphatic vessels _____

13. A tumor (-oma) of lymphatic tissue _____

14. Any disease (-pathy) of the lymph nodes _____

15. Enlargement (-megaly) of the spleen _____

16. Pertaining to (-ic) the thymus gland _____

17. Inflammation of a tonsil _____

Clinical Aspects of the Lymphatic System

Changes in the lymphatic system are often related to infection and may consist of inflammation and enlargement of the nodes, called **lymphadenitis**, or inflammation of the vessels, called **lymphangiitis**. Obstruction of lymphatic vessels because of surgical excision or infection results in tissue swelling, or **lymphedema** (see Box 9-4). Any neoplastic disease involving lymph nodes is termed **lymphoma**. These neoplastic disorders affect the white cells found in the lymphatic system, and they are discussed more fully in Chapter 10.

Terminology   Key Clinical Terms

Lymphatic Disorders

lymphadenitis lim-fad-e-NĪ-tis	Inflammation and enlargement of lymph nodes, usually as a result of infection
lymphangiitis lim-fan-jē-Ī-tis	Inflammation of lymphatic vessels as a result of bacterial infection. Appears as painful red streaks under the skin (also spelled *lymphangitis*)
lymphedema lim-fe-DĒ-ma	Swelling of tissues with lymph caused by obstruction or excision of lymphatic vessels (see Box 9-4)
lymphoma lim-FŌ-ma	Any neoplastic disease of lymphoid tissue

PASSport to Success® Go to the pronunciation glossary on the Student Resources to hear these words pronounced.

Box 9-4   Clinical Perspectives

Lymphedema: When Lymph Stops Flowing

Fluid balance in the body requires appropriate distribution of fluid among the cardiovascular system, lymphatic system, and the tissues. **Edema** occurs when the balance is tipped toward excess fluid in the tissues. Often, edema is due to heart failure. However, blockage of lymphatic vessels (with resulting fluid accumulation in the tissues) can cause another form of edema, called **lymphedema**. The clinical hallmark of lymphedema is chronic swelling of an arm or leg, whereas heart failure usually causes swelling of both legs.

Lymphedema may be either primary or secondary. Primary lymphedema is a rare congenital condition caused by abnormal development of lymphatic vessels. Secondary lymphedema, or acquired lymphedema, can develop as a result of trauma to a limb, surgery, radiation therapy, or infection of the lymphatic vessels (lymphangitis). One of the most common causes of lymphedema is the removal of axillary lymph nodes during mastectomy, which disrupts lymph flow from the adjacent arm. Lymphedema may also occur following prostate surgery.

Therapies that encourage the flow of fluid through the lymphatic vessels are useful in treating lymphedema. These therapies may include elevation of the affected limb, manual lymphatic drainage through massage, light exercise, and firm wrapping of the limb to apply compression. In addition, changes in daily habits can lessen the effects of lymphedema. For example, further blockage of lymph drainage can be prevented by wearing loose clothing and jewelry, carrying a purse or handbag on the unaffected arm, and not crossing the legs when sitting. Lymphangitis requires the use of appropriate antibiotics. Prompt treatment is necessary because, in addition to swelling, other complications include poor wound healing, skin ulcers, and increased risk of infection.

Terminology   Supplementary Terms

Normal Structure and Function

apical pulse	Pulse felt or heard over the heart's apex. It is measured in the fifth left intercostal space (between the ribs) about 8 to 9 cm from the midline
cardiac output	The amount of blood pumped from the right or left ventricle per minute
Korotkoff sounds ko-ROT-kof	Arterial sounds heard with a stethoscope during determination of blood pressure with a cuff
perfusion per-FŪ-zhun	The passage of fluid, such as blood, through an organ or tissue
precordium prē-KOR-dē-um	The anterior region over the heart and the lower part of the thorax; adjective: precordial
pulse pressure	The difference between systolic and diastolic pressure
stroke volume	The amount of blood ejected by the left ventricle with each beat
Valsalva maneuver val-SAL-va	Bearing down, as in childbirth or defecation, by attempting to exhale forcefully with the nose and throat closed. This action has an effect on the cardiovascular system

Symptoms and Conditions

bruit brwē	An abnormal sound heard in auscultation
cardiac tamponade tam-pon-ÃD	Pathologic accumulation of fluid in the pericardial sac. May result from pericarditis or injury to the heart or great vessels
ectopic beat ek-TOP-ik	A heartbeat that originates from some part of the heart other than the SA node
extrasystole eks-tra-SIS-tō-lē	Premature heart contraction that occurs separately from the normal beat and originates from a part of the heart other than the SA node
flutter	Very rapid (200 to 300 bpm) but regular contractions, as in the atria or the ventricles
hypotension hī-po-TEN-shun	A condition of lower-than-normal blood pressure
intermittent claudication claw-di-KĀ-shun	Pain in a muscle during exercise caused by inadequate blood supply. The pain disappears with rest
mitral valve prolapse	Movement of the mitral valve cusps into the left atrium when the ventricles contract
occlusive vascular disease	Arteriosclerotic disease of the vessels, usually peripheral vessels
palpitation pal-pi-TĀ-shun	A sensation of abnormally rapid or irregular heartbeat
pitting edema	Edema that retains the impression of a finger pressed firmly into the skin (Fig. 9-21)
polyarteritis nodosa nō-DŌ-sa	Potentially fatal collagen disease causing inflammation of small visceral arteries. Symptoms depend on the organ affected
Raynaud disease rā-NŌ	A disorder characterized by abnormal constriction of peripheral vessels in the arms and legs on exposure to cold
regurgitation rē-gur-ji-TĀ-shun	A backward flow, such as the backflow of blood through a defective valve
stasis STĀ-sis	Stoppage of normal flow, as of blood or urine. Blood stasis may lead to dermatitis and ulcer formation
subacute bacterial endocarditis (SBE)	Bacterial growth in a heart or valves previously damaged by rheumatic fever
tetralogy of Fallot fal-Ō	A combination of four congenital heart abnormalities: pulmonary artery stenosis, interventricular septal defect, displacement of the aorta to the right, and right ventricular hypertrophy

(continued)

Terminology	**Supplementary Terms** (continued)
thromboangiitis obliterans	Inflammation and thrombus formation resulting in occlusion of small vessels, especially in the legs. Most common in young men and correlated with heavy smoking. Thrombotic occlusion of leg vessels may lead to gangrene of the feet. Patients show a hypersensitivity to tobacco. Also called *Buerger disease*
vegetation	Irregular bacterial outgrowths on the heart valves; associated with rheumatic fever
Wolff–Parkinson–White syndrome (WPW)	A cardiac arrhythmia consisting of tachycardia and a premature ventricular beat caused by an alternative conduction pathway

Diagnosis

cardiac catheterization	Passage of a catheter into the heart through a vessel to inject a contrast medium for imaging, diagnosis, obtaining samples, or measuring pressure
central venous pressure (CVP)	Pressure in the superior vena cava
cineangiocardiography sin-e-an-jē-ō-kar-dē-OG-ra-fē	The photographic recording of fluoroscopic images of the heart and large vessels using motion picture techniques
Computed tomography angiography (CTA)	Method for imaging the interior of arteries using computed tomography; uses less dye and is less invasive than standard angiography
Doppler echocardiography	An imaging method used to study the rate and pattern of blood flow
heart scan	Imaging of the heart after injection of a radioactive isotope. The PYP (pyrophosphate) scan using technetium-99m (^{99m}Tc) is used to test for myocardial infarction because the isotope is taken up by damaged tissue. The MUGA (multigated acquisition) scan gives information on heart function
Holter monitor	A portable device that can record up to 24 hours of an individual's ECG readings during normal activity
homocysteine hō-mō-SIS-tēn	An amino acid in the blood that at higher-than-normal levels is associated with increased risk of cardiovascular disease
phlebotomist fle-BOT-ō-mist	Technician who specializes in drawing blood
phonocardiography fō-nō-kar-dē-OG-ra-fē	Electronic recording of heart sounds
plethysmography ple-thiz-MOG-ra-fē	Measurement of changes in the size of a part based on the amount of blood contained in or passing through it. Impedance plethysmography measures changes in electrical resistance and is used in the diagnosis of deep vein thrombosis
pulmonary capillary wedge pressure (PCWP)	Pressure measured by a catheter in a branch of the pulmonary artery. It is an indirect measure of pressure in the left atrium (see Box 9-2)
Swan–Ganz catheter	A cardiac catheter with a balloon at the tip that is used to measure pulmonary arterial pressure. It is flow guided through a vein into the right side of the heart and then into the pulmonary artery
transesophageal echocardiography (TEE)	Use of an ultrasound transducer placed endoscopically into the esophagus to obtain images of the heart
triglycerides trī-GLIS-er-īdz	Simple fats that circulate in the bloodstream
ventriculography ven-trik-ū-LOG-ra-fē	X-ray study of the heart's ventricles after introduction of an opaque dye by means of a catheter

Treatment and Surgical Procedures

atherectomy ath-er-EK-tō-mē	Removal of atheromatous plaque from the lining of a vessel. May be done by open surgery or through the vessel's lumen

(continued)

The Heart and Great Vessels > Write the name of each numbered part on the corresponding line of the answer sheet.

Aortic arch
Aortic valve
Apex
Ascending aorta
Brachiocephalic artery
Endocardium
Epicardium
Inferior vena cava
Interventricular septum
Left atrium
Left AV (mitral) valve
Left pulmonary artery (branches)

Left pulmonary veins
Left subclavian artery
Left ventricle
Myocardium
Pulmonary artery
Pulmonary valve
Right atrium
Right AV (tricuspid) valve
Right pulmonary artery
   (branches)
Right pulmonary veins
Right ventricle
Superior vena cava

1. _____

2. _____

3. _____

4. _____

5. _____

6. _____

7. _____

8. _____

9. _____

10. _____

11. _____

12. _____

13. _____

14. _____

15. _____

16. _____

17. _____

18. _____

19. _____

20. _____

21. _____

22. _____

23. _____

24. _____

25. _____

Blood high in oxygen
Blood low in oxygen

Chapter Review (continued)

Location of Lymphoid Tissue > Write the name of each numbered part on the corresponding line of the answer sheet:

Appendix   Spleen
Nodes   Thymus gland
Peyer patches (in intestine)   Tonsils

1. _____

2. _____

3. _____

4. _____

5. _____

6. _____

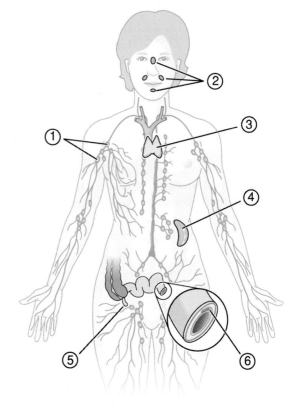

TERMINOLOGY

Matching > Match the following terms and write the appropriate letter to the left of each number:

_____ **1.** valve	**a.** vessel that empties into the right atrium
_____ **2.** vena cava	**b.** fibrous sac around the heart
_____ **3.** apex	**c.** structure that keeps fluid moving forward
_____ **4.** pericardium	**d.** central opening of a vessel
_____ **5.** lumen	**e.** lower pointed region of the heart

_____ **6.** thrombosis	**a.** ineffective quivering of muscle
_____ **7.** myocarditis	**b.** formation of a blood clot in a vessel
_____ **8.** infarction	**c.** inflammation of the heart muscle
_____ **9.** fibrillation	**d.** local deficiency of blood
_____ **10.** ischemia	**e.** local death of tissue

_____ **11.** atherosclerosis	**a.** twisted and swollen vessel
_____ **12.** varix	**b.** blockage
_____ **13.** occlusion	**c.** absence of a heartbeat
_____ **14.** asystole	**d.** localized dilatation of a vessel
_____ **15.** aneurysm	**e.** accumulation of fatty deposits

_____ **16.** VT	**a.** stroke
_____ **17.** CVA	**b.** a type of blood lipid
_____ **18.** HTN	**c.** rapid beat in the heart's lower chambers
_____ **19.** HDL	**d.** high blood pressure
_____ **20.** CABG	**e.** surgery to bypass a blocked vessel

Supplementary Terms

_____ **21.** diuretic
_____ **22.** regurgitation
_____ **23.** streptokinase
_____ **24.** atherectomy
_____ **25.** extrasystole

a. removal of plaque
b. drug that increases urinary output
c. premature contraction
d. drug used to dissolve blood clots
e. backward flow

9

Fill in the blanks:

26. Each upper receiving chamber of the heart is a(n) _____.

27. The microscopic vessels through which materials are exchanged between the blood and the tissues are the _____

_____.

28. The heart muscle is the _____.

29. The largest artery is the _____.

30. A sinus rhythm originates in the _____.

31. Blood returning to the heart from the systemic circuit enters the chamber called the _____.

32. The term *varicoid* pertains to a(n) _____.

33. The lymphoid organ in the chest is the _____.

34. A phlebotomist (*fle-BOT-ō-mist*) is one who drains blood from a(n) _____.

35. At its termination in the abdomen, the aorta divides into the right and left (see Fig. 9-5) _____

_____.

36. The large artery in the neck that supplies blood to the brain is the (see Fig. 9-5) _____.

37. The large vein that drains the lower body and empties into the heart is the (see Fig. 9-6) _____.

38. The right lymphatic duct and the thoracic duct drain into vessels called the (see Fig. 9-18) _____.

True–False > Examine the following statements. If the statement is true, write T in the first blank. If the statement is false, write F in the first blank and correct the statement by replacing the underlined word in the second blank.

39. The left AV valve is the <u>mitral</u> valve.   _____   _____

40. The <u>systemic circuit</u> pumps blood to the lungs.   _____   _____

41. An <u>artery</u> is a vessel that carries blood back to the heart.   _____   _____

42. <u>Diastole</u> is the relaxation phase of the heart cycle.   _____   _____

43. The <u>right ventricle</u> pumps blood into the aorta.   _____   _____

44. Blood returning from the lungs to the heart enters the <u>left</u> atrium.   _____   _____

45. The brachial artery supplies blood to the <u>leg</u>.   _____   _____

46. Peyer patches are in the <u>intestine</u>.   _____   _____

47. <u>Bradycardia</u> is a lower-than-average heart rate.   _____   _____

Chapter Review (continued)

Eliminations > In each of the sets below, underline the word that does not fit in with the rest and explain the reason for your choice:

48. SA node — Purkinje fibers — apex — AV node — AV bundle

_____

49. murmur — systolic — sphygmomanometer — mm Hg — diastolic

_____

50. U — S_1 — QRS — T — P

_____

51. thymus — spleen — cusp — tonsil — Peyer patches

_____

Define the following terms:

52. Avascular (*ā-VAS-kū-lar*) _____

53. Atriotomy (*ā-trē-OT-ō-mē*) _____

54. Splenectomy (*splē-NEK-tō-mē*) _____

55. Supraventricular (*sū-pra-ven-TRIK-ū-lar*) _____

56. Phlebectasis (*fleb-EK-ta-sis*) _____

Write words for the following definitions:

57. Physician who specializes in
study and treatment of the heart   _____

58. Suture (-rhaphy) of an artery   _____

59. Surgical fixation (-pexy) of the
spleen   _____

60. An instrument (-tome) for
incising a valve   _____

61. Stoppage (-stasis) of lymph flow   _____

62. Excision of a lymph node   _____

Use the root *aort/o* to write words with the following meanings:

63. Downward displacement (-ptosis)
of the aorta   _____

64. Narrowing (-stenosis) of the aorta   _____

65. Radiograph (-gram) of the aorta   _____

66. Before or in front of (pre-) the aorta   _____

Adjectives > Write the adjective form of the following words:

67. atrium   _____

68. thymus   _____

69. vein   _____

70. septum _____

71. sclerosis _____

72. spleen _____

Plurals > Write the plural form of the following words:

73. thrombus _____

74. varix _____

75. stenosis _____

76. septum _____

Write the meaning of the following abbreviations as they apply to the cardiovascular system:

77. AED _____

78. LVAD _____

79. DVT _____

80. VF _____

81. BBB _____

82. PCTA _____

Word Building > Write words for the following definitions using the word parts given.

-pathy   lymph/o   -oma   angi/o   -itis   aden/o   plasty

83. inflammation of a vessel _____

84. any disease of a lymph node _____

85. neoplasm involving the lymphatic system _____

86. plastic repair of a vessel _____

87. inflammation of a lymphatic vessel _____

88. any disease of a vessel _____

89. inflammation of a lymph node _____

90. neoplasm of a lymph node _____

91. tumor involving vessels _____

Word Analysis > Define the following words, and give the meaning of the word parts in each. Use a dictionary if necessary.

92. Endarterectomy (*end-ar-ter-EK-tō-mē*) _____

    a. end/o- _____

    b. arteri/o _____

    c. ecto- _____

    d. -tomy _____

Chapter Review (continued)

93. Telangiectasia (*tel-an-jē-ek-TĀ-zē-a*) _____

    a. tel- _____

    b. angi/o _____

    c. -ectasia _____

94. Lymphangiophlebitis (*lim-fan-jē-ō-fle-BĪ-tis*) _____

    a. lymph/o _____

    b. angi/o _____

    c. phleb/o _____

    d. -itis _____

PASSport to Success® Go to the word exercises on the Student Resources for additional review exercises.

Case Studies

▶ Case Study 9-1: PTCA and Echocardiogram

A.L., a 68-year-old woman, was admitted to the CCU with chest pain, dyspnea, diaphoresis, syncope, and nausea. She had taken three sublingual doses of nitroglycerin tablets within a 10-minute time span without relief before dialing 911. A previous stress test and thallium uptake scan suggested cardiac disease.

Her family history was significant for cardiovascular disease. Her father died at the age of 62 of an acute myocardial infarction. Her mother had bilateral carotid endarterectomies and a femoral–popliteal bypass procedure and died at the age of 72 of congestive heart failure. A.L.'s older sister died from a ruptured aortic aneurysm at the age of 65. A.L.'s ECG on admission showed tachycardia with a rate of 126 bpm with inverted T waves. A murmur was heard at S₁. Her skin color was dusky to cyanotic on her lips and fingertips. Her admitting diagnosis was possible coronary artery disease, acute myocardial infarction, and valvular disease.

Cardiac catheterization with balloon angioplasty (PTCA) was performed the next day. Significant stenosis of the left anterior descending coronary artery was shown and was treated with angioplasty and stent placement. Left ventricular function was normal.

Echocardiography, 2 days later, showed normal-sized left and enlarged right ventricular cavities. The mitral valve had normal amplitude of motion. The anterior and posterior leaflets moved in opposite directions during diastole. There was a late systolic prolapse

of the mitral leaflet at rest. The left atrium was enlarged. The impression of the study was mitral prolapse with regurgitation. Surgery was recommended.

▶ Case Study 9-2: Mitral Valve Replacement Operative Report

A.L. was transferred to the operating room, placed in a supine position, and given general endotracheal anesthesia. Her pericardium was entered longitudinally through a median sternotomy. The surgeon found that her heart was enlarged, with a dilated right ventricle. The left atrium was dilated. Preoperative transesophageal echocardiography revealed severe mitral regurgitation with severe posterior and anterior prolapse. Extracorporeal circulation was established. The aorta was cross-clamped, and cardioplegic solution (to stop the heartbeat) was given into the aortic root intermittently for myocardial protection.

The left atrium was entered via the interatrial groove on the right, exposing the mitral valve. The middle scallop of the posterior leaflet was resected. The remaining leaflets were removed to the areas of the commissures and preserved for the sliding plasty. The elongated chordae were shortened to better anchor the valve cusps. The surgeon slid the posterior leaflet across the midline and sutured it in place. A no. 30 annuloplasty ring was sutured in place with interrupted no. 2-0 Dacron suture. The valve was tested by inflating the ventricle with NSS and proved to be competent. The left atrium was closed with continuous no.

(continued)

Case Studies (continued)

4-0 Prolene suture. Air was removed from the heart. The cross-clamp was removed. Cardiac action resumed with normal sinus rhythm. After a period of cardiac recovery and attainment of normothermia, cardiopulmonary bypass was discontinued.

Protamine was given to counteract the heparin. Pacer wires were placed in the right atrium and ventricle. Silicone catheters were placed in the pleural and substernal spaces. The sternum and soft tissue wound was closed. A.L. recovered from her surgery and was discharged 6 days later.

CASE STUDY QUESTIONS

Write the word or phrase from the case study that means each of the following:

1. The state of profuse perspiration

   _____

2. Under the tongue _____

3. Test of cardiac function during physical exertion

   _____

4. Pertaining to both the heart and blood vessels

   _____

5. Excision of the inner lining along with atherosclerotic plaque from an artery (plural)

   _____

6. An abnormal heart sound _____

7. Bluish discoloration of the skin due to lack of oxygen

   _____

8. The noun form of stenotic _____

9. Between the atria _____

10. Below the sternum _____

Multiple choice. Select the best answer and write the letter of your choice to the left of each number:

_____ 11. The word transluminal means:
   a. across a wall
   b. between branches
   c. through an outer layer
   d. through a central opening
   e. across a valve

_____ 12. The term that means backflow, as of blood, is:
   a. infarction
   b. regurgitation
   c. amplitude
   d. prolapse
   e. tourniquet

_____ 13. The term for a narrowing of the bicuspid valve is:
   a. atrial prolapse
   b. pulmonic stenosis
   c. mitral stenosis
   d. mitral prolapse
   e. atrial stenosis

_____ 14. Blowout of a dilated segment of the main artery is:
   a. left anterior diastole
   b. peritoneal infarction
   c. coarctation of the aorta
   d. cardiac tamponade
   e. ruptured aortic aneurysm

_____ 15. Sternotomy is:
   a. incision into the sternum
   b. removal of the sternum
   c. narrowing of the sternum
   d. plastic repair of the sternum
   e. surgical fixation of the sternum

_____ 16. Extracorporeal circulation occurs:
   a. within the brain
   b. within the pericardium
   c. within the body
   d. in the legs
   e. outside the body

_____ 17. Protamine was given to counteract the action of the heparin. This drug action is described as:
   a. antagonistic
   b. synergy
   c. potentiating
   d. similation
   e. addiction

Abbreviations. Define the following abbreviations:

18. CCU _____

19. AMI _____

20. CAD _____

21. LAD _____

22. CHF _____

23. TEE _____

24. MVR _____

CHAPTER

10

Blood and Immunity

CHAPTER CONTENTS

OBJECTIVES

After study of this chapter you should be able to:

1. Describe the composition of the blood plasma.
2. Describe and give the functions of the three types of blood cells.
3. Label pictures of the blood cells.
4. Explain the basis of blood types.
5. Define immunity and list the possible sources of immunity.
6. Identify and use roots and suffixes pertaining to the blood and immunity.
7. Identify and use roots pertaining to blood chemistry.
8. List and describe the major disorders of the blood.
9. List and describe the major disorders of the immune system.
10. Describe the major tests used to study blood.
11. Interpret abbreviations used in blood studies.
12. Analyze several case studies involving the blood.

PRETEST

Multiple choice. Select the best answer and write the letter of your choice to the left of each number.

___ 1. Erythrocyte is the scientific name for a:

    a. white blood cell   c. red blood cell
    b. lymphocyte   d. muscle cell

___ 2. Leukocyte is the scientific name for a(n):

    a. platelet   c. white blood cell
    b. embolus   d. neuron

___ 3. Platelets, or thrombocytes, are
involved in:

    a. inflammation   c. immunity
    b. digestion   d. blood clotting

___ 4. The white blood cells active in
immunity are the:

    a. hematids   c. adipose cells
    b. lymphocytes   d. chondrocytes

___ 5. Substances produced by immune cells
that counteract microorganisms and
other foreign materials are called:

    a. antibodies   c. anticoagulants
    b. antigens   d. Rh factors

___ 6. A deficiency of hemoglobin results in
the disorder called:

    a. hypertension   c. anemia
    b. chromatosis   d. hemophilia

___ 7. A neoplastic overgrowth of white
blood cells is called:

    a. anemia   c. fibrosis
    b. leukemia   d. cystitis

10

Blood is the fluid that circulates through the vessels, bringing oxygen and nourishment to all cells and carrying away carbon dioxide and other waste products. The blood also distributes body heat and carries special substances, such as antibodies and hormones. Certain blood cells are a major component of the immune system, which protects against disease. This chapter thus includes a discussion of the immune system.

Blood

The total adult blood volume is about 5 L (5.2 quarts). Whole blood can be divided into two main components: the liquid portion, or **plasma** (55%), and **formed elements,** more commonly known as blood cells (45%) (Fig. 10-1).

Blood Plasma

Plasma is about 90% water. The remaining 10% contains nutrients, **electrolytes** (dissolved salts), gases, **albu-**min (a protein), clotting factors, antibodies, wastes, enzymes, and hormones. Laboratories test for a multitude of these substances in blood chemistry tests. The pH (relative acidity) of the plasma remains steady at about 7.4.

Blood Cells

The blood cells (Fig. 10-2) are **erythrocytes,** or red blood cells (RBCs); **leukocytes,** or white blood cells (WBCs); and **platelets,** also called **thrombocytes.** All blood cells are produced in red bone marrow. Some WBCs multiply in lymphoid tissue as well. Reference Box 10-1 summarizes the different types of blood cells; Box 10-2 discusses time-saving acronyms, such as RBC and WBC.

ERYTHROCYTES
The major function of erythrocytes is to carry oxygen to cells. This oxygen is bound to an iron-containing pigment in the cells called **hemoglobin.** Erythrocytes are small, disk-shaped cells with no nucleus (Fig. 10-3). Their

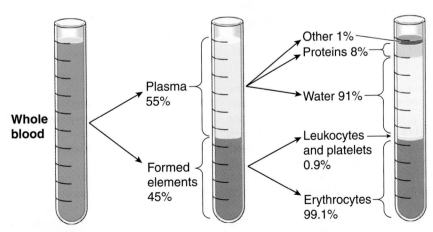

Figure 10-1 **Composition of whole blood.** Percentages show the relative proportions of the different components of plasma and formed elements.

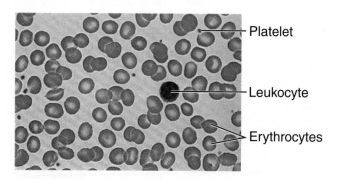

Figure 10-2 **Blood cells.** When viewed under a microscope, all three types of formed elements are visible.

Figure 10-3 **Erythrocytes (red blood cells).** The cells are seen under a scanning electron microscope, which gives a three-dimensional view.

Box 10-1   For Your Reference

Blood Cells

CELLS	NUMBER PER MICROLITER OF BLOOD	DESCRIPTION	FUNCTION
Erythrocyte (red blood cell)	5 million	Tiny (7 μm diameter), biconcave disk without nucleus (anuclear)	Carries oxygen bound to hemoglobin; also carries some carbon dioxide and buffers blood
Leukocyte (white blood cell)	5000 to 10,000	Larger than red cell with prominent nucleus that may be segmented (granulocyte) or unsegmented (agranulocyte); types vary in staining properties	Protects against pathogens. Destroys foreign matter and debris. Some are active in the immune system. Located in blood, tissues, and lymphatic system
Platelet (thrombocyte)	150,000 to 450,000	Fragment of large cell (megakaryocyte)	Hemostasis. Forms a platelet plug and starts blood clotting (coagulation)

Box 10-2   Focus on Words

Acronyms

Acronyms are abbreviations that use the first letters of the words in a name or phrase. They have become very popular because they save time and space in writing as the number and complexity of technical terms increases. Some examples that apply to studies of the blood are CBC (complete blood count) and RBC and WBC for red and white blood cells. Some other common acronyms are CNS (central nervous system), ECG (electrocardiogram) NIH (National Institutes of Health), and STI (sexually transmitted infection).

If the acronym has vowels and lends itself to pronunciation, it may be used as a word in itself, such as AIDS (acquired immunodeficiency syndrome); ELISA (enzyme-linked immunosorbent assay); *JAMA* (*Journal of the American Medical Association*); NSAID (nonsteroidal antiinflammatory drug), pronounced "en-sayd"; and CABG (coronary artery bypass graft), which inevitably becomes "cabbage." Few people even know that LASER is an acronym that means "light amplification by stimulated emission of radiation."

An acronym is usually introduced the first time a phrase appears in an article and is then used without explanation. If you have spent time searching back through an article in frustration for the meaning of an acronym, you probably wish, as does this author, that all the acronyms used and their meanings would be listed at the beginning of each article.

Figure 10-4 **Leukocytes (white blood cells).** The three types of granulocytes (*A–C*) have visible granules in the cytoplasm when stained. The two types of agranulocytes (*D* and *E*) do not show granules when stained.

concentration of about 5 million per microliter (mcL, μL) of blood makes them by far the most numerous of the blood cells. The hemoglobin that they carry averages 15 g/dL (100 mL) of blood. An RBC gradually wears out and dies in about 120 days, so these cells must be constantly replaced. Production of red cells in the bone marrow is regulated by the hormone **erythropoietin** (EPO), which is made in the kidneys.

LEUKOCYTES

WBCs all show prominent nuclei when stained (Fig. 10-4). They total about 5000 to 10,000/mcL, but their number may increase during infection. There are five types of leukocytes, which are identified by the size and appearance of the nucleus and by their staining properties:

- **Granulocytes**, or granular leukocytes, have visible granules in the cytoplasm when stained. A granulocyte has a segmented nucleus. There are three types of granulocytes, named for the kind of stain (dye) the granules take up:
  - **Neutrophils** stain weakly with both acidic and basic dyes.
  - **Eosinophils** stain strongly with acidic dyes.
  - **Basophils** stain strongly with basic dyes.
- **Agranulocytes** do not show visible granules when stained. An agranulocyte's nucleus is large and either round or curved. There are two types of agranulocytes:
  - **Lymphocytes** are the smaller agranulocytes.
  - **Monocytes** are the largest of all the WBCs.

WBCs protect against foreign substances. Some engulf foreign material by the process of **phagocytosis** (see Fig. 6-5); others function in the immune system. In diagnosis it is important to know not only the total number of leukocytes but also the relative number of each type, because these numbers can change in different disease conditions. Reference Box 10-3 gives the relative percentage and functions of the different white cell types.

The most numerous WBCs, neutrophils, are called *polymorphs* because of their various-shaped nuclei. They are also referred to as *segs*, *polys*, or *PMNs* (*poly*morphonuclear leukocytes). A **band cell**, also called a *stab cell*, is an immature neutrophil with a solid curved nucleus (Fig. 10-5). Large numbers of band cells in the blood indicate an active infection.

PLATELETS

The blood platelets (thrombocytes) are not complete cells, but fragments of large cells named **megakaryocytes**, which form in bone marrow (Fig. 10-6). They number from 200,000 to 400,000/mcL of blood. Platelets are important in **hemostasis**, the prevention of blood loss, which includes the process of blood clotting, or **coagulation**.

 PASSport to Success® See the animation *Hemostasis* on the Student Resources.

When a vessel is injured, platelets stick together to form a plug at the site. Substances released from the platelets and from damaged tissue then interact with clotting factors in the plasma to produce a wound-sealing clot.

Box 10-3   For Your Reference

White Blood Cells (Leukocytes)

TYPE OF CELL	RELATIVE PERCENTAGE (ADULT)	FUNCTION
GRANULOCYTES		
neutrophils NŪ-trō-fils	54% to 62%	phagocytosis
eosinophils ē-ō-SIN-ō-fils	1% to 3%	allergic reactions; defense against parasites
basophils BĀ-sō-fils	less than 1%	allergic reactions
AGRANULOCYTES		
lymphocytes LIM-fō-sītz	25% to 38%	immunity (T cells and B cells)
monocytes MON-ō-sītz	3% to 7%	phagocytosis

Clotting factors are inactive in the blood until an injury occurs. To protect against unwanted clot formation, 12 factors must interact before blood coagulates. The final reaction is the conversion of **fibrinogen** to threads of **fibrin** that trap blood cells and plasma to produce the clot (Fig. 10-7). The plasma that remains after blood coagulates is **serum**.

Blood Types

Genetically inherited proteins on the surface of RBCs determine blood type. More than 20 groups of these proteins have now been identified, but the most familiar are the ABO and Rh blood groups. The ABO system includes types A, B, AB, and O. The Rh types are Rh-positive (Rh^+) and Rh-negative (Rh^-).

A Mature neutrophil

B Band cell (immature neutrophil)

Figure 10-5 **Band cell.** (A) A mature neutrophil. (B) A band cell, or stab cell, is an immature neutrophil with a thick curved nucleus.

A Platelets

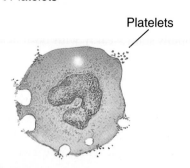

B Megakaryocyte

Figure 10-6 **Platelets (thrombocytes).** (A) Platelets seen in a blood smear under the microscope. (B) A megakaryocyte releases platelets.

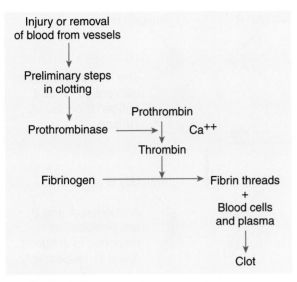

Figure 10-7 **Main steps in the formation of a blood clot.**

In giving blood transfusions, it is important to use blood that is the same type as the recipient's blood or a type to which the recipient will not have an immune reaction, as described below. Compatible blood types are determined by **cross-matching** (Fig. 10-8). When a blood sample is mixed separately with different antisera, its red cells will agglutinate (clump) with the antiserum that corresponds to its blood type.

Whole blood may be used to replace a large volume of blood lost, but in most cases requiring blood transfusion, a blood fraction such as packed red cells, platelets, plasma, or specific clotting factors is administered.

Immunity

Immunity is protection against disease. It includes defenses against harmful microorganisms, their products, or any other foreign substance. These defenses may be inborn or acquired during life (Fig. 10-9).

Innate Immunity

Innate defense mechanisms are inborn; they are based on the genetic makeup of the individual. Most of these defenses are physical mechanisms and are nonspecific (i.e., they protect against any intruder), and include:

- Unbroken skin, which acts as a barrier.
- Cilia, tiny cell projections that sweep impurities out of the body, as in the respiratory tract.
- Mucus that traps foreign material.

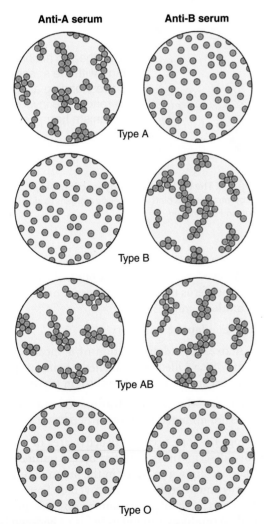

Figure 10-8 **Blood typing.** Labels at the top of each column denote the kind of antiserum added to the blood samples. Anti-A serum agglutinates red cells in type A blood, but anti-B serum does not. Anti-B serum agglutinates red cells in type B blood, but anti-A serum does not. Both sera agglutinate type AB blood cells, and neither serum agglutinates type O blood.

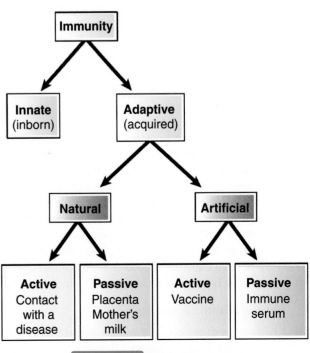

Figure 10-9 **Types of immunity.**

- Bactericidal body secretions, as found in tears, the skin, the digestive tract, and the reproductive tract.

- Reflexes, such as coughing and sneezing, which expel impurities.

- Lymphoid tissue, which filters impurities from blood and lymph, as described in Chapter 9.

- Phagocytes—cells that attack, ingest, and destroy foreign organisms.

Adaptive Immunity

Adaptive immunity is acquired during life and is specific, which means that it is directed toward a particular disease organism or other foreign substance. Thus, protection against measles, for example, will not protect against chickenpox or any other disease.

The specific immune response involves complex interactions between components of the lymphatic system and the blood. Any foreign particle, but mainly proteins, may act as an **antigen**, a substance that provokes an immune response. This response comes from two types of lymphocytes that circulate in the blood and lymphatic system:

- **T cells** (T lymphocytes) mature in the thymus gland. They are capable of attacking a foreign cell directly, producing *cell-mediated immunity*. **Macrophages**, descendants of monocytes, are important in the function of T cells. Macrophages take in and process foreign antigens. A T cell is activated when it contacts an antigen on a macrophage's surface in combination with some of the body's own proteins.

- **B cells** (B lymphocytes) mature in bone marrow. When they meet a foreign antigen, they multiply rapidly and mature into **plasma cells**. These cells produce **antibodies**, also called **immunoglobulins (Ig)**, that inactivate antigens (Fig. 10-10). Antibodies remain in the blood, often providing long-term immunity to the specific organism against which they were formed. Antibody-based immunity is referred to as *humoral immunity*.

TYPES OF ADAPTIVE IMMUNITY

Adaptive immunity may be acquired either naturally or artificially (see Fig. 10-9). In addition, each avenue for acquiring immunity may be either active or passive. In active immunity, a person makes his or her own antibodies in response to contact with an antigen. In passive immunity, an antibody, known as an immune serum, is transferred from an outside source. Immune sera may come from other people or from immunized animals. The portion of the blood plasma that contains antibodies is the **gamma globulin** fraction. The types of adaptive immunity are:

- Natural adaptive immunity

  - Active—from contact with a disease organism or other foreign antigen.

Antigen A   Antigen B

The invading organism with antigen A and antigen B on its cell surface.

Antibody A   Antibody B

Antibodies A and B are produced in response to antigens A and B, respectively.

Antibody bound to antigen

The specific antibodies bind with the specific corresponding antigens to render the invading organism harmless.

Figure 10-10 **The antigen–antibody reaction.** Antibodies produced by immune cells bind with specific antigens to aid in their inactivation and elimination.

- Passive—by transfer of antibodies from a mother to her fetus through the placenta or through the mother's milk.

- Artificial adaptive immunity

  - Active—by administration of a vaccine, which may be a killed or weakened organism, part of an organism, or an altered toxin (toxoid).

  - Passive—by administration of an immune serum obtained from other people or animals.

Immunology has long been a very active area of research. The above description is only the barest outline of the events that are known to occur in the immune response, and there is much still to be discovered. Some of the areas of research include **autoimmune diseases**, in which an individual produces antibodies to his or her own body tissues; hereditary and acquired immunodeficiency diseases; the relationship between cancer and immunity; and the development of techniques for avoiding rejection of transplanted tissue.

Terminology | Key Terms

Normal Structure and Function

Term	Definition
agranulocyte Ā-gran-ū-lō-sīt	A white blood cell that does not have visible granules in its cytoplasm. Agranulocytes include lymphocytes and monocytes (see Fig. 10-4)
albumin al-BŪ-min	A simple protein found in blood plasma
antibody AN-ti-bod-ē	A protein produced in response to, and interacting specifically with, an antigen
antigen AN-ti-jen	A substance that induces the formation of an antibody
B cell	A lymphocyte that matures in lymphoid tissue and is active in producing antibodies; B lymphocyte (LIM-fō-sīt)
band cell	An immature neutrophil with a nucleus in the shape of a band; also called a stab cell. Band cell counts are used to trace infections and other diseases (see Fig. 10-5)
basophil BĀ-sō-fil	A granular leukocyte that stains strongly with basic dyes; active in allergic reactions
blood blud	The fluid that circulates in the cardiovascular system (roots: hem/o, hemat/o)
coagulation kō-ag-ū-LĀ-shun	Blood clotting
cross-matching	Testing the compatibility of donor and recipient blood in preparation for a transfusion. Donor red cells are mixed with recipient serum, and red cells of the recipient are mixed with donor serum to look for an immunologic reaction. Similar tests are done on tissues before transplantation
electrolyte ē-LEK-trō-līt	A substance that separates into charged particles (ions) in solution; a salt. Term also applied to ions in body fluids
eosinophil ē-ō-SIN-ō-fil	A granular leukocyte that stains strongly with acidic dyes; active in allergic reactions and defense against parasites
erythrocyte e-RITH-rō-sīt	A red blood cell (roots: erythr/o, erythrocyt/o) (see Figs. 10-2 and 10-3)
erythropoietin (EPO) e-rith-rō-POY-e-tin	A hormone produced in the kidneys that stimulates red blood cell production in the bone marrow. This hormone is now made by genetic engineering for clinical use
fibrin FĪ-brin	The protein that forms a clot in the blood coagulation process
fibrinogen fī-BRIN-ō-jen	The inactive precursor of fibrin
formed elements	The cellular components of blood
gamma globulin GLOB-ū-lin	The fraction of the blood plasma that contains antibodies; given for passive transfer of immunity
granulocyte GRAN-ū-lō-sīt	A white blood cell that has visible granules in its cytoplasm. Granulocytes include neutrophils, basophils, and eosinophils (see Fig. 10-4)
hemoglobin (Hb, Hgb) HĒ-mō-glō-bin	The iron-containing pigment in red blood cells that transports oxygen
hemostasis hē-mō-STĀ-sis	The stoppage of bleeding
immunity	The state of being protected against a disease (root: immun/o)
immunoglobulin (Ig) im-ū-nō-GLOB-ū-lin	An antibody. Immunoglobulins fall into five classes, each abbreviated with a capital letter: IgG, IgM, IgA, IgD, IgE

(continued)

Terminology	Key Terms *(continued)*

Normal Structure and Function

leukocyte LŪ-kō-sīt	A white blood cell (roots: *leuk/o, leukocyt/o*)
lymphocyte LIM-fō-sīt	An agranular leukocyte active in immunity (T and B cells); found in both the blood and in lymphoid tissue (roots: *lymph/o, lymphocyt/o*)
megakaryocyte meg-a-KAR-ē-ō-sīt	A large bone marrow cell that fragments to release platelets
macrophage MAK-rō-faj	A phagocytic cell derived from a monocyte; usually located within the tissues. Macrophages process antigens for T cells
monocyte MON-ō-sīt	An agranular phagocytic leukocyte
neutrophil NŪ-trō-fil	A granular leukocyte that stains weakly with both acidic and basic dyes. The most numerous of the white blood cells. A type of phagocyte
phagocytosis fag-ō-sī-TŌ-sis	The engulfing of foreign material by white blood cells
plasma PLAZ-ma	The liquid portion of the blood
plasma cell	A mature form of a B cell that produces antibodies
platelet PLĀT-let	A formed element of the blood that is active in hemostasis; a thrombocyte (root: *thrombocyt/o*)
serum SĒR-um	The fraction of the plasma that remains after blood coagulation; it is the equivalent of plasma without its clotting factors (plural: sera, serums)
T cell	A lymphocyte that matures in the thymus gland and attacks foreign cells directly; T lymphocyte
thrombocyte THROM-bō-sīt	A blood platelet (root: *thrombocyt/o*)

PASSport to Success® — Go to the pronunciation glossary on the Student Resources to hear these words pronounced.

Word Parts Pertaining to Blood and Immunity

See Tables 10-1 to 10-3.

Table 10-1	Suffixes for Blood

Suffix	Meaning	Example	Definition of Example
-emia,* -hemia	condition of blood	polycythemia pol-ē-sī-THĒ-mē-a	increase of cells (cyt) in the blood
-penia	decrease in, deficiency of	cytopenia sī-tō-PĒ-nē-a	deficiency of cells in the blood
-poiesis	formation, production	hemopoiesis hē-mō-poy-Ē-sis	production of blood cells

*A shortened form of the root hem plus the suffix -ia.

EXERCISE **10-1**

Define the following terms:

1. hyperalbuminemia (*hī-per-al-bū-mi-NĒ-mē-a*) _____ excess albumin in the blood _____

2. hypoproteinemia (*hī-pō-prō-tēn-Ē-mē-a*) _____

3. leukocytopenia (*lū-kō-sī-tō-PĒ-nē-a*) _____

4. erythropoiesis (*e-rith-rō-poy-Ē-sis*) _____

5. toxemia (*tok-SĒ-mē-a*) _____

6. bacteremia (*bak-ter-Ē-mē-a*) _____

7. thrombocytopenia (*throm-bō-sī-tō-PĒ-nē-a*) _____

Use the suffix *-emia* to write words for the following definitions:

8. Presence of pus in the blood _____

9. Presence of viruses in the blood _____

10. Presence of excess white cells (leuk/o) in the blood _____

Many of the words relating to blood cells can be formed either with or without including the root *cyt/o*, as in erythropenia or erythrocytopenia, leukopoiesis or leukocytopoiesis. The remaining types of blood cells are designated by easily recognized roots such as *agranulocyt/o*, *monocyt/o*, *granul/o*, and so on (see Table 10-2).

Table 10-2   Roots for Blood and Immunity

Root	Meaning	Example	Definition of Example
myel/o	bone marrow	myelogenous *mī-e-LOJ-e-nus*	originating in bone marrow
hem/o, hemat/o	blood	hemopathy *hē-MOP-a-thē*	any disorder of blood
erythr/o, erythrocyt/o	red blood cell	erythroblast *e-RITH-rō-blast*	immature red blood cell
leuk/o, leukocyt/o	white blood cell	leukocytosis *lū-kō-sī-TŌ-sis*	increase in the number of leukocytes in the blood
lymph/o, lymphocyt/o	lymphocyte	lymphocytic *lim-fō-SĪT-ik*	pertaining to lymphocytes
thromb/o	blood clot	thrombolytic *throm-bō-LIT-ik*	dissolving a blood clot
thrombocyt/o	platelet, thrombocyte	thrombopoiesis *throm-bō-poy-Ē-sis*	formation of platelets
immun/o	immunity, immune system	immunization *im-ū-ni-ZĀ-shun*	production of immunity

EXERCISE **10-2**

Identify and define the root in the following words:

	Root	Meaning of Root
1. hematology (*hē-ma-TOL-ō-jē*)	_____	_____
2. panmyeloid (*pan-MĬ-e-loyd*)	_____	_____
3. prothrombin (*prō-THROM-bin*)	_____	_____
4. preimmunization (*prē-im-ū-ni-ZĀ-shun*)	_____	_____
5. ischemia (*is-KĒ-mē-a*)	_____	_____

Fill in the blanks:

6. Hemorrhage is a profuse flow (-rhage) of _____.

7. Myelofibrosis (*mi-e-lō-fĭ-BRO-sis*) is formation of fibrous tissue in _____.

8. Erythroclasis (*er-i-THROK-la-sis*) is the breaking (-clasis) of _____.

9. An immunocyte (*im-ū-nō-SĪT*) is a cell active in _____.

10. The term thrombocythemia (*throm-bō-sī-THĒ-mē-a*) refers to a blood increase in the number of _____.

11. Leukopoiesis (*lū-kō-poy-Ē-sis*) refers to the production of _____.

12. A hemocytometer (*hē-mō-sī-TOM-e-ter*) is a device for counting _____.

13. Lymphokines (*LIM-fō-kīnz*) are chemicals active in immunity that are produced by _____.

14. A hematoma (*hē-ma-TŌ-ma*) is a swelling caused by collection of _____.

Write a word for the following definitions:

15. Immature lymphocyte _____

16. Tumor of bone marrow _____

17. Decrease in red blood cells _____

18. Dissolving (-lysis) of a blood clot _____

19. Formation (-poiesis) of bone marrow _____

The suffix -*osis* added to a root for a type of cell means an increase in that type of cell in the blood. Use this suffix to write a word that means each of the following:

20. Increase in granulocytes in the blood _____ granulocytosis _____

21. Increase in lymphocytes in the blood _____

22. Increase in red blood cells _____

23. Increase in monocytes in the blood _____

24. Increase in platelets in the blood _____

Table 10-3	Roots for Chemistry		
Root	**Meaning**	**Example**	**Definition of Example**
azot/o	nitrogenous compounds	azoturia *āz-ō-TŪ-rē-a*	increased nitrogenous compounds in the urine (-uria)
calc/i	calcium (symbol Ca)	calcification *kal-si-fi-KĀ-shun*	deposition of calcium salts
ferr/o, ferr/i	iron (symbol Fe)	ferrous *FER-ous*	pertaining to or containing iron
sider/o	iron	sideroderma *sid-er-ō-DER-ma*	deposition of iron into the skin
kali	potassium (symbol K)	hyperkalemia* *hī-per-ka-LĒ-mē-a*	excess of potassium in the blood
natri	sodium (symbol Na)	natriuresis *nā-trē-ū-RĒ-sis*	excretion of sodium in the urine (ur/o)
ox/y	oxygen (symbol O)	hypoxia *hī-POK-sē-a*	deficiency of oxygen in the tissues

*The i in the root is dropped.

10

EXERCISE 10-3

Fill in the blanks:

1. A sideroblast (*SID-er-ō-blast*) is an immature cell containing _____.

2. The term *hypokalemia* (*hī-pō-ka-LĒ-mē-a*) refers to a blood deficiency of _____.

3. The bacterial species *Azotobacter* is named for its ability to metabolize _____.

4. Hypoxemia (*hī-pok-SĒ-mē-a*) is a blood deficiency of _____.

5. Ferritin (*FER-i-tin*) is a compound that contains _____.

6. A calcareous (*kal-KAR-ē-us*) substance contains _____.

Use the suffix *-emia* to form words with the following meanings:

7. Presence of potassium in the blood _____

8. Presence of nitrogenous compounds in the blood _____

9. Presence of sodium in the blood _____

10. Presence of calcium in the blood _____

Clinical Aspects of Blood

Anemia

Anemia is defined as an abnormally low amount of hemoglobin in the blood. Anemia may result from too few RBCs or from cells that are too small (microcytic) or have too little hemoglobin (hypochromic). Key tests in diagnosing anemia are blood counts, mean corpuscular volume (MCV), and mean corpuscular hemoglobin concentration (MCHC). (Reference Box 10-4 describes these and other blood tests. Box 10-5 has information on careers in hematology.)

The general symptoms of anemia include fatigue, shortness of breath, heart palpitations, pallor, and irritability. There are many different types of anemia, some

Box 10-4   For Your Reference

Common Blood Tests

TEST	ABBREVIATION	DESCRIPTION
red blood cell count	RBC	number of red blood cells per microliter of blood
white blood cell count	WBC	number of white blood cells per microliter of blood
differential count	Diff	relative percentage of the different types of leukocytes
hematocrit (Fig. 10-11)	Ht, Hct, crit	relative percentage of packed red cells in a given volume of blood
packed cell volume	PCV	hematocrit
hemoglobin	Hb, Hgb	amount of hemoglobin in g/dL (100 mL) of blood
mean corpuscular volume	MCV	volume of an average red cell
mean corpuscular hemoglobin	MCH	average weight of hemoglobin in red cells
mean corpuscular hemoglobin concentration	MCHC	average concentration of hemoglobin in red blood cells
erythrocyte sedimentation rate	ESR	rate of erythrocyte settling per unit of time; used to detect infection or inflammation
complete blood count	CBC	series of tests including cell counts, hematocrit, hemoglobin, and cell volume measurements

of which are caused by faulty production of red cells and others by loss or destruction of red cells.

ANEMIA DUE TO IMPAIRED PRODUCTION OF RED CELLS

- **Aplastic anemia** results from bone marrow destruction and affects all blood cells (pancytopenia). It may be caused by drugs, toxins, viruses, radiation, or bone marrow cancer. Aplastic anemia has a high mortality rate but has been treated successfully with bone marrow transplantation.

- **Nutritional anemia** may result from a deficiency of vitamin B_{12} or of folic acid, B vitamins needed for RBC development. Most commonly, it is caused by

Box 10-5   Health Professions

Careers in Hematology

Hematologists are physicians and other scientists who specialize in the study of blood and blood diseases. In medical practice, hematology is often combined with the study and treatment of blood cancers as the specialty hematology–oncology.

A hematology technician is usually a medical laboratory technician who specializes in blood studies. He or she may work in a clinical laboratory, blood banking, industry, or academic research. The job requires a BS or MS in biological science plus training in laboratory procedures, blood pathology, and testing methods. Hematology technicians perform a full range of blood studies for diagnosis of infections, allergies, anemia, leukemia, and other blood diseases. They also run tests to monitor anticoagulant therapy. They must be able to operate and maintain automated equipment used to analyze blood. In some cases, they may also draw blood or administer blood transfusions.

A phlebotomist draws blood for testing, transfusions, or research. The blood is often drawn from a vein (venipuncture), but may also be drawn from arteries and by skin puncture. Phlebotomists must be trained in sterile techniques and safety precautions to prevent the spread of infectious diseases. They must take specimens without harming the patient or interfering with medical care and must transport specimens to the proper laboratory. Educational requirements vary among states. Often, in-house training with certification by the National Phlebotomy Association is acceptable (www. nationalphlebotomy.org). Phlebotomists work in hospitals, laboratories, private physicians' offices, clinics, and blood banks.

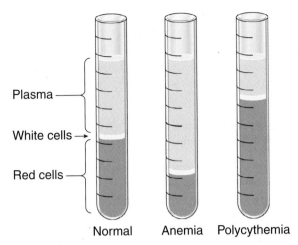

Plasma

White cells

Red cells

Normal   Anemia   Polycythemia

Figure 10-11 **Hematocrit.** The tube on the left shows a normal hematocrit. The middle tube shows that the percentage of red blood cells is low, indicating anemia. The tube on the right shows an excessively high percentage of red blood cells, as seen in polycythemia.

a deficiency of iron, needed to make hemoglobin (Fig. 10-12). Folic acid deficiency commonly appears in those with poor diet, in pregnant and lactating women, and in those who abuse alcohol. Iron-deficiency anemia results from poor diet, poor iron absorption, or blood loss. Both folic acid deficiency and iron deficiency respond to dietary supplementation.

- **Pernicious anemia** is a specific form of B_{12} deficiency. It results from the lack of **intrinsic factor** (IF), a substance produced in the stomach that aids in the intestinal absorption of B_{12}. Pernicious anemia must be treated with regular B_{12} injections.

- In **sideroblastic anemia**, there is adequate iron available, but the iron is not used properly to manufacture hemoglobin. This disorder may be hereditary or acquired, as by exposure to toxins or drug.

It may also be secondary to another disease. The excess iron precipitates out in immature red cells (normoblasts).

ANEMIA DUE TO LOSS OR DESTRUCTION OF RED CELLS

- **Hemorrhagic anemia** results from blood loss. This may be a sudden loss, as from injury, or loss from chronic internal bleeding, as from the digestive tract in cases of ulcers or cancer.

- **Thalassemia** is a hereditary disease that appears mostly in Mediterranean populations. A genetic mutation causes abnormal hemoglobin production and **hemolysis** (destruction) of red cells. Thalassemia is designated as α (alpha) or β (beta), according to the part of the molecule affected. Severe β thalassemia is also called **Cooley anemia** or *thalassemia major.*

- In **sickle cell anemia**, a mutation alters the hemoglobin molecule so that it precipitates when it gives up oxygen, distorting the RBCs into a crescent shape (Fig. 10-13). The altered cells block small blood vessels and deprive tissues of oxygen, an episode termed *sickle cell crisis.* The misshapen cells are also readily destroyed (hemolyzed). The disease predominates in black populations. Genetic carriers of the defect, those with one normal and one abnormal gene, show *sickle cell trait.* They usually have no symptoms, except when oxygen is low, such as at high altitudes. They can, however, pass the defective gene to offspring. Sickle cell anemia, as well as many other genetic diseases, can be diagnosed in carriers and in the fetus before birth.

Reticulocyte counts are useful in diagnosing the causes of anemia. Reticulocytes are immature RBCs that

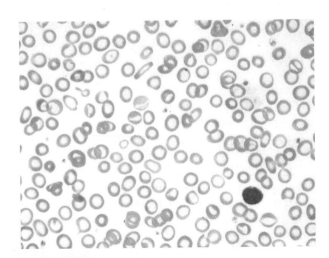

Figure 10-12 **Iron-deficiency anemia.** Red cells are small (microcytic) and are lacking in hemoglobin (hypochromic).

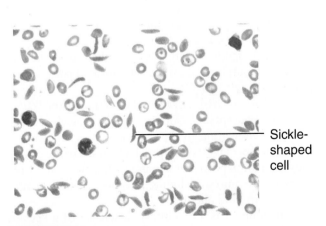

Sickle-shaped cell

Figure 10-13 **Sickle cell anemia.** A blood smear shows sickled red cells, which take on a crescent shape when they give up oxygen.

Box 10-6   Clinical Perspectives

Use of Reticulocytes in Diagnosis

As erythrocytes mature in the red bone marrow, they go through a series of stages in which they lose their nucleus and most other organelles, maximizing the space available for hemoglobin. In one of the last stages of development, small numbers of ribosomes and some rough endoplasmic reticulum remain in the cell and appear as a network, or reticulum, when stained. Cells at this stage are called *reticulocytes*. Reticulocytes leave the red bone marrow and enter the bloodstream, where they become fully mature erythrocytes in about 24 to 48 hours. The average number of red cells maturing through the reticulocyte stage at any given time is about 1% to 2%. Changes in these numbers can be used in diagnosing certain blood disorders.

When erythrocytes are lost or destroyed, as from chronic bleeding or some form of hemolytic anemia, red cell production is "stepped up" to compensate for the loss. Greater numbers of reticulocytes are then released into the blood before reaching full maturity, and counts increase to above normal. On the other hand, a decrease in the number of circulating

reticulocytes suggests a problem with red cell production, as in cases of deficiency anemias or suppression of bone marrow activity.

Reticulocytes. Erythrocytes show a network in a late stage of development.

---

normally appear as a small percentage of the total erythrocytes. An increase in the reticulocyte count indicates increased red cell formation, as in response to hemorrhage or cell destruction. A decrease in reticulocytes indicates a failure in red cell production, as caused by nutritional deficiency or aplastic anemia (see Box 10-6).

Coagulation Disorders

The most common cause of coagulation problems is a deficiency in the number of circulating platelets, a condition termed **thrombocytopenia**. Possible causes include aplastic anemia, infections, bone marrow cancer, and agents that destroy bone marrow, such as x-rays or certain drugs. This disorder results in bleeding into the skin and mucous membranes, variously described as **petechiae** (pinpoint spots), **ecchymoses** (bruises), and **purpura** (purple lesions).

In **disseminated intravascular coagulation (DIC)**, there is widespread clotting in the vessels, which obstructs circulation to the tissues. This is followed by diffuse hemorrhages as clotting factors are removed and the coagulation process is impaired. DIC may result from a variety of causes, including infection, cancer, hemorrhage, injury, and **allergy**.

Hemophilia is a hereditary deficiency of a specific clotting factor. It is a genetically sex-linked disease that is passed from mother to son. There is bleeding into the

tissues, especially into the joints (hemarthrosis). Hemophilia must be treated with transfusions of the necessary clotting factor.

Reference Box 10-7 lists tests done for these and other coagulation disorders.

Neoplasms

Leukemia is a neoplasm of WBCs. The rapidly dividing but incompetent white cells accumulate in the tissues and crowd out the other blood cells. The symptoms of leukemia include anemia, fatigue, easy bleeding, **splenomegaly**, and sometimes hepatomegaly (enlargement of the liver). The causes of leukemia are unknown but may include exposure to radiation or harmful chemicals, hereditary factors, and perhaps viral infection.

The two main categories of leukemia are determined by origin and the cells involved:

- Myelogenous leukemia originates in the bone marrow and involves mainly the granular leukocytes.

- Lymphocytic leukemia affects B cells and the lymphatic system, causing **lymphadenopathy** (lymph node disease) and adverse effects on the immune system.

Leukemias are further differentiated as acute or chronic based on clinical progress. Acute leukemia is the most

Box 10-7 | For Your Reference

Coagulation Tests

TEST	ABBREVIATION	DESCRIPTION
Activated partial thromboplastin time	APTT	Measures time required for clot formation; used to evaluate clotting factors and monitor heparin therapy
Bleeding time	BT	Measures capacity of platelets to stop bleeding after a standard skin incision
Partial thromboplastin time	PTT	Evaluates clotting factors; similar to APTT, but less sensitive
Prothrombin time	PT, Pro Time	Indirectly measures prothrombin; used to monitor anticoagulant therapy; also called Quick test
Thrombin time (thrombin clotting time)	TT (TCT)	Measures how quickly a clot forms

10

common form of cancer in young children. The acute forms are:

- Acute myeloblastic (myelogenous) leukemia (AML). The prognosis in AML is poor for both children and adults.

- Acute lymphoblastic (lymphocytic) leukemia (ALL). With treatment, the ALL remission rate is high.

The chronic forms of leukemia are:

- Chronic granulocytic leukemia, also called chronic myelogenous leukemia, affects young to middle-aged adults. Most cases show the **Philadelphia chromosome (Ph)**, an inherited anomaly in which part of chromosome 22 shifts to chromosome 9.

- Chronic lymphocytic leukemia (CLL), appears mostly in the elderly and is the most slowly growing form of the disease (Fig. 10-14).

Leukemia treatment includes chemotherapy, radiation therapy, and bone marrow transplantation. One advance in transplantation is the use of umbilical cord blood to replace blood-forming cells in bone marrow. This blood is more readily available than bone marrow and does not have to match as closely to avoid rejection.

Hodgkin disease is a disease of the lymphatic system that may spread to other tissues. It begins with enlarged but painless lymph nodes in the cervical (neck) region and then progresses to other nodes. A feature of Hodgkin disease is giant cells in the lymph nodes called **Reed–Sternberg cells** (Fig. 10-15). Symptoms include fever, night sweats, weight loss, and skin itching (pruritus). Persons of any age may be affected, but the disease predominates in young adults and those over age 50. Most cases can be cured with radiation and chemotherapy.

Non-Hodgkin lymphoma (NHL) is also a malignant enlargement of lymph nodes but does not show

Figure 10-14 **Chronic lymphocytic leukemia.** A blood smear shows an above-normal number of lymphocytes.

Figure 10-15 **Reed–Sternberg cell.** These cells are typical of Hodgkin disease.

Reed–Sternberg cells. It is more common than Hodgkin disease and has a higher mortality rate. Cases vary in severity and prognosis. It is most prevalent in the older adult population and in those with AIDS and other forms of immunodeficiency. NHL involves the T or B lymphocytes, and some cases may be related to infection with certain viruses. It requires systemic chemotherapy and, sometimes, bone marrow transplantation.

Multiple myeloma is a cancer of the blood-forming cells in bone marrow, mainly the plasma cells that produce antibodies. The disease causes anemia, bone pain, and bone weakening. Patients have a greater susceptibility to infection because of immunodeficiency. Abnormally high levels of calcium and protein in the blood often lead to kidney failure. Multiple myeloma is treated with radiation and chemotherapy, but the prognosis is generally poor.

Clinical Aspects of Immunity

Hypersensitivity

Hypersensitivity is a harmful overreaction of the immune system, commonly known as allergy. In cases of allergy, a person is more sensitive to a particular antigen than the average individual. Common **allergens** are pollen, animal dander, dust, and foods, but there are many more. A seasonal allergy to inhaled pollens is commonly called "hay fever." Responses may include itching, redness, or tearing of the eyes (conjunctivitis), skin rash, asthma, runny nose (rhinitis), sneezing, **urticaria** (hives), and **angioedema**, a reaction similar to hives but involving deeper layers of tissue.

An **anaphylactic reaction** is a severe generalized allergic response that can lead rapidly to death as a result of shock and respiratory distress. It must be treated by immediate administration of **epinephrine (adrenaline)** and maintenance of open airways. Oxygen, antihistamines, and corticosteroids may also be given. Common causes of anaphylaxis are drugs, especially penicillin and other antibiotics, vaccines, diagnostic chemicals, foods, and insect venom.

A **delayed hypersensitivity reaction** involves T cells and takes at least 12 hours to develop. A common example is the reaction to contact with plant irritants such as those of poison ivy and poison oak.

Immunodeficiency

The term **immunodeficiency** refers to any failure in the immune system. This may be congenital (present at birth) or acquired and may involve any components of the system. The deficiency may vary in severity but is always evidenced by an increased susceptibility to disease.

AIDS (acquired immunodeficiency syndrome) is acquired by infection with **HIV (human immunodeficiency virus)**, which attacks certain T cells. These cells have a specific surface attachment site, the CD4 receptor, for the virus. HIV is spread by sexual contact, use of contaminated needles, blood transfusions, and passage from an infected mother to a fetus. It leaves the host susceptible to opportunistic infections such as pneumonia caused by the fungus *Pneumocystis jirovicii*; thrush, an oral fungal infection caused by *Candida albicans*; and infection with *Cryptosporidium*, a protozoon that causes cramps and diarrhea. It also predisposes to **Kaposi sarcoma**, a once-rare form of skin cancer. AIDS may also induce autoimmunity or attack the nervous system.

AIDS is diagnosed and monitored by **CD4+ T lymphocyte counts**, a measure of cells with the HIV receptor. A count of less than 200/mcL of blood signifies severe immunodeficiency. HIV antibody levels and direct viral blood counts are also used to track the disease's course. At present there is no vaccine or cure for AIDS, but drugs can delay its progress.

Autoimmune Diseases

A disorder that results from an immune response to one's own tissues is classified as an autoimmune disease. The cause may be a failure in the immune system or a reaction to body cells that have been slightly altered by mutation or disease. The list of diseases that are believed to be caused, at least in part, by autoimmunity is long. Some, such as **systemic lupus erythematosus** (SLE), **systemic sclerosis** (scleroderma), and **Sjögren syndrome**, affect tissues in multiple systems. Others target more specific organs or systems. Examples are pernicious anemia, rheumatoid arthritis, Graves disease (of the thyroid), myasthenia gravis (a muscle disease), fibromyalgia syndrome (a musculoskeletal disorder), rheumatic heart disease, and glomerulonephritis (a kidney disease). These diseases are discussed in more detail in other chapters.

Terminology	Key Terms

Disorders

AIDS (acquired immunodeficiency syndrome)	Immune system failure caused by infection with HIV (human immunodeficiency virus). The virus infects certain T cells and thus interferes with immunity
allergen AL-er-jen	A substance that causes an allergic response
allergy AL-er-jē	Hypersensitivity
anaphylactic reaction an-a-fi-LAK-tik	An exaggerated allergic reaction to a foreign substance (root *phylaxis* means "protection"). It may lead to death caused by circulatory collapse, and respiratory distress if untreated. Also called *anaphylaxis*
anemia a-NĒ-mē-a	A deficiency in the amount of hemoglobin in the blood; may result from blood loss, malnutrition, a hereditary defect, environmental factors, and other causes (see Figs. 10-12 and 10-13)
angioedema an-jē-ō-e-DĒ-ma	A localized edema with large hives (wheals) similar to urticaria but involving deeper layers of the skin and subcutaneous tissue
aplastic anemia ā-PLAS-tik	Anemia caused by bone marrow failure resulting in deficient blood cell production, especially of red cells; pancytopenia
autoimmune disease aw-tō-i-MŪN	A condition in which the immune system produces antibodies against an individual's own tissues (prefix *auto* means "self")
Cooley anemia	A form of thalassemia (hereditary anemia) which affects production of the B (beta) hemoglobin chain; thalassemia major
delayed hypersensitivity reaction	An allergic reaction involving T cells that takes at least 12 hours to develop. Examples are various types of contact dermatitis, such as poison ivy or poison oak; the tuberculin reaction (test for TB); and rejections of transplanted tissue
disseminated intravascular coagulation (DIC)	Widespread clot formation in the microscopic vessels; may be followed by bleeding caused by depletion of clotting factors
ecchymosis ek-i-MŌ-sis	A collection of blood under the skin caused by leakage from small vessels (root *chym* means "juice")
hemolysis hē-MOL-i-sis	The rupture of red blood cells and the release of hemoglobin (adjective: hemolytic)
hemophilia hē-mō-FIL-ē-a	A hereditary blood disease caused by lack of a clotting factor and resulting in abnormal bleeding
HIV (human immunodeficiency virus)	The virus that causes AIDS
Hodgkin disease	A neoplastic disease of unknown cause that involves the lymph nodes, spleen, liver, and other tissues; characterized by the presence of giant Reed–Sternberg cells (see Fig. 10-15)
hypersensitivity	An immunologic reaction to a substance that is harmless to most people; allergy
immunodeficiency im-ū-nō-dē-FISH-en-sē	A congenital or acquired failure of the immune system to protect against disease
intrinsic factor	A substance produced in the stomach that aids in the intestinal absorption of vitamin B_{12}, necessary for the manufacture of red blood cells. Lack of intrinsic factor causes pernicious anemia
Kaposi sarcoma KAP-ō-sē	Cancerous lesion of the skin and other tissues, seen most often in patients with AIDS

10

(continued)

Terminology | Key Terms (continued)

leukemia lū-KĒ-mē-a	Malignant overgrowth of immature white blood cells; may be chronic or acute; may affect bone marrow (myelogenous leukemia) or lymphoid tissue (lymphocytic leukemia)
lymphadenopathy lim-fad-e-NOP-a-thē	Any disease of the lymph nodes
multiple myeloma mī-e-LŌ-ma	A tumor of the blood-forming tissue in bone marrow
non-Hodgkin lymphoma (NHL)	A widespread malignant disease of lymph nodes that involves lymphocytes. It differs from Hodgkin disease in that giant Reed–Sternberg cells are absent
Philadelphia chromosome (Ph)	An abnormal chromosome found in the cells of most individuals with chronic granulocytic (myelogenous) leukemia
pernicious anemia per-NISH-us	Anemia caused by failure of the stomach to produce intrinsic factor, a substance needed for the absorption of vitamin B_{12}. This vitamin is required for the formation of erythrocytes
petechiae pē-TĒ-kē-ē	Pinpoint, flat, purplish-red spots caused by bleeding within the skin or mucous membrane (singular: petechia)
purpura PUR-pū-ra	A condition characterized by hemorrhages into the skin, mucous membranes, internal organs, and other tissues (from Greek word meaning "purple"). Thrombocytopenic purpura is caused by a deficiency of platelets
sideroblastic anemia sid-e-rō-BLAS-tik	Anemia caused by inability to use available iron to manufacture hemoglobin. The excess iron precipitates in normoblasts (developing red blood cells)
Sjögren syndrome SHŌ-gren	An autoimmune disease involving dysfunction of the exocrine glands and affecting secretion of tears, saliva, and other body fluids. Deficiency leads to dry mouth, tooth decay, corneal damage, eye infections, and difficulty in swallowing
sickle cell anemia	A hereditary anemia caused by the presence of abnormal hemoglobin. Red blood cells become sickle shaped and interfere with normal blood flow to the tissues (see Fig. 10-13). Most common in black populations of West African descent
splenomegaly splē-nō-MEG-a-lē	Enlargement of the spleen
systemic lupus erythematosus LŪ-pus er-i-thē-ma-TŌ-sus	Inflammatory connective tissue disease affecting the skin and multiple organs. Patients are sensitive to light and may have a red butterfly-shaped rash over the nose and cheeks
systemic sclerosis	A diffuse connective tissue disease that may involve any system causing inflammation, degeneration, and fibrosis. Also called scleroderma because it causes thickening of the skin
thalassemia thal-a-SĒ-mē-a	A group of hereditary anemias mostly found in populations of Mediterranean descent (the name comes from the Greek word for "sea")
thrombocytopenia throm-bō-sī-tō-PĒ-nēa	A deficiency of thrombocytes (platelets) in the blood
urticaria ur-ti-KAR-ē-a	A skin reaction consisting of round, raised eruptions (wheals) with itching; hives

Diagnosis and Treatment

adrenaline a-DREN-a-lin	See epinephrine
CD4+ T lymphocyte count	A count of the T cells that have the CD4 receptors for the AIDS virus (HIV). A count of less than 200/mcL of blood signifies severe immunodeficiency
epinephrine ep-i-NEF-rin	A powerful stimulant produced by the adrenal gland and sympathetic nervous system. Activates the cardiovascular, respiratory, and other systems needed to meet stress. Used as a drug to treat severe allergic reactions and shock. Also called adrenaline

(continued)

Terminology	**Key Terms** (continued)

| reticulocyte counts
rē-TIK-ū-lō-sīt | Blood counts of reticulocytes, a type of immature red blood cell; reticulocyte counts are useful in diagnosis to indicate the rate of erythrocyte formation (see Box 10-6) |
| Reed–Sternberg cells
rēd-SHTERN-berg | Giant cells that are characteristic of Hodgkin disease. They usually have two large nuclei and are surrounded by a halo (see Fig. 10-15) |

Go to the pronunciation glossary on the Student Resources to hear these words pronounced.

Terminology	**Supplementary Terms**

Normal Structure and Function

agglutination *a-glū-ti-NĀ-shun*	The clumping of cells or particles in the presence of specific antibodies
bilirubin *bil-i-RŪ-bin*	A pigment derived from the breakdown of hemoglobin. It is eliminated by the liver in bile
complement *COM-ple-ment*	A group of plasma enzymes that interacts with antibodies
corpuscle *KOR-pus-l*	A small mass or body. A blood corpuscle is a blood cell
hemopoietic stem cell *hē-mō-poy-E-tik*	A primitive bone marrow cell that gives rise to all varieties of blood cells
heparin *HEP-a-rin*	A substance found throughout the body that inhibits blood coagulation; an anticoagulant
plasmin *PLAZ-min*	An enzyme that dissolves clots; also called *fibrinolysin*
thrombin *THROM-bin*	The enzyme derived from prothrombin that converts fibrinogen to fibrin

Symptoms and Conditions

agranulocytosis *ā-gran-ū-lō-sī-TŌ-sis*	A condition involving a decrease in the number of granulocytes in the blood; also called *granulocytopenia*
erythrocytosis *e-rith-rō-sī-TŌ-sis*	Increase in the number of red cells in the blood; may be normal, such as to compensate for life at high altitudes, or abnormal, such as in cases of pulmonary or cardiac disease
Fanconi syndrome *fan-KŌ-nē*	Congenital aplastic anemia that appears between birth and 10 years of age; may be hereditary or caused by damage before birth, as by a virus
graft-versus-host reaction (GVHR)	An immunologic reaction of transplanted lymphocytes against tissues of the host; a common complication of bone marrow transplantation
hairy cell leukemia	A form of leukemia in which cells have filaments, making them look "hairy"
hematoma *hē-ma-TŌ-ma*	A localized collection of blood, usually clotted, caused by a break in a blood vessel
hemolytic disease of the newborn (HDN)	Disease that results from incompatibility between the blood of a mother and her fetus, usually involving Rh factor. An Rh-negative mother produces antibody to an Rh-positive fetus that, in later pregnancies, will destroy the red cells of an Rh-positive fetus. The problem is usually avoided by treating the mother with antibodies to remove the Rh antigen; erythroblastosis fetalis

(continued)

Terminology	**Supplementary Terms** (continued)
hemosiderosis hē-mō-sid-er-Ō-sis	A condition involving the deposition of an iron-containing pigment (hemosiderin) mainly in the liver and the spleen. The pigment comes from hemoglobin released from disintegrated red blood cells
idiopathic thrombocytopenic purpura (ITP)	A clotting disorder caused by destruction of platelets that usually follows a viral illness. Causes petechiae and hemorrhages into the skin and mucous membranes
infectious mononucleosis mon-ō-nū-klē-Ō-sis	An acute infectious disease caused by Epstein–Barr virus (EBV). Characterized by fever, weakness, lymphadenopathy, hepatosplenomegaly, and atypical lymphocytes (resembling monocytes) (Fig. 10-16)
lymphocytosis lim-fō-sī-TŌ-sis	An increase in the number of circulating lymphocytes
myelodysplastic syndrome mī-e-lō-dis-PLAS-tik	Bone marrow dysfunction resulting in anemia and deficiency of neutrophils and platelets. May develop in time into leukemia; preleukemia
myelofibrosis mī-e-lō-fī-BRŌ-sis	Condition in which bone marrow is replaced with fibrous tissue
neutropenia nū-trō-PĒ-nē-a	A decrease in the number of neutrophils with increased susceptibility to infection. Causes include drugs, irradiation, and infection. May be a side effect of treatment for malignancy
pancytopenia pan-sī-tō-PĒ-nē-a	A decrease in all cells of the blood, as in aplastic anemia
polycythemia pol-ē-sī-THĒ-mē-a	Any condition in which there is a relative increase in the percent of red blood cells in whole blood. May result from excessive production of red cells because of oxygen lack, as caused by high altitudes, breathing obstruction, heart failure, or certain forms of poisoning. Apparent polycythemia results from concentration of the blood, as by dehydration
polycythemia vera pol-ē-sī-THĒ-mē-a VĒ-ra	A condition in which overactive bone marrow produces too many red blood cells. These interfere with circulation and promote thrombosis and hemorrhage. Treated by blood removal. Also called *erythremia, Vaquez–Osler disease*
septicemia sep-ti-SĒ-mē-a	Presence of microorganisms in the blood
spherocytic anemia sfēr-ō-SIT-ik	Hereditary anemia in which red blood cells are round instead of disk shaped and rupture (hemolyze) excessively
thrombotic thrombocytopenic purpura (TTP)	An often-fatal disorder in which multiple clots form in blood vessels
von Willebrand disease	A hereditary bleeding disease caused by lack of von Willebrand factor, a substance necessary for blood clotting

Diagnosis (see also Boxes 10-4 and 10-7)

Bence Jones protein	A protein that appears in the urine of patients with multiple myeloma
Coombs test	A test for detection of antibodies to red blood cells such as appear in cases of autoimmune hemolytic anemias
electrophoresis ē-lek-trō-fo-RĒ-sis	Separation of particles in a liquid by application of an electrical field; used to separate components of blood
ELISA	Enzyme-linked immunosorbent assay. A highly sensitive immunologic test used to diagnose HIV infection, hepatitis, and Lyme disease, among others
monoclonal antibody mon-ō-KLŌ-nal	A pure antibody produced in the laboratory; used for diagnosis and treatment
pH	A scale that measures the relative acidity or alkalinity of a solution. Represents the amount of hydrogen ion in the solution

(continued)

Terminology	**Supplementary Terms** (continued)

Schilling test *SHIL-ing*	Test used to determine absorption of vitamin B_{12} by measuring excretion of radioactive B_{12} in the urine. Used to distinguish pernicious from nutritional anemia
seroconversion *sē-rō-con-VER-zhun*	The appearance of antibodies in the serum in response to a disease or an immunization
Western blot assay	A very sensitive test used to detect small amounts of antibodies in the blood
Wright stain	A commonly used blood stain. Figure 10-2 shows blood cells stained with Wright stain

Treatment

anticoagulant *an-ti-kō-AG-ū-lant*	An agent that prevents or delays blood coagulation
antihistamine *an-ti-HIS-ta-mēn*	A drug that counteracts the effects of histamine and is used to treat allergic reactions
apheresis *af-e-RĒ-sis*	A procedure in which blood is withdrawn, a portion is separated and retained, and the remainder is returned to the donor. Apheresis may be used as a suffix with a root meaning the fraction retained, such as plasmapheresis, leukapheresis
autologous blood *aw-TOL-ō-gus*	A person's own blood. May be donated in advance of surgery and transfused if needed
cryoprecipitate *krī-ō-prē-SIP-i-tāt*	A sediment obtained by cooling. The fraction obtained by freezing blood plasma contains clotting factors
desensitization *dē-sen-si-ti-ZĀ-shun*	Treatment of allergy by small injections of the offending allergen. This causes an increase of antibody to destroy the antigen rapidly on contact
homologous blood *hō-MOL-ō-gus*	Blood from animals of the same species, such as human blood used for transfusion from one person to another. Blood used for transfusions must be compatible with the recipient's blood
immunosuppression *im-ū-nō-sū-PRESH-un*	Depression of the immune response. May be correlated with disease but also may be induced therapeutically to prevent rejection in cases of tissue transplantation
protease inhibitor *PRŌ-tē-ās*	An anti-HIV drug that acts by inhibiting an enzyme the virus needs to multiply

PASSport to Success® Go to the pronunciation glossary on the Student Resources to hear these words pronounced.

Figure 10-16 **Infectious mononucleosis.** Atypical lymphocytes characterize this viral disease.

Terminology Abbreviations

Ab	Antibody		ITP	Idiopathic thrombocytopenic purpura
Ag	Antigen		lytes	Electrolytes
AIDS	Acquired immunodeficiency syndrome		MCH	Mean corpuscular hemoglobin
ALL	Acute lymphoblastic (lymphocytic) leukemia		MCHC	Mean corpuscular hemoglobin concentration
AML	Acute myeloblastic (myelogenous) leukemia		mcL	Microliter
			MCV	Mean corpuscular volume
APTT	Activated partial thromboplastin time		MDS	Myelodysplastic syndrome
BT	Bleeding time		mEq	Milliequivalent
CBC	Complete blood count		NHL	Non-Hodgkin lymphoma
CLL	Chronic lymphocytic leukemia		PCV	Packed cell volume
CML	Chronic myelogenous leukemia		pH	Scale for measuring hydrogen ion concentration (acidity or alkalinity)
crit	Hematocrit			
DIC	Disseminated intravascular coagulation		Ph	Philadelphia chromosome
Diff	Differential count		PMN	Polymorphonuclear (neutrophil)
EBV	Epstein–Barr virus		poly	Neutrophil
ELISA	Enzyme-linked immunosorbent assay		polymorph	Neutrophil
EPO	Erythropoietin		PT	Pro time; prothrombin time
ESR	Erythrocyte sedimentation rate		PTT	Partial thromboplastin time
FFP	Fresh frozen plasma		RBC	Red blood cell; red blood (cell) count
Hb, Hgb	Hemoglobin		seg	Neutrophil
Hct, Ht	Hematocrit		SLE	Systemic lupus erythematosus
HDN	Hemolytic disease of the newborn		T(C)T	Thrombin (clotting) time
HIV	Human immunodeficiency virus		TTP	Thrombotic thrombocytopenic purpura
IF	Intrinsic factor		vWF	von Willebrand factor
Ig	Immunoglobulin		WBC	White blood cell; white blood (cell) count

Chapter Review

LABELING EXERCISE

Blood Cells > Write the name of each numbered part on the corresponding line of the answer sheet.

Erythrocyte
Leukocyte
Platelet

1. _____

2. _____

3. _____

Leukocytes (White Blood Cells)

Write the name of each numbered part on the corresponding line of the answer sheet.

Basophil   Monocyte
Eosinophil   Neutrophil
Lymphocyte

Leukocytes (white blood cells)

1
2
3

4   5

1. _____

2. _____

3. _____

4. _____

5. _____

10

Terminology > Match the following terms and write the appropriate letter to the left of each number:

_____ **1.** hemolysis
_____ **2.** prothrombin
_____ **3.** antibody
_____ **4.** megakaryocyte
_____ **5.** thrombolytic

a. substance active in blood clotting
b. cell that produces platelets
c. destruction of red blood cells
d. able to dissolve a blood clot
e. substance active in an immune response

_____ **6.** calcitonin
_____ **7.** natriuresis
_____ **8.** ferric
_____ **9.** siderosis
_____ **10.** azoturia

a. pertaining to iron
b. hormone involved in the metabolism of calcium
c. urinary excretion of sodium
d. urinary excretion of nitrogenous compounds
e. condition involving iron deposits

_____ **11.** thalassemia
_____ **12.** purpura
_____ **13.** hypersensitivity
_____ **14.** hemophilia
_____ **15.** hemostasis

a. allergy
b. hereditary form of anemia
c. stoppage of blood flow
d. hereditary clotting disorder
e. bleeding into the tissues

_____ **16.** pH
_____ **17.** HIV
_____ **18.** ALL
_____ **19.** PCV
_____ **20.** CBC

a. hematocrit
b. scale for measuring acidity or alkalinity
c. laboratory test of blood
d. a form of leukemia
e. virus that causes an immunodeficiency disease

Supplementary Terms

_____ **21.** electrophoresis
_____ **22.** heparin
_____ **23.** apheresis
_____ **24.** ELISA
_____ **25.** bilirubin

a. separation of blood and use of components
b. pigment that comes from hemoglobin
c. anticoagulant
d. method for separating components of a solution
e. sensitive immunologic test

Fill in the blanks:

26. The engulfing of foreign material by white cells is called _____.

27. The iron-containing pigment in red blood cells that carries oxygen is called _____.

28. A substance that separates into ions in solution is a(n) _____.

29. The cell fragments active in blood clotting are the _____.

30. A hemocytometer is used to count _____.

31. Oxyhemoglobin is hemoglobin combined with _____.

32. A hematoma is a localized collection of _____.

33. A disorder involving lack of hemoglobin in the blood is _____.

34. A myeloma is a neoplasm that involves the _____.

True–False > Examine the following statements. If the statement is true, write T in the first blank. If the statement is false, write F in the first blank and correct the statement by replacing the underlined word in the second blank.

35. A platelet is also called a <u>monocyte</u>.   _____   _____

36. A plasma cell produces <u>antibodies</u>.   _____   _____

37. The liquid that remains after blood coagulates is called <u>serum</u>.   _____   _____

38. Blood that does not react with either A or B antiserum is <u>type O</u>.   _____   _____

39. A band cell is an immature <u>monocyte</u>.   _____   _____

40. The root kali- pertains to <u>potassium</u>.   _____   _____

The suffixes *-ia*, *-osis*, and *-hemia* all denote an increase in the type of cell indicated by the word root. Define the following terms:

41. leukocytosis (*lū-kō-sī-TŌ-sis*) _____

42. eosinophilia (*ē-ō-sin-ō-FIL-ē-a*) _____

43. erythrocytosis (*e-rith-rō-sī-TŌ-sis*) _____

44. thrombocythemia (*throm-bō-sī-THĒ-mē-a*) _____

45. neutrophilia (*nū-trō-FIL-ē-a*) _____

46. monocytosis (*mon-ō-sī-TŌ-sis*) _____

Write a word for each of the following:

47. An immature red blood cell   _____

48. A decrease in the number of platelets (thrombocytes) in the blood   _____

49. Presence of pus in the blood   _____

50. Specialist in the study of immunity   _____

51. Profuse flow of blood   _____

Adjectives > Use the ending *-ic* to write the adjective form of the following words:

52. septicemia   _____

53. lymphocyte   _____

54. basophil   _____

55. hemolysis   _____

56. thrombosis   _____

57. leukemia   _____

Define each of the following:

58. viremia   _____

59. neutropenia   _____

60. myelotoxin   _____

61. autoimmunity   _____

62. hypoxemia   _____

Eliminations > In each of the sets below, underline the word that does not fit in with the rest and explain the reason for your choice:

63. fibrin — thrombin — thrombolysis — prothrombin — fibrinogen

_____

64. Diff — Hct — MCV — EPO — MCH

_____

65. eosinophil — reticulocyte — monocyte — basophil — lymphocyte

_____

66. allergy — hypersensitivity — gamma globulin — urticaria — anaphylaxis

_____

Word Building > Write a word for the following definitions using the word parts given.

-penia   -blast   leuk/o   -oid   -poiesis   myel/o   gen   -emia   -ic   -oma   cyt/o

67. pertaining to a white blood cell   _____

68. an immature white blood cell   _____

69. pertaining to bone marrow   _____

70. originating in bone marrow   _____

71. an immature bone marrow cell   _____

72. neoplastic overgrowth of white cells in the blood   _____

73. deficiency of white cells in the blood   _____

74. cancer of bone marrow   _____

75. formation of white blood cells   _____

76. pertaining to bone marrow cells   _____

Chapter Review *(continued)*

Word Analysis > Define the following words, and give the meaning of the word parts in each. Use a dictionary if necessary.

77. Pancytopenia (*pan-sī-tō-PĒ-nē-a*) _____

    a. pan- _____

    b. cyt/o _____

    c. -penia _____

78. Polycythemia (*pol-ē-sī-THĒ-mē-a*) _____

    a. poly- _____

    b. cyt/o _____

    c. hem/o _____

    d. -ia _____

79. Anisochromia (*an-ī-sō-KRŌ-mē-a*) _____

    a. an- _____

    b. iso- _____

    c. chrom/o _____

    d. -ia _____

80. myelodysplastic (*mī-e-lō-dis-PLAS-tic*) _____

    a. myel/o _____

    b. dys- _____

    c. plast(y) _____

    d. -ic _____

PASSport to Success®   Go to the word exercises on the Student Resources for additional review exercises.

Case Studies

► Case Study 10-1: Latex Allergy

M.R., a 36-year-old certified registered nurse anesthetist (CRNA), was diagnosed 7 years ago with latex allergy. She first noticed that contact dermatitis developed when she wore powdered latex gloves. Tachycardia, hypotension, bronchospasm, urticaria, and rhinitis soon developed with contact or proximity to latex in surgery. She had one frightening episode of anaphylaxis. Her allergy is of the type I hypersensitivity, IgE T cell-mediated latex allergy, which was diagnosed by both a radioallergosorbent test (RAST) and a skin-prick test.

M.R. avoids all contact with any natural rubber latex in her home and at work. She can work only in a pediatric OR because they are latex free, since many children with congenital disorders are allergic to latex. She wears a medical alert bracelet, uses a bronchodilator inhaler at the first symptom of bronchospasm, and carries a syringe of epinephrine at all times.

(continued)

Case Studies (continued)

➤ Case Study 10-2: Blood Replacement

C.L., a 16-year-old girl, sustained a ruptured liver when she hit a tree while sledding. Emergency surgery was needed to stop the internal bleeding. During surgery, the ruptured segment of the liver was removed and the laceration was sutured with a heavy, absorbable suture on a large smooth needle. Before surgery, her hemoglobin was 10.2 g/dL, but the reading decreased to 7.6 g/dL before hemostasis was attained. Cell salvage, or autotransfusion, was set up. In this procedure, the free blood was suctioned from her abdomen and mixed with an anticoagulant (heparin). The RBCs were washed in a sterile centrifuge with NSS and transfused back to her through tubing fitted with a filter. She also received six units of homologous, leukocyte-reduced whole blood, five units of fresh frozen plasma, and two units of platelets. During the surgery, the CRNA repeatedly tested her Hgb and Hct as well as prothrombin time and partial thromboplastin time to monitor her clotting mechanisms.

C.L. is B positive. Fortunately, there was enough B-positive blood in the hospital blood bank for her surgery. The lab informed her surgeon that they had two units of B-negative and six units of O-negative blood, which she could have received safely if she needed more blood during the night. However, her hemoglobin level increased to 12 g/dL, and she was stable during her recovery. She was monitored for DIC and pulmonary emboli.

➤ Case Study 10-3: Myelofibrosis

A.Y., a 52-year-old kindergarten teacher, had myelofibrosis that had been in remission for 25 years. She had seen her hematologist regularly and had had routine blood testing since the age of 27. After several weeks of fatigue, idiopathic joint and muscle aching, weakness, and a frightening episode of syncope, she saw her hematologist for evaluation. Her hemoglobin was 9.0 g/dL and her hematocrit was 29%. Concerned that she was having an exacerbation, her doctor scheduled a bone marrow aspiration, and the results were positive for myelofibrosis.

A.Y. went through a 6-month therapy regimen of iron supplements in the form of ferrous sulfate tablets and received weekly vitamin B_{12} injections. Interferon was given every other week in addition to erythropoiesis therapy, which was unsuccessful. She was treated for presumed aplastic anemia. During treatment, splenomegaly developed, which compromised her abdominal organs and pulmonary function. She continued to lose weight, and her hemoglobin dropped as low as 6.0 g/dL. Weekly transfusions of packed RBCs did not improve her hemoglobin and hematocrit.

After a regimen of high-dose chemotherapy to shrink the fibers in her bone marrow and a splenectomy, A.Y. received a stem cell transplant. The stem cells were obtained from blood donated by her brother, who was a perfect immunologic match. After a 6-month period of

recovery in a protected environment, required because of her immunocompromised state, A.Y. returned home and has been free of disease symptoms for over 1 year.

CASE STUDY QUESTIONS

Multiple choice. Select the best answer and write the letter of your choice to the left of each number:

_____ 1. The natural latex protein in latex gloves may act as a(n):
   a. antibody
   b. allergen
   c. lymphocyte
   d. purpura
   e. immunocyte

_____ 2. Urticaria is commonly called:
   a. rhinitis
   b. dermatitis
   c. hives
   d. ELISA
   e. congenital

_____ 3. The cells involved in a T cell-mediated allergic response are:
   a. basophils
   b. monocytes
   c. antigen
   d. T lymphocytes
   e. B cells

_____ 4. Anaphylaxis, a life-threatening physiological response, is an extreme form of:
   a. remission
   b. hypersensitivity
   c. hemostasis
   d. exacerbation
   e. homeostasis

_____ 5. The common name for epinephrine is:
   a. heparin
   b. adrenaline
   c. cortisone
   d. apheresis
   e. antihistamine

_____ 6. The removal of part of the liver is called:
   a. partial hepatectomy
   b. hepatomegaly
   c. resection of the liver
   d. a and b
   e. a and c

_____ 7. The unit for hemoglobin measurement (g/dL) means:
   a. grams in decimal point
   b. grains in a decathlon
   c. drops in 50 cc
   d. grams in 100 mL
   e. grains in deciliter

(continued)

Case Studies (continued)

_____ 8. Heparin, an anticoagulant, is a drug that:
   a. increases the rate of blood clotting
   b. takes the place of fibrin
   c. supports thrombin
   d. interferes with blood clotting
   e. makes blood thinner than water

_____ 9. The RBCs were washed with NSS. This means: the _____ were washed with _____.
   a. reticulocytes, heparin
   b. red blood cells, nutritional solution
   c. erythrocytes, normal saline solution
   d. reticulocytes, normal simple solution
   e. red blood cells, heparin

_____ 10. Autotransfusion is transfusion of autologous blood, that is, the patient's own blood. Homologous blood is taken from:
   a. another human
   b. synthetic chemicals
   c. plasma with clotting factors
   d. an animal with similar antibodies as humans
   e. IV fluid with electrolytes

_____ 11. Patients who lose a significant amount of blood may lose clotting ability. Effective therapy in such cases would be replacement of:
   a. IV solution with electrolytes
   b. iron supplements
   c. platelets
   d. heparin
   e. packed RBCs

_____ 12. C.L.'s blood type is B positive. The best blood for her to receive is:
   a. positive
   b. negative
   c. AB positive
   d. B negative
   e. B positive

_____ 13. Myelofibrosis, like aplastic anemia, is a disease in which there is:
   a. overgrowth of RBCs
   b. destruction of the bone marrow
   c. dangerously high hemoglobin and hematocrit
   d. absence of bone marrow
   e. lymphatic tissue in the bone marrow

_____ 14. Erythropoiesis is:
   a. production of blood
   b. production of red cells
   c. production of plasma
   d. destruction of white cells
   e. destruction of platelets

_____ 15. The "ferrous" in ferrous sulfate represents:
   a. electrolytes
   b. RBCs
   c. iron
   d. oxygen
   e. B vitamins

_____ 16. Hemoglobin and hematocrit values pertain to:
   a. leukocytes
   b. immune response
   c. granulocytes
   d. red blood cells
   e. fibrinogen

_____ 17. Splenomegaly is:
   a. prolapse of the spleen
   b. movement of the spleen
   c. enlargement of the lymph glands
   d. destruction of the bone marrow
   e. enlargement of the spleen

_____ 18. The stem cells A.Y. received were expected to develop into new:
   a. spleen cells
   b. bone marrow cells
   c. hemoglobin
   d. abdominal organs
   e. cartilage

_____ 19. A.Y.'s health was compromised because the high-dose chemotherapy caused:
   a. immunodeficiency
   b. electrolyte imbalance
   c. anoxia
   d. Rh incompatibility
   e. autoimmunity

Abbreviations. Define the following abbreviations:

20. Ig _____

21. Hgb _____

22. Hct _____

23. FFP _____

24. PT _____

25. PTT _____

26. DIC _____

The Respiratory System

CHAPTER 11

CHAPTER CONTENTS

OBJECTIVES

After study of this chapter you should be able to:

1. Explain the roles of oxygen and carbon dioxide in the body and describe how each is carried in the blood.
2. Label a diagram of the respiratory tract and briefly explain the function of each part.
3. Describe the mechanism of breathing, including the roles of the diaphragm and phrenic nerve.
4. Identify and use word parts pertaining to the respiratory system.
5. Discuss the major disorders of the respiratory system.
6. Define medical terms related to breathing and diseases of the respiratory system.
7. List and define 10 volumes and capacities commonly used to measure pulmonary function.
8. Interpret abbreviations commonly used with reference to the respiratory system.
9. Analyze several case studies pertaining to diseases that affect respiration.

PRETEST

Multiple choice. Select the best answer and write the letter of your choice to the left of each number.

___ 1. The gas that is supplied to tissues by the respiratory system is:

    a. oxygen   c. sulfur
    b. neon   d. carbon dioxide

___ 2. The gas that is eliminated by the respiratory system is:

    a. chlorine   c. hydrogen
    b. carbon dioxide   d. fluoride

___ 3. The air sacs through which gases are exchanged in the lungs are the:

    a. trachea   c. bursae
    b. alveoli   d. bronchi

___ 4. The structure that holds the vocal cords is the:

    a. larynx   c. uvula
    b. tongue   d. tonsils

___ 5. The tubes that carry air from the trachea into the lungs are the:

    a. arteries   c. veins
    b. nares   d. bronchi

___ 6. The dome-shaped muscle under the lungs is the:

    a. palate   c. hiatus
    b. diaphragm   d. esophagus

___ 7. The membrane around the lungs is the:

    a. peritoneum   c. pleura
    b. mucosa   d. mediastinum

___ 8. A term for inflammation of the lungs is:

    a. pneumonia   c. pleuritis
    b. bronchitis   d. laryngitis

The main function of the respiratory system is to provide **oxygen** to body cells for energy metabolism and to eliminate **carbon dioxide**, a byproduct of metabolism. Because these gases must be carried to and from the cells in the blood, the respiratory system works closely with the cardiovascular system to accomplish gas exchange (Fig. 11-1). This activity has two phases:

- External gas exchange occurs between the outside atmosphere and the blood.

- Internal gas exchange occurs between the blood and the tissues.

External exchange takes place in the **lungs**, located in the thoracic cavity. The remainder of the respiratory tract consists of a series of passageways that conduct air to and from the lungs. No gas exchange occurs in these regions. Refer to Figure 11-2 as you read the following description of the respiratory tract.

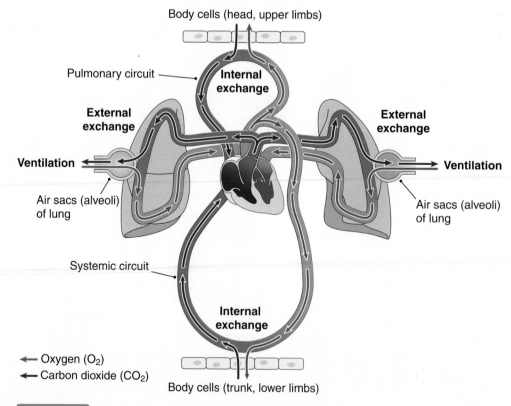

Figure 11-1 **Respiration.** In ventilation, gases are moved into and out of the lungs. In external exchange, gases move between the air sacs (alveoli) of the lungs and the blood. In internal exchange, gases move between the blood and body cells. The circulation transports gases in the blood.

In the bones of the skull and face near the nose are air-filled cavities lined with mucous membrane that drain into the nasal cavity. These chambers lighten the bones and provide resonance for speech production. These cavities, called **sinuses**, are named specifically for the bones in which they are located, such as the sphenoid, ethmoid, and maxillary sinuses. Together, because they are near the nose, these cavities are referred to as the paranasal sinuses (see Fig. 11-2).

The Pharynx

Inhaled air passes into the throat, or pharynx, where it mixes with air that enters through the mouth and also with food destined for the digestive tract. The pharynx is divided into three regions, which are shown in Figure 11-2:

- The nasopharynx is the superior portion located behind the nasal cavity.
- The oropharynx is the middle portion located behind the mouth.
- The laryngeal pharynx is the inferior portion located behind the **larynx**.

The tonsils, lymphoid tissue described in Chapter 10, are in the region of the pharynx (Fig. 11-3):

- The **palatine tonsils** are on either side of the soft palate in the oropharynx.
- The single pharyngeal tonsil, commonly known as the **adenoids**, is in the nasopharynx.

Figure 11-2 **The respiratory system.** (A) Overview. (B) Enlarged section of lung tissue showing the relationship between the alveoli (air sacs) and the blood capillaries.

Upper Respiratory Passageways

The upper respiratory passageways consist of the **nose** and **pharynx** (throat). Air can also be exchanged through the mouth, but there are fewer mechanisms for cleansing the air taken in by this route.

The Nose

Air enters through the nose, where it is warmed, filtered, and moistened as it passes over the hair-covered mucous membranes of the nasal cavity. Cilia—microscopic hairlike projections from the cells that line the nose—sweep dirt and foreign material toward the throat for elimination. Material that is eliminated from the respiratory tract by coughing or clearing the throat is called **sputum**. Receptors for the sense of smell are located within bony side projections of the nasal cavity called **turbinate bones,** or conchae.

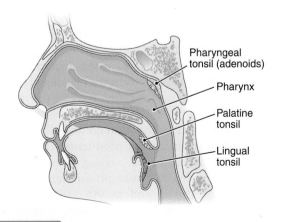

Figure 11-3 **The tonsils.** All of the tonsils are located in the vicinity of the pharynx (throat).

Tonsillectomy: A Procedure Reconsidered

Tonsillitis, a bacterial infection of the tonsils, is a common childhood illness. In years past, surgical removal of the infected tonsils was a standard procedure, as tonsillectomy was thought to prevent severe infections like strep throat. Because tonsils were thought to have little function, surgeons often removed infected tonsils—even healthy tonsils, in order to prevent tonsillitis later. With the discovery that tonsils play an important immune function, the number of tonsillectomies performed in the United States dropped dramatically, reaching an all-time low in the 1980s.

Today, although many cases of tonsillitis are successfully treated with appropriate antibiotics, tonsillectomy is becoming more frequent; in fact, it is the second most common surgical procedure among American children. Surgery is considered if an infection recurs, or if enlarged tonsils make swallowing or breathing difficult. Many tonsillectomies are performed in children to treat obstructive sleep apnea, a condition in which the child stops breathing for a few seconds at a time during sleep. Recent studies suggest that tonsillectomy may also be beneficial for children suffering from otitis media (middle ear infection), because bacteria infecting the tonsils may travel to this region of the ear.

Most tonsillectomies are performed by electrocautery, a technique that uses an electrical current to burn the tonsils away from the throat. Now that this operation is becoming more common, surgeons are developing new techniques. For example, coblation tonsillectomy uses radio waves to break down tonsillar tissue. Studies suggest that this procedure results in a faster recovery, fewer complications, and decreased postoperative pain compared with electrocautery.

- The lingual tonsils are small mounds of lymphoid tissue at the posterior of the tongue.

Opinions on the advisability of removing the tonsils have changed over time, as described in Box 11-1.

Lower Respiratory Passageways and Lungs

Air moves from the pharynx into the larynx, commonly called the voice box, because it contains the **vocal cords**. The larynx is at the top of the **trachea**, commonly called the windpipe, which conducts air into the bronchial system toward the lungs.

The Larynx

The larynx is shaped by nine cartilages, the most prominent of which is the anterior thyroid cartilage that forms the "Adam's apple" (Fig. 11-4). The small leaf-shaped cartilage at the top of the larynx is the **epiglottis**. When one swallows, the epiglottis covers the opening of the larynx and helps to prevent food from entering the respiratory tract.

The larynx contains the vocal cords, folds of tissue that are important in speech production (Fig. 11-5). Vibrations produced by air passing over the vocal cords form the basis for voice production, although portions of the throat and mouth are needed for proper speech articulation. The opening between the vocal cords is the **glottis** (the epiglottis is above the glottis).

The Trachea

The trachea is a tube reinforced with C-shaped rings of cartilage to prevent its collapse (you can feel these rings if you press your fingers gently against the front of your throat). Cilia in the trachea's lining move impurities up toward the throat, where they can be eliminated by swallowing or by **expectoration**, coughing them up.

The trachea is contained in a region known as the **mediastinum**, which consists of the space between the lungs together with the organs contained in this space (see Fig. 11-2). In addition to the trachea, the mediastinum contains the heart, esophagus, large vessels, and other tissues.

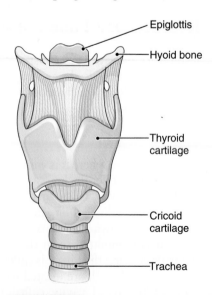

Figure 11-4 **The larynx, anterior view.**

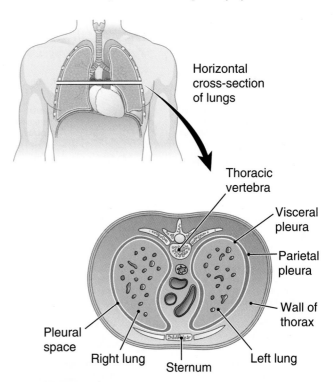

Figure 11-6 **The pleura.** A transverse section through the lungs shows the parietal and visceral layers of the pleura.

Figure 11-5 **The vocal cords, superior view.** (*A*) The glottis in closed position. (*B*) The glottis in open position.

The Bronchial System

At its lower end, the trachea divides into a right and a left main stem **bronchus**; these enter the lungs. The right bronchus is shorter and wider; it divides into three secondary bronchi in the right lung. The left bronchus divides into two branches that supply the left lung. Further divisions produce an increasing number of smaller tubes that supply air to smaller subdivisions of lung tissue. As the air passageways progress through the lungs, the cartilage in the walls gradually disappears and is replaced by smooth (involuntary) muscle.

The smallest of the conducting tubes, the **bronchioles**, carry air into the microscopic air sacs, the **alveoli**, through which gases are exchanged between the lungs and the blood. It is through the ultrathin walls of the alveoli and their surrounding capillaries that oxygen diffuses into the blood and carbon dioxide diffuses out of the blood for elimination (see Fig. 11-2).

The Lungs

The cone-shaped lungs occupy the major portion of the thoracic cavity. The right lung is larger and divided into three lobes. The left lung, which is smaller, to accommodate the heart, is divided into two lobes. The lobes are further subdivided to correspond to divisions of the bronchial network.

A double membrane, the **pleura**, covers the lungs and lines the thoracic cavity (Fig. 11-6). There are two pleural layers:

- The parietal pleura, the outer layer, is attached to the wall of the thoracic cavity.

- The visceral pleura, the inner layer, is attached to the surface of the lungs.

The very narrow, fluid-filled space between the two layers is the **pleural space**. The moist pleural membranes slide easily over each other within the chest cavity, allowing the lungs to expand during breathing.

Breathing

Air is moved into and out of the lungs by the process of breathing, technically called **pulmonary ventilation**. This consists of a steady cycle of **inspiration** (inhalation) and **expiration** (exhalation), separated by a period of rest. Breathing is normally regulated unconsciously by centers in the brainstem. These centers adjust the rate and rhythm of breathing according to changes in the blood's composition, especially the concentration of carbon dioxide.

PASSport to Success®   See the *Pulmonary Ventilation* animation on the Student Resources to view this process in action.

Inspiration

The breathing cycle begins when the **phrenic nerve** stimulates the **diaphragm** to contract and flatten, enlarging the chest cavity. At the same time, external intercostal muscles between the ribs elevate and expand the rib cage. A resulting decrease in pressure within the thorax causes air to flow into the lungs (Fig. 11-7). Muscles of the neck and thorax are used in addition for forceful inhalation.

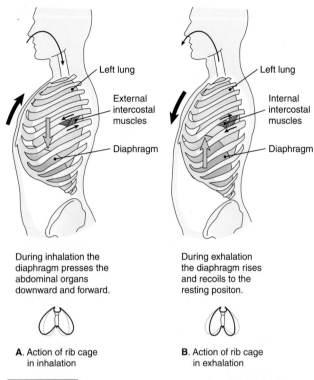

During inhalation the diaphragm presses the abdominal organs downward and forward.

During exhalation the diaphragm rises and recoils to the resting positon.

A. Action of rib cage in inhalation

B. Action of rib cage in exhalation

Figure 11-7 **Pulmonary ventilation.** (*A*) In inhalation, the diaphragm lowers and the external intercostals elevate the rib cage. (*B*) In exhalation, the diaphragm rises and the internal intercostals draw the ribs downward.

The measure of how easily the lungs expand under pressure is **compliance**. Fluid produced in the lungs, known as **surfactant**, aids in compliance by reducing surface tension within the alveoli.

Expiration

Expiration occurs as the breathing muscles relax and the elastic lungs spring back to their original size. Increased pressure in the smaller thorax forces air out of the lungs. In forceful exhalation, the internal intercostal muscles contract to lower the rib cage, and the abdominal muscles contract, pressing internal organs upward against the diaphragm.

Gas Transport

Oxygen is carried in the blood bound to **hemoglobin** in red blood cells. The oxygen is released to the cells as needed. Carbon dioxide is carried in several ways but is mostly converted to **carbonic acid**. The amount of carbon dioxide that is exhaled is important in regulating the blood's acidity or alkalinity, based on the amount of carbonic acid that is formed. Dangerous shifts in blood pH can result from exhalation of too much or too little carbon dioxide.

Terminology   Key Terms

Normal Structure and Function

adenoids AD-e-noyds	Lymphoid tissue located in the nasopharynx; the pharyngeal tonsils
alveoli al-VĒ-ō-lī	The tiny air sacs in the lungs through which gases are exchanged between the atmosphere and the blood in respiration (singular: alveolus). An alveolus, in general, is a small hollow or cavity; the term also applies to the bony socket for a tooth
bronchiole BRONG-kē-ōl	One of the smaller subdivisions of the bronchial tubes (root: *bronchiol*)
bronchus BRONG-kus	One of the larger air passageways in the lungs. The bronchi begin as two branches of the trachea and then subdivide within the lungs (plural: bronchi) (root: *bronch*)
carbon dioxide (CO$_2$)	A gas produced by energy metabolism in cells and eliminated through the lungs
carbonic acid kar-BON-ik	An acid formed when carbon dioxide dissolves in water; H$_2$CO$_3$
compliance kom-PLĪ-ans	A measure of how easily the lungs expand under pressure. Compliance is reduced in many types of respiratory disorders
diaphragm DĪ-a-fram	The dome-shaped muscle under the lungs that flattens during inspiration (root: *phren/o*)
epiglottis ep-i-GLOT-is	A leaf-shaped cartilage that covers the larynx during swallowing to prevent food from entering the trachea
expectoration ek-spek-to-RĀ-shun	The act of coughing up material from the respiratory tract; also the material thus released; sputum

(continued)

Terminology   Key Terms (continued)

expiration *ek-spi-RĀ-shun*	The act of breathing out or expelling air from the lungs; exhalation
glottis *GLOT-is*	The opening between the vocal cords
hemoglobin *HĒ-mō-glō-bin*	The iron-containing pigment in red blood cells that transports oxygen
inspiration *in-spi-RĀ-shun*	The act of drawing air into the lungs; inhalation
larynx *LAR-inks*	The enlarged, superior portion of the trachea that contains the vocal cords (root: *laryng/o*)
lung	A cone-shaped, spongy respiratory organ contained within the thorax (roots: *pneum, pulm*)
mediastinum *mē-dē-as-TĪ-num*	The space between the lungs together with the organs contained in this space
nose *nōz*	The organ of the face used for breathing and for housing receptors for the sense of smell; includes an external portion and an internal nasal cavity (roots: *nas/o, rhin/o*)
oxygen (O₂) *OK-si-jen*	The gas needed by cells to release energy from food during metabolism
palatine tonsils *PAL-a-tīn*	The paired masses of lymphoid tissue located on either side of the oropharynx; usually meant when the term *tonsils* is used alone
pharynx *FAR-inks*	The throat; a common passageway for food entering the esophagus and air entering the larynx (root: *pharyng/o*)
phrenic nerve *FREN-ik*	The nerve that activates the diaphragm (root: *phrenic/o*)
pleura *PLŪR-a*	A double-layered membrane that lines the thoracic cavity (parietal pleura) and covers the lungs (visceral pleura) (root: *pleur/o*)
pleural space	The thin, fluid-filled space between the two layers of the pleura; pleural cavity
pulmonary ventilation *PUL-mō-nār-ē* *ven-ti-LĀ-shun*	The movement of air into and out of the lungs
sinus *SĪ-nus*	A cavity or channel; the paranasal sinuses are located near the nose and drain into the nasal cavity
sputum *SPŪ-tum*	The substance released by coughing or clearing the throat; expectoration. It may contain a variety of material from the respiratory tract
surfactant *sur-FAK-tant*	A substance that decreases surface tension within the alveoli and eases lung expansion
trachea *TRĀ-kē-a*	The air passageway that extends from the larynx to the bronchi (root: *trache/o*)
turbinate bones *TUR-bi-nāt*	The bony projections in the nasal cavity that contain receptors for the sense of smell. Also called conchae (KON-kē)
vocal cords *VŌ-kal*	Membranous folds on either side of the larynx that are important in speech production. Also called vocal folds

11

Go to the pronunciation glossary on the Student Resources to hear these words pronounced.

Word Parts Pertaining to the Respiratory System

See Tables 11-1 to 11-3.

Table 11-1   Suffixes for Respiration

Suffix	Meaning	Example	Definition of Example
-pnea	breathing	orthopnea or-THOP-nē-a	breathing difficulty that is relieved by assuming an upright (ortho-) position
-oxia*	level of oxygen	hypoxia hī-POK-sē-a	decreased amount of oxygen in the tissues
-capnia*	level of carbon dioxide	hypercapnia hī-per-KAP-nē-a	increased carbon dioxide in the tissues
-phonia	voice	dysphonia dis-FŌ-nē-a	difficulty in speaking

*When referring to levels of oxygen and carbon dioxide in the blood, the suffix -emia is used, as in hypoxemia, hypercapnemia.

EXERCISE 11-1

Use the suffix -pnea to form words with the following meanings:

1. lack of breathing   _____apnea_____

2. painful or difficult breathing   _____

3. easy, normal (eu-) breathing   _____

4. slow (brady-) rate of breathing   _____

Use the ending -pneic to write the adjective form of the above words:

5.   _____apneic_____

6.   _____

7.   _____

8.   _____

Use the suffixes in Table 11-1 to write a word for each of the following definitions:

9. lack of voice   _____

10. decreased carbon dioxide in the tissues   _____

11. lack of (an-) oxygen in the tissues   _____

12. normal levels of carbon dioxide in the tissues   _____

TB symptoms include fever, weight loss, weakness, cough, and **hemoptysis**, the coughing up of blood-containing sputum. Laboratories study sputum samples to isolate, stain, and identify infectious organisms. Accumulation of exudate in the alveoli may result in consolidation of lung tissue.

The **tuberculin test** is a test for tuberculosis infection. The test material, tuberculin, is made from byproducts of the tuberculosis organism. PPD (purified protein derivative) is the form of tuberculin commonly used.

BCG vaccine is used worldwide to help to prevent TB; it is not used routinely in the United States because the incidence of TB is relatively low and also because it invalidates the tuberculin test. (The vaccine is named for Calmette and Guérin, discoverers of the avirulent mycobacterium strain it contains.)

INFLUENZA

Influenza ("flu") is a viral respiratory disease associated with chills, fever, headaches, muscular aches, and cold-like symptoms. It usually resolves in several days, but severe forms of influenza have caused fatal pandemics, most recently in 1918, 1957, and 1968. The virus can mutate readily and spread among animals, such as birds or pigs, and humans.

Because influenza viruses change so rapidly, scientists must prepare vaccines against the strains most likely to cause an epidemic in any given year. The virus strains are grouped into categories A to C, with A the most severe and C the least. They are further designated H and N with numbers, such as H3N2, H5N1. The H and N represent surface proteins that the virus uses to infect a host.

Medical personnel combat influenza with vaccines, isolation of infected populations, destruction of infected animals, and antiviral medications.

COMMON COLD

More than 200 viruses are known to cause the common cold. About one half of these are rhinoviruses, and the others include adenoviruses and coronaviruses. The symptoms, known to all, are sneezing, **acute rhinitis**, which is inflammation of the nasal passageways with copious secretion of watery mucus, tearing of the eyes, and congestion. The infection may spread from the nose and throat to the sinuses, middle ear, and lower respiratory tract.

Cold viruses are mostly spread by airborne virus-filled droplets released by an infected person's coughs and sneezes. Frequent hand washing and not touching one's hands to any part of the face are good preventive measures.

The disorder usually resolves in about a week. Because colds are caused by viruses, antibiotics do not cure them. Rest, fluid intake, symptomatic treatment, and time work best. The large variety of cold viruses and their frequent mutation have prevented the development of an effective vaccine.

Box 11-3 has some history on terminology related to respiratory infections and other disorders.

Emphysema

Emphysema is a chronic disease associated with over-expansion and destruction of the alveoli. Common causes are exposure to cigarette smoke and other forms of pollution as well as chronic infection. Emphysema is the main disorder included under the heading of **chronic obstructive pulmonary disease (COPD)** (also called COLD, chronic obstructive lung disease). Other conditions included in this category are asthma, chronic **bronchitis**, and **bronchiectasis**.

Asthma

Asthma attacks result from narrowing of the bronchial tubes. This constriction, along with edema (swelling) of the bronchial linings, inflammation, and mucus accumulation, results in wheezing, extreme **dyspnea** (difficulty in breathing), and **cyanosis**.

Box 11-3	Focus on Words

Don't Breathe a Word

Some laypersons' terms for respiratory symptoms and conditions are so old-fashioned and quaint that you might see them today only in Victorian novels. Catarrh (*ka-TAR*) is an old word for an upper respiratory infection with much mucus production. Quinsy (*KWIN-zē*) referred to a sore throat or tonsillar abscess. Consumption was tuberculosis, and dropsy referred to generalized edema. The grip meant influenza, which we more often abbreviate as "flu."

Some unscientific words are still in use. These include whooping cough for pertussis, croup for laryngeal spasm, cold sore or fever blister for a herpes lesion, and phlegm for sputum.

Many people use informal terms instead of scientific words to describe their symptoms. Health professionals should be familiar with the slang or colloquialisms that patients might use so that they can better communicate with them.

Asthma is most common in children. Although its causes are uncertain, a main factor is irritation caused by allergy. Heredity may also play a role. Treatment of asthma includes:

- removal of allergens
- administration of bronchodilators to widen the airways
- administration of corticosteroids to reduce inflammation

PASSport to Success® The animation *Asthma* on the Student Resources reviews information on breathing and describes asthma.

Pneumoconiosis

Chronic irritation and inflammation caused by dust inhalation is termed **pneumoconiosis**. This is an occupational hazard seen mainly in people working in mining and stoneworking industries. Different forms of pneumoconiosis are named for the specific type of dust inhaled: silicosis (silica or quartz), anthracosis (coal dust), asbestosis (asbestos fibers).

Although the term *pneumoconiosis* is limited to conditions caused by inhalation of inorganic dust, lung irritation may also result from inhalation of organic dusts, such as textile or grain dusts.

Lung Cancer

Lung cancer is the leading cause of cancer-related deaths in both men and women. The incidence of lung cancer has increased steadily over the past 50 years, especially in women. Cigarette smoking is a major risk factor in this as well as other types of cancer. The most common form of lung cancer is squamous carcinoma, originating in the lining of the bronchi (bronchogenic). Lung cancer usually cannot be detected early, and it metastasizes rapidly. The overall long-term survival rate is low.

Methods used to diagnose lung cancer include radiographic studies, computed tomography (CT) scans, and sputum examination for cancer cells. Physicians can use a **bronchoscope** to examine the airways and to collect tissue samples for study. They may also take samples by surgical or needle biopsies.

Respiratory Distress Syndrome

Respiratory distress syndrome (RDS) of the newborn, also called *hyaline membrane disease*, occurs in premature infants and is the most common cause of death in this group. It results from a lack of lung surfactant, which reduces compliance. **Acute respiratory distress syndrome (ARDS)**, also known as *shock lung*, may result from trauma, allergic reactions, infection, and other causes. It involves edema that can lead to respiratory failure and death if untreated.

Cystic Fibrosis

Cystic fibrosis (CF) is the most common fatal hereditary disease among white children. The flawed gene that causes CF affects glandular secretions by altering chloride transport across cell membranes. Thickening of bronchial secretions leads to infection and other respiratory disorders. Other mucus-secreting glands, sweat glands, and the pancreas are also involved, causing electrolyte imbalance and digestive disturbances.

CF is diagnosed by the increased amounts of sodium and chloride in the sweat. Geneticists also can identify the gene that causes CF by DNA analysis. There is no cure at present for CF. Patients are treated to relieve their symptoms, as by postural drainage, aerosol mists, bronchodilators, antibiotics, and mucolytic (mucus-dissolving) agents.

Sudden Infant Death Syndrome

Sudden infant death syndrome (SIDS), also called "crib death," is the unexplained death of a seemingly healthy infant under 1 year of age. Death usually occurs during sleep, leaving no signs of its cause. Neither autopsy nor careful investigation of family history and circumstances of death provides any clues.

Certain maternal conditions during pregnancy are associated with an increased risk of SIDS, although none is a sure predictor. These include cigarette smoking, age under 20, low weight gain, anemia, illegal drug use, and reproductive or urinary tract infections.

Some practices that have reduced the incidence of SIDS are:

- Place the baby on its back (supine) for sleep ("back to sleep").
- Keep the baby in a smoke-free environment.
- Use a firm, flat baby mattress.
- Don't overheat the baby.

Pleural Disorders

Pleurisy, also called pleuritis, is an inflammation of the pleura, usually associated with infection. Pain is the common symptom of pleurisy. Because this pain is intensified by breathing or coughing as the inflamed membranes move, breathing becomes rapid and shallow. Analgesics and antiinflammatory drugs are used to treat the symptoms of pleurisy.

As a result of injury, infection, or weakness in the pleural membrane, substances may accumulate between the layers of the pleura. When air or gas collects in this space, the condition is termed **pneumothorax** (Fig. 11-10). Compression may cause collapse of the lung, termed **atelectasis**.

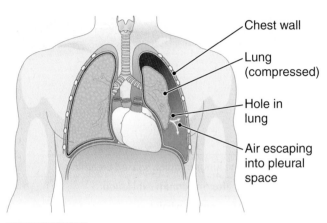

Chest wall

Lung
(compressed)

Hole in
lung

Air escaping
into pleural
space

Figure 11-10 **Pneumothorax.** Injury to lung tissue allows air to leak into the pleural space and put pressure on the lung.

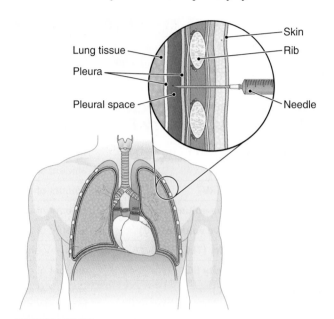

Lung tissue

Pleura

Pleural space

Skin

Rib

Needle

Figure 11-12 **Thoracentesis.** A needle is inserted into the pleural space.

In **pleural effusion**, other materials accumulate in the pleural space (Fig. 11-11). Depending on the substance involved, these are described as **empyema** (pus), also termed **pyothorax; hemothorax** (blood); or **hydrothorax** (fluid). Causes of these conditions include injury, infection, heart failure, and pulmonary embolism. **Thoracentesis**, needle puncture of the chest to remove fluids (Fig. 11-12), or fusion of the pleural membranes (pleurodesis) may be required. A chest tube may be inserted to remove air and fluid from the pleural space.

Diagnosis of Respiratory Disorders

In addition to chest radiographs, CT scans, and magnetic resonance imaging (MRI) scans, methods for diagnosing respiratory disorders include **lung scans**, bronchoscopy, and tests of pleural fluid removed by thoracentesis. **Arterial blood gases (ABGs)** are used to evaluate gas exchange in the lungs by measuring carbon dioxide, oxygen, bicarbonate, and pH in an arterial blood sample. **Pulse oximetry** is routinely used to measure the oxygen saturation of arterial blood by means of an oximeter, a simple device placed on a thin part of the body, usually the finger or the ear (Fig. 11-13).

Pulmonary function tests are used to assess breathing, usually by means of a **spirometer**. They measure the volumes of air that can be moved into or out of the lungs with different degrees of effort. Often used to monitor treatment in cases of allergy, asthma, emphysema, and other respiratory conditions, they are also used to measure progress in smoking cessation. The main volumes and capacities measured in these tests are summarized in reference Box 11-4 and illustrated in Figure 11-14. A capacity is the sum of two or more volumes.

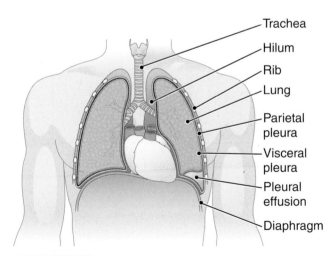

Trachea

Hilum

Rib

Lung

Parietal
pleura

Visceral
pleura

Pleural
effusion

Diaphragm

Figure 11-11 **Pleural effusion.** An abnormal volume of fluid collects in the pleural space.

Figure 11-13 **Pulse oximetry.** The oximeter measures the oxygen saturation of arterial blood.

Box 11-4

For Your Reference

Volumes and Capacities (Sums of Volumes) Used in Pulmonary Function Tests

VOLUME OR CAPACITY	DEFINITION
tidal volume (TV)	amount of air breathed into or out of the lungs in quiet, relaxed breathing
residual volume (RV)	amount of air that remains in the lungs after maximum exhalation
expiratory reserve volume (ERV)	amount of air that can be exhaled after a normal exhalation
inspiratory reserve volume (IRV)	amount of air that can be inhaled above a normal inspiration
total lung capacity (TLC)	total amount of air that can be contained in the lungs after maximum inhalation
inspiratory capacity (IC)	amount of air that can be inhaled after normal exhalation
vital capacity (VC)	amount of air that can be expelled from the lungs by maximum exhalation after maximum inhalation
functional residual capacity (FRC)	amount of air remaining in the lungs after normal exhalation
forced expiratory volume (FEV)	volume of gas exhaled with maximum force within a given interval of time; the time interval is shown as a subscript, such as FEV_1 (1 second), FEV_3 (3 seconds)
forced vital capacity (FVC)	the volume of gas exhaled as rapidly and completely as possible after a complete inhalation

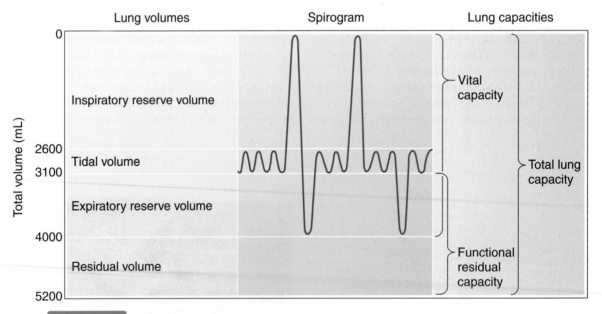

Figure 11-14 **A spirogram.** A spirometer produces a tracing of lung volumes and capacities (sums of volumes).

See Box 11-5 for information on respiratory therapists, who perform many of these tests.

Box 11-5   **Health Professions**

Careers in Respiratory Therapy

Respiratory therapists and respiratory therapy technicians specialize in evaluating and treating breathing disorders. Respiratory therapists evaluate the severity of their clients' conditions by taking complete histories and testing respiratory function with specialized equipment. Based on their findings, and in consultation with a physician, therapists design and implement individualized treatment plans, which may include oxygen therapy and chest physiotherapy. They also educate clients on the use of ventilators and other medical devices. Respiratory therapy technicians assist in carrying out evaluations and treatments.

To perform their duties, both types of practitioners need a thorough scientific background. Most respiratory therapists in the United States receive their training from an accredited college or university and take a national licensing exam. Respiratory therapists and technicians work in a variety of settings, such as hospitals, nursing-care facilities, and private clinics. For additional information about careers in respiratory therapy, contact the American Association for Respiratory Care at www.aarc.org.

Terminology | Key Terms

11

Disorders

acidosis *as-i-DŌ-sis*	Abnormal acidity of body fluids. Respiratory acidosis is caused by abnormally high carbon dioxide levels
acute respiratory distress syndrome (ARDS)	Pulmonary edema that can lead rapidly to fatal respiratory failure; causes include trauma, aspiration into the lungs, viral pneumonia, and drug reactions; shock lung
acute rhinitis *rī-NĪ-tis*	Inflammation of the nasal mucosa with sneezing, tearing, and profuse secretion of watery mucus, as seen in the common cold
alkalosis *al-ka-LŌ-sis*	Abnormal alkalinity of body fluids. Respiratory alkalosis is caused by abnormally low carbon dioxide levels
aspiration *as-pi-RĀ-shun*	The accidental inhalation of food or other foreign material into the lungs. Also means the withdrawal of fluid from a cavity by suction
asthma *AZ-ma*	A disease characterized by dyspnea and wheezing caused by spasm of the bronchial tubes or swelling of their mucous membranes
atelectasis *at-e-LEK-ta-sis*	Incomplete expansion of a lung or part of a lung; lung collapse. May be present at birth (as in respiratory distress syndrome) or be caused by bronchial obstruction or compression of lung tissue (prefix *atel/o* means "imperfect")
bronchiectasis *brong-kē-EK-ta-sis*	Chronic dilatation of a bronchus or bronchi
bronchitis *brong-KĪ-tis*	Inflammation of a bronchus
chronic obstructive pulmonary disease (COPD)	Any of a group of chronic, progressive, and debilitating respiratory diseases, which includes emphysema, asthma, bronchitis, and bronchiectasis
cyanosis *sī-a-NŌ-sis*	Bluish discoloration of the skin caused by lack of oxygen in the blood (adjective: cyanotic) (see Fig. 3-4)

(continued)

Terminology	Key Terms (continued)
cystic fibrosis (CF) *SIS-tik fī-BRŌ-sis*	An inherited disease that affects the pancreas, respiratory system, and sweat glands. Characterized by mucus accumulation in the bronchi causing obstruction and leading to infection
diphtheria *dif-THĒR-ī-a*	Acute infectious disease, usually limited to the upper respiratory tract, characterized by the formation of a surface pseudomembrane composed of cells and coagulated material
dyspnea *dysp-NĒ-a*	Difficult or labored breathing, sometimes with pain; "air hunger"
emphysema *em-fi-SĒ-ma*	A chronic pulmonary disease characterized by enlargement and destruction of the alveoli
empyema *em-pī-Ē-ma*	Accumulation of pus in a body cavity, especially the pleural space; pyothorax
hemoptysis *hē-MOP-ti-sis*	The spitting of blood from the mouth or respiratory tract (*ptysis* means "spitting")
hemothorax *hē-mō-THOR-aks*	Presence of blood in the pleural space
hydrothorax *hī-drō-THOR-aks*	Presence of fluid in the pleural space
hyperventilation *hī-per-ven-ti-LĀ-shun*	Increased rate and depth of breathing; increase in the amount of air entering the alveoli
hypoventilation *hī-pō-ven-ti-LĀ-shun*	Decreased rate and depth of breathing; decrease in the amount of air entering the alveoli
influenza *in-flū-EN-za*	An acute, contagious respiratory infection causing fever, chills, headache, and muscle pain; "flu"
pertussis *per-TUS-is*	An acute, infectious disease characterized by a cough ending in a whooping inspiration; whooping cough
pleural effusion *PLŪR-al e-FŪ-zhun*	Accumulation of fluid in the pleural space. The fluid may contain blood (hemothorax) or pus (pyothorax or empyema)
pleurisy *PLŪR-i-sē*	Inflammation of the pleura; pleuritis. A symptom of pleurisy is sharp pain on breathing
pneumoconiosis *nū-mō-kō-nē-Ō-sis*	Disease of the respiratory tract caused by inhalation of dust particles. Named more specifically by the type of dust inhaled, such as silicosis, anthracosis, asbestosis
pneumonia *nū-MŌ-nē-a*	Inflammation of the lungs generally caused by infection. May involve the bronchioles and alveoli (bronchopneumonia) or one or more lobes of the lung (lobar pneumonia)
pneumonitis *nū-mō-NĪ-tis*	Inflammation of the lungs; may be caused by infection, asthma, allergy, or inhalation of irritants
pneumothorax *nū-mō-THOR-aks*	Accumulation of air or gas in the pleural space. May result from injury or disease or may be produced artificially to collapse a lung
pyothorax *pī-ō-THOR-aks*	Accumulation of pus in the pleural space; empyema
respiratory distress syndrome (RDS)	A respiratory disorder that affects premature infants born without enough surfactant in the lungs. It is treated with respiratory support and surfactant administration
sudden infant death syndrome (SIDS)	The sudden and unexplained death of an apparently healthy infant; crib death
tuberculosis *tū-ber-kū-LŌ-sis*	An infectious disease caused by the tubercle bacillus, *Mycobacterium tuberculosis*. Often involves the lungs but may involve other parts of the body as well. Miliary (*MIL-ē-ar-ē*) tuberculosis is an acute generalized form of the disease with formation of minute tubercles that resemble millet seeds

(continued)

Terminology Key Terms (continued)

Diagnosis

arterial blood gases (ABGs)	The concentrations of gases, specifically oxygen and carbon dioxide, in arterial blood. Reported as the partial pressure (P) of the gas in arterial (a) blood, such as Pao_2 or $Paco_2$. These measurements are important in measuring acid–base balance
bronchoscope *BRONG-kō-skōp*	An endoscope used to examine the tracheobronchial passageways. Also allows access for tissue biopsy or removal of a foreign object (see Fig. 7-7)
lung scan	Study based on the accumulation of radioactive isotope in lung tissue. A *ventilation scan* measures ventilation after inhalation of radioactive material. A *perfusion scan* measures blood supply to the lungs after injection of radioactive material. Also called a pulmonary scintiscan
pulse oximetry *ok-SIM-e-trē*	Determination of the oxygen saturation of arterial blood by means of a photoelectric apparatus (oximeter), usually placed on the finger or the ear; reported as SpO_2 in percent (see Fig. 11-13)
pulmonary function tests	Tests done to assess breathing, usually by spirometry
spirometer *spī-ROM-e-ter*	An apparatus used to measure breathing volumes and capacities; record of test is a spirogram (see Fig. 11-14)
thoracentesis *thor-a-sen-TĒ-sis*	Surgical puncture of the chest for removal of air or fluids, such as may accumulate after surgery or as a result of injury, infection, or cardiovascular problems. Also called thoracocentesis (see Fig. 11-12)
tuberculin test *tū-BER-kū-lin*	A skin test for tuberculosis. Tuberculin, the test material made from products of the tuberculosis organism, is injected below the skin or inoculated with a four-pronged device (tine test)

Go to the pronunciation glossary on the Student Resources to hear these words pronounced.

Terminology Supplementary Terms

Normal Structure and Function

carina *ka-RĪ-na*	A projection of the lowest tracheal cartilage that forms a ridge between the two bronchi. Used as a landmark for endoscopy. Any ridge or ridgelike structure (from a Latin word that means "keel")
hilum *HĪ-lum*	An anatomic depression in an organ where vessels and nerves enter
nares *NĀ-rēz*	The external openings of the nose; the nostrils (singular: naris)
nasal septum	The partition that divides the nasal cavity into two parts (root *sept/o* means "septum")

Symptoms and Conditions

anoxia *an-OK-sē-a*	Lack or absence of oxygen in the tissues; often used incorrectly to mean hypoxia
asphyxia *as-FIK-sē-a*	Condition caused by inadequate intake of oxygen; suffocation (literally "lack of pulse")

(continued)

Terminology	**Supplementary Terms** (continued)
Biot respirations *bē-Ō*	Deep, fast breathing interrupted by sudden pauses; seen in spinal meningitis and other central nervous system disorders
bronchospasm *BRONG-kō-spazm*	Narrowing of the bronchi caused by smooth muscle spasms; common in cases of asthma and bronchitis
Cheyne–Stokes respiration *chān-stōks*	A repeating cycle of gradually increased and then decreased respiration followed by a period of apnea; caused by depression of the breathing centers in the brainstem; seen in cases of coma and in terminally ill patients
cor pulmonale *kor pul-mō-NĀ-lē*	Enlargement of the heart's right ventricle caused by disease of the lungs or pulmonary blood vessels
coryza *kō-RĪ-za*	Acute inflammation of the nasal passages with profuse nasal discharge; acute rhinitis
croup *krūp*	A childhood disease usually caused by a viral infection that involves upper airway inflammation and obstruction. Croup is characterized by a barking cough, difficulty breathing, and laryngeal spasm
deviated septum	A shifted nasal septum; may require surgical correction
epiglottitis *ep-i-glo-TĪ-tis*	Inflammation of the epiglottis that may lead to upper airway obstruction. Commonly seen in croup (also spelled *epiglottiditis*)
epistaxis *ep-i-STAK-sis*	Hemorrhage from the nose; nosebleed (Greek -*staxis* means "dripping")
fremitus *FREM-i-tus*	A vibration, especially as felt through the chest wall on palpation
Kussmaul respiration *KOOS-mawl*	Rapid and deep gasping respiration without pause; characteristic of severe acidosis
pleural friction rub	A sound heard on auscultation that is produced by the rubbing together of the two pleural layers; a common sign of pleurisy
rales *rahlz*	Abnormal chest sounds heard when air enters small airways or alveoli containing fluid; usually heard during inspiration; singular: rale (*rahl*). Also called crackles
rhonchi *RONG-kī*	Abnormal chest sounds produced in airways with accumulated fluids; more noticeable during expiration (singular: rhonchus)
stridor *STRĪ-dor*	A harsh, high-pitched sound caused by obstruction of an upper air passageway
tussis *TUS-is*	A cough. An antitussive drug is one that relieves or prevents coughing
wheeze	A whistling or sighing sound caused by narrowing of a respiratory passageway

Disorders

byssinosis *bis-i-NŌ-sis*	Obstructive airway disease caused by reaction to the dust in unprocessed plant fibers
sleep apnea *AP-nē-a*	Intermittent periods of breathing cessation during sleep. Central sleep apnea arises from failure of the brainstem to stimulate breathing. Obstructive sleep apnea results from airway obstruction during deep sleep, as from obesity or enlarged tonsils
small cell carcinoma	A highly malignant type of bronchial tumor involving small, undifferentiated cells; "oat cell" carcinoma

Diagnosis

Mantoux test *man-TOO*	A test for tuberculosis in which PPD (tuberculin) is injected into the skin. The test does not differentiate active from inactive cases

(continued)

Terminology	**Supplementary Terms** (continued)	

mediastinoscopy *mē-dē-as-ti-NOS-kō-pē*	Examination of the mediastinum by means of an endoscope inserted through an incision above the sternum
plethysmograph *ple-THIZ-mō-graf*	An instrument that measures changes in gas volume and pressure during respiration
pneumotachometer *nū-mō-tak-OM-e-ter*	A device for measuring air flow
thoracoscopy *thor-a-KOS-kō-pē*	Examination of the pleural cavity through an endoscope; pleuroscopy
tine test	A test for tuberculosis in which PPD (tuberculin) is introduced into the skin with a multi-pronged device. The test does not differentiate active from inactive cases

Treatment

aerosol therapy	Treatment by inhalation of a drug or water in spray form
continuous positive airway pressure (CPAP)	Use of a mechanical respirator to maintain pressure throughout the respiratory cycle in a patient who is breathing spontaneously
extubation	Removal of a previously inserted tube
intermittent positive pressure breathing (IPPB)	Use of a ventilator to inflate the lungs at intervals under positive pressure during inhalation
intermittent positive pressure ventilation (IPPV)	Use of a mechanical ventilator to force air into the lungs while allowing for passive exhalation
nasal cannula *KAN-ū-la*	A two-pronged plastic device inserted into the nostrils for delivery of oxygen (Fig. 11-15)
orthopneic position *or-thop-NĒ-ik*	An upright or semiupright position that aids breathing
positive end-expiratory pressure (PEEP)	Use of a mechanical ventilator to increase the volume of gas in the lungs at the end of exhalation, thus improving gas exchange
postural drainage *POS-tū-ral*	Use of body position to drain secretions from the lungs by gravity. The patient is placed so that secretions will move passively into the larger airways for elimination
thoracic gas volume (TGV, V_{TG})	The volume of gas in the thoracic cavity calculated from measurements made with a body plethysmograph

Surgery

adenoidectomy *ad-e-noyd-EK-tō-mē*	Surgical removal of the adenoids
intubation *in-tū-BĀ-shun*	Insertion of a tube into a hollow organ, such as into the larynx or trachea for entrance of air (Fig. 11-16). Patients may be intubated during surgery for administration of anesthesia or to maintain an airway. Endotracheal intubation may be used as an emergency measure when airways are blocked
lobectomy *lō-BEK-tō-mē*	Surgical removal of a lobe of the lung or of another organ
pneumoplasty *NŪ-mō-plas-tē*	Plastic surgery of the lung. In reduction pneumoplasty, nonfunctional portions of the lung are removed, as in cases of advanced emphysema
tracheotomy *trā-kē-OT-ō-mē*	Incision of the trachea through the neck, usually to establish an airway in cases of tracheal obstruction
tracheostomy *trā-kē-OS-tō-mē*	Surgical creation of an opening into the trachea to form an airway or to prepare for the insertion of a tube for ventilation (Fig. 11-17); also the opening thus created

11

(continued)

Terminology Supplementary Terms (continued)

Drugs

antihistamine *an-ti-HIS-ta-mēn*	Agent that prevents responses mediated by histamine, such as allergic and inflammatory reactions
antitussive *an-ti-TUS-iv*	Drug that prevents or relieves coughing
asthma maintenance drug	Agent used to prevent asthma attacks and for chronic treatment of asthma
bronchodilator *brong-kō-DĪ-lā-tor*	Drug that relieves bronchial spasm and widens the bronchi
corticosteroid *kor-ti-kō-STĒR-oyd*	Hormone from the adrenal cortex; used to reduce inflammation
decongestant *dē-kon-JES-tant*	Agent that reduces congestion or swelling
expectorant *ek-SPEK-tō-rant*	Agent that aids in removal of bronchopulmonary secretions
isoniazid (INH) *ī-sō-NĪ-a-zid*	Drug used to treat tuberculosis
leukotriene antagonist *lū-kō-TRĪ-ēn*	Drug that prevents or reduces inflammation by inhibiting leukotrienes, substances made in white blood cells that promote inflammation; they also constrict the bronchi and increase mucus production; used in asthma treatment
mucolytic *mū-kō-LIT-ik*	Agent that loosens mucus to aid in its removal

PASSport to Success® Go to the pronunciation glossary on the Student Resources to hear these words pronounced.

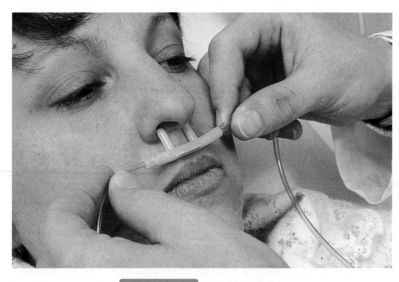

Figure 11-15 **A nasal cannula.**

Intranasal intubation

A

Oral intubation

B

Figure 11-16 **Endotracheal intubation.** (*A*) Nasal endotracheal catheter in proper position. (*B*) Oral endotracheal intubation.

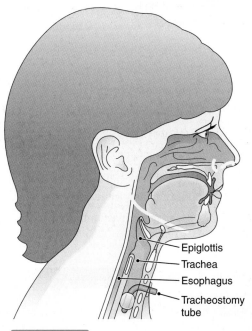

Figure 11-17 **A tracheostomy tube in place.**

Terminology | Abbreviations

ABG(s)	Arterial blood gas(es)		**HPS**	*Hantavirus* pulmonary syndrome
AFB	Acid-fast bacillus (usually *Mycobacterium tuberculosis*)		**IC**	Inspiratory capacity
			INH	Isoniazid
ARDS	Acute respiratory distress syndrome; shock lung		**IPPB**	Intermittent positive pressure breathing
			IPPV	Intermittent positive pressure ventilation
ARF	Acute respiratory failure		**IRV**	Inspiratory reserve volume
BCG	Bacillus Calmette–Guérin (tuberculosis vaccine)		**LLL**	Left lower lobe (of lung)
			LUL	Left upper lobe (of lung)
BS	Breath sounds		**MEFR**	Maximal expiratory flow rate
C	Compliance		**MMFR**	Maximum midexpiratory flow rate
CF	Cystic fibrosis		**O$_2$**	Oxygen
CO$_2$	Carbon dioxide		**Paco$_2$**	Arterial partial pressure of carbon dioxide
COLD	Chronic obstructive lung disease		**Pao$_2$**	Arterial partial pressure of oxygen
COPD	Chronic obstructive pulmonary disease		**PCP**	*Pneumocystis* pneumonia
CPAP	Continuous positive airway pressure		**PEEP**	Positive end-expiratory pressure
CXR	Chest radiograph, chest x-ray		**PEFR**	Peak expiratory flow rate
DTaP	Diphtheria, tetanus, acellular pertussis (vaccine)		**PFT**	Pulmonary function test(s)
			PIP	Peak inspiratory pressure
ERV	Expiratory reserve volume		**PND**	Paroxysmal nocturnal dyspnea
FEV	Forced expiratory volume		**PPD**	Purified protein derivative (tuberculin)
FRC	Functional residual capacity		**R**	Respiration
FVC	Forced vital capacity			

(continued)

Terminology Abbreviations (continued)

RDS	Respiratory distress syndrome		**T & A**	Tonsils and adenoids; tonsillectomy and adenoidectomy
RLL	Right lower lobe (of lung)		**TB**	Tuberculosis
RML	Right middle lobe (of lung)		**TGV**	Thoracic gas volume
RSV	Respiratory syncytial virus		**TLC**	Total lung capacity
RUL	Right upper lobe (of lung)		**TV**	Tidal volume
RV	Residual volume		**URI**	Upper respiratory infection
SARS	Severe acute respiratory syndrome		**VC**	Vital capacity
SIDS	Sudden infant death syndrome		V_{TG}	Thoracic gas volume
SpO_2	Oxygen percent saturation			

Chapter Review

LABELING EXERCISE

The Respiratory System > Write the name of each numbered part on the corresponding line of the answer sheet.

Alveolar duct   Mediastinum
Alveoli   Nasal cavity
Capillaries   Nasopharynx
Diaphragm   Oropharynx
Epiglottis   Right bronchus
Esophagus   Right lung
Frontal sinus   Sphenoidal sinus
Laryngeal pharynx   Terminal bronchiole
Larynx and vocal cords   Trachea
Left lung

1. _____

2. _____

3. _____

4. _____

5. _____

6. _____

7. _____

8. _____

9. _____

10. _____   15. _____

11. _____   16. _____

12. _____   17. _____

13. _____   18. _____

14. _____   19. _____

101. pneumoconiosis (*nū-mō-kō-nē-Ō-sis*) _____

   a. pneum/o _____

   b. coni/o _____

   c. -sis _____

 Go to the word exercises on the Student Resources for additional review exercises.

Case Studies

▶ Case Study 11-1: Preoperative Testing in a Patient With Asthma

A.D., 15 years old, was seen in the preadmission testing unit in preparation for her elective spinal surgery. She has a history of mild asthma since age 4, with at least one attack per week. In an acute attack, she will have mild dyspnea, diffuse wheezing, yet an adequate air exchange that responds to bronchodilators. She was sent to pulmonary health services for a consult with a specialist and pulmonary function studies to clear her for surgery. The anesthesiologist reviewed the pulmonologist's report.

Her prebronchodilator spirometry showed a mild reduction in vital capacity but with a moderate to severe decrease in FEV_1 and FEV_1/FVC ratio. After bronchodilator administration, there was a mild but insignificant improvement in FEV_1. The postbronchodilator FEV_1 was 55% of predicted and was considered moderately abnormal. The flow volume loops and spirographic curves were consistent with airflow obstruction.

▶ Case Study 11-2: Giant Cell Sarcoma of the Lung

L.E., a 68-year-old man, was admitted to the pulmonary unit with chest pain on inspiration, dyspnea, and diaphoresis. He had smoked 1–1/2 packs of cigarettes per day for 52 years and had quit 3 months ago. L.E. was retired from the advertising industry and admitted to occasional alcohol use. He was treated for primary giant cell sarcoma of the left lung 3 years ago with a lobectomy of the left lung followed by radiation and chemotherapy.

Physical examination was unremarkable except for a thoracotomy scar in the left hemithorax,

decreased breath sounds, and dullness to percussion of the left base. There was no hemoptysis. Radionucleotide bone scan showed increased activity in the left upper posterior hemithorax. Chest and upper abdomen CT scan showed findings compatible with recurrent sarcoma of the left hemithorax. Abnormal mediastinal nodes were evident. Thoracentesis was attempted but did not yield fluid. L.E. was scheduled for a left thoracoscopy, mediastinoscopy, and biopsy.

▶ Case Study 11-3: Terminal Dyspnea

N.A., a 76-year-old woman, was in the ICU in the terminal stage of multisystem organ failure. She had been admitted to the hospital for bacterial pneumonia, which had not resolved with antibiotic therapy. She had a 20-year history of COPD. She was not conscious and was unable to breathe on her own. Her ABGs were abnormal, and she was diagnosed with refractory ARDS. The decision was made to support her breathing with endotracheal intubation and mechanical ventilation. After 1 week and several unsuccessful attempts to wean her from the ventilator, the pulmonologist suggested a permanent tracheostomy and family consideration of continuing or withdrawing life support. Her physiologic status met the criteria of remote or no chance for recovery.

N.A.'s family discussed her condition and decided not to pursue aggressive life-sustaining therapies. N.A. was assigned DNR status. After the written orders were read and signed by the family, the endotracheal tube, feeding tube, pulse oximeter, and ECG electrodes were removed and a morphine IV drip was started with prn boluses ordered to promote comfort and relieve pain and other symptoms of dying. The family sat with N.A. for many hours while her breaths became shallow with

(continued)

Case Studies *(continued)*

Cheyne–Stokes respirations. She died surrounded by her family with the hospital chaplain.

CASE STUDY QUESTIONS

Multiple choice. Select the best answer and write the letter of your choice to the left of each number:

_____ 1. The root *spir/o*, as in *spirometry*, means:
   a. turbulence
   b. breathing
   c. twisted
   d. air quality
   e. saturation

_____ 2. The root *pulmon*, as in *pulmonary*, means:
   a. chest
   b. air
   c. lung
   d. breath sound
   e. blood vessel

_____ 3. Hemoptysis is:
   a. drooping eyelids
   b. discoloration of skin
   c. blue nail beds
   d. spitting of blood
   e. acute leukemia

_____ 4. Dyspnea could NOT be described as:
   a. difficulty breathing
   b. eupnea
   c. air hunger
   d. orthopnea
   e. Cheyne–Stokes respirations

_____ 5. Pulse oximetry is used to measure:
   a. forced expiratory volume
   b. tidal volume
   c. end-tidal CO_2
   d. oxygen saturation of blood
   e. positive end-expiratory pressure

_____ 6. An endotracheal tube is placed:
   a. under the trachea
   b. beyond the carina
   c. within the bronchus
   d. around the airway
   e. within the trachea

Write words from the case histories with the following meanings:

7. Whistling breath sounds due to narrowing of the breathing passageways

   _____

8. A drug that enlarges the lumen of the bronchi

   _____

9. Removal of a lobe

   _____

10. Profuse sweating

   _____

11. Surgical incision of the chest

   _____

12. Endoscopic examination of the chest cavity

   _____

13. Half of the chest

   _____

14. Endoscopic examination of the space between the lungs

   _____

15. Movement of air into and out of the lungs

   _____

Abbreviations. Define the following abbreviations:

16. COPD _____

17. FVC _____

18. ABG _____

19. ARDS _____

20. DNR _____

The Digestive System

CHAPTER CONTENTS

OBJECTIVES

After study of this chapter you should be able to:

1. Explain the function of the digestive system.
2. Label a diagram of the digestive tract, and describe the function of each part.
3. Label a diagram of the accessory organs, and explain the role of each in digestion.
4. Identify and use the roots pertaining to the digestive system.
5. Describe the major disorders of the digestive system.
6. Define medical terms used in reference to the digestive system.
7. Interpret abbreviations used in referring to the gastrointestinal system.
8. Analyze case studies concerning gastroenterology.

PRETEST

Multiple choice. Select the best answer and write the letter of your choice to the left of each number.

___ 1. An organic catalyst is a(n):

  a. sugar   c. saliva
  b. nucleic acid   d. enzyme

___ 2. The organ that carries food from the pharynx to the stomach is the:

  a. trachea   c. esophagus
  b. larynx   d. intestine

___ 3. The word root for the stomach is:

  a. gastr/o   c. ren/o
  b. hepat/o   d. cardi/o

___ 4. The main portion of the large intestine is the:

  a. stomach   c. colon
  b. appendix   d. rectum

___ 5. The word root *enter/o* refers to the:

   a. intestine   c. kidney
   b. heart   d. gallbladder

___ 6. The wavelike action that moves substances through an organ is called:

   a. pulmonary   c. parotid
   b. peristalsis   d. mastication

___ 7. The process of moving digested nutrients from the intestine into the circulation is called:

   a. digestion   c. absorption
   b. egestion   d. lymphedema

___ 8. The organ that secretes bile is the:

   a. kidney   c. liver
   b. spleen   d. stomach

___ 9. Cholecystitis is inflammation of the:

   a. gallbladder   c. diaphragm
   b. throat   d. small intestine

The function of the digestive system is to prepare food for intake by body cells. Nutrients must be broken down by mechanical and chemical means into molecules that are small enough to be absorbed into the circulation. Within cells, the nutrients are used for energy and for rebuilding vital cell components.

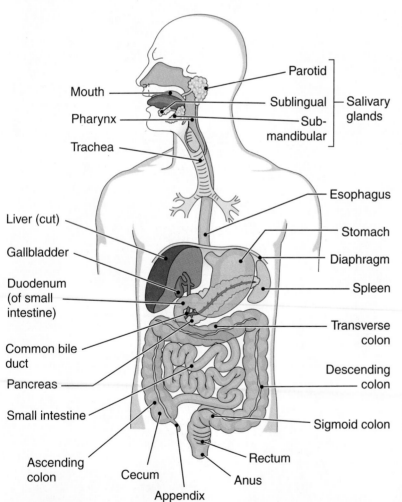

Figure 12-1 **Digestive system.** Some divisions of the small and large intestine are shown. The accessory organs are the salivary glands, liver, gallbladder, and pancreas. The trachea, diaphragm, and spleen are shown for reference.

Digestion

Digestion takes place in the digestive tract proper, which extends from the **mouth** to the **anus** (Fig. 12-1). **Peristalsis**, wavelike contractions of the organ walls, moves food through the digestive tract and also moves undigested waste material out of the body. Also contributing to digestion are several accessory organs that release secretions into the digestive tract.

Enzymes are needed throughout the digestive process. These compounds are organic catalysts that speed the rate of food's chemical breakdown. The names of most enzymes can be recognized by the ending *-ase*.

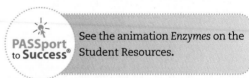

See the animation *Enzymes* on the Student Resources.

The Digestive Tract

The digestive tract, also known as the alimentary canal or gastrointestinal (GI) tract, is essentially a long tube modified into separate organs with special functions (see Fig. 12-1). Reference Box 12-1 summarizes the activities of the digestive organs described below.

Box 12-1 — For Your Reference

Organs of the Digestive Tract

ORGAN	DIGESTIVE ACTIONS
Mouth	Used to bite and chew food. Mixes food with saliva, which contains salivary amylase, an enzyme that begins the digestion of starch. Shapes food into small portions, which the tongue pushes into the pharynx
Pharynx	Swallows food by reflex action and moves it into the esophagus
Esophagus	Moves food into the stomach by peristalsis
Stomach	Stores food; churns to mix food with water and digestive juices. Secretes protein-digesting hydrochloric acid (HCl) and the enzyme pepsin
Small intestine	Secretes enzymes. Receives secretions from the accessory organs, which digest and neutralize food. Site of most digestion and absorption of nutrients into the circulation
Large intestine	Forms, stores, and eliminates undigested waste material

The Mouth to the Stomach

Digestion begins in the mouth (Fig. 12-2), also called the oral cavity. Here food is chewed into small bits by the teeth. There are 32 teeth in a complete adult set, including incisors and canines to bite food and molars for grinding. The structural features of a molar tooth and its surrounding tissue are shown in Figure 12-3. The **palate** is the roof of the mouth; the anterior portion (hard palate) is formed by bone, and the posterior part (soft palate) is made of soft tissue. The fleshy **uvula**, used in speech production, hangs from the soft palate. Dental hygienists help in care of the mouth and teeth. Box 12-2 has information on careers in dental hygiene.

In the process of chewing, or **mastication**, the tongue, lips, cheeks, and palate also help to break up food and mix it with **saliva**, a secretion that moistens the food and begins starch digestion. The salivary glands (see Fig. 12-1) secrete saliva into the mouth and are considered to be accessory digestive organs.

Portions of moistened food are moved toward the **pharynx** (throat), where swallowing reflexes push it into the **esophagus**. Peristalsis moves the food through the esophagus and into the **stomach**. At its distal end, where

12

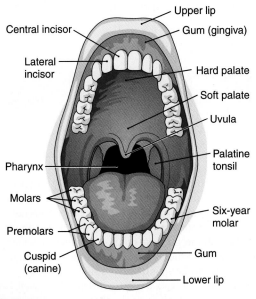

Figure 12-2 **The mouth.** The teeth, pharynx, tonsils, and other structures in the oral cavity are shown.

Labels: Central incisor, Lateral incisor, Pharynx, Molars, Premolars, Cuspid (canine), Upper lip, Gum (gingiva), Hard palate, Soft palate, Uvula, Palatine tonsil, Six-year molar, Gum, Lower lip

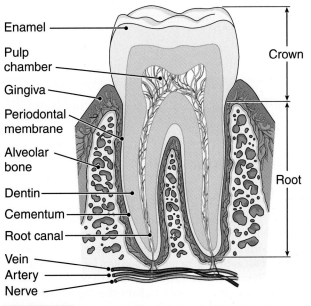

Figure 12-3 **A molar tooth.** The bony socket, gingiva, blood vessels, and nerve supply are shown, as well as portions of the tooth.

Labels: Enamel, Pulp chamber, Gingiva, Periodontal membrane, Alveolar bone, Dentin, Cementum, Root canal, Vein, Artery, Nerve, Crown, Root

Box 12-2 Health Professions

Dental Hygienist

Dental hygienists are concerned with dental health mainte-nance and preventive dental care. They examine patients' teeth and gums; take and develop dental x-rays; and clean the teeth, using hand, rotary, and ultrasonic instruments to remove deposits, such as calculus, stains, and plaque. They may also apply fluorides to prevent cavities. They work inde-pendently or along with a dentist to administer anesthesia, finish fillings and restorations, remove sutures, or assist in periodontal (gum) treatment. Dental hygienists must be informed about safety concerning x-ray equipment, anesthe-sia, and infectious diseases. They wear safety glasses, surgical masks, and gloves to protect themselves and their patients. A major component of the dental hygienist's work is patient education for maintenance of good oral health. They may give instruction on diet and proper dental care, such as flossing and brushing the teeth.

Most dental hygiene programs award an associate degree; some offer a certificate, bachelor's, or master's degree. The higher degrees are required for research, teaching, or practice in public or school health facilities. The curriculum includes aca-demic and health-oriented sciences, material on the legal aspects of dental hygiene practice, and clinical training. After graduation, dental hygienists must be licensed in their states by passing a clinical examination and a written examination administered by the American Dental Association's (ADA's) Joint Commission on National Dental Examinations.

Almost all hygienists work in dental offices. One advan-tage of this field is scheduling flexibility and the opportunity for part-time work. Job prospects are good; dental hygiene is among the fastest growing occupations. Benefits vary with place of employment. For additional information, contact the American Dental Hygienists' Association at www.adha.org.

---

it joins the stomach, the esophagus has muscle tissue that contracts to keep stomach contents from refluxing (flow-ing backward). This **lower esophageal sphincter (LES)** is also called the "cardiac sphincter" because it lies above the cardia of the stomach, the region around its upper opening.

In the stomach, food is further broken down as it is churned and mixed with secretions containing the enzyme pepsin and powerful hydrochloric acid (HCl), both of which break down proteins. The partially digested food then passes through the stomach's lower portion, the **pylorus**, into the **intestine**.

The Small Intestine

Food leaving the stomach enters the **duodenum**, the first portion of the **small intestine**. As the food continues through the **jejunum** and **ileum**, the small intestine's remaining sections, digestion is completed (see Box 12-3). The digestive substances active in the small intestine include enzymes from the intestine itself and products from accessory organs that secrete into the duodenum.

The digested nutrients, as well as water, minerals, and vitamins, are absorbed into the circulation, aided by small projections in the intestinal lining called **villi** (Fig. 12-4).

Box 12-3 Focus on Words

Homonyms

Homonyms are words that sound alike but have different meanings. One must know the context in which they are used in order to understand the intended meaning. For example, the ilium is the upper portion of the pelvis, but the ileum is the last portion of the small intestine. Different adjectives are pre-ferred for each, iliac for the first and ileal for the second.

The word *meiosis* refers to the type of cell division that halves the chromosomes to form the gametes, but miosis means abnormal contraction of the pupil. Both words come from the Greek word that means a decrease.

Similar-sounding names lead to some funny misspellings. The large bone of the upper arm is the humerus, but this bone is often written as humorous. The vagus nerve (cranial nerve X) is named with a root that means "wander," as in the words vague and vagabond, because this nerve branches to many of the internal organs. Students often write the name as if it had some relation to the famous gambling city in Nevada.

Homonyms may have a more serious side as well. Drug names may sound or look so similar that clinicians could con-fuse them, leading to dangerous situations.

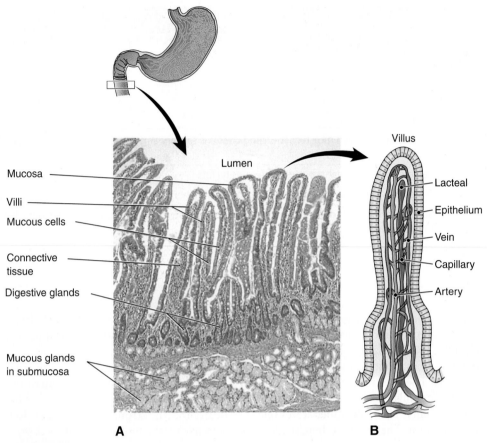

Figure 12-4 **Intestinal villi.** (*A*) Microscopic view of the small intestine's lining showing villi and glands that secrete mucus and digestive juices. The lumen is the central opening. (*B*) An intestinal villus. Each villus has blood vessels and a lacteal (lymphatic capillary) for nutrient absorption.

Each villus has blood capillaries to absorb nutrients into the bloodstream and lymphatic capillaries, or **lacteals**, to absorb small molecules of digested fats into the lymph. These fats join the blood when lymph flows into the bloodstream near the heart.

The Large Intestine

Any food that has not been digested, along with water and digestive juices, passes into the **large intestine**. This part of the digestive tract begins in the lower right region of the abdomen with a small pouch, the **cecum**, to which the **appendix** is attached. (The appendix does not aid in digestion, but contains lymphatic tissue and may function in immunity.) The large intestine continues as the **colon**, a name that is often used alone to mean the large intestine, because the colon constitutes such a large portion of that organ. The colon travels upward along the right side of the abdomen as the ascending colon, crosses below the stomach as the transverse colon, then continues down the left side of the abdomen as the descending colon. As food is pushed through the colon, water is reabsorbed and stool or **feces** is formed. This waste material passes into the S-shaped **sigmoid colon** and is stored in the **rectum** until eliminated through the anus.

The Accessory Organs

The salivary glands, which secrete into the mouth, are the first accessory organs to act on food. They secrete an enzyme (salivary amylase) that begins starch digestion. The remaining accessory organs are in the abdomen and secrete into the duodenum (Fig. 12-5). The **liver** is a

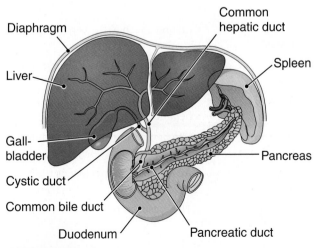

Figure 12-5 **Accessory organs of digestion.** The organs and ducts are shown. The diaphragm and spleen are shown for reference.

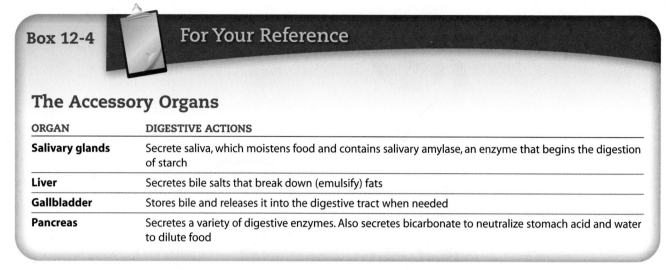

Box 12-4 — For Your Reference

The Accessory Organs

ORGAN	DIGESTIVE ACTIONS
Salivary glands	Secrete saliva, which moistens food and contains salivary amylase, an enzyme that begins the digestion of starch
Liver	Secretes bile salts that break down (emulsify) fats
Gallbladder	Stores bile and releases it into the digestive tract when needed
Pancreas	Secretes a variety of digestive enzymes. Also secretes bicarbonate to neutralize stomach acid and water to dilute food

large gland with many functions. A major activity is to process blood, removing toxins and converting nutrients into new compounds. A special circulatory pathway, the **hepatic portal system,** carries blood to the liver from the other abdominal organs. The liver functions in digestion by secreting **bile,** which emulsifies fats, that is, breaks them down into smaller units. The **gallbladder** stores bile until it is needed in digestion. The common hepatic duct from the liver and the cystic duct from the gallbladder merge to form the **common bile duct,** which empties into the duodenum.

The **pancreas** produces a mixture of digestive enzymes that is delivered into the duodenum through the pancreatic duct. It also secretes large amounts of bicarbonate, which neutralizes the strong stomach acid. Reference Box 12-4 summarizes the functions of the accessory organs.

Terminology — Key Terms

Normal Structure and Function

anus Ā-nus	The distal opening of the digestive tract (root: an/o)
appendix a-PEN-diks	An appendage; usually means the narrow tube of lymphatic tissue attached to the cecum, the vermiform (wormlike) appendix
bile bīl	The fluid secreted by the liver that emulsifies fats and aids in their absorption (roots: chol/e, bili)
cecum SĒ-kum	A blind pouch at the beginning of the large intestine (root: cec/o)
colon KŌ-lon	The major portion of the large intestine; extends from the cecum to the rectum and is formed by ascending, transverse, and descending portions (roots: col/o, colon/o)
common bile duct	The duct that carries bile into the duodenum; formed by the union of the cystic duct and the common hepatic duct (root: choledoch/o)
duodenum dū-ō-DĒ-num	The first portion of the small intestine (root: duoden/o)
enzyme en-zīm	An organic catalyst; speeds the rate of chemical reactions
esophagus ē-SOF-a-gus	The muscular tube that carries food from the pharynx to the stomach

(continued)

Terminology	**Key Terms** (continued)
feces *FĒ-sēz*	The waste material eliminated from the intestine (adjective: fecal); stool
gallbladder	A sac on the undersurface of the liver that stores bile (root: *cholecyst/o*)
hepatic portal system	A special circulatory pathway that brings blood directly from the abdominal organs to the liver for processing (also called simply the *portal system*). The vessel that enters the liver is the hepatic portal vein (portal vein)
ileum *IL-ē-um*	The terminal portion of the small intestine (root: *ile/o*)
intestine *in-TES-tin*	The portion of the digestive tract between the stomach and the anus. It consists of the small intestine and large intestine. It functions in digestion, absorption, and elimination of waste (root: *enter/o*). The bowel (*BOW-el*)
jejunum *je-JŪ-num*	The middle portion of the small intestine (root: *jejun/o*)
lacteal *lak-TĒL*	A lymphatic capillary in a villus of the small intestine. Lacteals absorb digested fats into the lymph
large intestine *in-TES-tin*	The terminal portion of the digestive tract, consisting of the cecum, colon, rectum, and anus. It stores and eliminates undigested waste material (feces)
liver *LIV-er*	The large gland in the upper right abdomen. In addition to many other functions, it secretes bile needed for digestion and absorption of fats (root: *hepat/o*)
lower esophageal sphincter (LES) *ē-sof-a-JĒ-al SFINK-ter*	Muscle tissue at the distal end of the esophagus (gastroesophageal junction) that prevents stomach contents from refluxing into the esophagus. Also called the cardiac sphincter
mastication *mas-ti-KĀ-shun*	Chewing
mouth	The oral cavity; contains the tongue and teeth. Used to take in and chew food, mix it with saliva, and move it toward the throat to be swallowed
palate *PAL-at*	The roof of the mouth; the partition between the mouth and nasal cavity. Consists of an anterior portion formed by bone, the hard palate, and a posterior portion formed of tissue, the soft palate (root: *palat/o*)
pancreas *PAN-krē-as*	A large, elongated gland posterior to the stomach. It produces hormones that regulate sugar metabolism and also produces digestive enzymes (root: *pancreat/o*)
peristalsis *per-i-STAL-sis*	Wavelike contractions of an organ's walls; moves material through an organ or duct
pharynx *FAR-inks*	The throat; a common passageway for food entering the esophagus and air entering the larynx (root: *pharyng/o*)
pylorus *pī-LOR-us*	The stomach's distal opening into the duodenum (root: *pylor/o*). The opening is controlled by a ring of muscle, the pyloric sphincter
rectum *REK-tum*	The distal portion of the large intestine. It stores and eliminates undigested waste (roots: *rect/o*, *proct/o*)
saliva *sa-LĪ-va*	The clear secretion released into the mouth that moistens food and contains a starch-digesting enzyme (root: *sial/o*). Saliva is produced by three pairs of glands: the parotid, submandibular, and sublingual glands (see Fig. 12-1)
sigmoid colon	Distal S-shaped portion of the large intestine located between the descending colon and the rectum
small intestine *in-TES-tin*	The portion of the intestine between the stomach and the large intestine; comprised of the duodenum, jejunum, and ileum. Accessory organs secrete into the small intestine, and almost all digestion and absorption occur there

12

(continued)

Terminology	Key Terms (continued)	

stomach STUM-ak	A muscular saclike organ below the diaphragm that stores food and secretes juices that digest proteins (root: *gastr/o*)
uvula Ū-vū-la	The fleshy mass that hangs from the soft palate; aids in speech production (literally "little grape") (root: *uvul/o*)
villi VIL-ī	Tiny projections in the lining of the small intestine that absorb digested foods into the circulation (singular: villus)

PASSport to Success® — Go to the pronunciation glossary on the Student Resources to hear these words pronounced.

Roots Pertaining to the Digestive System

See Tables 12-1 to 12-3.

Table 12-1	Roots for the Mouth		
Root	**Meaning**	**Example**	**Definition of Example**
bucc/o	cheek	buccoversion *buk-kō-VER-zhun*	turning toward the cheek
dent/o, dent/i	tooth, teeth	edentulous *ē-DEN-tū-lus*	without teeth
odont/o	tooth, teeth	periodontics *per-ē-ō-DON-tiks*	dental specialty that deals with the study and treatment of the tissues around the teeth
gingiv/o	gum (gingiva)	gingivectomy *jin-ji-VEK-tō-mē*	excision of gum tissue
gloss/o	tongue	glossoplegia *glos-ō-PLĒ-jē-a*	paralysis (-plegia) of the tongue
lingu/o	tongue	orolingual *or-ō-LING-gwal*	pertaining to the mouth and tongue
gnath/o	jaw	prognathous *PROG-na-thus*	having a projecting jaw
labi/o	lip	labium *LĀ-bē-um*	lip or liplike structure
or/o	mouth	circumoral *sir-kum-OR-al*	around the mouth
stoma, stomat/o	mouth	xerostomia *zē-rō-STŌ-mē-a*	dryness (xero-) of the mouth
palat/o	palate	palatine *PAL-a-tīn*	pertaining to the palate (also palatal)
sial/o	saliva, salivary gland, salivary duct	sialogram *sī-AL-ō-gram*	radiograph of the salivary glands and ducts
uvul/o	uvula	uvulotome *Ū-vū-lō-tōm*	instrument (-tome) for incising the uvula

EXERCISE **12-1**

Use the adjective suffix -al to write a word that has the same meaning as the following:

1. pertaining to the mouth   oral _____

2. pertaining to the lip _____

3. pertaining to the cheek _____

4. pertaining to the teeth _____

5. pertaining to the gums _____

6. pertaining to the tongue _____

Fill in the blanks:

7. The oropharynx is the part of the pharynx that is located behind the _____.

8. A dentifrice (DEN-ti-fris) is an agent used to clean the _____.

9. An orthodontist (or-thō-DON-tist) specializes in straightening (ortho-) of the _____.

10. Micrognathia (mī-krō-NĀ-thē-a) is excessive smallness of the _____.

11. Stomatoplasty (STŌ-ma-tō-plas-tē) is any plastic repair of the _____.

12. Hemiglossal (hem-ī-GLOS-al) means pertaining to one half of the _____.

13. A sialolith (sī-AL-ō-lith) is a stone formed in a _____ gland or duct.

Define the following words:

14. extrabuccal (eks-tra-BUK-al) _____

15. sublingual (sub-LING-gwal) _____

16. labiodental (lā-bē-ō-DEN-tal) _____

17. gingivitis (jin-ji-VĪ-tis) _____

18. uvuloptosis (ū-vū-lop-TŌ-sis) _____

19. hypoglossal (hī-pō-GLOS-al) _____

20. palatorrhaphy (pal-at-OR-a-fē) _____

12

Table 12-2	Roots for the Digestive Tract (Except the Month)		
Root	**Meaning**	**Example**	**Definition of Example**
esophag/o	esophagus	esophageal* ē-sof-a-JĒ-al	pertaining to the esophagus
gastr/o	stomach	gastroparesis gas-trō-pa-RĒ-sis	partial paralysis (paresis) of the stomach
pylor/o	pylorus	pyloroplasty pī-LOR-ō-plas-tē	plastic repair of the pylorus
enter/o	intestine	dysentery DIS-en-ter-ē	infectious disease of the intestine
duoden/o	duodenum	duodenostomy dū-ō-de-NOS-tō-mē	surgical creation of an opening into the duodenum

(continued)

Table 12-2	Continued		
jejun/o	jejunum	jejunectomy je-jū-NEK-tō-mē	excision of the jejunum
ile/o	ileum	ileitis il-ē-Ī-tis	inflammation of the ileum
cec/o	cecum	cecoptosis sē-kop-TŌ-sis	downward displacement of the cecum
col/o, colon/o	colon	coloclysis kō-lō-KLĪ-sis	irrigation (-clysis) of the colon
sigmoid/o	sigmoid colon	sigmoidoscope sig-MOY-dō-skōp	an endoscope for examining the sigmoid colon
rect/o	rectum	rectocele REK-tō-sēl	hernia of the rectum
proct/o	rectum	proctopexy PROK-tō-pek-sē	surgical fixation of the rectum
an/o	anus	perianal per-ē-Ā-nal	around the anus

*Note addition of e before -al.

EXERCISE **12-2**

Use the adjective suffix -ic to write a word for the following definitions:

1. pertaining to the stomach   _____ gastric _____

2. pertaining to the intestine   _____

3. pertaining to the pylorus   _____

4. pertaining to the colon   _____

Use the adjective suffix -*al* to write a word for the following definitions:

5. pertaining to the duodenum   _____ duodenal _____

6. pertaining to the jejunum   _____

7. pertaining to the ileum   _____

8. pertaining to the cecum   _____

9. pertaining to the anus   _____

Write a word for the following definitions:

10. inflammation of the esophagus   _____

11. surgical fixation of the stomach   _____

12. study of the stomach and intestines   _____

13. endoscopic examination of the duodenum   _____

14. downward displacement of the pylorus   _____

15. surgical creation of an opening into the jejunum   _____

16. excision of the ileum   _____

17. pertaining to the anus and rectum   _____

Use the root *col/o* to write a word for the following definitions:

18. inflammation of the colon _____

19. surgical creation of an opening into the colon _____

20. surgical fixation of the colon _____

21. surgical puncture of the colon _____

Use the root *colon/o* to write a word for the following definitions:

22. any disease of the colon _____

23. endoscopic examination of the colon _____

Two organs of the digestive tract or even two parts of the same organ may be surgically connected by a passage (anastomosis) after removal of damaged tissue. Such a procedure is named for the connected organs plus the ending -*stomy*. Use two roots plus the suffix -*stomy* to write a word for the following definitions:

24. surgical creation of a passage between the esophagus and stomach _____ esophagogastrostomy _____

25. surgical creation of a passage between the stomach and intestine _____

26. surgical creation of a passage between the stomach and the jejunum _____

27. surgical creation of a passage between the duodenum and the ileum _____

28. surgical creation of a passage between the sigmoid colon and the rectum (proct/o) _____

Table 12-3	Roots for the Accessory Organs		
Root	Meaning	Example	Definition of Example
hepat/o	liver	hepatocyte *HEP-a-tō-sīt*	a liver cell
bili	bile	biliary *BIL-ē-ar-ē*	pertaining to the bile or bile ducts
chol/e, chol/o	bile, gall	cholestasis *kō-lē-STĀ-sis*	stoppage of bile flow
cholecyst/o	gallbladder	cholecystogram *kō-lē-SIS-tō-gram*	radiograph of the gallbladder
cholangi/o	bile duct	cholangioma *kō-lan-jē-Ō-ma*	cancer of the bile ducts
choledoch/o	common bile duct	choledochal *kō-LED-o-kal*	pertaining to the common bile duct
pancreat/o	pancreas	pancreatotropic *pan-krē-at-ō-TROP-ik*	acting on the pancreas

EXERCISE 12-3

Use the suffix -*ic* to write a word for the following definitions:

1. pertaining to the liver _____

2. pertaining to the gallbladder _____

3. pertaining to the pancreas _____

Use the suffix *-graphy* to write a word for the following definitions:

4. radiographic study of the pancreas

_____

5. radiographic study of the bile ducts

_____

6. radiographic study of the gallbladder

_____

7. radiographic study of the liver

_____

Use the suffix *-lithiasis* to write a word for the following definitions:

8. condition of having a stone in the common bile duct _____

9. condition of having a stone in the pancreas _____

Fill in the blanks:

10. Inflammation of the liver is called _____

11. The word biligenesis (*bil-i-JEN-e-sis*) means the formation of _____.

12. A cholelith (*KŌ-lē-lith*) is a(n) _____.

13. Choledochotomy (*kō-led-o-KOT-o-mē*) is incision of the _____.

14. Cholecystorrhaphy (*kō-lē-sis-TOR-a-fē*) is suture of the _____.

15. Hepatomegaly (*hep-a-tō-MEG-a-lē*) is enlargement of the _____.

16. Cholangitis (*kō-lan-JĪ-tis*) is inflammation of a(n) _____.

17. Pancreatolysis (*pan-krē-a-TOL-i-sis*) is dissolving of the _____.

Clinical Aspects of the Digestive System

Digestive Tract

INFECTION

A variety of organisms can infect the GI tract, from viruses and bacteria to protozoa and worms. In the mouth, bacterial infection contributes to tooth decay, or **caries**. It may cause a mild gum infection (gingivitis) or more extensive involvement of the deeper tissues and bony support around the tooth (peridontitis). Infections of the stomach or intestine may produce short-lived upsets with **gastroenteritis, nausea, diarrhea**, and **emesis** (vomiting). Other infectious diseases of the GI tract, such as typhoid, cholera, and dysentery, are more serious, even fatal.

Appendicitis results from infection of the appendix, often secondary to its obstruction. Surgery is necessary to avoid rupture and **peritonitis**, infection of the peritoneal cavity.

ULCERS

An ulcer is a lesion of the skin or a mucous membrane marked by inflammation and tissue damage. Ulcers caused by the damaging action of gastric, or peptic, juices on the lining of the GI tract are termed **peptic ulcers**. Most peptic ulcers appear in the first portion of the duodenum. The origins of such ulcers are not completely known, although infection with a bacterium, *Helicobacter pylori*, has been identified as a major cause. Heredity and stress may be factors, as well as chronic inflammation and exposure to damaging drugs, such as aspirin and other NSAIDs, or to irritants in food and drink.

Current ulcer treatment includes the administration of antibiotics to eliminate *H. pylori* infection and use of drugs that inhibit gastric acid secretion. Ulcers may lead to hemorrhage or to perforation of the digestive tract wall.

Ulcers can be diagnosed by **endoscopy** (Fig. 12-6, Box 12-5) and by radiographic study of the GI tract

Figure 12-6   Endoscopy. A patient undergoing gastroscopy is shown.

Box 12-5   Clinical Perspectives

Endoscopy

Modern medicine has made great strides toward looking into the body without resorting to surgery. The endoscope, an instrument that is inserted through a body opening or small incision, has allowed the noninvasive examination of passageways, hollow organs, and body cavities. The first endoscopes were rigid lighted telescopes that could be inserted only a short distance into the body. Today, physicians can navigate the twists and turns of the digestive tract using long fiberoptic endoscopes composed of flexible, light-transmitting bundles of glass or plastic.

Physicians can detect structural abnormalities, ulcers, inflammation, and tumors in the GI tract endoscopically. In addition, they use endoscopes to remove fluid or tissue samples for testing. Some surgery can even be done with an endoscope, such as polyp removal from the colon or sphincter expansion. Endoscopy can also be used to examine and operate on joints (arthroscopy), the bladder (cystoscopy), respiratory passages (bronchoscopy), and the abdominal cavity (laparoscopy).

A "virtual colonoscopy" uses computerized x-rays to generate detailed images of the colon. This method can provide an adequate screening for most people, although a small percentage might then need a standard colonoscopy for further assessment or surgery. Capsular endoscopy, a recent technological advance, has made examination of the GI tract even easier. It uses a pill-sized camera that a patient can swallow! As the camera moves through the digestive tract, it transmits video images to a data recorder worn on the patient's belt.

using a contrast medium, usually barium sulfate. A **barium study** can reveal a variety of GI disorders in addition to ulcers, including tumors and obstructions. A barium swallow is used for study of the pharynx and esophagus; an upper GI series examines the esophagus, stomach, and small intestine.

CANCER

Cancer of the mouth generally involves the lips or tongue. Smoking is a major risk factor in these cases. **Leukoplakia,** white patches on mucous membranes, often resulting from smoking or other irritants, is an early sign of cancer in up to 25% of cases. The most common sites for GI tract cancer are the colon and rectum. Together these colorectal cancers rank among the most frequent causes of cancer deaths in the United States in both men and women. A diet low in fiber and calcium and high in fat is a major risk factor in colorectal cancer. Heredity is also a factor, as is chronic inflammation of the colon (colitis). **Polyps** (growths) in the intestine often become cancerous and should be removed. Polyps can be identified and even removed by endoscopy.

One sign of colorectal cancer is bleeding into the intestine, which can be detected by testing the stool for blood. Because this blood may be present in very small amounts, it is described as **occult** ("hidden") **blood.** Colorectal cancers are staged according to **Dukes classification,** ranging from A to C according to severity.

Examiners can observe the intestine's interior with various endoscopes named for the specific area in which they are used, such as proctoscope (rectum), sigmoidoscope (sigmoid colon), and colonoscope (colon) (Fig. 12-7).

12

A   **B**

Figure 12-7 **Colonoscopy.** (*A*) Sigmoidoscopy. The flexible fiberoptic endoscope is advanced past the proximal sigmoid colon and then into the descending colon. (*B*) Endoscopic image of the cecum, the first portion of the large intestine.

In some cases of cancer, and for other reasons as well, it may be necessary to surgically remove a portion of the GI tract and create a **stoma** (opening) on the abdominal wall for elimination of waste. Such **ostomy** surgery (Fig. 12-8) is named for the organ involved, such as ileostomy (ileum) or colostomy (colon). When an **anastomosis** (connection) is formed between two organs of the tract, both organs are included in naming, such as gastroduodenostomy (stomach and duodenum) or coloproctostomy (colon and rectum).

OBSTRUCTIONS

A hernia is the protrusion of an organ through an abnormal opening. The most common type is an inguinal hernia, described in Chapter 14 (see Fig. 14-7). In a **hiatal hernia,** part of the stomach moves upward into the chest cavity through the space (hiatus) in the diaphragm where the esophagus passes through (see Fig. 6-7). Often this condition produces no symptoms, but it may result in chest pain, **dysphagia** (difficulty in swallowing), or reflux (backflow) of stomach contents into the esophagus.

In **pyloric stenosis,** the opening between the stomach and small intestine is too narrow. This usually occurs in infants, and in boys more often than in girls. A sign of pyloric stenosis is projectile vomiting. Surgery may be needed to correct it.

Other types of obstruction include **intussusception** (Fig. 12-9), slipping of an intestinal segment into a part below it; **volvulus,** twisting of the intestine (see Fig. 12-9B); and **ileus,** intestinal obstruction often caused by lack of peristalsis.

Hemorrhoids are varicose veins in the rectum associated with pain, bleeding, and, in some cases, rectal prolapse.

A

B

C

Figure 12-8 **Ostomy surgery.** Various locations are shown. The shaded portions represent the bowel sections that have been removed or are inactive. (A) Sigmoid colostomy. (B) Transverse colostomy. (C) Ileostomy.

A

B

Figure 12-9 **Intestinal obstruction.** (A) Intussusception. (B) Volvulus, showing counterclockwise twist.

GASTROESOPHAGEAL REFLUX DISEASE

Gastroesophageal reflux disease (GERD) refers to reflux of gastric juices into the esophagus due to weakness at the gastroesophageal junction, specifically the LES (lower esophageal sphincter). These acidic secretions irritate the lining of the esophagus and even the throat and mouth if propelled upward by **regurgitation**. A GERD symptom commonly known as **heartburn**, an upward-radiating burning sensation behind the sternum, does not involve the heart, but is experienced in the area near the heart.

GERD symptoms are more likely to occur after meals when the stomach is full, when one is lying or bending down, and with hiatal hernia, obesity, and pregnancy. Treatment includes weight reduction if needed; elevating the head of the bed 4 to 6 in.; avoidance of irritating foods; and drugs to reduce gastric acid secretion. Surgery to repair an incompetent LES might be needed.

INFLAMMATORY INTESTINAL DISEASE

Two similar diseases are included under the heading of inflammatory bowel disease (IBD):

- **Crohn disease** is a chronic inflammation of the intestinal wall, usually in the ileum and colon, causing pain, diarrhea, abscess, and often formation of an abnormal passageway, or **fistula**.

- **Ulcerative colitis** involves a continuous inflammation of the colon's lining that begins in the rectum and extends proximally (Fig. 12-10).

Both forms of IBD occur mainly in adolescents and young adults and show a hereditary pattern. They originate with an abnormal immunologic response, perhaps to the normal intestinal flora, along with autoimmunity. Treatment is with antiinflammatory agents, immunosuppressants, and frequently surgery to remove damaged portions of the colon.

Figure 12-10 Ulcerative colitis. Prominent erythema and ulceration of the colon begin in the ascending colon and are most severe in the rectosigmoid area.

Figure 12-11 Lower gastrointestinal series. Barium enema shows lesions of enteritis (*straight arrows*) and thickened mucosa (*curved arrows*).

Celiac disease is characterized by the inability to absorb foods containing gluten, a protein found in wheat and some other grains. It affects the upper part of the small intestine and originates with an excess immune response to gluten. Mucosal inflammation diminishes the intestinal villi and interferes with absorption. Celiac disease is treated with a gluten-free diet.

Diverticulitis most commonly affects the colon. Diverticula are small pouches in the intestinal wall that commonly appear with age. The presence of these pouches is termed **diverticulosis**, which has been attributed to a diet low in fiber. Collection of waste and bacteria in these sacs leads to diverticulitis, which is accompanied by pain and sometimes bleeding. Diverticula can be seen by radiographic studies of the lower GI tract using barium as a contrast medium, a so-called *barium enema* (Fig. 12-11). Although there is no cure, diverticulitis is treated with diet, stool softeners, and drugs (antispasmodics) to reduce motility.

Accessory Organs

HEPATITIS

In the United States and other industrialized countries, **hepatitis** is most often caused by viral infection. More than five types of hepatitis virus have now been identified. Vaccines are available for hepatitis A and hepatitis B.

- Hepatitis A virus (HAV) is the most common hepatitis virus. It is spread by fecal–oral contamination, often by food handlers, and in crowded, unsanitary conditions. It may also be acquired by eating contaminated food, especially seafood.

- Hepatitis B virus (HBV) is spread by blood and other body fluids. It may be transmitted sexually, by sharing injection needles, and by close interpersonal contact. Infected individuals may become carriers of the disease. Most patients recover, but the disease may be serious, even fatal, and may lead to liver cancer.

- Hepatitis C is spread through blood and blood products or by close contact with an infected person.

- Hepatitis D, the delta virus, is highly pathogenic but infects only those already infected with hepatitis B.

- Hepatitis E, like HAV, is spread by contaminated food and water. It has caused epidemics in Asia, Africa, and Mexico.

The name *hepatitis* simply means "inflammation of the liver," but this disease also causes necrosis (death) of liver cells. Hepatitis also may be caused by other infections and by drugs and toxins. Liver function tests performed on blood serum are important in diagnosis.

Jaundice, or **icterus**, is a symptom of hepatitis and other diseases of the liver and biliary system (Fig. 12-12). It appears as yellowness of the skin, whites of the eyes, and mucous membranes due to the presence of bile pigments, mainly **bilirubin**, in the blood.

CIRRHOSIS

Cirrhosis is a chronic liver disease characterized by **hepatomegaly**, edema, **ascites** (fluid in the abdomen), and jaundice. Disease progression leads to internal bleeding, and brain damage caused by changes in the blood's composition. One complication of cirrhosis is **portal hypertension**, increased pressure in the hepatic portal system, the vessels that carry blood from the other abdominal organs to the liver. Portal hypertension causes **splenomegaly** and the formation of varices (varicose veins) in the distal esophagus with possible hemorrhage. The main cause of cirrhosis is the excess consumption of alcohol.

PASSport to Success® The animation, *The Liver in Health and Disease*, on the Student Resources reviews liver function and illustrates cirrhosis.

GALLSTONES

Cholelithiasis refers to the presence of stones in the gallbladder or bile ducts, which is usually associated with **cholecystitis**, inflammation of the gallbladder. Cholelithiasis is characterized by **biliary colic** (pain) in the right upper quadrant (RUQ), nausea, and vomiting.

Most gallstones are composed of cholesterol, an ingredient of bile. They form more commonly in women than in men and are promoted by conditions that increase estrogen, as this hormone raises the cholesterol level in bile. These predisposing conditions include pregnancy, use of oral contraceptives, and obesity. Oddly, the rapid weight loss that follows stomach reduction surgery to treat morbid obesity commonly leads to gallstones because of changes in bile production and cholesterol precipitation in the bile. Drugs may dissolve gallstones, but often the cure is removal of the gallbladder in a **cholecystectomy**. Originally, this procedure required an extensive incision, but now the gallbladder is almost always removed laparoscopically through a small abdominal slit. Following gallbladder removal, bile flows directly into the duodenum through the common bile duct.

Ultrasonography, radiography, and magnetic resonance imaging are used to diagnosis gallstones (Fig. 12-13). **Endoscopic retrograde cholangiopancreatography (ERCP)** (Fig. 12-14) is a technique for viewing the pancreatic and bile ducts and for performing certain techniques to relieve obstructions. Contrast medium is injected into the biliary system from the duodenum before imaging.

Figure 12-12 **Jaundice.** Yellowish discoloration due to bile pigments in the blood is seen in the eye.

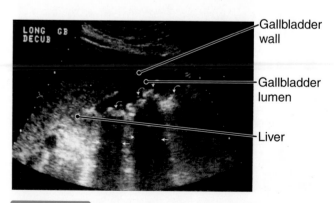

Figure 12-13 **Cholelithiasis (gallstones).** Sonogram shows dense gallstones (curved arrows). Shadows appear (between the straight arrows) because the sound waves cannot penetrate the stones (calculi).

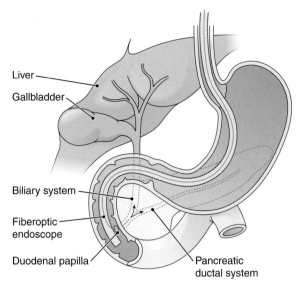

Liver
Gallbladder
Biliary system
Fiberoptic endoscope
Duodenal papilla
Pancreatic ductal system

Figure 12-14 **Endoscopic retrograde cholangiopancreatography (ERCP).** A contrast medium is injected into the pancreatic and bile ducts in preparation for radiography.

PANCREATITIS

Pancreatitis, or inflammation of the pancreas, may result from alcohol abuse, drug toxicity, bile obstruction, infections, and other causes. Blood tests in acute pancreatitis show increased levels of the enzymes amylase and lipase. Glucose and bilirubin levels may also be elevated. Often the disease subsides with only symptomatic treatment.

Terminology	Key Terms

Disorders

appendicitis a-pen-di-SĪ-tis	Inflammation of the appendix
ascites a-SĪ-tēz	Accumulation of fluid in the abdominal cavity; a form of edema. May be caused by heart disease, lymphatic or venous obstruction, cirrhosis, or changes in blood plasma composition
biliary colic BIL-ē-ar-ē KOL-ik	Acute abdominal pain caused by gallstones in the bile ducts
bilirubin bil-i-RŪ-bin	A pigment released in the breakdown of hemoglobin from red blood cells; mainly excreted by the liver in bile
caries KAR-ēz	Tooth decay
celiac disease SĒ-lē-ak	Inability to absorb foods containing gluten, a protein found in wheat and some other grains; caused by an excess immune response to gluten
cholecystitis kō-lē-sis-TĪ-tis	Inflammation of the gallbladder
cholelithiasis kō-lē-li-THĪ-a-sis	The condition of having stones in the gallbladder; also used to refer to stones in the common bile duct
cirrhosis sir-RŌ-sis	Chronic liver disease with degeneration of liver tissue
Crohn disease krōn	A chronic inflammatory disease of the gastrointestinal tract usually involving the ileum and colon
diarrhea dī-a-RĒ-a	The frequent passage of watery bowel movements
diverticulitis dī-ver-tik-ū-LĪ-tis	Inflammation of diverticula (small pouches) in the wall of the digestive tract, especially in the colon

(continued)

Terminology	**Key Terms** (continued)

diverticulosis dī-ver-tik-ū-LŌ-sis	The presence of diverticula, especially in the colon
dysphagia dis-FĀ-jē-a	Difficulty in swallowing
emesis EM-e-sis	Vomiting
fistula FIS-tū-la	An abnormal passageway between two organs or from an organ to the body surface, such as between the rectum and anus (anorectal fistula)
gastroenteritis gas-trō-en-ter-Ī-tis	Inflammation of the stomach and intestine
gastroesophageal reflux disease (GERD) gas-trō-ē-sof-a-JĒ-al	Condition caused by reflux of gastric juices into the esophagus resulting in heartburn, regurgitation, inflammation, and possible damage to the esophagus; caused by weakness of the lower esophageal sphincter (LES)
heartburn HART-burn	A warm or burning sensation felt behind the sternum and radiating upward. Commonly associated with gastroesophageal reflux. Medical name is pyrosis (pyr/o means "heat")
hemorrhoids HEM-ō-royzd	Varicose veins in the rectum associated with pain, bleeding, and sometimes rectal prolapse; piles
hepatitis hep-a-TĪ-tis	Inflammation of the liver; commonly caused by a viral infection
hepatomegaly hep-a-tō-MEG-a-lē	Enlargement of the liver
hiatal hernia hī-Ā-tal	A protrusion of the stomach through the opening (hiatus) in the diaphragm through which the esophagus passes (see Fig. 6-7)
icterus IK-ter-us	Jaundice
ileus IL-ē-us	Intestinal obstruction. May be caused by lack of peristalsis (adynamic, paralytic ileus) or by contraction (dynamic ileus). Intestinal matter and gas may be relieved by insertion of a drainage tube
intussusception in-tu-su-SEP-shun	Slipping of one intestinal segment into another part below it. Occurs mainly in male infants in the ileocecal region (see Fig. 12-9A). May be fatal if untreated for more than 1 day
jaundice JAWN-dis	A yellowish color of the skin, mucous membranes, and whites of the eye caused by bile pigments in the blood (from French jaune meaning "yellow"). The main pigment is bilirubin, a byproduct of erythrocyte destruction (see Fig. 12-12)
leukoplakia lū-kō-PLĀ-kē-ah	White patches on mucous membranes, as on the tongue or cheeks, often resulting from smoking or other irritants; may be precancerous
nausea NAW-zha	An unpleasant sensation in the upper abdomen that often precedes vomiting. Typically occurs in digestive upset, motion sickness, and sometimes early pregnancy
occult blood o-KULT	Blood present in such small amounts that it can be detected only microscopically or chemically; in the feces, a sign of intestinal bleeding (occult means "hidden")
pancreatitis pan-krē-a-TĪ-tis	Inflammation of the pancreas
peptic ulcer PEP-tik UL-ser	A lesion in the mucous membrane of the esophagus, stomach, or duodenum caused by the action of gastric juice
peritonitis per-i-tō-NĪ-tis	Inflammation of the peritoneum, the membrane that lines the abdominal cavity and covers the abdominal organs. May result from perforation of an ulcer, ruptured appendix, or reproductive tract infection, among other causes
polyp POL-ip	A tumor that grows on a stalk and bleeds easily

(continued)

Terminology	Key Terms *(continued)*

portal hypertension	An abnormal pressure increase in the hepatic portal system. May be caused by cirrhosis, infection, thrombosis, or a tumor
pyloric stenosis *pī-LOR-ik*	Narrowing of the opening between the stomach and the duodenum; pylorostenosis
regurgitation *rē-gur-ji-TĀ-shun*	A backward flowing, such as the backflow of undigested food
splenomegaly *splē-nō-MEG-a-lē*	Enlargement of the spleen
ulcerative colitis *UL-ser-a-tiv kō-LĪ-tis*	Chronic ulceration of the rectum and colon; the cause is unknown, but may involve autoimmunity
volvulus *VOL-vū-lus*	Twisting of the intestine resulting in obstruction. Usually involves the sigmoid colon and occurs most often in children and in the elderly. May be caused by congenital malformation, a foreign body, or adhesion. Failure to treat immediately may result in death (see Fig. 12-9B)

Diagnosis and Treatment

anastomosis *a-nas-to-MŌ-sis*	A passage or communication between two vessels or organs. May be normal or pathologic, or may be created surgically
barium study	Use of barium sulfate as a liquid contrast medium for fluoroscopic or radiographic study of the digestive tract. Can show obstruction, tumors, ulcers, hiatal hernia, and motility disorders, among other conditions
cholecystectomy *kō-lē-sis-TEK-tō-mē*	Surgical removal of the gallbladder
Dukes classification	A system for staging colorectal cancer based on degree of bowel wall penetration and lymph node involvement; severity is graded from A to C
endoscopy *en-DOS-kō-pē*	Use of a fiberoptic endoscope for direct visual examination. GI studies include esophagogastroduodenoscopy, proctosigmoidoscopy (rectum and distal colon), and colonoscopy (all regions of the colon) (see Figs. 12-6 and 12-7)
ERCP	Endoscopic retrograde cholangiopancreatography; a technique for viewing the pancreatic and bile ducts and for performing certain techniques to relieve obstructions. Contrast medium is injected into the biliary system from the duodenum before radiographs are taken (see Fig. 12-14)
ostomy *OS-tō-mē*	An opening into the body; generally refers to an opening created for elimination of body waste. Also refers to the operation done to create such an opening (see stoma)
stoma *STŌ-ma*	A surgically created opening to the body surface or between two organs (literally "mouth") (see Fig. 12-8)

12

PASSport to Success® Go to the pronunciation glossary on the Student Resources to hear these words pronounced.

Terminology	**Supplementary Terms**

Normal Structure and Function

bolus BŌ-lus	A mass, such as the rounded mass of food that is swallowed
cardia KAR-dē-a	The part of the stomach near the esophagus, named for its closeness to the heart
chyme kīm	The semiliquid partially digested food that moves from the stomach into the small intestine
defecation def-e-KĀ-shun	The evacuation of feces from the rectum
deglutition deg-lū-TISH-un	Swallowing
duodenal bulb dū-ō-DĒ-nal	The part of the duodenum near the pylorus; the first bend (flexure) of the duodenum
duodenal papilla dū-ō-DĒ-nal pa-PIL-la	The raised area where the common bile duct and pancreatic duct enter the duodenum (see Fig. 12-14); papilla of Vater (FA-ter)
greater omentum ō-MEN-tum	A fold of the peritoneum that extends from the stomach over the abdominal organs
hepatic flexure he-PAT-ik FLEK-shur	The right bend of the colon, forming the junction between the ascending colon and the transverse colon (see Fig. 12-1)
ileocecal valve il-ē-ō-SĒ-kal	A valvelike structure between the ileum of the small intestine and the cecum of the large intestine
mesentery MES-en-ter-ē	The portion of the peritoneum that folds over and supports the intestine
mesocolon mes-ō-KŌ-lon	The portion of the peritoneum that folds over and supports the colon
papilla of Vater	See duodenal papilla
peritoneum per-i-tō-NĒ-um	The serous membrane that lines the abdominal cavity and supports the abdominal organs
rugae RŪ-jē	The large folds in the stomach's lining seen when the stomach is empty
sphincter of Oddi OD-ē	The muscular ring at the opening of the common bile duct into the duodenum
splenic flexure SPLEN-ik FLEK-shur	The left bend of the colon, forming the junction between the transverse colon and the descending colon (see Fig. 12-1)

Disorders

achalasia ak-a-LĀ-zē-a	Failure of a smooth muscle to relax, especially the lower esophageal sphincter, so that food is retained in the esophagus
achlorhydria ā-klor-HĪ-drē-a	Lack of hydrochloric acid in the stomach; opposite is hyperchlorhydria
anorexia an-ō-REK-sē-a	Loss of appetite. Anorexia nervosa is a psychologically induced refusal or inability to eat (adjectives: anorectic, anorexic)
aphagia a-FĀ-jē-a	Inability to swallow or difficulty in swallowing; refusal or inability to eat
aphthous ulcer AF-thus	An ulcer in a mucous membrane, as in the mouth
Barrett syndrome	Lower esophageal ulcer resulting from chronic esophagitis, often with constriction caused by mucosal changes; may be premalignant. Also called Barrett esophagus

(continued)

Terminology	**Supplementary Terms** (continued)
bruxism *BRUK-sizm*	Clenching and grinding of the teeth, usually during sleep
bulimia *bū-LIM-ē-a*	Excessive, insatiable appetite. A disorder characterized by overeating followed by induced vomiting, diarrhea, or fasting
cachexia *ka-KEK-sē-a*	Profound ill health, malnutrition, and wasting
cheilosis *kī-LŌ-sis*	Cracking at the corners of the mouth, often caused by B vitamin deficiency (root *cheil/o* means "lip")
cholestasis *kō-lē-STA-sis*	Stoppage of bile flow
constipation *con-sti-PĀ-shun*	Infrequency or difficulty in defecation and the passage of hard, dry feces
dyspepsia *dis-PEP-sē-a*	Poor or painful digestion
eructation *e-ruk-TĀ-shun*	Belching
familial adenomatous polyposis (FAP) *fa-MIL-ē-al ad-e-NŌ-ma-tus pol-i-PŌ-sis*	A heredity condition in which multiple polyps form in the colon and rectum, predisposing to colorectal cancer
flatulence *FLAT-ū-lens*	Condition of having gas or air in the GI tract
flatus *FLĀ-tus*	Gas or air in the gastrointestinal tract; gas or air expelled through the anus
hematemesis *hē-ma-TEM-e-sis*	Vomiting of blood
irritable bowel syndrome (IBS)	A chronic stress-related disease characterized by diarrhea, constipation, and pain associated with rhythmic intestinal contractions. Mucous colitis; spastic colon
megacolon *meg-a-KŌ-lon*	An extremely dilated colon. Usually congenital but may occur in acute ulcerative colitis
melena *MEL-ē-na*	Black tarry feces resulting from blood in the intestines. Common in newborns. May also be a sign of gastrointestinal bleeding
obstipation *ob-sti-PĀ-shun*	Extreme constipation
pernicious anemia *per-NISH-us*	A form of anemia caused by the stomach's failure to secrete intrinsic factor, a substance needed for the absorption of vitamin B$_{12}$
pilonidal cyst *pī-lō-NĪ-dal*	A dermal cyst in the sacral region, usually at the top of the cleft between the buttocks. May become infected and begin to drain
thrush	Fungal infection of the mouth and/or throat caused by *Candida*; appears as mucosal white patches or ulcers
Vincent disease *VIN-sent*	Severe gingivitis with necrosis associated with the bacterium *Treponema vincentii*; necrotizing ulcerative gingivitis; trench mouth

Diagnosis and Treatment

appendectomy *ap-en-DEK-tō-mē*	Surgical removal of the appendix
bariatrics *bar-ē-AT-riks*	The branch of medicine concerned with prevention and control of obesity and associated diseases (from Greek *baros*, meaning "weight")

12

(continued)

Terminology Supplementary Terms *(continued)*

Billroth operations	Gastrectomy with anastomosis of the stomach to the duodenum (Billroth I) or to the jejunum (Billroth II) (Fig. 12-15)
gastric bypass surgery	Division of the stomach and anastomosis of its upper part to the small intestine (jejunum) to reduce nutrient absorption (Fig. 12-16); used to treat morbid obesity. Other surgical methods are used for this purpose, including partition of the stomach with rows of staples (gastric stapling)
gavage *ga-VAHZH*	Process of feeding through a nasogastric tube into the stomach
lavage *la-VAJ*	Washing out of a cavity; irrigation
manometry *man-OM-e-trē*	Measurement of pressure; pertaining to the GI tract, measurement of pressure in the portal system as a sign of obstruction
Murphy sign	Inability to take a deep breath when fingers are pressed firmly below the right arch of the ribs (below the liver). Signifies gallbladder disease
nasogastric (NG) tube *nā-zō-GAS-trik*	Tube that is passed through the nose into the stomach (Fig. 12-17). May be used for emptying the stomach, administering medication, giving liquids, or sampling stomach contents
parenteral hyperalimentation *pa-REN-ter-al*	Complete intravenous feeding for one who cannot take in food. Total parenteral nutrition (TPN)
percutaneous endoscopic gastrostomy (PEG) tube	Tube inserted into the stomach for long-term feeding (Fig. 12-18)
vagotomy *vā-GOT-ō-mē*	Interruption of vagal nerve impulses to reduce stomach secretions in the treatment of gastric ulcer. Originally done surgically but may also be done with drugs

Drugs

antacid *ant-AS-id*	Agent that counteracts acidity, usually gastric acidity
antidiarrheal *an-ti-dī-a-RĒ-al*	Drug that treats or prevents diarrhea by reducing intestinal motility or absorbing irritants and soothing the intestinal lining
antiemetic *an-tē-e-MET-ik*	Agent that relieves or prevents nausea and vomiting
antiflatulent *an-ti-FLAT-ū-lent*	Agent that prevents or relieves flatulence
antispasmodic *an-ti-spas-MOD-ik*	Agent that relieves spasm, usually of smooth muscle
emetic *e-MET-ik*	An agent that causes vomiting
histamine H_2 antagonist	Drug that decreases secretion of stomach acid by interfering with the action of histamine at H_2 receptors. Used to treat ulcers and other gastrointestinal problems. H_2-receptor blocking agent
laxative *LAK-sa-tiv*	Agent that promotes elimination from the large intestine. Types include stimulants, substances that retain water (hyperosmotics), stool softeners, and bulk-forming agents
proton pump inhibitor (PPI)	Agent that inhibits gastric acid secretion by blocking the transport of hydrogen ions (protons) into the stomach

Go to the pronunciation glossary on the Student Resources to hear these words pronounced.

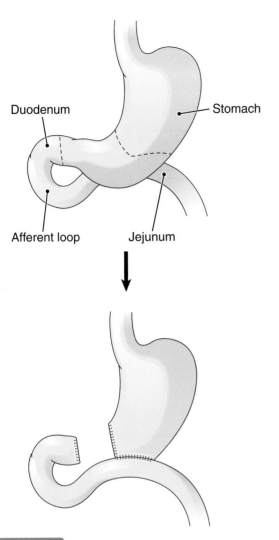

Duodenum

Stomach

Afferent loop   Jejunum

Figure 12-15 **Gastrojejunostomy (Billroth II operation).** The dotted lines show the portion removed.

Stomach

Surgical staples

Figure 12-16 **Gastric bypass.** For treatment of morbid obesity, a small pouch is created in the stomach to limit food intake. The pouch is attached to the jejunum in a gastrojejunostomy to bypass the stomach and reduce nutrient absorption.

12

Nasogastric tube

Splenic impression on descending colon

A

B

Figure 12-17 **A nasogastric (NG) tube.** (*A*) Diagram showing an NG tube in place. (*B*) Abdominal radiograph showing an NG tube. The filter (*arrow*) shown in the inferior vena cava is meant to trap emboli that might originate in the lower extremities and pelvis.

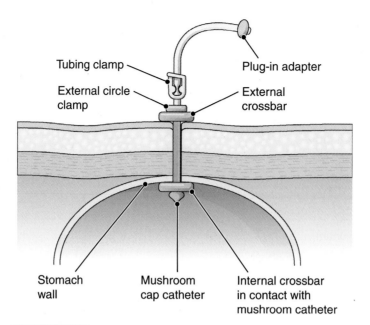

Tubing clamp

Plug-in adapter

External circle clamp

External crossbar

Stomach wall

Mushroom cap catheter

Internal crossbar in contact with mushroom catheter

Figure 12-18 **Percutaneous endoscopic gastrostomy (PEG) tube.** The tube is shown in place in the stomach.

Terminology   Abbreviations

BE	Barium enema (for radiographic study of the colon)	HCl	Hydrochloric acid
BM	Bowel movement	IBD	Inflammatory bowel disease
CBD	Common bile duct	IBS	Irritable bowel syndrome
ERCP	Endoscopic retrograde cholangiopancreatography	LES	Lower esophageal sphincter
FAP	Familial adenomatous polyposis	NG	Nasogastric (tube)
GERD	Gastroesophageal reflux disease	N & V	Nausea and vomiting
GI	Gastrointestinal	N/V/D	Nausea, vomiting, and diarrhea
HAV	Hepatitis A virus	PONV	Postoperative nausea and vomiting
HBV	Hepatitis B virus	PPI	Proton pump inhibitor
HCV	Hepatitis C virus	TPN	Total parenteral nutrition
HDV	Hepatitis D virus	UGI	Upper gastrointestinal (radiograph series)
HEV	Hepatitis E virus		

Chapter Review

LABELING EXERCISE

The Digestive System > Write the name of each numbered part on the corresponding line of the answer sheet.

Anus
Ascending colon
Cecum
Descending colon
Duodenum (of small intestine)
Esophagus
Gallbladder
Liver
Mouth
Pancreas

Parotid salivary gland
Pharynx
Rectum
Sigmoid colon
Small intestine
Stomach
Sublingual salivary gland
Submandibular salivary
   gland
Transverse colon

1. _____

2. _____

3. _____

4. _____

5. _____

6. _____

7. _____

8. _____

9. _____

10. _____

11. _____

12. _____

13. _____

14. _____

15. _____

16. _____

17. _____

18. _____

19. _____

Chapter Review *(continued)*

Accessory Organs of Digestion > Write the name of each numbered part on the corresponding line of the answer sheet.

Common bile duct   Gallbladder
Common hepatic duct   Liver
Cystic duct   Pancreas
Diaphragm   Pancreatic duct
Duodenum   Spleen

1. _____

2. _____

3. _____

4. _____

5. _____

6. _____

7. _____

8. _____

9. _____

10. _____

TERMINOLOGY

Matching > Match the following terms and write the appropriate letter to the left of each number:

_____ **1.** sublingual   **a.** lymphatic capillary
_____ **2.** emetic   **b.** pertaining to the lip
_____ **3.** labial   **c.** substance that induces vomiting
_____ **4.** agnathia   **d.** hypoglossal
_____ **5.** lacteal   **e.** absence of the jaw

_____ **6.** icterus   **a.** terminal portion of the small intestine
_____ **7.** colocentesis   **b.** wavelike muscular contractions
_____ **8.** ileum   **c.** organic catalyst
_____ **9.** peristalsis   **d.** surgical puncture of the colon
_____ **10.** enzyme   **e.** jaundice

_____ **11.** leukoplakia   **a.** a type of liver disease
_____ **12.** cirrhosis   **b.** pertaining to the common bile duct
_____ **13.** cholangiectasis **c.** crushing of a biliary calculus
_____ **14.** choledochal   **d.** dilatation of a bile duct
_____ **15.** cholelithotripsy **e.** white patches on a mucous membrane

Supplementary Terms

_____ **16.** peritoneum   **a.** part of the stomach near the esophagus
_____ **17.** cardia   **b.** chewing
_____ **18.** deglutition   **c.** serous membrane in the abdomen
_____ **19.** bolus   **d.** swallowing
_____ **20.** mastication   **e.** a mass, as of food

_____ **21.** gavage   **a.** inability to eat
_____ **22.** bruxism   **b.** partially digested food
_____ **23.** aphagia   **c.** malnutrition and wasting
_____ **24.** cachexia   **d.** feeding through a tube
_____ **25.** chyme   **e.** tooth grinding

Fill in the blanks:

26. The hepatic portal system carries blood to the _____.

27. The organ that stores bile is the _____.

28. The blind pouch at the beginning of the colon is the _____.

29. Glossorrhaphy is suture of the _____.

30. The palatine tonsils are located on either side of the _____.

31. Dentin is the main substance of a(n) _____.

32. From its name you might guess that the buccinator muscle is in the _____.

33. An enterovirus is a virus that infects the _____.

34. The anticoagulant heparin is found throughout the body, but it is named for its presence in the _____.

35. The substance cholesterol is named for its chemical composition (sterol) and for its presence in _____.

Write a word for the following definitions:

36. a dentist who specializes in treating the tissues around the teeth _____

37. surgical excision of the stomach _____

38. surgical repair of the palate _____

39. narrowing of the pylorus _____

40. inflammation of the pancreas _____

41. medical specialist who treats diseases of the stomach and intestine _____

42. surgical creation of an opening into the colon _____

43. surgical creation of a passage between the stomach and the duodenum _____

44. within (intra-) the liver _____

Plurals > Write the plural form of the following words:

45. diverticulum   _____

46. gingiva   _____

47. calculus   _____

48. anastomosis   _____

True–False > Examine the following statements. If the statement is true, write T in the first blank. If the statement is false, write F in the first blank and correct the statement by replacing the underlined word in the second blank.

49. The epigastrium is the region of the abdomen <u>below</u> the stomach.   _____   _____

50. The middle portion of the small intestine is the <u>duodenum</u>.   _____   _____

51. Polysialia is the excess secretion of <u>bile</u>.   _____   _____

52. The cystic duct carries bile to and from the <u>gallbladder</u>.   _____   _____

53. The appendix is attached to the <u>cecum</u>.   _____   _____

54. The common hepatic duct and the cystic duct merge to form the <u>common bile duct</u>.   _____   _____

12

Eliminations > In each of the sets below, underline the word that does not fit in with the rest and explain the reason for your choice:

55. gingiva — villus — palate — uvula — incisor

_____

56. spleen — cecum — colon — rectum — anus

_____

57. pancreas — gallbladder — liver — pylorus — salivary glands

_____

58. diarrhea — emesis — nausea — regurgitation — amylase

_____

Write the meaning of the following abbreviations:

59. TPN _____

60. GERD _____

61. GI _____

62. HCl _____

63. PEG (tube) _____

64. HAV _____

Word Building > Write a word for the following definitions using the word parts provided.

-al   cec/o   r   -pexy   -cele   proct/o   -itis   -rhaphy   ile/o

65. inflammation of the cecum   _____

66. suture of the rectum   _____

67. fixation of the ileum   _____

68. hernia of the rectum   _____

69. pertaining to the ileum and cecum _____

70. fixation of the cecum   _____

71. inflammation of the rectum   _____

72. suture of the ileum   _____

73. inflammation of the ileum   _____

Word Analysis > Define each of the following words, and give the meaning of the word parts in each. Use a dictionary if necessary.

74. myenteric (*mī-en-TER-ik*) _____

    a. my/o _____

    b. enter/o _____

    c. -ic _____

75. cholescintigraphy *(kō-lē-sin-TIG-ra-fē)* _____

   a. chole _____

   b. scinti _____ spark (radiation) _____

   c. -graphy _____

76. parenteral *(pa-REN-ter-al)* _____

   a. par(a) _____

   b. enter/o _____

   c. -al _____

PASSport to Success®

Go to the word exercises on the Student Resources for additional review exercises.

Case Studies

▶ Case Study 12-1: Cholecystectomy

G.L., a 42-year-old obese Caucasian woman, entered the hospital with nausea and vomiting, flatulence and eructation, a fever of 100.5°F, and continuous right upper quadrant (RUQ) and subscapular pain. Examination on admission showed rebound tenderness in the RUQ with a positive Murphy sign. Her skin, nails, and conjunctivae were yellowish, and she reported frequent clay-colored stools. Her leukocyte count was 16,000. An ERCP and ultrasound of the abdomen suggested many small stones in her gallbladder and possibly the common bile duct. Her diagnosis was cholecystitis with cholelithiasis.

A laparoscopic cholecystectomy was attempted, with an intraoperative cholangiogram and common bile duct exploration. Because of G.L.'s size and some unexpected bleeding, visualization was difficult and the procedure was converted to an open approach. Small stones and granular sludge were irrigated from her common duct, and the gallbladder was removed. She had a T-tube inserted into the duct for bile drainage; this tube was removed on the second postoperative day. An NG tube in place before and during the surgery was also removed on day 2. She was discharged on the fifth postoperative day with a prescription for prn pain medication.

▶ Case Study 12-2: Surgical Pathology Report

Gross Description: The specimen is received in formalin labeled "ruptured duodenal diverticula" and consists of enteric tissue measuring approximately 6.3 × 2.8 × 0.7 cm. The serosal surface is markedly dull in appearance and fibrotic. The mucosal surface is hemorrhagic. Representative sections are taken for microscopic examination.

Microscopic Description: Sectioned slide shows segments of duodenal tissues with areas of gangrenous change in the bowel wall, and acute and chronic inflammatory infiltrates. There are chronic and focal acute inflammatory cell infiltrates with hemorrhage in the mesenteric fatty tissue. There are areas of acute inflammatory exudates noted in the fatty tissue. Histopathologic changes are consistent with ruptured duodenal diverticula.

▶ Case Study 12-3: Colonoscopy with Biopsy

S.M., a 24-year-old man, had a recent history of lower abdominal pain with frequent loose mucoid stools. He described symptoms of occasional dysphagia, dyspepsia, nausea, and aphthous ulcers of his tongue and buccal mucosa. A previous barium enema examination showed some irregularities in the sigmoid and rectal segments of his large bowel. Stool samples for culture, ova, and parasites were negative. His tentative diagnosis was irritable bowel syndrome.

He followed a lactose-free, low-residue diet and took Imodium to reduce intestinal motility. His gastroenterologist recommended a colonoscopy. After a 2-day regimen of a soft to clear liquid diet, laxatives, and an enema the morning of the procedure, he reported to the endoscopy unit. He was transported to the

12

(continued)

Case Studies (continued)

procedure room. ECG electrodes, a pulse oximeter sensor, and a blood pressure cuff were applied for monitoring, and an IV was inserted in S.M.'s right arm. An IV bolus of Demerol and a bolus of Versed were given, and S.M. was positioned on his left side. The colonoscope was gently inserted through the anal sphincter and advanced proximally. S.M. was instructed to take a deep breath when the scope approached the splenic flexure and the hepatic flexure to facilitate comfortable passage.

The physician was able to advance past the ileocecal valve, examining the entire length of the colon. Ulcerated granulomatous lesions were seen throughout the colon, with a concentration in the sigmoid segment. Many biopsy specimens were taken. The mucosa of the distal ileum was normal. Pathology examination of the biopsy samples was expected to establish a diagnosis of IBD.

CASE STUDY QUESTIONS

Multiple choice. Select the best answer and write the letter of your choice to the left of each number:

_____ 1. Flatulence and eructation represent:
  a. regurgitation of chyme
  b. distention of the esophagus
  c. passage of gas or air from the GI tract
  d. muscular movement of the alimentary tract
  e. sounds heard only by abdominal auscultation

_____ 2. The Murphy sign is tested for:
  a. under the ribs on the left
  b. near the spleen
  c. in the lower right abdomen
  d. under the ribs on the right
  e. in the lower left abdomen

_____ 3. The NG tube is inserted through the _____ and terminates in the _____.
  a. nose/stomach
  b. nostril/gallbladder
  c. glottis/nephron
  d. anus/cecum
  e. Nissen/glottis

_____ 4. Enteric tissue is found in the:
  a. gallbladder
  b. stomach
  c. esophagus
  d. liver
  e. intestine

_____ 5. The mucosal surface of a digestive organ is the:
  a. outer surface
  b. medulla
  c. cortex
  d. inner surface
  e. central opening

_____ 6. Diverticula are:
  a. small pouches in the wall of the colon
  b. communications between two organs
  c. ducts in the liver
  d. intestinal obstructions
  e. polyps in the intestine

_____ 7. Dysphagia and dyspepsia are difficulty or pain with:
  a. chewing and intestinal motility
  b. speaking and motility
  c. swallowing and digestion
  d. breathing and absorption
  e. swallowing and nutrition

_____ 8. The buccal mucosa is in the:
  a. nostril, medial side
  b. mouth, inside of the cheek
  c. greater curvature of the stomach
  d. lesser curvature near the duodenum
  e. base of the tongue

_____ 9. A gastroenterologist is a physician who specializes in study of:
  a. respiration and pathology
  b. mouth and teeth
  c. stomach, intestines, and related structures
  d. musculoskeletal system
  e. nutritional and weight loss diets

_____ 10. The splenic and hepatic flexures are bends in the colon near the:
  a. liver and splanchnic vein
  b. common bile duct and biliary tree
  c. spleen and appendix
  d. spleen and liver
  e. mesenteric vessels and liver

_____ 11. Intestinal motility refers to:
  a. chewing
  b. peristalsis
  c. absorption
  d. antiemetics
  e. ascites

_____ 12. A colonoscopy is:
  a. a radiograph of the small intestine
  b. an endoscopic study of the esophagus
  c. an upper endoscopy with biopsy
  d. a type of barium enema
  e. an endoscopic examination of the large bowel

_____ 13. The ileocecal valve is:
  a. part of a colonoscope
  b. at the distal ileum
  c. in the pylorus
  d. at the proximal ileum
  e. near the liver

(continued)

Case Studies (continued)

Write the meaning of each of the following abbreviations:

14. ERCP _____

15. RUQ _____

16. NG _____

17. IBD _____

Give the word or words in the case studies with each of the following meanings:

18. pertaining to the first part of the small intestine

_____

19. pertaining to the membrane that supports the intestine

_____

20. localized

_____

21. fluid that escapes from blood vessels as a result of inflammation

_____

22. hidden or microscopic blood

_____

23. jaundice

_____

24. drug that treats nausea and vomiting

_____

25. presence of stones in the gallbladder

_____

26. endoscopic surgery of the gallbladder

_____

27. inflammation of the gallbladder

_____

28. radiographic study of the gallbladder and biliary system

_____

29. ring of muscle that regulates the distal opening of the colon

_____

30. surgical excision of tissue for pathology examination

_____

12

The Urinary System

CHAPTER CONTENTS

OBJECTIVES

After study of this chapter you should be able to:

1. Label a diagram of the urinary tract and follow the flow of urine through the body.
2. Label diagrams of the kidney and the urinary bladder.
3. Identify the portions of the nephron, and explain how each functions in urine formation.
4. Explain the relationship between the kidney and the blood circulation.
5. Identify and use the roots pertaining to the urinary system.
6. Describe the major disorders of the urinary system.
7. Define medical terms commonly used in reference to the urinary system.
8. Interpret abbreviations used in reference to the urinary system.
9. Analyze several case studies pertaining to urinary disorders.

PRETEST

Multiple choice. Select the best answer and write the letter of your choice to the left of each number.

___ 1. The organ that forms urine is the:

    a. gallbladder   c. bladder
    b. cystic duct   d. kidney

___ 2. The tube that carries urine out of the body is the:

    a. pylorus   c. urethra
    b. appendix   d. peristalsis

___ 3. The hormone erythropoietin stimulates production of:

    a. red blood cells   c. leukocytes
    b. platelets   d. saliva

___ 4. Micturition is the scientific term for:

    a. urination   c. breathing
    b. digestion   d. retention

___ 5. With reference to the urinary system, the root *cyst/o* means:

    a. ureter   c. urinary stasis
    b. urinary bladder   d. kidney

___ 6. Nephritis is inflammation of the:

    a. liver   c. bladder
    b. intestine   d. kidney

___ 7. Separation of substances by passage through a membrane is termed:

    a. centrifugation   c. deglutition
    b. absorption   d. dialysis

___ 8. A substance that promotes urinary output is a(n):

    a. hypertensive   c. channel blocker
    b. diuretic   d. enzyme

The urinary system excretes metabolic waste. In forming and eliminating urine, it also regulates the composition, volume, and acid–base balance (pH) of body fluids. In several ways, kidney activity affects the circulation. The urinary system is thus of critical importance in maintaining homeostasis, the state of internal balance. As shown in Figure 13-1, the urinary system consists of:

- Two kidneys, the organs that form urine
- Two ureters, which transport urine from the kidneys to the bladder
- The urinary bladder, which stores and eliminates urine
- The urethra, which carries urine out of the body

The Kidneys

The **kidneys** are the organs that form **urine** from substances filtered out of the blood. In addition to metabolic wastes, urine contains water and ions, so its formation is important in regulating the blood's volume and composition. In addition, the kidneys produce two substances that act on the circulatory system:

- **Erythropoietin (EPO)**, a hormone that stimulates red blood cell production in the bone marrow.
- **Renin**, an enzyme that functions to raise blood pressure. It activates a blood component called **angiotensin**, which causes constriction of the blood vessels. The drugs known as ACE inhibitors (angiotensin-converting enzyme inhibitors) lower blood pressure by interfering with the production of angiotensin.

Location and Structure of the Kidneys

The kidneys are located behind the peritoneum in the lumbar region. On the top of each kidney rests an adrenal gland. The kidney is encased in a capsule of fibrous connective tissue overlaid with fat. An outermost

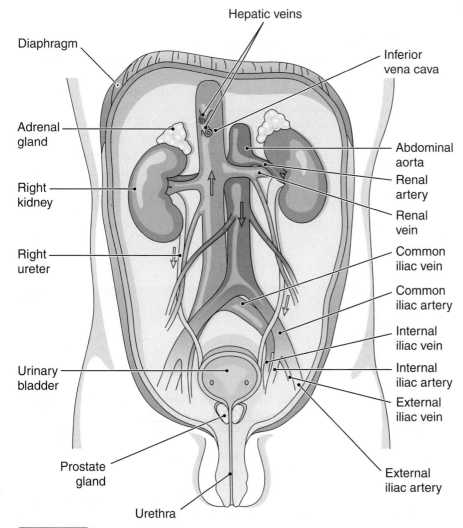

Figure 13-1 **The urinary system.** The male system is shown, with associated and nearby blood vessels.

13

273

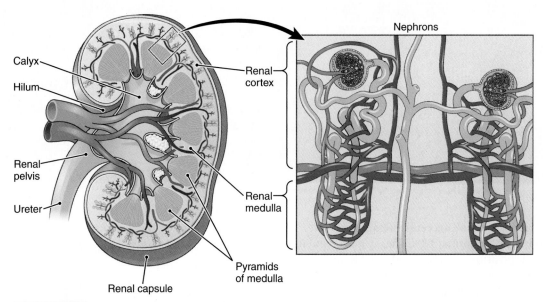

Figure 13-2 **The kidney.** (*Left*) A longitudinal section through the kidney shows its internal structure. The hilum is the point where blood vessels and ducts connect with the kidney. (*Right*) An enlarged diagram of nephrons. Each kidney contains more than 1 million nephrons.

layer of connective tissue supports the kidney and anchors it to the body wall.

If you look inside the kidney (Fig. 13-2), you will see that it has an outer region, the **renal cortex**, and an inner region, the **renal medulla** (see Box 13-1). The medulla is divided into triangular sections, the **renal pyramids**. These pyramids have a lined appearance because they are made up of the loops and collecting tubules of the **nephrons**, the kidney's functional units. Each collecting tubule empties into a urine-collecting area called a **calyx** (from the Latin word meaning "cup"). Several of the smaller minor calices merge to form a major calyx. The major calices then unite to form the **renal pelvis**, the upper funnel-shaped portion of the **ureter**.

The Nephrons

The tiny working units of the kidneys are the nephrons (Fig. 13-3). These microscopic structures are basically a single tubule coiled and folded into various shapes. The tubule begins with a cup-shaped **glomerular** (Bowman) **capsule**, which is part of the nephron's blood-filtering device. The tubule then folds into the proximal convoluted tubule, straightens out to form the nephron loop (loop of Henle), coils again into the distal convoluted tubule, and then finally straightens out to form a collecting duct.

Blood Supply to the Kidney

Blood enters the kidney through a renal artery, a short branch of the abdominal aorta. This vessel subdivides

---

Box 13-1   Focus on Words

Words That Serve Double Duty

Some words appear in more than one body system to represent different structures. The medulla of the kidney is the inner portion of the organ. Other organs, such as the adrenal gland, ovary, and lymph nodes, may also be divided into a central medulla and outer cortex. But *medulla* means "marrow," and this term is also applied to the bone marrow, to the spinal cord, and to the part of the brain that connects with the spinal cord, the medulla oblongata.

A ventricle is a chamber. There are ventricles in the brain and in the heart. The word *fundus* means the back part or base

of an organ. The uterus has a fundus, the upper rounded portion farthest from the cervix, as does the stomach. The fundus of the eye, examined for signs of diabetes and glaucoma, is the innermost layer, where the retina is located. A macula is a spot. There is a macula in the eye, which is the point of sharpest vision. There is also a macula in the ear, which contains receptors for equilibrium.

In interpreting medical terminology, it is often important to know the context in which a word is used.

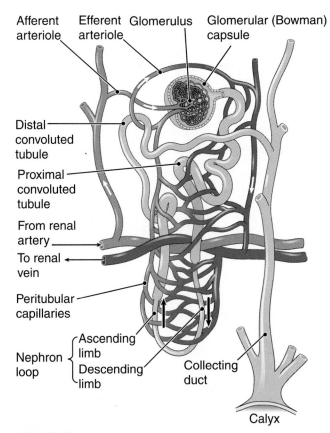

Afferent arteriole — Efferent arteriole — Glomerulus — Glomerular (Bowman) capsule

Distal convoluted tubule

Proximal convoluted tubule

From renal artery

To renal vein

Peritubular capillaries

Nephron loop { Ascending limb / Descending limb }

Collecting duct

Calyx

Figure 13-3 **A nephron and its blood supply.** The nephron regulates the proportion of water, waste, and other materials in urine according to the body's constantly changing needs. A nephron consists of a glomerular capsule, convoluted tubules, the nephron loop (loop of Henle), and a collecting duct. Blood filtration occurs through the glomerulus in the glomerular capsule. Materials that enter the nephron can be returned to the blood through the surrounding peritubular capillaries.

into smaller vessels as it branches throughout the kidney tissue, until finally blood is brought into the glomerular capsule and circulated through a cluster of capillaries, called a **glomerulus**, within the capsule.

Blood leaves the kidney by a series of vessels that finally merge to form the renal vein, which empties into the inferior vena cava.

Urine Formation

As blood flows through the glomerulus, blood pressure forces materials through the glomerular wall and through the wall of the glomerular capsule into the nephron. The fluid that enters the nephron, the **glomerular filtrate**, consists mainly of water, electrolytes, soluble wastes, nutrients, and toxins. The main waste material is **urea**, the nitrogenous (nitrogen-containing) byproduct of protein metabolism. The filtrate should not contain any cells or proteins, such as albumin.

The waste material and the toxins must be eliminated, but most of the water, electrolytes, and nutrients

must be returned to the blood or we would rapidly starve and dehydrate. This return process, termed **tubular reabsorption**, occurs through the peritubular capillaries that surround the nephron.

As the filtrate flows through the nephron, other processes further regulate its composition and pH. The filtrate's concentration is also adjusted under the effects of a pituitary hormone. **Antidiuretic hormone (ADH)** promotes reabsorption of water, thus concentrating the filtrate. The final filtrate, now called urine, flows into the collecting tubules to be eliminated. A **diuretic** is a substance that promotes increased urinary output, or **diuresis**. Diuretic drugs are used in treating hypertension and heart failure to decrease fluid volume and reduce the heart's workload (see Chapter 9).

> **PASSport to Success®** The animation *Renal Function* on the Student Resources shows the process of urine formation in action.

Transport and Removal of Urine

Urine is drained from the renal pelvis and carried by the left and right ureters to the **urinary bladder** (Fig. 13-4), where it is stored. As the bladder fills, it expands upward from a stable triangle at its base. This triangle, the **trigone**, is marked by the ureteral openings and the urethral opening below (see Fig. 13-4). The trigone's stability prevents urine from refluxing into the ureters.

Fullness stimulates a reflex contraction of the bladder muscle and expulsion of urine through the **urethra**.

Ureter — Smooth muscle

Openings of ureters — Trigone

Internal urethral sphincter — Prostate — Urethra

External urethral sphincter

Figure 13-4 **The urinary bladder.** The interior of the male bladder is shown. The trigone is a triangular region in the bladder floor marked by the openings of the ureters and the urethra. The urethra travels through the prostate gland in the male.

13

The female urethra is short (4 cm [1.5 in.]) and carries only urine. The male urethra is longer (20 cm [8 in.]) and carries both urine and semen.

The voiding (release) of urine, technically called **micturition** or **urination**, is regulated by two sphincters (circular muscles) that surround the urethra. The superior muscle, the internal urethral sphincter, is around the entrance to the urethra and functions involuntarily; the inferior muscle, the external urethral sphincter, is under conscious control.

Terminology	Key Terms

Normal Structure and Function

antidiuretic hormone (ADH) *an-ti-dī-ū-RET-ik*	A hormone released from the pituitary gland that causes water reabsorption in the kidneys, thus concentrating the urine
angiotensin *an-jē-ō-TEN-sin*	A substance that increases blood pressure; activated in the blood by renin, an enzyme produced by the kidneys
calyx *KĀ-liks*	A cuplike cavity in the pelvis of the kidney; also calix (plural: calices) (roots: *cali, calic*)
diuresis *dī-ū-RĒ-sis*	Excretion of urine; usually meaning increased urinary excretion
diuretic *dī-ū-RET-ik*	A substance that increases the excretion of urine; pertaining to diuresis
diuresis *dī-ū-RĒ-sis*	Increased excretion of urine
erythropoietin (EPO) *e-rith-rō-POY-e-tin*	A hormone produced by the kidneys that stimulates red blood cell production in the bone marrow
glomerular capsule *glō-MER-ū-lar KAP-sūl*	The cup-shaped structure at the beginning of the nephron that surrounds the glomerulus and receives material filtered out of the blood; Bowman (*BŌ-man*) capsule
glomerular filtrate *glō-MER-ū-lar FIL-trāt*	The fluid and dissolved materials that filter out of the blood and enter the nephron through the glomerular capsule
glomerulus *glō-MER-ū-lus*	The cluster of capillaries within the glomerular capsule (plural: glomeruli) (root: *glomerul/o*)
kidney *KID-nē*	An organ of excretion (roots: *ren/o, nephr/o*); the two kidneys filter the blood and form urine, which contains metabolic waste products and other substances as needed to regulate the water, electrolyte, and pH balance of body fluids
micturition *mik-tū-RISH-un*	The voiding of urine; urination
nephron *NEF-ron*	A microscopic functional unit of the kidney; working with blood vessels, the nephron filters the blood and balances the composition of urine
renal cortex *RĒ-nal KOR-tex*	The kidney's outer portion; contains portions of the nephrons
renal medulla *me-DUL-la*	The kidney's inner portion; contains portions of the nephrons and ducts that transport urine toward the renal pelvis
renal pelvis *PEL-vis*	The expanded upper end of the ureter that receives urine from the kidney; Greek root *pyel/o* means "basin"
renal pyramid *PIR-a-mid*	A triangular structure in the renal medulla; composed of the nephrons' loops and collecting ducts
renin *RĒ-nin*	An enzyme produced by the kidneys that activates angiotensin in the blood

(continued)

Terminology	**Key Terms** (continued)
trigone TRĪ-gŏn	A triangle at the base of the bladder formed by the openings of the two ureters and the urethra (see Fig. 13-4)
tubular reabsorption TŪB-ŭ-lar rē-ab-SORP-shun	The return of substances from the glomerular filtrate to the blood through the peritubular capillaries
urea ū-RĒ-a	The main nitrogenous (nitrogen-containing) waste product in the urine
ureter Ū-rē-ter	The tube that carries urine from the kidney to the bladder (root: *ureter/o*)
urethra ū-RĒ-thra	The tube that carries urine from the bladder to the outside of the body (root: *urethr/o*)
urinary bladder ū-ri-NAR-ē BLAD-der	The organ that stores and eliminates urine excreted by the kidneys (roots: *cyst/o, vesic/o*)
urination ū-ri-NĀ-shun	The voiding of urine; micturition
urine Ū-rin	The fluid excreted by the kidneys. It consists of water, electrolytes, urea, other metabolic wastes, and pigments. A variety of other substances may appear in urine in cases of disease (root: *ur/o*)

PASSport to Success® Go to the pronunciation glossary on the Student Resources to hear these words pronounced.

Roots Pertaining to the Urinary System

See Tables 13-1 and 13-2.

| Table 13-1 | Roots for the Kidney |

Root	Meaning	Example	Definition of Example
ren/o	kidney	suprarenal sū-pra-RĒ-nal	above the kidney
nephr/o	kidney	nephrosis nef-RŌ-sis	any noninflammatory disease condition of the kidney
glomerul/o	glomerulus	juxtaglomerular juks-ta-glō-MER-ū-lar	near the glomerulus
pyel/o	renal pelvis	pyelectasis pī-e-LEK-ta-sis	dilatation of the renal pelvis
cali/o, calic/o	calyx	caliceal kal-i-SĒ-al	pertaining to a renal calyx (note addition of *e*); also spelled calyceal

13

EXERCISE **13-1**

Use the root *ren/o* to write a word for the following:

1. behind (post-) the kidney _____ postrenal _____

2. before or in front of (pre-) the kidney _____

3. between the kidneys _____

4. around the kidneys _____

Use the root *nephr/o* to write a word for the following:

5. study of the kidney _____

6. any disease of the kidney _____

7. poisonous or toxic to the kidney _____

8. softening of the kidney _____

9. surgical removal of the kidney _____

Use the appropriate root to write a word for the following:

10. inflammation of a glomerulus _____

11. dilatation of a renal calyx _____

12. plastic repair of the renal pelvis _____

13. radiograph of the renal pelvis _____

14. radiographic study (-graphy) of the kidney _____

15. incision of a renal calyx _____

16. hardening of a glomerulus _____

17. inflammation of the renal pelvis and kidney _____

Table 13-2	**Roots for the Urinary Tract (Except the Kidney)**		
Root	**Meaning**	**Example**	**Definition of Example**
ur/o	urine, urinary tract	urosepsis ū-ro-SEP-sis	generalized infection that originates in the urinary tract
urin/o	urine	nocturia nok-TŪ-rē-a	urination during the night (noct/i)
ureter/o	ureter	ureterostenosis ū-rē-ter-ō-ste-NŌ-sis	narrowing of the ureter
cyst/o	urinary bladder	cystocele SIS-tō-sēl	hernia of the urinary bladder
vesic/o	urinary bladder	intravesical in-tra-VES-i-kal	within the urinary bladder
urethr/o	urethra	urethrotome ū-RĒ-thrō-tōm	instrument for incising the urethra

EXERCISE **13-2**

Use the root *ur/o* to write a word for the following:

1. study of the urinary tract _____

2. radiography of the urinary tract _____

3. a urinary calculus (stone) _____

4. presence of urinary waste products in the blood _____

The root *ur/o-* is used in the suffix *-uria*, which means "condition of urine or of urination." Use *-uria* to write a word for the following:

5. lack of urine _____ anuria _____

6. painful or difficult urination _____

7. formation of excess (poly-) urine _____

8. presence of cells in the urine _____

9. presence of blood (hemat/o) in the urine _____

The suffix *-uresis* means "urination." Use *-uresis* to write a word for the following:

10. increased excretion of urine _____ diuresis _____

11. lack of urination _____

12. excretion of sodium (natri-) in the urine _____

13. excretion of potassium (kali-) in the urine _____

The adjective ending for the above words is *-uretic*, as in *diuretic* (pertaining to diuresis) and *natriuretic* (pertaining to the excretion of sodium in the urine).

Use the appropriate root to write a word for the following:

14. surgical fixation of the urethra _____

15. surgical creation of an opening in the ureter _____

16. a ureteral calculus _____

17. endoscopic examination of the urethra _____

Use the root *cyst/o* to write a word for the following:

18. inflammation of the urinary bladder _____

19. surgical fixation of the urinary bladder _____

20. an instrument for examining the interior of the bladder _____

21. incision of the bladder _____

Use the root *vesic/o* to write a word for the following:

22. above the urinary bladder _____

23. pertaining to the urethra and bladder _____

Define the following terms:

24. cystalgia (sis-TAL-jē-a) _____

25. ureterotomy (ū-rē-ter-OT-ō-mē) _____

26. transurethral (trans-ū-RĒ-thral) _____

27. uropoiesis (ū-rō-poy-Ē-sis) _____

13

Clinical Aspects of the Urinary System

Infections

Organisms that infect the urinary tract generally enter through the urethra and ascend toward the bladder, producing **cystitis**. Untreated, the infection can ascend even further into the urinary tract. The infecting organisms are usually colon bacteria carried in feces, particularly *Escherichia coli*. Although urinary tract infections (UTIs) do occur in men, they appear more commonly in women because the female urethra is shorter than the male urethra and its opening is closer to the anus. Poor toilet habits and **urinary stasis** are contributing factors. In the hospital, UTIs may result from procedures involving the urinary system, especially **catheterization**, in which a tube is inserted into the bladder to withdraw urine (Fig. 13-5). Less frequently, UTIs originate in the blood and descend through the urinary system.

An infection that involves the kidney and renal pelvis is termed **pyelonephritis**. As in cystitis, signs of this condition include **dysuria**, painful or difficult urination, and the presence of bacteria and pus in the urine, **bacteriuria** and **pyuria**, respectively.

Urethritis is inflammation of the urethra, generally associated with sexually transmitted infections such as gonorrhea and chlamydial infections (see Chapter 14).

Glomerulonephritis

Although the name simply means inflammation of the glomeruli and kidney, **glomerulonephritis** is a specific disorder that follows an immunologic reaction. It is usually a response to infection in another system, commonly a streptococcal infection of the respiratory tract or a skin infection. It may also accompany autoimmune diseases such as lupus erythematosus. The symptoms are hypertension, edema, and **oliguria**, the passage of small amounts of urine. This urine is highly concentrated. Because of damage to kidney tissue, blood and proteins escape into the nephrons, causing **hematuria**, blood in the urine, and **proteinuria**, protein in the urine. Blood cells may also form into small molds of the kidney tubule, called **casts**, which can be found in the urine. Most patients recover fully from glomerulonephritis, but in some cases, especially among the elderly, the disorder may lead to chronic renal failure (CRF) or end-stage renal disease (ESRD). In such cases, urea and other nitrogenous compounds accumulate in the blood, a condition termed **uremia**. These compounds affect the central nervous system, causing irritability, loss of appetite, stupor, and other symptoms. There is also electrolyte imbalance and **acidosis**.

Nephrotic Syndrome

Glomerulonephritis is one cause of **nephrotic syndrome**, a disease in which the glomeruli become overly permeable and allow the loss of proteins. Other possible causes of nephrotic syndrome are renal vein thrombosis, diabetes, systemic lupus erythematosus, toxins, or any other condition that damages the glomeruli.

Nephrotic syndrome is marked by proteinuria and **hypoproteinemia**, low blood protein. The low plasma protein level affects capillary exchange and results in edema. There is also an increase in blood lipids, as the liver compensates for lost protein by releasing lipoproteins.

Acute Renal Failure

Injury, shock, exposure to toxins, infections, and other renal disorders may cause damage to the nephrons, resulting in acute renal failure (ARF). There is rapid loss of kidney function with oliguria and accumulation of nitrogenous wastes in the blood. Failure of the kidneys to eliminate potassium leads to **hyperkalemia**, along with other electrolyte imbalances and acidosis (see Box 13-2). When destruction (necrosis) of kidney tubules is involved, the condition may be referred to as acute tubular necrosis (ATN).

Renal failure may lead to a need for kidney **dialysis** or, ultimately, **renal transplantation**. Dialysis refers to the movement of substances across a semipermeable membrane; it is a method used to eliminate harmful or unnecessary substances from the body when the kidneys are impaired or have been removed (Fig. 13-6). Two approaches are used:

- In **hemodialysis**, blood is cleansed by passage over a membrane surrounded by fluid (dialysate) that draws out unwanted substances. Most people on hemodialysis are treated for 4 hours three times a week in a dialysis center. Some patients are able to use simpler

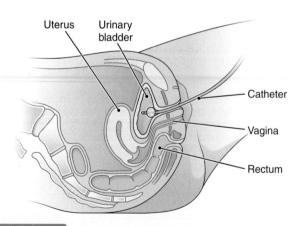

Figure 13-5 **An indwelling (Foley) catheter.** The catheter is shown in place in the female bladder.

Box 13-2   Clinical Perspectives

Sodium and Potassium: Causes and Consequences of Imbalance

Sodium and potassium concentrations in body fluids are important measures of water and electrolyte balance. An excess of sodium in body fluids is termed **hypernatremia**, taken from the Latin name for sodium, *natrium*. This condition accompanies dehydration and severe vomiting and may cause hypertension, edema, convulsions, and coma. **Hyponatremia**, a sodium deficiency in body fluids, can come from water intoxication (overhydration), heart failure, kidney failure, cirrhosis of the liver, pH imbalance, or endocrine disorders. It can cause muscle weakness, hypotension, confusion, shock, convulsions, and coma.

The term **hyperkalemia** is taken from the Latin name for potassium, *kalium*. It refers to excess potassium in body fluids, which may result from kidney failure, dehydration, and other causes. Its signs and symptoms include nausea, vomiting, muscular weakness, and severe cardiac arrhythmias. **Hypokalemia**, or low potassium in body fluids, may result from taking diuretics that cause potassium to be lost along with water. It may also result from pH imbalance or secretion of too much aldosterone from the adrenal cortex, resulting in potassium excretion. Hypokalemia causes muscle fatigue, paralysis, confusion, hypoventilation, and cardiac arrhythmias.

machines at home for daily dialysis. Box 13-3 has information on careers in hemodialysis treatment.

- In **peritoneal dialysis**, fluid is introduced into the peritoneal cavity. The fluid, along with waste products, is periodically withdrawn and replaced (Fig. 13-7). Fluid may be exchanged at intervals throughout the day in continuous ambulatory peritoneal dialysis (CAPD) or during the night in continuous cyclic peritoneal dialysis (CCPD).

Urinary Stones

Urinary lithiasis (presence of stones) may be related to infection, irritation, diet, or hormone imbalances that lead to increased calcium in the blood. Most urinary calculi (stones) are made up of calcium salts, but they may be composed of other materials as well. Causes of stone formation include dehydration, infection, abnormal pH of urine, urinary stasis, and metabolic imbalances. The stones generally form in the kidney and may move to the

Figure 13-6 **A hemodialysis system.** In hemodialysis, a cellophane membrane separates the blood compartment from the dialysis fluid compartment. This membrane is porous enough to allow all of the constituents except the plasma proteins (PRO) and blood cells (WBC, RBC) to diffuse between the two compartments.

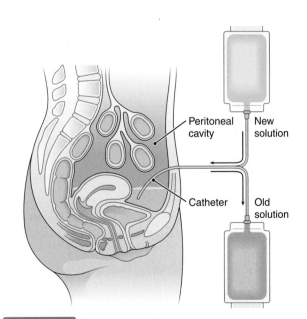

Figure 13-7 **Peritoneal dialysis.** The peritoneum, a semipermeable membrane richly supplied with small blood vessels, lines the peritoneal cavity. Waste products diffuse from the network of blood vessels into the dialysate in the peritoneal cavity.

13

Box 13-3 | **Health Professions**

Hemodialysis Technician

A hemodialysis technician, also called a renal technician or a nephrology technician, specializes in the safe and effective delivery of renal dialysis therapy to patients suffering from kidney failure. Before treatment begins, the technician prepares the dialysis solutions and ensures that the dialysis machine is clean, sterile, and in proper working order. The technician measures and records the patient's weight, temperature, and vital signs, inserts a catheter into the patient's arm, and connects the dialysis machine to it. During dialysis, the technician monitors the patient for adverse reactions and guards against any equipment malfunction. After the treatment is completed, the technician again measures and records the patient's weight, temperature, and vital signs. To perform these duties, hemodialysis technicians need a thorough scientific and clinical training. Most technicians in the United States receive their training from a college or technical school, and many states require that the technician be certified.

Hemodialysis technicians work in a variety of settings, such as hospitals, clinics, and patients' homes. As populations age, the incidence of kidney disease is expected to rise, as will the need for hemodialysis. For more information about this career, contact the National Association of Nephrology Technicians (NANT) at <www.dialysistech.net>

bladder (Fig. 13-8). This results in great pain, termed **renal colic,** and obstruction that can promote infection and cause **hydronephrosis,** collection of urine in the renal pelvis (Fig. 13-9).

Because they are radiopaque, stones can usually be seen on simple radiographs of the abdomen. Stones may dissolve and pass out of the body on their own. If not, they may be removed surgically, in a **lithotomy,** or by endoscopy. External shock waves are used to crush stones in the urinary tract in a procedure called extracorporeal (outside the body) shock-wave **lithotripsy** (crushing of stones).

Cancer

Carcinoma of the bladder has been linked to occupational exposure to chemicals, parasitic infections, and cigarette smoking. A key symptom is sudden, painless hematuria. Often the cancer can be seen by viewing the bladder lining with a **cystoscope** (Fig. 13-10).

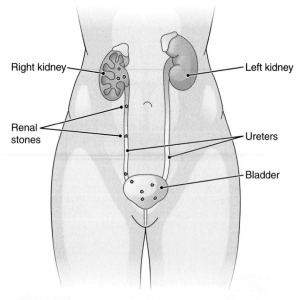

Figure 13-8 **Calculus formation in the urinary tract.** Various possible sites of calculus (stone) formation are shown.

Figure 13-9 **Hydronephrosis.** Urinary tract obstruction has led to dilation of the ureter, renal pelvis, and calices.

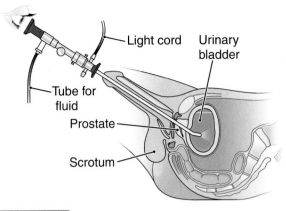

Figure 13-10 **Cystoscopy.** A lighted cystoscope is introduced through the urethra into the bladder of a male subject. Sterile fluid is used to inflate the bladder. Cystoscopes are used to examine the bladder, take biopsy specimens, and remove tumors.

Figure 13-11 **Ileal conduit.** In this surgery, the ureters are vented to the body surface through the ileum when the bladder is removed or nonfunctional.

This instrument can also be used to biopsy tissue for study.

If treatment is not effective in permanently removing the tumor, a **cystectomy** (removal of the bladder) may be necessary. In this case, the ureters must be vented elsewhere, such as directly to the body surface through the ileum in an **ileal conduit** (Fig. 13-11), or to some other portion of the intestine.

Cancer may also involve the kidney and renal pelvis. Additional means for diagnosing cancer and other urinary tract disorders include ultrasound, computed tomography scans, and radiographic studies such as **intravenous urography (IVU)** (Fig. 13-12), also called **intravenous pyelography (IVP)**, and **retrograde pyelography**.

Urinalysis

Urinalysis (UA) is a simple and widely used method for diagnosing urinary tract disorders. It may also reveal disturbances in other systems when abnormal byproducts are eliminated in the urine. In a routine UA, the urine is grossly examined for color and turbidity (a sign that bacteria are present); **specific gravity (SG)** (a measure of concentration) and pH are recorded; tests are performed for chemical components such as glucose, ketones, and hemoglobin; and the urine is examined microscopically for cells, crystals, and casts. In more detailed tests, drugs, enzymes, hormones, and other metabolites may be analyzed and bacterial cultures may be performed.

- Right and left renal pelves
- Ureteropelvic junction
- Left ureter
- Right ureter
- Urinary bladder

Figure 13-12 **Intravenous urogram.** The image shows the renal pelves, ureters, and urinary bladder.

13

Terminology | Key Terms

Disorders

acidosis *as-i-DŌ-sis*	Excessive acidity of body fluids
bacteriuria *bak-tē-rē-Ū-rē-a*	Presence of bacteria in the urine
cast	A solid mold of a renal tubule found in the urine
cystitis *sis-TĪ-tis*	Inflammation of the urinary bladder, usually as a result of infection
dysuria *dis-Ū-rē-a*	Painful or difficult urination
glomerulonephritis *glō-mer-ū-lō-nef-RĪ-tis*	Inflammation of the kidney primarily involving the glomeruli. The acute form usually occurs after an infection elsewhere in the body; the chronic form varies in cause and usually leads to renal failure
hematuria *hē-mat-Ū-rē-a*	Presence of blood in the urine
hydronephrosis *hī-drō-nef-RŌ-sis*	Collection of urine in the renal pelvis caused by obstruction; causes distention and renal atrophy (see Fig. 13-9)
hypokalemia *hī-pō-ka-LĒ-mē-a*	Deficiency of potassium in the blood
hyponatremia *hī-pō-na-TRĒ-mē-a*	Deficiency of sodium in the blood
hypoproteinemia *hī-pō-prō-tē-NĒ-mē-a*	Decreased amount of protein in the blood; may by caused by kidney damage resulting in protein loss
hyperkalemia	Excess amount of potassium in the blood
hypernatremia	Excess amount of sodium in the blood
nephrotic syndrome *nef-ROT-ik*	Condition that results from glomerular damage leading to loss of protein in the urine (proteinuria). There is low plasma protein (hypoproteinemia), edema, and increased blood lipids as the liver releases lipoproteins. Also called nephrosis
oliguria *ol-ig-Ū-rē-a*	Elimination of small amounts of urine
proteinuria *prō-tē-NŪ-rē-ā*	Presence of protein, mainly albumin, in the urine
pyelonephritis *pī-e-lō-ne-FRĪ-tis*	Inflammation of the renal pelvis and kidney, usually caused by infection
pyuria *pī-Ū-rē-a*	Presence of pus in the urine
renal colic *KOL-ik*	Radiating pain in the region of the kidney associated with the passage of a stone
uremia *ū-RĒ-mē-a*	Presence of toxic levels of urea and other nitrogenous substances in the blood as a result of renal insufficiency
urethritis *ū-rē-THRĪ-tis*	Inflammation of the urethra, usually due to infection
urinary stasis *STĀ-sis*	Stoppage of urine flow; urinary stagnation

(continued)

Terminology   Key Terms (continued)

Diagnosis and Treatment

catheterization *kath-e-ter-i-ZĀ-shun*	Introduction of a tube into a passage, such as through the urethra into the bladder for withdrawal of urine (see Fig. 13-5)
cystoscope *SIS-tō-skōp*	An instrument for examining the interior of the urinary bladder. Also used for removing foreign objects, for surgery, and for other forms of treatment
dialysis *dī-AL-i-sis*	Separation of substances by passage through a semipermeable membrane. Dialysis is used to rid the body of unwanted substances when the kidneys are impaired or missing. The two forms of dialysis are hemodialysis and peritoneal dialysis
hemodialysis *hē-mō-dī-AL-i-sis*	Removal of unwanted substances from the blood by passage through a semipermeable membrane (see Fig. 13-6)
intravenous pyelography (IVP) *pī-e-LOG-ra-fē*	Intravenous urography (see Fig. 13-12)
intravenous urography (IVU) *u-ROG-ra-fē*	Radiographic visualization of the urinary tract after intravenous administration of a contrast medium that is excreted in the urine; also called excretory urography or intravenous pyelography, although the latter is less accurate because the procedure shows more than just the renal pelvis
lithotripsy *LITH-ō-trip-sē*	Crushing of a stone
peritoneal dialysis *per-i-tō-NĒ-al dī-AL-i-sis*	Removal of unwanted substances from the body by introduction of a dialyzing fluid into the peritoneal cavity followed by removal of the fluid (see Fig. 13-7)
retrograde pyelography *RET-rō-grād pī-e-LOG-ra-fē*	Pyelography in which the contrast medium is injected into the kidneys from below, by way of the ureters
specific gravity (SG)	The weight of a substance compared with the weight of an equal volume of water. The specific gravity of normal urine ranges from 1.015 to 1.025. This value may increase or decrease in disease
urinalysis (UA) *ū-ri-NAL-i-sis*	Laboratory study of the urine. Physical and chemical properties and microscopic appearance are included

Surgery

cystectomy *sis-TEK-tō-mē*	Surgical removal of all or part of the urinary bladder
ileal conduit *IL-ē-al KON-dū-it*	Diversion of urine by connection of the ureters to an isolated segment of the ileum. One end of the segment is sealed, and the other drains through an opening in the abdominal wall (see Fig. 13-11). A procedure used when the bladder is removed or nonfunctional. Also called ileal bladder
lithotomy *lith-OT-ō-mē*	Incision of an organ to remove a stone (calculus)
renal transplantation	Surgical implantation of a donor kidney into a patient

13

PASSport to Success®   Go to the pronunciation glossary on the Student Resources to hear these words pronounced.

Terminology   Supplementary Terms

Normal Structure and Function

aldosterone *al-DOS-ter-ōn*	A hormone secreted by the adrenal gland that regulates electrolyte excretion by the kidneys
clearance	The volume of plasma that the kidneys can clear of a substance per unit of time; renal plasma clearance
creatinine *krē-AT-in-in*	A nitrogenous byproduct of muscle metabolism. An increase in blood creatinine is a sign of renal failure
detrusor muscle *dē-TRŪ-sor*	The muscle in the bladder wall
glomerular filtration rate (GFR)	The amount of filtrate formed per minute by both kidneys
maximal transport capacity (Tm)	The maximum rate at which a given substance can be transported across the renal tubule; tubular maximum
renal corpuscle *KOR-pus-l*	The glomerular capsule and the glomerulus considered as a unit; the filtration device of the kidney

Symptoms and Conditions

anuresis *an-ū-RĒ-sis*	Lack of urination
anuria *an-Ū-rē-a*	Lack of urine formation
azotemia *az-ō-TĒ-mē-a*	Presence of increased nitrogenous waste, especially urea, in the blood
azoturia *az-ō-TŪ-rē-a*	Presence of increased nitrogenous compounds, especially urea, in the urine
cystocele *SIS-tō-sēl*	Herniation of the bladder into the vagina (see Fig. 15-11); vesicocele
dehydration *dē-hī-DRĀ-shun*	Excessive loss of body fluids
diabetes insipidus *dī-a-BĒ-tēz in-SIP-id-us*	A condition caused by inadequate production of antidiuretic hormone, resulting in excessive excretion of dilute urine and extreme thirst
enuresis *en-ū-RĒ-sis*	Involuntary urination, usually at night; bed-wetting
epispadias *ep-i-SPĀ-dē-as*	A congenital condition in which the urethra opens on the dorsal surface of the penis as a groove or cleft; anaspadias
glycosuria *glī-kō-SŪ-rē-a*	Presence of glucose in the urine, as in cases of diabetes mellitus
horseshoe kidney	A congenital union of the lower poles of the kidneys, resulting in a horseshoe-shaped organ (Fig. 13-13)
hydroureter *hī-drō-ū-RĒ-ter*	Distention of the ureter with urine due to obstruction
hypospadias *hī-pō-SPĀ-dē-as*	A congenital condition in which the urethra opens on the undersurface of the penis or into the vagina (Fig. 13-14)

(continued)

Terminology	**Key Terms** (continued)
hypovolemia hī-pō-vō-LĒ-mē-a	A decrease in blood volume
incontinence in-KON-tin-ens	Inability to retain urine. Incontinence may originate with a neurologic disorder, trauma to the spinal cord, weakness of the pelvic muscles, urinary retention, or impaired bladder function. Term also applies to inability to retain semen or feces
neurogenic bladder nū-rō-JEN-ik	Any bladder dysfunction that results from a central nervous system lesion
nocturia nok-TŪ-rē-a	Excessive urination at night (noct/o means "night")
pitting edema	Edema in which the skin, when pressed firmly with the finger, will maintain the depression produced (see Fig. 9-21)
polycystic kidney disease pol-ē-SIS-tik	A hereditary condition in which the kidneys are enlarged and contain many cysts (Fig. 13-15)
polydipsia pol-ē-DIP-sē-a	Excessive thirst
polyuria pol-ē-Ū-rē-a	Elimination of large amounts of urine, as in diabetes mellitus
retention of urine	Accumulation of urine in the bladder because of an inability to urinate
staghorn calculus	A kidney stone that fills the renal pelvis and calices to give a "staghorn" appearance (Fig. 13-16)
ureterocele ū-RĒ-ter-ō-sēl	A cystlike dilation of the ureter near its opening into the bladder. Usually results from a congenital narrowing of the ureteral opening (Fig. 13-17)
urinary frequency	A need to urinate often without an increase in average output
urinary urgency	Sudden need to urinate
water intoxication in-tok-si-KĀ-shun	Excess intake or retention of water with decrease in sodium concentration. May result from excess drinking, excess ADH, or replacement of a large amount of body fluid with pure water. Causes an imbalance in the cellular environment, with edema and other disturbances
Wilms tumor	A malignant kidney tumor that usually appears in children before the age of 5 years

Diagnosis

anion gap AN-ī-on	A measure of electrolyte imbalance
blood urea nitrogen (BUN)	Nitrogen in the blood in the form of urea. An increase in BUN indicates an increase in nitrogenous waste products in the blood and renal failure
clean-catch specimen	A urine sample obtained after thorough cleansing of the urethral opening and collection in midstream to minimize the chance of contamination
cystometrography sis-tō-me-TROG-ra-fē	A study of bladder function in which the bladder is filled with fluid or air and the pressure exerted by the bladder muscle at varying degrees of filling is measured. The tracing recorded is a cystometrogram
protein electrophoresis (PEP)	Laboratory study of urinary proteins; used to diagnose multiple myeloma, systemic lupus erythematosus, and lymphoid tumor
urinometer ū-ri-NOM-e-ter	Device for measuring the specific gravity of urine

13

(continued)

Terminology	Key Terms (continued)

Treatment

indwelling Foley catheter	A urinary tract catheter with a balloon at one end that prevents the catheter from leaving the bladder (see Fig. 13-5)
lithotrite LITH-ō-trīt	Instrument for crushing a bladder stone

PASSport to Success®   Go to the pronunciation glossary on the Student Resources to hear these words pronounced.

Figure 13-13 Horseshoe kidney. The photograph shows the kidneys fused at the poles.

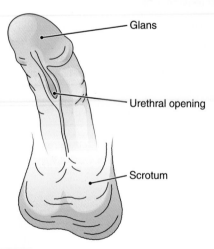

Glans

Urethral opening

Scrotum

Figure 13-14 Hypospadias. The urethra is shown opening on the ventral surface of the penis.

Figure 13-15 Adult polycystic disease. The kidney is enlarged and the active tissue is almost entirely replaced by cysts of varying size. (*Left*) Surface view. (*Right*) Longitudinal section.

Figure 13-16 **Staghorn calculus.** The kidney shows hydronephrosis and stones that are casts of the dilated calices.

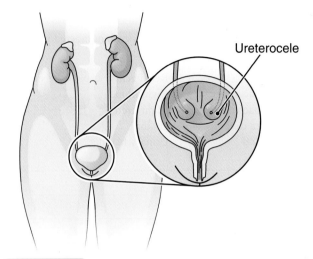

Figure 13-17 **Ureterocele.** The ureter bulges into the bladder. The resulting obstruction causes urine to reflux into the ureter (hydroureter) and renal pelvis (hydronephrosis).

Terminology   Abbreviations

ACE	Angiotensin-converting enzyme		GFR	Glomerular filtration rate
ADH	Antidiuretic hormone		GU	Genitourinary
ARF	Acute renal failure		IVP	Intravenous pyelography
ATN	Acute tubular necrosis		IVU	Intravenous urography
BUN	Blood urea nitrogen		K	Potassium
CAPD	Continuous ambulatory peritoneal dialysis		KUB	Kidney–ureter–bladder (radiography)
CCPD	Continuous cyclic peritoneal dialysis		Na	Sodium
CMG	Cystometrography; cystometrogram		PEP	Protein electrophoresis
CRF	Chronic renal failure		SG	Specific gravity
EPO	Erythropoietin		Tm	Maximal transport capacity
ESRD	End-stage renal disease		UA	Urinalysis
ESWL	Extracorporeal shock-wave lithotripsy		UTI	Urinary tract infection

13

Chapter Review

LABELING EXERCISE

Urinary System > Write the name of each numbered part on the corresponding line of the answer sheet.

Abdominal aorta   Renal artery
Adrenal gland   Renal vein
Common iliac artery   Right kidney
Common iliac vein   Right ureter
Inferior vena cava   Urethra
Prostate gland   Urinary bladder

1. _____

2. _____

3. _____

4. _____

5. _____

6. _____

7. _____

8. _____

9. _____

10. _____

11. _____

12. _____

Chapter Review *(continued)*

The Kidney > Write the name of each numbered part on the corresponding line of the answer sheet.

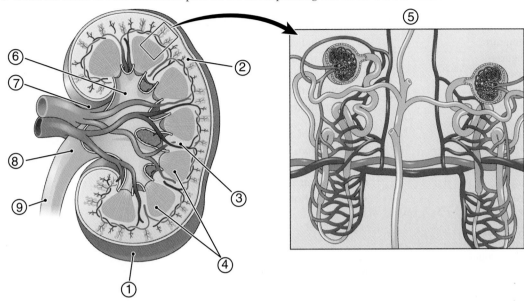

Calyx   Renal medulla
Hilum   Renal pelvis
Nephrons   Renal cortex
Pyramids of medulla   Ureter
Renal capsule

1. _____   6. _____

2. _____   7. _____

3. _____   8. _____

4. _____   9. _____

5. _____

The Urinary Bladder > Write the name of each numbered part on the corresponding line of the answer sheet.

External urethral sphincter   Smooth muscle
Internal urethral sphincter   Trigone
Openings of ureters   Ureter
Prostate   Urethra

1. _____

2. _____

3. _____

4. _____

5. _____

6. _____

7. _____

8. _____

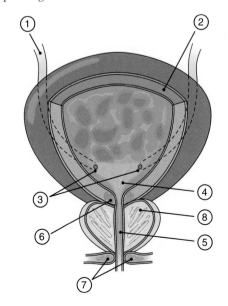

13

Chapter Review (continued)

TERMINOLOGY

Matching > Match the following terms and write the appropriate letter to the left of each number:

_____	**1.** hematuria	**a.**	abnormal color of urine
_____	**2.** oliguria	**b.**	pus in the urine
_____	**3.** chromaturia	**c.**	elimination of small amounts of urine
_____	**4.** albuminuria	**d.**	blood in the urine
_____	**5.** pyuria	**e.**	proteinuria
_____	**6.** trigone	**a.**	absence of a bladder
_____	**7.** catheterization	**b.**	stagnation, as of urine
_____	**8.** stasis	**c.**	deficiency of urine
_____	**9.** acystia	**d.**	triangle at the base of the bladder
_____	**10.** uropenia	**e.**	introduction of a tube

Supplementary Terms

_____	**11.** aldosterone	**a.**	urination during the night
_____	**12.** diabetes insipidus	**b.**	condition caused by lack of ADH
_____	**13.** incontinence	**c.**	nitrogenous metabolic waste
_____	**14.** nocturia	**d.**	hormone that regulates electrolytes
_____	**15.** creatinine	**e.**	inability to retain urine
_____	**16.** anuresis	**a.**	excessive thirst
_____	**17.** epispadias	**b.**	bed-wetting
_____	**18.** polydipsia	**c.**	presence of excess nitrogenous waste in the urine
_____	**19.** enuresis	**d.**	congenital misplacement of the ureteral opening
_____	**20.** azoturia	**e.**	lack of urination

Fill in the blanks:

21. A microscopic working unit of the kidney is called a(n) _____.

22. The cluster of capillaries within the glomerular capsule is the _____.

23. An enzyme released by the kidneys that acts to increase blood pressure _____.

24. Micturition is the scientific term for _____.

25. Laboratory study of the urine is a(n) _____.

26. The main nitrogenous waste product in urine is _____.

True–False > Examine the following statements. If the statement is true, write T in the first blank. If the statement is false, write F in the first blank and correct the statement by replacing the underlined word in the second blank.

27. A reniform structure is shaped like the <u>bladder.</u>   _____   _____

28. Pyelitis is inflammation of the <u>renal pelvis.</u>   _____   _____

29. A nephrotropic substance acts on the <u>kidney.</u>   _____   _____

30. The outer portion of the kidney is the <u>medulla.</u>   _____   _____

31. The tube that carries urine out of the body is the <u>ureter.</u>   _____   _____

32. EPO stimulates the production of <u>red blood cells.</u>   _____   _____

33. A lithotomy is an incision to remove a <u>calculus.</u>   _____   _____

34. Kaliuresis refers to the excretion of <u>sodium</u> in the urine.   _____   _____

Chapter Review (continued)

Define the following words:

35. pararenal (*par-a-RĒ-nal*) _____

36. dysuria (*dis-Ū-rē-a*) _____

37. nephrotoxic (*nef-rō-TOK-sik*) _____

38. juxtaglomerular (*juks-ta-glō-MER-ū-lar*) _____

39. calicectomy (*kal-i-SEK-tō-mē*) _____

40. urethrostenosis (*ū-rē-thrō-ste-NŌ-sis*) _____

Write a word for the following definitions:

41. dilatation of the renal pelvis and calices _____

42. softening of a kidney (nephr/o) _____

43. excision of the bladder (cyst/o) _____

44. any disease of the kidney (nephr/o) _____

45. radiograph of the bladder (cyst/o) and urethra _____

46. plastic repair of a ureter and renal pelvis _____

47. inflammation of the renal pelvis and the kidney _____

48. surgical creation of an opening between a ureter and the sigmoid colon _____

Eliminations > In each of the sets below, underline the word that does not fit in with the rest and explain the reason for your choice:

49. capsule — cast — pyramid — nephron — cortex

_____

50. nephron loop — distal convoluted tubule — glomerular capsule — calyx — proximal convoluted tubule

_____

51. ileal conduit — specific gravity — dialysis — cystoscopy — lithotripsy

_____

Opposites > Write a word that means the opposite of the following:

52. hydration _____

53. hypervolemia _____

54. diuretic _____

55. hyponatremia _____

56. uresis _____

Adjectives > Write the adjective form of the following:

57. calyx _____

58. urology _____

59. uremia _____

13

Chapter Review (continued)

60. diuresis   _____

61. nephrosis   _____

62. ureter   _____

63. urethra   _____

Plurals > Write the plural form of the following:

64. pelvis   _____

65. calyx   _____

66. glomerulus _____

Word Building > Write a word for the following definitions using the word parts given.

graph-   ren/o   -al   intra-   vesic/o   -y   ur/o   inter-   lith   log   supra-

67. radiographic study of the urinary tract   _____

68. pertaining to the kidney   _____

69. within the kidney   _____

70. radiographic study of the kidney   _____

71. within the bladder   _____

72. above the kidney   _____

73. study of the urinary tract   _____

74. between the kidneys   _____

75. pertaining to the bladder   _____

76. a urinary tract stone   _____

Write the meaning of the following abbreviations:

77. IVP _____

78. ADH _____

79. EPO _____

80. IVU _____

81. Na _____

82. GFR _____

83. UA _____

Word Analysis > Define the following words, and give the meaning of the word parts in each. Use a dictionary if necessary.

84. hemodialysis (*hē-mō-dī-AL-i-sis*)_____

   a. hem/o _____

   b. dia- _____

   c. lysis _____

EXERCISE **14-1**

Define the following words:

1. seminal (SEM-i-*nal*) _____

2. orchialgia (*or-kē-AL-jē-a*) _____

3. oscheoplasty (*os-kē-ō-PLAS-tē*) _____

4. epididymectomy (*ep-i-did-i-MEK-tō-mē*) _____

5. prostatodynia (*pros-ta-tō-DIN-ē-a*) _____

6. testopathy (*tes-TOP-a-thē*) _____

7. orchiepididymitis (*or-kē-ep-i-did-i-MĪ-tis*) _____

Use the root *orchi/o* to write a word for the following definitions. Each is also written with the root *orchid/o*.

8. surgical fixation of a testis _____

9. plastic repair of a testis _____

10. incision of a testis _____

Use the root *spermat/o* to write a word for the following definitions:

11. a sperm-forming cell _____

12. destruction (-lysis) of sperm _____

13. excessive discharge (-rhea) of semen _____

14. formation (-genesis) of spermatozoa _____

15. condition of having sperm in the urine (-uria) _____

The ending *-spermia* means "condition of sperm or semen." Add a prefix to *-spermia* to form a word for the following definitions:

16. lack of semen _____

17. presence of blood in the semen _____

18. deficiency of (olig/o) semen _____

19. presence of pus in the semen _____

Write a word for the following definitions:

20. excision of the ductus deferens _____

21. tumor of the scrotum _____

22. suture of the vas deferens _____

23. excision of the prostate gland _____

24. radiographic study of a seminal vesicle _____

25. inflammation of a seminal vesicle _____

26. incision of the epididymis _____

14

Clinical Aspects of the Male Reproductive System

Infection

Most infections of the male reproductive tract are **sexually transmitted infections (STIs)**, listed in Box 14-2. The most common STI in the United States is caused by the bacterium *Chlamydia trachomatis*, which mainly causes **urethritis** in males. This same organism also causes lymphogranuloma venereum, an STI associated with lymphadenopathy, which occurs most commonly in tropical regions. Both forms of these chlamydial infections respond to treatment with antibiotics.

Gonorrhea is caused by *Neisseria gonorrhoeae*, the gonococcus (GC). Infection usually centers in the urethra, causing urethritis with burning, a purulent discharge, and dysuria. Untreated, the disease can spread through the reproductive system. Gonorrhea is treated with antibiotics, but gonococci can rapidly develop resistance to these drugs.

Another common STI is herpes infection, caused by a virus. Other STIs are discussed in Chapter 15.

Box 14-2	**For Your Reference**

Sexually Transmitted Infections

DISEASE	ORGANISM	DESCRIPTION
BACTERIAL		
chlamydial infection	*Chlamydia trachomatis* types D to K	Ascending infection of reproductive and urinary tracts. May spread to pelvis in women, causing pelvic inflammatory disease (PID)
lymphogranuloma venereum	*Chlamydia trachomatis* type L	General infection with swelling of inguinal lymph nodes; scarring of genital tissue
gonorrhea	*Neisseria gonorrhoeae*; gonococcus (GC)	Inflammation of reproductive and urinary tracts. Urethritis in men. Vaginal discharge and cervical inflammation (cervicitis) in women, leading to pelvic inflammatory disease (PID). Possible systemic infection. May spread to newborns. Treated with antibiotics
bacterial vaginosis	*Gardnerella vaginalis*	Vaginal infection with foul-smelling discharge
syphilis	*Treponema pallidum* (a spirochete)	Primary stage: chancre (lesion); secondary stage: systemic infection and syphilitic warts; tertiary stage: degeneration of other systems. Cause of spontaneous abortions, stillbirths, and fetal deformities. Treated with antibiotics
VIRAL		
AIDS (acquired immuno-deficiency syndrome)	HIV (human immunodeficiency virus)	An often fatal disease that infects T cells of the immune system, weakening the host and leading to other diseases
genital herpes	herpes simplex virus (HSV)	Painful genital lesions. In women, may be a risk factor in cervical carcinoma. Often fatal infections of newborns. No cure at present
hepatitis B	hepatitis B virus (HBV)	Causes liver inflammation, which may be acute or may develop into a chronic carrier state. Linked to liver cancer
condyloma acuminatum (genital warts)	human papillomavirus (HPV)	Benign genital warts. In women, predisposes to cervical dysplasia and carcinoma. A vaccine against the most prevalent strains is available
PROTOZOAL		
trichomoniasis	*Trichomonas vaginalis*	Vaginitis. Green, frothy discharge with itching; pain on intercourse (dyspareunia); and painful urination (dysuria)

Mumps is a nonsexually transmitted viral disease that can infect the testes and lead to **sterility**. Other microorganisms can infect the reproductive tract as well, causing urethritis, **prostatitis**, **orchitis**, or **epididymitis**.

Benign Prostatic Hyperplasia

As men age, the prostate gland commonly enlarges, a condition known as **benign prostatic hyperplasia (BPH)**. Although not cancerous, this overgrown tissue can press on the urethra near the bladder and interfere with urination. Urinary retention, infection, and other complications may follow if an obstruction is not corrected.

Medications to relax smooth muscle in the prostate and bladder neck are used to treat the symptoms of BPH. Alpha-adrenergic blocking agents interfere with sympathetic nervous stimulation in these regions to improve urinary flow rate. One example is tamsulosin (Flomax). Because testosterone stimulates enlargement of the prostate, drugs that interfere with prostatic testosterone activity may slow progress of the disorder. One example is finasteride (Proscar). A herbal remedy that seems to act in this same manner is an extract of the berries of the saw palmetto, a low-growing palm tree. Saw palmetto has been found to delay the need for surgery in some cases of BPH.

In advanced cases of BPH, removal of the prostate, or **prostatectomy**, may be required. When this is performed through the urethra, the procedure is called a transurethral resection of the prostate (TURP) (Fig. 14-5A). The prostate may also be cut in a transurethral incision of the prostate (TUIP) to reduce pressure on the urethra (Fig. 14-5B). Surgeons also use a laser beam or heat to destroy prostatic tissue. BPH is diagnosed by digital rectal examination (DRE) or imaging studies.

Cancer

CANCER OF THE PROSTATE

Prostatic cancer is the most common malignancy in men in the United States. Only lung cancer and colon cancer cause more cancer-related deaths in men who are past middle age. Blood levels of a protein produced by prostatic cells increase in cases of prostatic cancer. This prostate-specific antigen (PSA) is used, along with palpation and DREs, to screen for prostate cancer and to assess the results of treatment.

The TNM system for staging prostate cancer includes the following categories:

- T_1: tumor not palpable by rectal examination; detected by biopsy or abnormal PSA
- T_2: tumor palpable and confined to the prostate
- T_3: tumor has spread locally beyond the prostate
- M: distant metastases

Treatment methods include surgery (prostatectomy), radiation, inhibition of male hormones (androgens), which stimulate prostatic growth, and chemotherapy. Radiation is usually delivered by implantation of radioactive seeds. Another approach is termed "watchful waiting" or deferred therapy, which consists of monitoring without therapy. Choice of this option is based on a man's age, tumor invasiveness, and the probability that an untreated tumor will result in harm to a patient during his lifetime.

TESTICULAR CANCER

Cancer of the testis represents less than 1% of cancer in adult males. It usually appears between the ages of 25

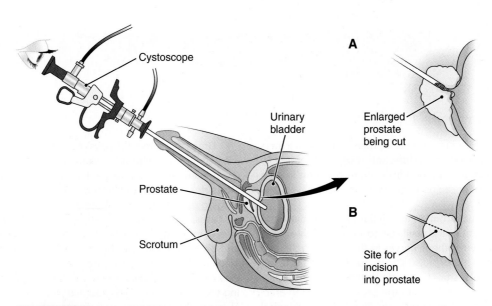

Figure 14-5 Prostate surgery procedures. (*A*) Transurethral resection of the prostate (TURP). Portions of the prostate are removed at the bladder opening. (*B*) Transurethral incision of the prostate (TUIP). One or two incisions are made in the prostate to reduce pressure on the urethra.

and 45 years and shows no sign of genetic inheritance. This cancer typically originates in germ cells and can spread to abdominal lymph nodes. More than half of testicular tumors release markers that can be detected in the blood. Treatment may include removal of the testis (orchiectomy), radiation, and chemotherapy.

Cryptorchidism

It is fairly common that one or both testes will fail to descend into the scrotum by the time of birth (Fig. 14-6). This condition is termed **cryptorchidism**, literally hidden (crypt/o) testis (orchid/o). The condition usually corrects itself within the first year of life. If not, it must be corrected surgically to avoid sterility and an increased risk of cancer.

Infertility

An inability or a diminished ability to reproduce is termed **infertility**. Its causes may be hereditary, hormonal, disease related, or the result of exposure to chemical or physical agents. The most common causes of infertility are STIs. A total inability to produce offspring may be termed sterility. Men may be voluntarily sterilized by cutting and sealing the vas deferens on both sides in a **vasectomy** (see Fig. 15-5).

ERECTILE DYSFUNCTION

Erectile dysfunction, also called **impotence**, is the male lack of ability to perform intercourse because of failure to initiate or maintain an erection until ejaculation. About 10% to 20% of such cases are psychogenic—that is, caused by emotional factors, such as stress, depression, or emotional trauma. More often, erectile dysfunction has a physical cause, which may be:

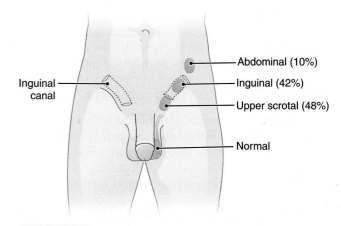

Figure 14-6 **Cryptorchidism.** The testis fails to descend into the scrotum. In most cases, the testis is retained in the upper part of the scrotal sac or in the inguinal canal. The percentages of different locations are shown.

- A vascular disorder, such as arteriosclerosis, varicose veins, or damage caused by diabetes
- A neurologic problem, as caused by a tumor, trauma, the effects of diabetes, or damage caused by radiation or surgery
- A side effect of a drug, such as an antihypertensive agent, antiulcer medication, or an appetite suppressant

Drugs that are used to treat erectile dysfunction work by dilating arteries in the penis to increase blood flow to that organ. Nondrug approaches include corrective surgery, vacuum pumps to draw blood into the penis, penile injections to dilate blood vessels, and penile prostheses. Box 14-3 has more information on erectile dysfunction.

Box 14-3   **Clinical Perspectives**

Treating Erectile Dysfunction

Approximately 25 million American men and their partners are affected by **erectile dysfunction (ED),** the inability to achieve an erection. Although ED is more common in men over the age of 65, it can occur at any age and can have many causes.

Erection results from an interaction between the autonomic nervous system and penile blood vessels. Sexual arousal stimulates parasympathetic nerves in the penis to release a compound called nitric oxide (NO). This substance activates an enzyme in vascular smooth muscle that promotes vasodilation, increasing blood flow into the penis and causing erection. Physical factors that cause ED prevent these physiological changes.

Drugs that target the physiologic mechanisms of erection are helping men who suffer from ED. These include sildenafil (trade name, Viagra), vardenafil (Levitra), and tadalafil (Cialis). These drugs prevent the breakdown of vasodilators, thus prolonging the effects of NO. Although effective in about 80% of ED cases, these drugs can cause some relatively minor side effects, including headache, nasal congestion, stomach upset, and blue-tinged vision. They should never be used by men who are taking nitrate drugs to treat angina. Because nitrates elevate NO levels, taking them with drugs for ED and prolonging the effects of NO can cause life-threatening hypotension. They are also contraindicated in men with low blood pressure and heart failure.

Inguinal Hernia

The inguinal canal, through which the testis descends, may represent a weakness in the abdominal wall that can lead to a hernia. In the most common form of **inguinal hernia** (Fig. 14-7), an abdominal organ, usually the intestine, enters the inguinal canal and may extend into the scrotum. This is an indirect, or external, inguinal hernia. In a direct, or internal, inguinal hernia, the organ protrudes through the abdominal wall into the scrotum. If blood supply to the organ is cut off, the hernia is said to be *strangulated*. Surgery to correct a hernia is a **herniorrhaphy**.

Physician assistants aid in patient care in all medical and surgical fields. Box 14-4 describes careers in this specialty.

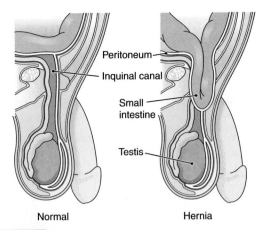

Normal   Hernia

Figure 14-7 **Inguinal hernia.** Weakness in the abdominal wall allows the intestine or other abdominal contents to protrude into the inguinal canal. The hernial sac is a continuation of the peritoneum.

Box 14-4 **Health Professions**

Physician Assistant

Physician assistants (PAs) practice medicine under the supervision of physicians and surgeons. They are trained in diagnosis, therapy, and preventive health care. They are also licensed to treat minor injuries. In almost all states, they are permitted to prescribe medications. Depending on the work setting, they may also manage a practice and supervise other medical personnel. In medically underserved areas, they may work independently most of the time and confer with physicians as needed. Many PAs work in general, pediatric, or family medicine practices. If they specialize in surgery, they may provide patient care before and after an operation or assist in surgery.

A PA must complete a formal educational program, usually requiring at least 2 years and including clinical training.

Most PA candidates enter their programs with a bachelor's degree and clinical experience either in the military or some other allied health field. They receive an associate degree or higher, and must be licensed by passing a national exam. They may also become certified (PA-C) through the National Commission on Certification of Physician Assistants (NCCPA) and maintain that certification by continuing education. The job outlook is very good, especially as telecommunication increases the ease of consultations and hospitals need to add staffing to compensate for shorter medical residents' shifts. For additional information, contact the American Academy of Physician Assistants at www.aapa.org.

Terminology **Key Terms**

Disorders

benign prostatic hyperplasia (BPH)	Nonmalignant enlargement of the prostate; frequently develops with age; also called benign prostatic hypertrophy
cryptorchidism *krip-TOR-kid-izm*	Failure of the testis to descend into the scrotum (see Fig. 14-6)
epididymitis *ep-i-did-i-MĪ-tis*	Inflammation of the epididymis. Common causes are UTIs and STIs
erectile dysfunction *e-REK-til dis-FUNK-shun*	A lack of ability to perform intercourse in males because of failure to initiate or maintain an erection until ejaculation; impotence
impotence *IM-pō-tens*	Erectile dysfunction

14

(continued)

Terminology   Key Terms (continued)

infertility *in-fer-TIL-i-tē*	Decreased capacity to produce offspring
inguinal hernia *ING-gwin-al*	Protrusion of the intestine or other abdominal organ through the inguinal canal (see Fig. 14-7) or through the wall of the abdomen into the scrotum
orchitis *or-KĪ-tis*	Inflammation of a testis. May be caused by injury, mumps virus, or other infections
prostatitis *pros-ta-TĪ-tis*	Inflammation of the prostate gland. Often appears with UTI, STI, and a variety of other stresses
sexually transmitted infection (STI)	Infection spread through sexual activity (see Box 14-2); also called sexually transmitted disease (STD) and formerly venereal (*ve-NĒR-ē-al*) disease (VD) (from Venus, the goddess of love)
sterility *ste-RIL-i-tē*	Complete inability to produce offspring
urethritis *ū-rē-THRĪ-tis*	Inflammation of the urethra; often caused by gonorrhea and chlamydial infections

Surgery

herniorrhaphy *her-nē-OR-a-fē*	Surgical repair of a hernia
prostatectomy *pros-ta-TEK-tō-mē*	Surgical removal of the prostate
vasectomy *va-SEK-tō-mē*	Excision of the vas deferens. Usually done bilaterally to produce sterility (see Fig. 15-5). May be accomplished through the urethra (transurethral resection)

 PASSport to Success® Go to the pronunciation glossary on the Student resources to hear these words pronounced.

Terminology   Supplementary Terms

Normal Structure and Function

emission *ē-MISH-un*	The discharge of semen
genitalia *jen-i-TĀL-ē-a*	The organs concerned with reproduction, divided into internal and external components
insemination *in-sem-i-NĀ-shun*	Introduction of semen into a woman's vagina
orgasm *OR-gazm*	A state of physical and emotional excitement, especially that which occurs at the climax of sexual intercourse
phallus *FAL-us*	The penis

(continued)

| **Terminology** | **Supplementary Terms** (continued) |

Disorders

balanitis *bal-a-NĪ-tis*	Inflammation of the glans penis and mucous membrane beneath it (root *balan/o* means "glans penis")
bladder neck obstruction (BNO)	Blockage of urine flow at the outlet of the bladder. The common cause is benign prostatic hyperplasia
hydrocele *HĪ-drō-sēl*	The accumulation of fluid in a saclike cavity, especially within the covering of the testis or spermatic cord (Fig. 14-8)
phimosis *fī-MŌ-sis*	Narrowing of the prepuce's opening so that the foreskin cannot be pushed back over the glans penis
priapism *PRĪ-a-pizm*	Abnormal, painful, continuous erection of the penis, as may be caused by drugs or specific damage to the spinal cord
seminoma *sem-i-NŌ-ma*	A tumor of the testis
spermatocele *SPER-ma-tō-sēl*	An epididymal cyst containing spermatozoa (see Fig. 14-8)
varicocele *VAR-i-kō-sēl*	Enlargement of the veins of the spermatic cord (see Fig. 14-8)

Diagnosis and Treatment

brachytherapy *brak-ē-THER-a-pē*	Radiation therapy by placement of encapsulated radiation sources, such as seeds, directly into a tumor or nearby tissue (from Greek *brachy-*, meaning "short")
castration *kas-TRĀ-shun*	Surgical removal of the testes or ovaries. Hormones and drugs can inhibit the gonads, to produce functional castration
Gleason tumor grade *GLĒ-son*	A system for assessing the severity of cancerous changes in the prostate; reported as a Gleason score
Whitmore–Jewett staging *WIT-mōr–JEW-et*	A method for staging prostatic tumors; and alternate to TNM staging

PASSport to Success® Go to the pronunciation glossary on the Student resources to hear these words pronounced.

14

Figure 14-8 **Scrotal abnormalities.** (*A*) Normal. (*B*) Hydrocele. (*C*) Varicocele. (*D*) Spermatocele.

Terminology   Abbreviations

AIDS	Acquired immunodeficiency syndrome		**NGU**	Nongonococcal urethritis
BNO	Bladder neck obstruction		**PSA**	Prostate-specific antigen
BPH	Benign prostatic hyperplasia (hypertrophy)		**STD**	Sexually transmitted disease
DRE	Digital rectal examination		**STI**	Sexually transmitted infection
ED	Erectile dysfunction		**TPUR**	Transperineal urethral resection
FSH	Follicle-stimulating hormone		**TSE**	Testicular self-examination
GC	Gonococcus		**TUIP**	Transurethral incision of prostate
GU	Genitourinary		**TURP**	Transurethral resection of prostate
HBV	Hepatitis B virus		**UG**	Urogenital
HIV	Human immunodeficiency virus		**UTI**	Urinary tract infection
HSV	Herpes simplex virus		**VD**	Venereal disease (sexually transmitted infection)
LH	Luteinizing hormone		**VDRL**	Venereal Disease Research Laboratory (test for syphilis)

Chapter Review

LABELING EXERCISE

Male Reproductive System > Write the name of each numbered part on the corresponding line of the answer sheet.

Anus

Bulbourethral (Cowper) gland

Ductus (vas) deferens

Ejaculatory duct

Epididymis

Glans penis

Kidney

Penis

Peritoneal cavity

Prepuce (foreskin)

Prostate

Rectum

Scrotum

Seminal vesicle

Testis

Ureter

Urethra

Urinary bladder

1. _____

2. _____

3. _____

4. _____

5. _____

6. _____

7. _____

8. _____

9. _____

10. _____

11. _____

12. _____

13. _____

14. _____

15. _____

16. _____

17. _____

18. _____

14

Chapter Review *(continued)*

TERMINOLOGY

Matching > Match the following terms and write the appropriate letter to the left of each number:

———	**1.** gonad	**a.**	a reproductive cell
———	**2.** meiosis	**b.**	overgrowth of tissue
———	**3.** gamete	**c.**	gland located below the bladder in males
———	**4.** hyperplasia	**d.**	cell division that forms the gametes
———	**5.** prostate	**e.**	sex gland

———	**6.** glans	**a.**	excision of the ductus deferens
———	**7.** coitus	**b.**	erectile dysfunction
———	**8.** impotence	**c.**	surgical removal of the foreskin
———	**9.** vasectomy	**d.**	end of the penis
———	**10.** circumcision	**e.**	sexual intercourse

Supplementary Terms

———	**11.** priapism	**a.**	reproductive organs
———	**12.** phallus	**b.**	prolonged erection of the penis
———	**13.** genitalia	**c.**	tumor of the testis
———	**14.** phimosis	**d.**	narrowing of the foreskin opening
———	**15.** seminoma	**e.**	the penis

———	**16.** spermatocele	**a.**	inflammation of the glans penis
———	**17.** balanitis	**b.**	a form of radiation treatment
———	**18.** castration	**c.**	discharge of semen
———	**19.** emission	**d.**	removal of the testes
———	**20.** brachytherapy	**e.**	epididymal cyst

Fill in the blanks:

21. The male gonad is the _____.

22. The sac that holds the testis is the _____.

23. The thick fluid that transports spermatozoa is _____.

24. The main male sex hormone is _____.

25. The channel through which the testis descends is the _____.

26. The coiled tube that stores sperm cells on the surface of the testis is the _____.

Define the following terms:

27. vasorrhaphy (*vas-OR-a-fē*) _____

28. anorchism (*an-OR-kizm*) _____

29. oscheoma (*os-kē-Ō-ma*) _____

30. vesiculotomy (*ve-sik-ū-LOT-ō-mē*) _____

31. prostatometer (*pros-ta-TOM-e-ter*) _____

32. hemospermia (*hē-mō-SPER-mē-a*) _____

Write a word for the following definitions:

33. surgical incision of the prostate _____

34. stone in the scrotum _____

35. surgical fixation of the testis _____

36. plastic repair of the scrotum _____

37. surgical creation of an opening _____
between two parts of a cut
ductus deferens (done to
reverse a vasectomy)

True–False > Examine the following statements. If the statement is true, write T in the first blank. If the statement is false, write F in the first blank and correct the statement by replacing the underlined word in the second blank.

38. Any male sex hormone is an <u>androgen.</u>   _____   _____

39. The adjective *oscheal* refers to the <u>seminal vesicle.</u>   _____   _____

40. The spirochete *Treponema pallidum* causes <u>syphilis.</u>   _____   _____

41. Herpes simplex is a <u>virus.</u>   _____   _____

42. The <u>ureter</u> carries both urine and semen in males.   _____   _____

43. FSH and LH are produced by the <u>pituitary gland.</u>   _____   _____

44. Spermatogenesis begins at <u>puberty.</u>   _____   _____

Eliminations > In each of the sets below, underline the word that does not fit in with the rest and explain the reason for your choice:

45. bulbourethral gland — prostate — testis — spermatic cord — seminal vesicle

_____

46. FSH — semen — testosterone — androgen — LH

_____

47. condyloma acuminatum — gonorrhea — hernia — AIDS — herpes

_____

Adjectives > Write the adjective form of the following words:

48. semen _____

49. prostate _____

50. penis _____

51. urethra _____

52. scrotum _____

14

Chapter Review *(continued)*

Write the meaning of the following abbreviations:

53. HBV _____

54. STI _____

55. TSE _____

56. GC _____

57. PSA _____

58. GU _____

Word Building > Write a word for the following definitions using the word parts provided.

-ar   -tomy   -graphy   -genesis   spermat/o   vas/o   -plasty   -itis   -ic   -cyte   -lysis   vesicul/o

59. plastic repair of the ductus deferens   _____

60. destruction of sperm cells   _____

61. pertaining to the seminal vesicle   _____

62. x-ray study of the vas deferens   _____

63. inflammation of the seminal vesicle   _____

64. pertaining to spermatozoa   _____

65. cell that develops into a sperm cell   _____

66. incision of the ductus deferens   _____

67. formation of spermatozoa   _____

68. radiographic study of the seminal vesicle   _____

Word Analysis > Define the following words, and give the meaning of the word parts in each. Use a dictionary if necessary.

69. hydrocelectomy (*hi-drō-sē-LEK-tō-mē*) _____

   a. hydr/o _____

   b. -cele _____

   c. ecto- _____

   d. tom/o _____

   e. -y _____

70. spermicidal (*sper-mi-SĪ-dal*) _____

   a. sperm/i _____

   b. -cide _____

   c. -al _____

71. cryptorchidism (*krip-TOR-kid-izm*) _____

   a. crypt- _____

   b. orchid/o _____

   c. -ism _____

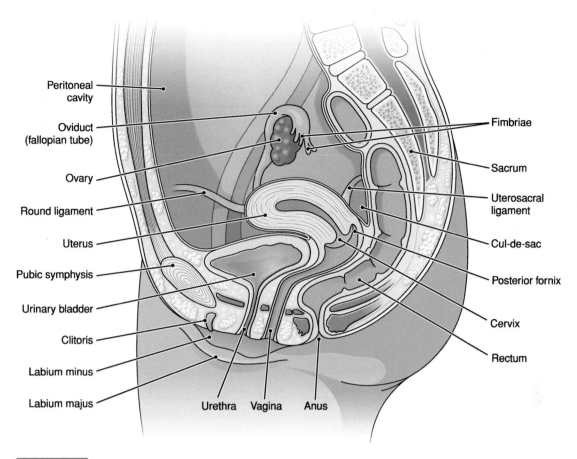

Peritoneal cavity
Oviduct (fallopian tube)
Ovary
Round ligament
Uterus
Pubic symphysis
Urinary bladder
Clitoris
Labium minus
Labium majus
Urethra   Vagina   Anus
Fimbriae
Sacrum
Uterosacral ligament
Cul-de-sac
Posterior fornix
Cervix
Rectum

Figure 15-1 **Female reproductive system.** The system is seen in sagittal section along with some adjacent structures.

fundus, a triangular cavity, and a lower narrow **cervix** that projects into the **vagina.** The recess around the cervix in the superior vagina is the **fornix.** At the posterior cervix, the peritoneum dips downward to form a blind pouch, or **cul-de-sac** (from French, meaning "bottom of the bag"), the lowest point of the peritoneal cavity.

The innermost layer of the uterine wall, the **endometrium,** has a rich blood supply. It receives the fertilized ovum and becomes part of the **placenta** during pregnancy. The endometrium is shed during the menstrual period if no fertilization occurs. The muscle layer of the uterine wall is the **myometrium.**

The vagina is a muscular tube that receives the penis during intercourse, functions as a birth canal, and transports the menstrual flow out of the body (see Fig. 15-1).

The External Genital Organs

All of the external female genitalia together are called the **vulva** (Fig. 15-2). This includes the large outer **labia majora** and small inner **labia minora** that enclose the vaginal and urethral openings. The **clitoris,** anterior to the urethral opening, is similar in origin to the penis and responds to sexual stimulation.

In both males and females, the region between the thighs, from the external genital organs to the anus, is the **perineum.** During childbirth, an incision may be

made between the vagina and the anus to facilitate birth and prevent the tearing of tissue, a procedure called an *episiotomy.* (This procedure is actually a perineotomy, as the root *episi/o* means "vulva.")

The Mammary Glands

The **mammary glands,** or breasts, are composed mainly of glandular tissue and fat (Fig. 15-3). Their purpose is to provide nourishment for the newborn. The milk secreted by the glands is carried in ducts to the nipple.

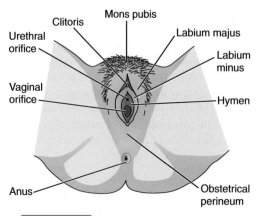

Clitoris
Mons pubis
Urethral orifice
Labium majus
Labium minus
Vaginal orifice
Hymen
Anus
Obstetrical perineum

Figure 15-2 **The external female genitalia.**

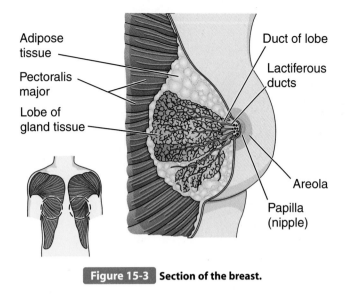

Figure 15-3 Section of the breast.

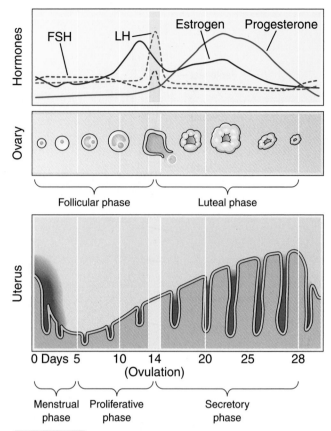

Figure 15-4 **The menstrual cycle.** (*Top*) Before ovulation on day 14, the follicle is ripening in the ovary; after ovulation, the follicle becomes the corpus luteum. (*Bottom*) Changes in the uterine endometrium during the menstrual cycle.

The Menstrual Cycle

Female reproductive activity normally begins during puberty with **menarche**, the first menstrual period. Each month, the menstrual cycle is controlled, as is male reproductive activity, by hormones from the anterior pituitary gland.

Follicle-stimulating hormone (FSH) begins the cycle by causing the ovum to ripen in the ovarian follicle (Fig. 15-4). The follicle secretes **estrogen**, a hormone that starts endometrial development in preparation for the fertilized egg.

A second pituitary hormone, **luteinizing hormone (LH)**, triggers ovulation and conversion of the follicle to the **corpus luteum**. This structure, left behind in the ovary, secretes **progesterone** and estrogen, which further the endometrial growth. If no fertilization occurs, hormone levels decline, and the endometrium sloughs off in the process of **menstruation**.

The average menstrual cycle lasts 28 days, with the first day of menstruation taken as day 1 and ovulation occurring on about day 14. Throughout the cycle, estrogen and progesterone feed back to the pituitary to regulate the production of FSH and LH. Hormonal birth control methods act by supplying estrogen and progesterone, which inhibit the pituitary and prevent ovulation, while not interfering with menstruation.

Figure 15-4 shows changes occurring simultaneously in the ovary and uterus during the course of one menstrual cycle under the effects of pituitary and ovarian hormones.

Menopause

Menopause is the cessation of monthly menstrual cycles. This generally occurs between the ages of 45 and 55 years. Reproductive hormone levels decline, and ovarian egg cells gradually degenerate. Some women experience unpleasant symptoms, such as hot flashes, headaches, insomnia, mood swings, and urinary problems. There is also some atrophy of the reproductive tract, with vaginal dryness. Most importantly, the decline in estrogen levels is associated with bone weakening (osteoporosis).

Hormone replacement therapy (HRT) has been used to alleviate menopausal symptoms. This treatment usually consists of administering estrogen in combination with progestin (*prō-JES-tin*), a synthetic progesterone given to minimize the risk of endometrial cancer. Estrogen replacement reduces bone loss associated with aging. Concerns about HRT safety, however, have caused reconsideration of this therapy beyond the early postmenopausal years. Studies with the most widely used form of HRT showed an increased risk of endometrial cancer, breast cancer, heart disease, and blood clots with extended use. Studies are ongoing on HRT safety and the use of estrogen alone for women who have no uterus.

Aside from HRT, antidepressants and vitamin E may help to relieve menopausal symptoms; locally applied estrogen and moisturizers relieve vaginal dryness. Nonhormonal drugs that increase bone density are also available if needed. As always, exercise and a balanced diet with adequate calcium are important in maintaining health throughout life.

Contraception

Contraception is the use of artificial methods to prevent fertilization of the ovum or its implantation in the uterus. Temporary methods of birth control function to:

- Block sperm penetration of the uterus (e.g., condom, diaphragm)
- Prevent implantation of the fertilized egg (e.g., intrauterine device, or IUD)
- Prevent ovulation (e.g., hormones). Hormonal methods differ in dosage and route of delivery, such as oral intake (the "birth control pill"), injection, skin patch, and vaginal ring.

The so-called "morning after pill" is intended for emergency contraception. It considerably reduces the chance of pregnancy if taken within 72 hours after unprotected sexual intercourse. One such product, Plan B, consists of two progestin doses taken 12 hours apart.

Surgical sterilization provides the most effective and usually permanent contraception. In males, this procedure is a vasectomy; in females, surgical sterilization is a **tubal ligation**, in which oviducts are cut and tied on both sides (Fig. 15-5). Laparoscopic surgery through the abdominal wall is the preferred method for performing the procedure (Fig. 15-6).

RU486 (mifepristone) is more widely used for birth control in other countries than in the United States. It terminates an early pregnancy by blocking progesterone, causing the endometrium to break down. Technically, RU486 is an abortion-causing agent (abortifacient), not a contraceptive.

Box 15-1 describes the main contraceptive methods currently in use. Each has advantages and disadvantages over other methods, but they are listed roughly in order of decreasing effectiveness.

Box 15-1   For Your Reference

Main Methods of Birth Control Currently in Use

METHOD	DESCRIPTION
SURGICAL	
Vasectomy/tubal ligation	Cutting and tying the tubes that carry the gametes
HORMONAL	
Birth control pills	Estrogen and progestin or progestin alone taken orally to prevent ovulation
Birth control shot	Injection of synthetic progesterone every 3 months to prevent ovulation
Birth control patch	Adhesive patch placed on body that administers estrogen and progestin through the skin; left on for 3 weeks and removed for a fourth week
Birth control ring	Flexible ring inserted into vagina that releases hormones internally; left in place for 3 weeks and removed for a fourth week
BARRIER	
Male condom	Sheath that fits over erect penis and prevents release of semen
Diaphragm (with spermicide)	Rubber cap that fits over cervix and prevents sperm entrance
Contraceptive sponge (with spermicide)	Soft, disposable foam disk containing spermicide, which is moistened with water and inserted into vagina
Intrauterine device (IUD)	Metal or plastic device inserted into uterus through vagina; prevents fertilization and implantation by release of copper or birth control hormones
OTHER	
Spermicide	Chemicals used to kill sperm; best when used in combination with a barrier method
Fertility awareness	Abstinence during fertile part of cycle as determined by menstrual history, basal body temperature, or quality of cervical mucus

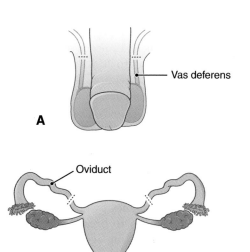

Figure 15-5 **Sterilization.** (*A*) Vasectomy. (*B*) Tubal ligation.

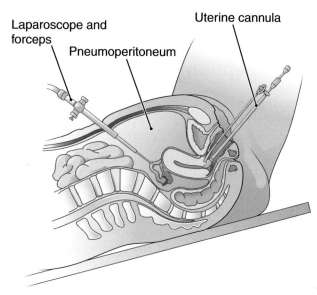

Figure 15-6 **Laparoscopic sterilization.** The peritoneal cavity is inflated (pneumoperitoneum) and the oviducts are cut laparoscopically through a small incision.

Terminology   Key Terms

FEMALE REPRODUCTIVE SYSTEM

Normal Structure and Function

cervix SER-viks	Neck. Usually means the lower narrow portion (neck) of the uterus (root: *cervic/o*); cervix uteri (*U-ter-ī*)
clitoris KLIT-o-ris	A small erectile body anterior to the urethral opening that is similar in origin to the penis (roots: *clitor/o, clitorid/o*)
contraception kon-tra-SEP-shun	The prevention of pregnancy
corpus luteum KOR-pus LŪ-tē-um	The small yellow structure that develops from the ovarian follicle after ovulation and secretes progesterone and estrogen
cul-de-sac kul-di-SAK	A blind pouch, such as the recess between the rectum and the uterus; the rectouterine pouch or pouch of Douglas (see Fig. 15-1)
endometrium en-dō-MĒ-trē-um	The inner lining of the uterus
estrogen ES-trō-jen	A group of hormones that produce female characteristics and prepare the uterus for the fertilized egg. The most active of these is estradiol
fallopian tube fa-LŌ-pē-an	See oviduct
fimbriae FIM-brē-ē	The long fingerlike extensions of the oviduct that wave to capture the released ovum (see Fig. 15-1) (singular: *fimbria*)
follicle-stimulating hormone (FSH)	A hormone secreted by the anterior pituitary that acts on the gonads. In the female, it stimulates ripening of ova in the ovary
fornix FOR-niks	An archlike space, such as the space between the uppermost wall of the vagina and the cervix (see Fig. 15-1); from Latin meaning "arch"

(continued)

Terminology	Key Terms (continued)

graafian follicle *GRAF-ē-an*	See ovarian follicle
labia majora *LĀ-bē-a ma-JOR-a*	The two large folds of skin that form the sides of the vulva (root *labi/o* means "lip") (singular: labium majus)
labia minora *LĀ-bē-a mī-NOR-a*	The two small folds of skin within the labia majora (singular: labium minus)
luteinizing hormone (LH) *LŪ-tē-in-ī-zing*	A hormone secreted by the anterior pituitary that acts on the gonads. In the female, it stimulates ovulation and corpus luteum formation
mammary gland *MAM-a-rē*	A specialized gland capable of secreting milk in the female (roots: *mamm/o*, *mast/o*); the breast
menarche *men-AR-kē*	The first menstrual period, which normally occurs during puberty
menopause *MEN-ō-pawz*	Cessation of menstrual cycles in the female
menstruation *men-strū-Ā-shun*	The cyclic discharge of blood and mucosal tissues from the lining of the nonpregnant uterus (roots: *men/o*, *mens*); menstrual period, menses (*MEN-sez*)
myometrium *mī-ō-MĒ-trē-um*	The muscular wall of the uterus
ovarian follicle *ō-VAR-ē-an FOL-i-kel*	The cluster of cells in which the ovum ripens in the ovary. Also called graafian (*GRAF-ē-an*) follicle
ovary *Ō-va-rē*	A female gonad (roots: *ovari/o*, *oophor/o*)
oviduct *O-vi-dukt*	A tube extending from the upper lateral portion of the uterus that carries the ovum to the uterus (root: *salping/o*). Also called fallopian (*fa-LŌ-pē-an*) or uterine tube
ovulation *ov-ū-LĀ-shun*	The release of a mature ovum from the ovary (from *ovule*, meaning "little egg")
ovum *Ō-vum*	The female gamete or reproductive cell (roots: *oo*, *ov/o*) (plural: ova)
perineum *per-i-NĒ-um*	The region between the thighs from the external genitalia to the anus (root: *perine/o*)
progesterone *prō-JES-ter-ōn*	A hormone produced by the corpus luteum and the placenta that maintains the endometrium for pregnancy
tubal ligation *lī-GĀ-shun*	Surgical constriction of the oviducts to produce sterilization (see Figs. 15-5 and 15-6)
uterus *Ū-ter-us*	The organ that receives the fertilized egg and maintains the developing offspring during pregnancy (roots: *uter/o*, *metr*, *hyster/o*) (see Box 15-2)
vagina *va-JĪ-na*	The muscular tube between the cervix and the vulva (roots: *vagin/o*, *colp/o*)
vulva *VUL-va*	The external female genital organs (roots: *vulv/o*, *episi/o*)

PASSport to Success®   Go to the pronunciation glossary on the Student Resources to hear these words pronounced.

Box 15-2   Focus on Words

Crazy Ideas

Most women would be shocked and surprised to learn the origin of the root hyster/o, used for the uterus. It comes from the same root as the words hysterical and hysterics and was based on the very old belief that the womb was the source of mental disturbances in women.

A similar history lies at the origin of the word hypochondriac, a term for someone who has imaginary illnesses. The hypochondriac regions are in the upper portions of the abdomen, an area that the ancients believed was the seat of mental disorders.

Roots Pertaining to the Female Reproductive System

See Tables 15-1 to 15-3.

Table 15-1   Roots for Female Reproduction and the Ovaries

Root	Meaning	Example	Definition of Example
gyn/o, gynec/o*	woman	gynecology gī-ne-KOL-ō-jē	study of women's diseases
men/o, mens	month, menstruation	premenstrual prē-MEN-strŭ-al	before a menstrual period
oo	ovum, egg cell	oocyte Ō-ō-sīt	cell that gives rise to an ovum
ov/o, ovul/o	ovum, egg cell	anovulatory an-OV-ū-la-tōr-ē	absence of egg ripening or of ovulation
ovari/o	ovary	ovariopexy ō-var-ē-ō-PEK-sē	surgical fixation of an ovary
oophor/o	ovary	oophorectomy ō-of-ō-REK-tō-mē	excision of an ovary

*This root may also be pronounced with a soft g, as in jin-e-KOL-ō-jē.

EXERCISE 15-1

Define the following words:

1. gynecopathy (ji-ne-KOP-a-thē) _____

2. intermenstrual (in-ter-MEN-strŭ-al) _____

3. oogenesis (ō-ō-JEN-e-sis) _____

4. ovulation (ov-ū-LĀ-shun) _____

5. ovarian (ō-VAR-ē-an) _____

6. oophoritis (ō-of-ō-RĪ-tis) _____

Write a word for the following definitions:

7. a physician who specializes in the treatment of women's diseases _____

8. pertaining to ovulation _____

9. profuse bleeding (-rhagia) at the time of menstruation _____

The word *menorrhea* means "menstruation." Add a prefix to *menorrhea* to form words for the following definitions:

10. painful or difficult menstruation _____

11. absence of menstruation _____

12. scanty menstrual flow

Use the root *ovari/o* to write words for the following:

13. rupture of an ovary _____

14. surgical puncture of an ovary _____

15. hernia of an ovary _____

Use the root *oophor/o* to write words for the following:

16. incision of an ovary _____

17. malignant tumor of the ovary _____

Table 15-2   Roots for the Oviducts, Uterus, and Vagina

Root	Meaning	Example	Definition of Example
salping/o	oviduct, tube	salpingoplasty *sal-PING-ō-plas-tē*	plastic repair of an oviduct
uter/o	uterus	intrauterine *in-tra-Ū-ter-in*	within the uterus
metr/o, metr/i	uterus	metrorrhea *mē-trō-RĒ-a*	abnormal uterine discharge
hyster/o	uterus	hysterotomy *his-ter-OT-ō-mē*	incision of the uterus
cervic/o	cervix, neck	endocervical *en-dō-SER-vi-kal*	pertaining to the lining of the cervix
vagin/o	vagina	vaginometer *vaj-i-NOM-e-ter*	instrument for measuring the vagina
colp/o	vagina	colpostenosis *kol-pō-sten-Ō-sis*	narrowing of the vagina

---

EXERCISE 15-2

Define the following terms:

1. intracervical (*in-tra-SER-vi-kal*) _____

2. uterovesical (*ū-ter-ō-VES-i-kal*) _____

3. salpingectomy (*sal-pin-JEK-tō-mē*) _____

4. colpodynia (*kol-pō-DIN-ē-a*) _____

5. vaginoplasty (*vaj-i-nō-PLAS-tē*) _____

6. metromalacia (*mē-trō-ma-LĀ-shē-a*) _____

7. hysteroscopy (*his-ter-OS-kō-pē*) _____

Write words for the following:

8. surgical fixation of an oviduct _____

9. radiographic study of the oviduct _____

The root *salping/o* is taken from the word *salpinx*, which means "tube." Add a prefix to *salpinx* to write a word for the following:

10. Collection of fluid in an oviduct _____

11. Presence of pus in an oviduct _____

Note how the roots *salping/o* and *oophor/o* are combined to form salpingo-oophoritis (inflammation of an oviduct and ovary). Write a word for the following:

12. surgical removal of an oviduct and ovary _____

Use the roots indicated to write words for the following:

13. surgical fixation of the uterus (hyster/o) _____

14. prolapse of the uterus (metr/o) _____

15. through the cervix _____

16. narrowing of the uterus (metr/o) _____

17. radiograph of the uterus (hyster/o) and oviducts _____

18. pertaining to the uterus (uter/o) _____

19. hernia of the vagina (colp/o) _____

20. inflammation of the vagina (vagin/o) _____

Table 15-3   Roots for the Female Accessory Structures

Root	Meaning	Example	Definition of Example
vulv/o	vulva	vulvar *VUL-var*	pertaining to the vulva
episi/o	vulva	episiotomy *e-piz-ē-OT-ō-mē*	incision of the vulva
perine/o	perineum	perineal *per-i-NĒ-al*	pertaining to the perineum
clitor/o, clitorid/o	clitoris	clitorectomy *klī-tō-REK-tō-mē*	excision of the clitoris
mamm/o	breast, mammary gland	mammoplasty *mam-ō-PLAS-tē*	plastic surgery of the breast
mast/o	breast, mammary gland	amastia *a-MAS-tē-a*	absence of the breasts

---

EXERCISE 15-3

Write a word for the following:

1. any disease of the vulva (vulv/o) _____

2. suture of the vulva (episi/o) _____

3. pertaining to the vagina (vagin/o) and perineum _____

4. inflammation of the clitoris _____

5. radiograph of the breast (mamm/o) _____

6. inflammation of the breast (mast/o) _____

7. excision of the breast _____

Clinical Aspects of Female Reproduction

Infection

The major organisms that cause sexually transmitted infections in both men and women are given in Box 14-2.

Genital herpes is a presently incurable viral infection that affects over 25% of adults in the United States. Once infection occurs, the virus lives in the nervous system, causing intermittent outbreaks that may include genital sores, itching, burning, and urinary problems. The virus is easily spread to sexual partners even if there are no active signs of the disease. Pregnant women can pass the virus to their babies during delivery, resulting in possible disabilities and even death. Some basic hygiene measures and condom use can reduce viral spread.

A fungus that infects the vulva and vagina is *Candida albicans*, causing **candidiasis**. The resultant **vaginitis**, inflammation of the vagina, causes itching and release of a thick, white, cheesy discharge. Pregnancy, diabetes mellitus, and use of antibiotics, steroids, or birth control pills predispose to this infection. If the infection is recurrent, the patient's partner should be treated to prevent reinfections. Antifungal agents (mycostatics) are used in treatment.

Pelvic inflammatory disease (PID) is the spread of infection from the reproductive organs into the pelvic cavity. It is most often caused by the gonorrhea organism or by chlamydia, although bacteria normally living in the reproductive tract may also be responsible when conditions allow. PID is a serious disorder that may result in septicemia or shock. Inflammation of the oviducts, called **salpingitis**, may close off these tubes and cause infertility.

Fibroids

A **fibroid** is a benign smooth muscle tumor usually occurring in the uterine wall, the myometrium (Fig. 15-7). This type of growth, technically called a **leiomyoma**, is one of the most common uterine disorders, but it usually causes no symptoms and requires no treatment. Fibroids may, however, cause heavy menstrual bleeding (menorrhagia), and rectal or bladder pressure. Treatments include:

- Suppression of hormones that stimulate fibroid growth

- Surgical removal of the fibroids (myomectomy)

- Surgical removal of the uterus, or **hysterectomy**

- Uterine fibroid embolization (UFE), a method that has reduced the need for hysterectomies. A specially trained radiologist uses a catheter to inject small synthetic particles into a uterine artery. These particles then block blood supply to the fibroid causing it to shrink.

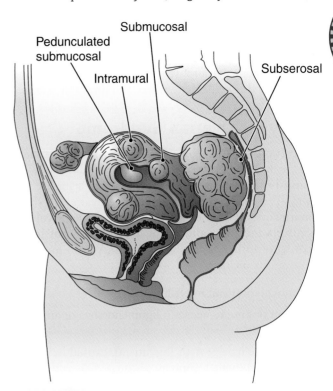

Figure 15-7 **Uterine leiomyomas (fibroids).** Various possible locations are shown. They may be within the uterine wall (intramural), below the mucous membrane (submucosal), on a stalk (pedunculated), or below the outer serous membrane (subserosal). One tumor is shown compressing the urinary bladder and another the rectum.

Endometriosis

Growth of endometrial tissue outside the uterus is termed **endometriosis**. Commonly the ovaries, oviducts, peritoneum, and other pelvic organs are involved. Stimulated by normal hormones, the endometrial tissue causes inflammation, fibrosis, and adhesions in surrounding areas. The results may be pain, **dysmenorrhea** (painful or difficult menstruation), and infertility. Laparoscopy is used to diagnose endometriosis and also to remove the abnormal tissue.

Menstrual Disorders

Menstrual abnormalities include flow that is too scanty (oligomenorrhea) or too heavy (menorrhagia) and the absence of monthly periods (amenorrhea). Dysmenorrhea, when it occurs, usually begins at the start of menstruation and lasts 1 to 2 days. Together these disorders are classified as dysfunctional uterine bleeding (DUB). These responses may be caused by hormone imbalances, systemic disorders, or uterine problems. They are most common in adolescence or near menopause. At other times they are often related to life changes and emotional upset.

Premenstrual syndrome (PMS) describes symptoms that appear during the menstrual cycle's second half and includes emotional changes, fatigue, bloating, headaches, and appetite changes. Possible causes of PMS have been under study. Symptoms may be relieved by hormone therapy, antidepressants, or antianxiety medications. Exercise, dietary control, rest, and relaxation strategies may also be helpful. Avoiding caffeine and taking vitamin E supplements may relieve breast tenderness; one should also drink adequate water and limit salt intake.

Polycystic Ovarian Syndrome

Polycystic ovarian syndrome (PCOS) is discussed here because the first-described symptoms of this disorder were enlarged ovaries with multiple cysts. These signs are not always present in PCOS, although the ovaries do show abnormalities. PCOS is an endocrine disorder involving increased androgen and estrogen secretion that interferes with normal secretion of pituitary FSH and LH. Some effects include:

- anovulation and infertility
- scant or absent menses (oligomenorrhea or amenorrhea)
- excessive hair growth (hirsutism), caused by excess androgen (male hormone)
- resistance to insulin, a hormone that lowers blood sugar, resulting in symptoms of diabetes mellitus
- obesity

PCOS is treated with hormones to regulate hormonal imbalance, drugs to increase responsiveness to insulin, weight reduction (estrogen is produced in adipose tissue), and sometimes partial removal of the ovaries.

Cancer of the Female Reproductive Tract

ENDOMETRIAL CANCER

Cancer of the endometrium is the most common cancer of the female reproductive tract. Women at risk should have biopsies taken regularly because endometrial cancer is not always detected by **Pap (Papanicolaou) smear**. Treatment consists of hysterectomy (removal of the uterus) (Fig. 15-8) and sometimes radiation therapy. A small percentage of cases occur after endometrial overgrowth (hyperplasia). This tissue can be removed by **dilation and curettage (D&C)**, in which the cervix is widened and the lining of the uterus is scraped with a curette.

CERVICAL CANCER

Almost all patients with cervical cancer have been infected with human papillomavirus (HPV), a virus that causes genital warts. Incidence is also related to high sexual activity and other sexually transmitted viral infections, such as herpes.

In the 1940s and 1950s, the synthetic steroid DES (diethylstilbestrol) was given to prevent miscarriages. A small percentage of daughters born to women treated with this drug have shown an increased risk for cancer

Figure 15-8 **Reproductive surgery.** A hysterectomy is surgical removal of the uterus. Removal of the ovary (oophorectomy) and oviduct (salpingectomy) may also be required either unilaterally or bilaterally.

of the cervix and vagina. These women need to be examined regularly.

Cervical carcinoma is often preceded by abnormal growth (dysplasia) of the epithelial cells lining the cervix. Growth is graded as CIN I, II, or III, depending on the depth of tissue involved. CIN stands for cervical intraepithelial neoplasia. Diagnosis of cervical cancer is by a Pap smear, examination with a **colposcope**, and biopsy. In a **cone biopsy** (Fig. 15-9), a cone-shaped piece of tissue

Cone biopsy

Figure 15-9 **Cone biopsy of the uterine cervix.**

is removed from the lining of the cervix for study. Often in the procedure, all of the abnormal cells are removed as well.

OVARIAN CANCER

Cancer of the ovary has a high mortality rate because it usually causes no distinct early symptoms and there is no accurate routine screening test yet available. Women may overlook the vague possible signs of ovarian cancer, such as bloating, change in bowel habits, backache, urinary changes, abnormal bleeding, weight loss, and fatigue. Often by the time of diagnosis, the tumor has invaded the pelvis and abdomen. Removal of the ovaries (**oophorectomy**) and oviducts (**salpingectomy**) along with the uterus is required (see Fig. 15-8, in addition to chemotherapy and radiation therapy.

Breast Cancer

Carcinoma of the breast is second only to lung cancer in causing cancer-related deaths among women in the United States. This cancer metastasizes readily through the lymph nodes and blood to other sites such as the lung, liver, bones, and ovaries.

DIAGNOSIS

Palpation is a simple first step in breast cancer diagnosis. Regular breast self-examination (BSE) is of utmost importance, because most breast cancers are discovered by women themselves.

Mammography, which provides two-dimensional x-ray images of the breast, is still the standard diagnostic procedure for breast cancer (Fig. 15-10). After the age of 40, women should have mammograms yearly. In digital mammography, x-ray images are stored on computers instead of on film. These images can be manipulated electronically to aid interpretation. They are more easily stored and retrieved or sent to other medical facilities.

Ultrasound and MRI studies are adjuncts to mammography. Ultrasound can show whether a lump seen on mammography is simply a benign cyst. MRI with a contrast medium can show abnormal blood vessel formation signifying a tumor.

Any suspicious breast tissue must be biopsied by needle aspiration or surgical excision for further study. In a **stereotactic biopsy**, a physician uses a computer-guided imaging system to locate suspicious tissue and remove samples with a needle. This method is less invasive than surgical biopsy.

Ductal carcinoma in situ (DCIS) is a form of breast cancer that arises from an overgrowth of the cells lining a milk duct. It is initially confined to the duct, that is, it does not invade nearby tissue or metastasize, and it usually can be detected in its early stages.

TREATMENT

Treatment of breast cancer is usually some form of **mastectomy**, or removal of breast tissue:

- In a radical mastectomy, the entire breast is removed. Underlying muscle and axillary lymph nodes (in the armpit) are also removed.

- In a modified radical mastectomy, the breast and lymph nodes are removed, but muscles are left in place.

- In a segmental mastectomy, or "lumpectomy," just the tumor itself is removed. When the tumor is small and surgery is followed by additional treatment, this procedure gives survival rates as high as those with more radical surgeries.

Surgeons can assess the extent of tumor spread and conserve lymphatic tissue using a **sentinel-node biopsy**. A

Figure 15-10 **Mammograms.** (*A*) Normal mammogram, left breast. (*B*) Mammogram of right breast showing lesions (*arrows*). In mammograms, fat tissue appears gray; breast tissue, calcium deposits, and benign or cancerous tumors appear white.

dye or radioactive tracer identifies the first lymph nodes that receive lymph from a tumor. Study of possible tumor spread to these "sentinel nodes" guides further treatment.

Often after breast surgery, a patient receives chemotherapy and/or radiation therapy. It is now possible in some cases to deliver radiation to just the tumor area (brachytherapy) instead of irradiating the whole breast. A radiation source is delivered through catheters or implanted in the breast tissue for a short time.

Progress in breast cancer treatment involves genetic studies and tumor analysis that allows therapy more specific to each particular case. About 8% of these cancers are linked to a defective gene (*BRCA1* or *BRCA2*) that is transmitted within families. Women with these genetic predispositions can be screened more carefully or treated prophylactically.

Some types of specific drug treatments for breast cancer, which may be given in combination, are:

- Drugs that block estrogen production or block estrogen receptors in breast tissue if a tumor responds to this hormone
- Drugs that inhibit tumor growth factors
- Drugs that inhibit growth of blood vessels that supply the tumor (antiangiogenesis agents)

These and other anticancer drugs are described in more detail in the list of supplementary terms.

Terminology Key Terms

FEMALE REPRODUCTIVE SYSTEM

Disorders

candidiasis kan-di-DĪ-a-sis	Infection with the fungus *Candida*, a common cause of vaginitis
dysmenorrhea DIS-men-ō-rē-a	Painful or difficult menstruation. A common disorder that may be caused by infection, use of an intrauterine device, endometriosis, overproduction of prostaglandins, or other factors
endometriosis en-dō-mē-trē-Ō-sis	Growth of endometrial tissue outside the uterus, usually in the pelvic cavity
fibroid FĪ-broyd	Benign tumor of smooth muscle (see leiomyoma)
leiomyoma lī-ō-mī-Ō-ma	Benign tumor of smooth muscle, usually in the uterine wall (myometrium). In the uterus, may cause bleeding and pressure on the bladder or rectum. Also called fibroid or myoma (see Fig. 15-7)
pelvic inflammatory disease (PID)	Condition caused by the spread of infection from the reproductive tract into the pelvic cavity. Commonly caused by sexually transmitted gonorrhea and chlamydial infections
salpingitis sal-pin-JĪ-tis	Inflammation of the oviduct; typically caused by urinary tract infection or sexually transmitted infection. Chronic salpingitis may lead to infertility or ectopic pregnancy (development of the fertilized egg outside of the uterus)
vaginitis vaj-i-NĪ-tis	Inflammation of the vagina

Diagnosis and Treatment

colposcope KOL-pō-skōp	Instrument for examining the vagina and cervix
cone biopsy	Removal of a cone of tissue from the cervical lining for cytologic examination; also called conization (see Fig. 15-9)
dilation and curettage (D&C) kū-re-TAJ	Procedure in which the cervix is dilated (widened) and the uterine lining is scraped with a curette
hysterectomy his-ter-EK-tō-mē	Surgical removal of the uterus. Most commonly done because of tumors. Often the oviducts and ovaries are removed as well (see Fig. 15-8)
mammography mam-OG-ra-fē	Radiographic study of the breast for the detection of breast cancer

(continued)

Terminology   Key Terms *(continued)*

mastectomy *mas-TEK-tō-mē*	Excision of the breast to eliminate malignancy
oophorectomy *ō-of-ō-REK-tō-mē*	Excision of an ovary (see Fig. 15-8)
Pap smear	Study of cells collected from the cervix and vagina for early detection of cancer. Also called Papanicolaou smear or Pap test
salpingectomy *sal-pin-JEK-tō-mē*	Surgical removal of the oviduct (see Fig. 15-8)
sentinel-node biopsy *SEN-ti-nel*	Biopsy of the first lymph nodes to receive drainage from a tumor; used to determine spread of cancer in planning treatment
stereotactic biopsy *ster-ē-ō-TAK-tik*	Needle biopsy using a computer-guided imaging system to locate suspicious tissue and remove samples for study

PASSport to Success®

Go to the pronunciation glossary on the Student Resources to hear these words pronounced.

Terminology   Supplementary Terms

FEMALE REPRODUCTIVE SYSTEM

Normal Structure and Function

adnexa *ad-NEK-sa*	Appendages, such as the adnexa uteri—the ovaries, oviducts, and uterine ligaments
areola *a-RĔ-ō-la*	A pigmented ring, such as the dark area around the nipple of the breast
greater vestibular gland *ves-TIB-ū-lar*	A small mucus-secreting gland on the side of the vestibule (see below) near the vaginal opening. Also called Bartholin (BAR-to-lin) gland (see Fig. 15-12)
hymen *HĪ-men*	A fold of mucous membrane that partially covers the entrance of the vagina
mons pubis *monz PŪ-bis*	The rounded, fleshy elevation anterior to the pubic joint that is covered with hair after puberty
oocyte *Ō-ō-sīt*	An immature ovum
perimenopause *per-i-MEN-ō-pawz*	The period immediately before and after menopause; begins at the time of irregular menstrual cycles and ends 1 year after the last menstrual period; averages 3 to 4 years
vestibule *VES-ti-būl*	The space between the labia minora that contains the openings of the urethra, vagina, and ducts of the greater vestibular glands

Disorders

cystocele *SIS-tō-sēl*	Herniation of the urinary bladder into the wall of the vagina (Fig. 15-11)

(continued)

Terminology   Supplementary Terms (continued)

dyspareunia dis-par-Ū-nē-a	Pain during sexual intercourse
fibrocystic disease of the breast fī-brō-SIS-tik	A condition in which there are palpable lumps in the breasts, usually associated with pain and tenderness. These lumps or "thickenings" change with the menstrual cycle and must be distinguished from malignant tumors by diagnostic methods
hirsutism HIR-sū-tizm	Excess hair growth
leucorrhea lū-kō-RĒ-a	White or yellowish discharge from the vagina. Infection and other disorders may change the amount, color, or odor of the discharge
microcalcification mī-krō-kal-si-fi-KĀ-shun	Small deposit of calcium that appears as a white spot on mammograms. Most microcalcifications are harmless, but some might indicate breast cancer
prolapse of the uterus	Downward displacement of the uterus with the cervix sometimes protruding from the vagina
rectocele REK-tō-sēl	Herniation of the rectum into the wall of the vagina; also called proctocele (see Fig. 15-11)

Diagnosis and Treatment

culdocentesis kul-dō-sen-TĒ-sis	Puncture of the vaginal wall to sample fluid from the rectouterine space for diagnosis
episiorrhaphy e-pis-ē-OR-a-fē	Suture of the vulva or suture of the perineum cut in an episiotomy (incision to ease childbirth)
laparoscopy lap-a-ROS-kō-pē	Endoscopic examination of the abdomen; may include surgical procedures, such as tubal ligation (see Fig. 15-5)
myomectomy mī-ō-MEK-tō-mē	Surgical removal of a uterine leiomyoma (fibroid, myoma)
speculum SPEK-ū-lum	An instrument used to enlarge the opening of a passage or cavity to allow examination (see Fig. 7-13)
teletherapy tel-e-THER-a-pē	Delivery of radiation to a tumor from an external beam source, as compared to implantation of radioactive material (brachytherapy) or systemic administration of radionuclide

Drugs

aromatase inhibitor (AI) a-RŌ-ma-tās	Agent that inhibits estrogen production; used for postmenopausal treatment of breast cancers that respond to estrogen. Examples are exemestane (Aromasin), anastrozole (Arimidex), and letrozole (Femara)
bisphosphonate bis-FOS-fō-nāt	Agent used to prevent and treat osteoporosis; increases bone mass by decreasing bone turnover. Examples are alendronate (Fosamax) and risedronate (Actonel)
HER2 inhibitor	Drug used to treat breast cancers that show excess receptors (HER2) for human epidermal growth factor. Example is trastuzumab (Herceptin)
paclitaxel pak-li-TAKS-el	Antineoplastic agent derived from yew trees used mainly in treatment of breast and ovarian cancer; Taxol
selective estrogen receptor modulator (SERM)	Drug that acts on estrogen receptors. Examples are tamoxifen (Nolvadex) and raloxifene (Evista), which is also used to prevent bone loss after menopause

PASSport to Success® Go to the pronunciation glossary on the Student Resources to hear these words pronounced.

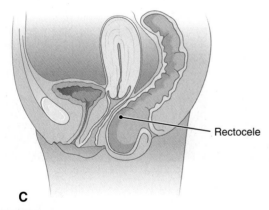

Figure 15-11 **Herniation into the vagina.** (*A*) Normal. (*B*) Cystocele. (*C*) Rectocele.

Terminology	Abbreviations

Female Reproductive System

AI	Aromatase inhibitor
BRCA1	Breast cancer gene 1
BRCA2	Breast cancer gene 2
BSE	Breast self-examination
BSO	Bilateral salpingo-oophorectomy
BV	Bacterial vaginosis
CIN	Cervical intraepithelial neoplasia
D&C	Dilation and curettage
DCIS	Ductal carcinoma in situ
DES	Diethylstilbestrol
DUB	Dysfunctional uterine bleeding
FSH	Follicle-stimulating hormone
GC	Gonococcus (cause of gonorrhea)
GYN	Gynecology
HPV	Human papillomavirus
HRT	Hormone replacement therapy
IUD	Intrauterine device
LH	Luteinizing hormone
NGU	Nongonococcal urethritis
PCOS	Polycystic ovarian syndrome
PID	Pelvic inflammatory disease
PMS	Premenstrual syndrome
SERM	Selective estrogen receptor modulator
STD	Sexually transmitted disease
STI	Sexually transmitted infection
TAH	Total abdominal hysterectomy
TSS	Toxic shock syndrome
UFE	uterine fibroid embolization
VD	Venereal disease (sexually transmitted disease)

Pregnancy and Birth

Fertilization and Early Development

Penetration of an ovulated egg cell by a spermatozoon results in fertilization (Fig. 15-12). This union normally occurs in the oviduct. The nuclei of the sperm and egg cells fuse, restoring the chromosome number to 46 and forming a **zygote**. As the zygote travels through the oviduct toward the uterus, it divides rapidly. Within 6 to

7 days, the fertilized egg reaches the uterus and implants into the endometrium, and the **embryo** begins to develop.

During the first 8 weeks of growth, all of the major body systems are established. Embryonic tissue produces **human chorionic gonadotropin (hCG)**, a hormone that keeps the corpus luteum functional in the ovary to maintain the endometrium. (The presence of hCG in urine is the basis for the most commonly used tests for pregnancy.) After 2 months, placental hormones take over this function and the corpus luteum degenerates. At this time, the embryo becomes a **fetus** (Fig. 15-13).

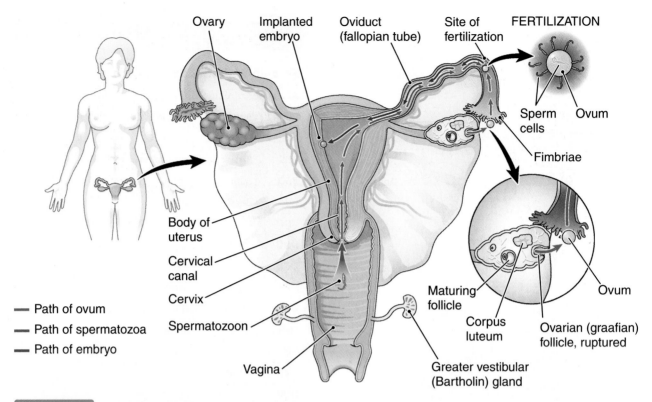

Ovary Implanted embryo Oviduct (fallopian tube) Site of fertilization FERTILIZATION

Sperm cells Ovum

Fimbriae

Body of uterus

Cervical canal

Cervix

Spermatozoon

— Path of ovum
— Path of spermatozoa
— Path of embryo

Maturing follicle

Corpus luteum

Ovum

Ovarian (graafian) follicle, ruptured

Vagina

Greater vestibular (Bartholin) gland

Figure 15-12 **Ovulation and fertilization.** Arrows show the pathway of spermatozoa and ovum. Fertilization occurs in the oviduct, after which the zygote implants in the uterine lining.

Figure 15-13 **Human development.** Human embryos and an early fetus are shown. (A) Implantation in the uterus 7 to 8 days after conception. (B) Embryo at 32 days. (C) At 37 days. (D) At 41 days. (E) Fetus at 12 to 15 weeks.

Review the animation *Ovulation and Fertilization* on the Student Resources.

The Placenta

During development, the fetus is nourished by the placenta, an organ formed from the embryo's outermost layer, the **chorion**, and the endometrium, the innermost layer of the uterus (Fig. 15-14). Here, exchanges take place between the bloodstreams of the mother and the fetus through fetal capillaries.

The **umbilical cord** contains the blood vessels that link the fetus to the placenta. Fetal blood is carried to the placenta in two umbilical arteries. While traveling through the placenta, the blood picks up nutrients and oxygen and gives up carbon dioxide and metabolic waste. Replenished blood is carried from the placenta to the fetus in a single umbilical vein.

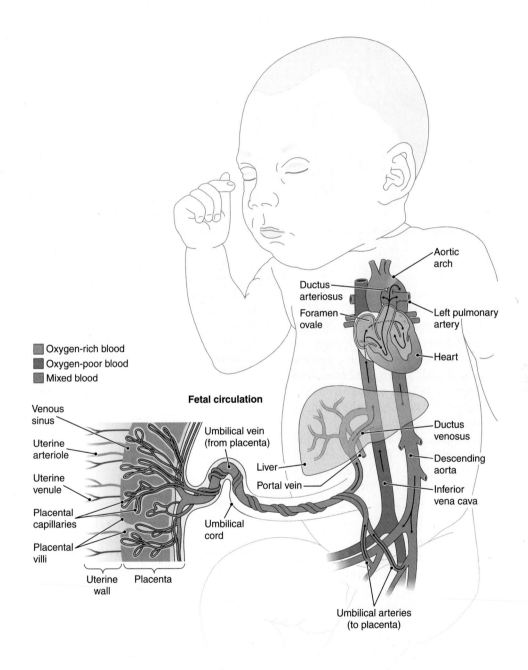

Figure 15-14 **Fetal circulation.** A section of the placenta is also shown. Colors show relative oxygen content of blood.

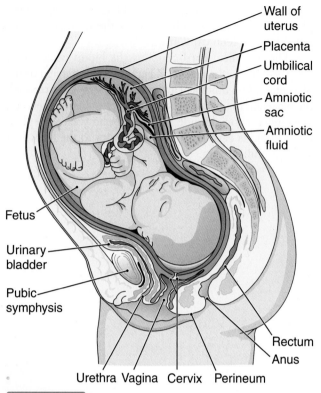

Wall of uterus
Placenta
Umbilical cord
Amniotic sac
Amniotic fluid
Fetus
Urinary bladder
Pubic symphysis
Rectum
Anus
Urethra Vagina Cervix Perineum

Figure 15-15 **Midsagittal section of a pregnant uterus with intact fetus.**

See the animation *Fetal Circulation* on the Student Resources for a demonstration of fetal circulatory adaptations.

Although the bloodstreams of the mother and the fetus do not mix, and all exchanges take place through capillaries, some materials do manage to get through the placenta in both directions. For example, some viruses, such as HIV and **rubella**, as well as drugs, alcohol, and other harmful substances are known to pass from the mother to the fetus; fetal proteins can enter the mother's blood and cause immunologic reactions.

During **gestation** (the period of development), the fetus is cushioned and protected by fluid contained in the **amniotic sac** (amnion) (Fig. 15-15), commonly called the "bag of waters." This sac ruptures at birth.

Fetal Circulation

The fetus has several adaptations that serve to bypass the lungs, which are not needed to oxygenate the blood. When blood coming from the placenta enters the right atrium, the **foramen ovale**, a small hole in the septum between the atria, allows some of the blood to go directly into the left atrium, thus bypassing the pulmonary artery. Further, blood pumped out of the right ventricle can shunt directly into the aorta through a short vessel, the **ductus arteriosus**, which connects the pulmonary artery with the descending aorta (see Fig. 15-14). Both of these passages close off at birth when the pulmonary circuit is established. Their failure to close taxes the heart and may require medical attention.

Childbirth

The length of pregnancy, from fertilization of the ovum to birth, is about 38 weeks, or 266 days. In practice, it is calculated as approximately 280 days or 40 weeks from the first day of the last menstrual period (LMP). For study purposes, pregnancy is divided into 3-month periods (trimesters), during which defined changes can be observed in the fetus.

Childbirth, or **parturition**, occurs in three stages:

1. onset of regular uterine contractions and dilation of the cervix
2. expulsion of the fetus
3. delivery of the placenta and fetal membranes

The third stage of childbirth is followed by contraction of the uterus and control of bleeding. The factors that start labor are not completely understood, but it is clear that the hormone **oxytocin** from the posterior pituitary gland and other hormones called **prostaglandins** are involved. Box 15-3 has career information on midwives and other birth assistants.

The term **gravida** refers to a pregnant woman. The term **para** refers to a woman who has given birth. This means the production of a viable infant (500 g or more or over 20 weeks' gestation) regardless of whether the infant is alive at birth or whether the birth is single or multiple. Prefixes are added to both terms to indicate the number of pregnancies or births, such as:

- nulli-   none
- primi-   one
- secundi-   two
- tri- or terti-   three
- quadri-   four
- multi-   two or more

Alternatively, a number can be added after the term to indicate events, such as gravida 1, para 3, etc.

Lactation

The secretion of milk from the breasts, called **lactation**, is started by the hormone prolactin from the anterior pituitary gland, as well as hormones from the placenta. The baby's suckling then stimulates milk release. The pituitary hormone oxytocin is needed for this release or "letdown" of milk. For the first few days after delivery, only **colostrum** is produced. This has a slightly different composition than milk, but like the milk, it has protective antibodies.

Box 15-3 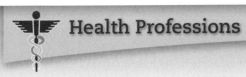 **Health Professions**

Nurse-Midwives and Other Birth Assistants

A midwife is someone, not a physician and traditionally a woman, who assists women in childbirth. The name literally means "with woman," and the practice is termed midwifery (*mid-WĪF-rē* or *mid-WIF-er-ē*). A certified nurse-midwife (CNM) is a graduate nurse who takes special training in midwifery leading to a certificate or master's degree. CNMs assist women in labor, delivery, and postpartum care as well as provide routine gynecologic care. The practice is legal throughout the United States, but states vary in their requirements and restrictions. Most grant CNMs some prescription-writing privileges and mandate insurance reimbursement for their services. Most CNMs work in hospitals, but they may also work in private practice, birth centers, and homes, usually in cooperation with an obstetrician.

A certified midwife (CM) can enter specialized training with a high-school diploma. Education in social sciences, health sciences, and nursing practices leads to a certificate or degree in midwifery. A CM may assist alone at a birth, but is trained to detect complications and obtain medical assistance if needed.

CMs are licensed by states, which may require prior examination of the mother by a physician or qualified nurse and supervision by an obstetrician. States also may place limitations on the cases CMs can handle based on medical conditions. The American College of Nurse-Midwives at www.acnm.org has information on this career.

A birth assistant is someone who works with families during pregnancy, through labor, and after delivery. Birth assistants may help with early labor at home, give care between home and the hospital, and provide continuity and support throughout the hospital stay. A "doula" may or may not assist at a birth, but helps a mother and her family for some time after the birth. The name comes from Greek and refers to the most important female servant in the household, who probably assisted the lady of the house in childbearing. Both doulas and birth assistants have professional associations that set standards for training and certification. For more information visit www.dona.org.

Terminology Key Terms

PREGNANCY AND BIRTH

Normal Structure and Function

amniotic sac *am-nē-OT-ik*	The membranous sac filled with fluid that holds the fetus; also called amnion (root: *amnio*)
chorion *KOR-ē-on*	The outermost layer of the embryo that, with the endometrium, forms the placenta (adjective: chorionic)
colostrum *kō-LOS-trum*	Breast fluid that is secreted in the first few days after giving birth, before milk is produced
ductus arteriosus *DUK-tus ar-tēr-ē-Ō-sus*	A fetal blood vessel that connects the pulmonary artery with the descending aorta, thus allowing blood to bypass the lungs
embryo *EM-brē-ō*	The stage in development between the zygote and the fetus, extending from the second through the eighth week of growth in the uterus (root: *embry/o*); adjective: embryonic
fertilization *fer-ti-li-ZĀ-shun*	The union of an ovum and a spermatozoon
fetus *FĒ-tus*	The developing child in the uterus from the third month to birth (root: *fet/o*); adjective: fetal
foramen ovale *fō-RĀ-men ō-VĀ-lē*	A small hole in the interatrial septum in the fetal heart that allows blood to pass directly from the right to the left side of the heart
gestation *jes-TĀ-shun*	The period of development from conception to birth
gravida *GRAV-i-da*	Pregnant woman

(continued)

Terminology | Key Terms (continued)

human chorionic gonadotropin (hCG) *kor-ē-ON-ik GŌ-na-dō-trō-pin*	A hormone secreted by the embryo early in pregnancy that maintains the corpus luteum so that it will continue to secrete hormones
lactation *lak-TĀ-shun*	The secretion of milk from the mammary glands
oxytocin *ok-sē-TŌ-sin*	A pituitary hormone that stimulates contractions of the uterus. It also stimulates release ("letdown") of milk from the breasts
para	Woman who has produced a viable infant. Multiple births are considered as single pregnancies
parturition *par-tū-RI-shun*	Childbirth (root: *nat/i*); labor (root: *toc/o*)
placenta *pla-SEN-ta*	The organ, composed of fetal and maternal tissues, that nourishes and maintains the developing fetus
prostaglandins *PROS-ta-glan-dinz*	A group of hormones with varied effects, including the stimulation of uterine contractions
umbilical cord *um-BIL-i-kal*	The structure that connects the fetus to the placenta. It contains vessels that carry blood between the mother and the fetus
zygote *ZĪ-gōt*	The fertilized ovum

PASSport to Success® Go to the pronunciation glossary on the Student Resources to hear these words pronounced.

Roots Pertaining to Pregnancy and Birth

See Table 15-4.

Table 15-4 | Roots Pertaining to Pregnancy and Birth

Root	Meaning	Example	Definition of Example
amnio	amnion, amniotic sac	diamniotic *dī-am-nē-OT-ik*	showing two amniotic sacs
embry/o	embryo	embryonic *em-brē-ON-ik*	pertaining to the embryo
fet/o	fetus	fetometry *fē-TOM-e-trē*	measurement of a fetus
toc/o	labor	dystocia *dis-TŌ-sē-ā*	difficult labor
nat/i	birth	neonate *NĒ-ō-nāt*	newborn
lact/o	milk	lactose *LAK-tōs*	sugar (-ose) found in milk
galact/o	milk	galactogogue *ga-LAK-tō-gog*	agent that promotes (-agogue) the flow of milk
gravida	pregnant woman	nulligravida *nul-i-GRAV-i-da*	woman who has never (nulli-) been pregnant
para	woman who has given birth	multipara *mul-TIP-a-ra*	woman who has given birth two or more times

Figure 15-19 A myelomeningocele.

A **carrier** of a genetic disorder is an individual who has a genetic defect that does not appear but that can be passed to offspring. Laboratory tests can identify carriers of some genetic disorders.

Teratogens are factors that cause malformations in the developing fetus. These include infections—such as rubella (German measles), herpes simplex, and syphilis—alcohol, drugs, chemicals, and radiation. The fetus is most susceptible to teratogenic effects during the first 3 months of pregnancy.

Examples of developmental disorders are **atresia** (absence or closure of a normal body opening), **anencephaly** (absence of a brain), **cleft lip**, **cleft palate**, and congenital heart disease. **Spina bifida** is incomplete closure of the spine, through which the spinal cord and its membranes may project (Fig. 15-18). This usually occurs in the lumbar region. If there is no hernia-

Figure 15-21 **Amniocentesis.** A sample is removed from the amniotic sac. Cells and fluid are tested for fetal abnormalities.

tion of tissue, the condition is spina bifida occulta. Protrusion of the meninges through the opening is a meningocele; in a myelomeningocele, both the spinal cord and membranes herniate through the defect, as seen in Figures 15-18D and 15-19. Note that folic acid, a B vitamin, can prevent embryonic spinal malformations, known as neural tube defects. This vitamin is found in vegetables, liver, legumes and seeds, but it is now added to some commercial foods, including cereals and breads, to provide young women with this vitamin early on in case they become pregnant.

Diagnosis of Congenital Disorders

Many congenital disorders can now be detected before birth. Ultrasonography (Fig. 15-20), in addition to its use for monitoring pregnancies and determining fetal sex, can also reveal certain fetal abnormalities. In **amniocentesis** (Fig. 15-21), a sample is withdrawn from the amniotic cavity with a needle. The fluid obtained is analyzed for chemical abnormalities. The cells are grown in the laboratory and tested for biochemical disorders. A **karyotype** is prepared to study the genetic material (see Fig. 4-10).

In **chorionic villus sampling (CVS)**, small amounts of the membrane around the fetus are obtained through the cervix for analysis. This can be done at 8 to 10 weeks of pregnancy, in comparison with 14 to 16 weeks for amniocentesis.

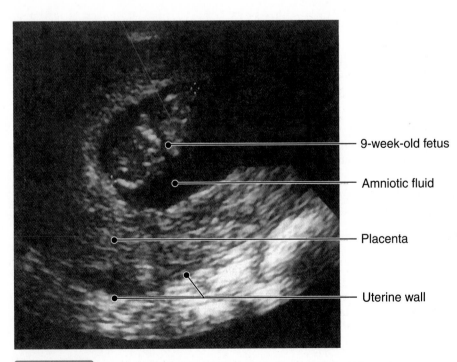

— 9-week-old fetus

— Amniotic fluid

— Placenta

— Uterine wall

Figure 15-20 **Sonogram.** This transvaginal sonogram shows a 9-week-old fetus.

Terminology | Key Terms

PREGNANCY AND BIRTH

Disorders

abortion a-BOR-shun	Termination of a pregnancy before the fetus is capable of surviving outside the uterus, usually at 20 weeks or 500 g. May be spontaneous or induced. A spontaneous abortion is commonly called a miscarriage
anencephaly an-en-SEF-a-lē	Congenital absence of a brain
atresia a-TRĒ-zē-a	Congenital absence or closure of a normal body opening
carrier	An individual who has an unexpressed genetic defect that can be passed to his or her children
cleft lip	A congenital separation of the upper lip
cleft palate	A congenital split in the roof of the mouth
congenital disorder kon-GEN-i-tal	A disorder that is present at birth. May be developmental or hereditary (familial)
eclampsia e-KLAMP-sē-a	Convulsions and coma occurring during pregnancy or after delivery and associated with the conditions of pregnancy-induced hypertension (see below); adjective: eclamptic
ectopic pregnancy ek-TOP-ik	Development of the fertilized ovum outside the body of the uterus. Usually occurs in the oviduct (tubal pregnancy) but may occur in other parts of the reproductive tract or abdominal cavity (see Fig. 15-16)
hemolytic disease of the newborn (HDN)	Disease that results from Rh incompatibility between the blood of a mother and her fetus. An Rh-negative mother produces antibody to Rh-positive fetal red cells that enter her circulation. These antibodies can destroy Rh-positive fetal red cells in a later pregnancy unless the mother is treated with antibodies to remove the Rh antigen. Formerly called erythroblastosis fetalis
mastitis mas-TĪ-tis	Inflammation of the breast, usually associated with the early weeks of breastfeeding
mutation mū-TĀ-shun	A change in the genetic material of the cell. Most mutations are harmful. If the change appears in the sex cells, it can be passed to future generations
placental abruption ab-RUP-shun	Premature separation of the placenta; abruptio placentae
placenta previa PRĒ-vē-a	Placental attachment in the lower portion of the uterus instead of the upper portion, as is normal. May result in hemorrhage late in pregnancy
pregnancy-induced hypertension (PIH)	A toxic condition of late pregnancy associated with hypertension, edema, and proteinuria that, if untreated, may lead to eclampsia. Also called preeclampsia (prē-e-KLAMP-sē-a) and toxemia of pregnancy
rubella rū-BEL-la	German measles. The virus can cross the placenta and cause fetal abnormalities, such as eye defects, deafness, heart abnormalities, and mental retardation. The virus is most damaging during the first trimester
spina bifida SPĪ-na BIF-i-da	A congenital defect in the closure of the spinal column through which the spinal cord and its membranes may project (see Figs. 15-18 and 15-19)
teratogen ter-AT-ō-jen	A factor that causes developmental abnormalities in the fetus (root terat/o means "malformed fetus"); adjective: teratogenic

Diagnosis and Treatment

amniocentesis am-nē-ō-sen-TĒ-sis	Transabdominal puncture of the amniotic sac to remove amniotic fluid for testing. Tests on the cells and fluid obtained can reveal congenital abnormalities, blood incompatibility, and sex of the fetus (see Fig. 15-21)

(continued)

Terminology **Key Terms** (continued)

chorionic villus sampling (CVS)	Removal of chorionic cells through the cervix for prenatal testing. Can be done earlier in pregnancy than amniocentesis
dilatation and evacuation (D&E)	Widening of the cervix and removal of conception products by suction
karyotype *KAR-ē-ō-tīp*	A picture of cellular chromosomes arranged in order of decreasing size; can reveal abnormalities in the chromosomes themselves or in their number or arrangement (root *kary/o* means "nucleus") (see Fig. 4-10)
ultrasonography *ul-tra-so-NOG-ra-fē*	The use of high-frequency sound waves to produce a photograph of an organ or tissue (see Fig. 15-20). Used in obstetrics to diagnose pregnancy, multiple births, and abnormalities and also to study and measure the fetus. The image obtained is a sonogram or ultrasonogram

PASSport to Success®   Go to the pronunciation glossary on the Student Resources to hear these words pronounced.

Terminology **Supplementary Terms**

PREGNANCY AND BIRTH

Normal Structure and Function

afterbirth	The placenta and membranes delivered after birth of a child
antepartum *an-tē-PAR-tum*	Before childbirth, with reference to the mother
Braxton–Hicks contractions	Light uterine contractions that occur during pregnancy and increase in frequency and intensity during the third trimester. They strengthen the uterus for delivery
chloasma *klō-AZ-ma*	Brownish pigmentation that appears on the face during pregnancy; melasma
fontanel *fon-tan-EL*	A membrane-covered space between cranial bones in the fetus that later becomes ossified; a soft spot. Also spelled fontanelle
intrapartum *in-tra-PAR-tum*	Occurring during childbirth
linea nigra *LIN-ē-a NĪ-gra*	A dark line on the abdomen from the umbilicus to the pubic region that may appear late in pregnancy
lochia *LŌ-kē-a*	The mixture of blood, mucus, and tissue discharged from the uterus after childbirth
meconium *me-KŌ-nē-um*	The first feces of the newborn
peripartum *per-i-PAR-tum*	Occurring during the end of pregnancy or the first few months after delivery, with reference to the mother
postpartum	After childbirth, with reference to the mother
premature	Describing an infant born before the organ systems are fully developed; immature
preterm	Occurring before the 37th week of gestation; describing an infant born before the 37th week of gestation
puerperium *pū-er-PĒR-ē-um*	The first 42 days after childbirth, during which the mother's reproductive organs usually return to normal (root *puer* means "child")

(continued)

Terminology Supplementary Terms (continued)

striae atrophicae *STRĪ-ē a-TRŌ-fi-kē*	Pinkish or gray lines that appear where skin has been stretched, as in pregnancy; stretch marks, striae gravidarum
umbilicus *um-bi-LĪ-kus*	The scar in the middle of the abdomen that marks the attachment point of the umbilical cord to the fetus; the navel
vernix caseosa *VER-niks kā-sē-Ō-sa*	The cheeselike deposit that covers and protects the fetus (literally "cheesy varnish")

Disorders

cephalopelvic disproportion *sef-a-lō-PEL-vik*	The condition in which the head of the fetus is larger than the mother's pelvic outlet; also called fetopelvic disproportion
choriocarcinoma *kor-ē-ō-kar-si-NŌ-ma*	A rare malignant neoplasm composed of placental tissue
galactorrhea *ga-lak-tō-RĒ-a*	Excessive secretion of milk or continued milk production after breastfeeding has ceased. Often results from excess prolactin secretion and may signal a pituitary tumor
hydatidiform mole *hī-da-TID-i-form*	A benign overgrowth of placental tissue. The placenta dilates and resembles grapelike cysts. The neoplasm may invade the uterine wall, causing rupture. Also called hydatid mole
hydramnios *hī-DRAM-nē-os*	An excess of amniotic fluid; also called polyhydramnios
oligohydramnios *ol-i-gō-hī-DRAM-nē-os*	A deficiency of amniotic fluid
patent ductus arteriosus (PDA) *PĀ-tent DUK-tus ar-tē-rē-Ō-sus*	Persistence of the ductus arteriosus after birth so that blood continues to shunt from the pulmonary artery to the aorta
puerperal infection *pū-ER-per-al*	Infection of the genital tract after delivery

Diagnosis and Treatment

abortifacient *a-bor-ti-FĀ-shent*	Agent that induces abortion
alpha-fetoprotein (AFP) *AL-fa fē-tō-PRŌ-tēn*	A fetal protein that may be elevated in amniotic fluid and maternal serum in cases of certain fetal disorders
Apgar score *AP-gar*	A system of rating an infant's physical condition immediately after birth. Five features are rated as 0, 1, or 2 at 1 and 5 minutes after delivery, and sometimes thereafter. The maximum possible score at each test interval is 10. Infants with low scores require medical attention
artificial insemination (AI)	Placement of active semen into the vagina or cervix for the purpose of impregnation. The semen can be from a husband, partner, or donor
cesarean section *se-ZAR-ē-an*	Incision of the abdominal wall and uterus for delivery of a fetus
endometrial ablation *ab-LĀ-shun*	Selective destruction of the endometrium for therapeutic purpose; done to relieve excessive menstrual bleeding (menorrhagia)
extracorporeal membrane oxygenation (ECMO) *eks-tra-kor-PŌ-rē-al*	A technique for pulmonary bypass in which deoxygenated blood is removed, passed through a circuit that oxygenates the blood, and then returned. Used for selected newborn and pediatric patients in respiratory failure with an otherwise good prognosis

(continued)

Terminology | Supplementary Terms (continued)

in vitro fertilization (IVF)	Clinical procedure for achieving fertilization when it cannot be accomplished naturally. An oocyte (immature ovum) is removed, fertilized in the laboratory, and placed as a zygote into the uterus or fallopian tube (ZIFT, zygote intrafallopian transfer). Alternatively, an ovum can be removed and placed along with sperm cells into the fallopian tube (GIFT, gamete intrafallopian transfer) (see Box 15-4)
obstetrics ob-STET-riks	The branch of medicine that treats women during pregnancy, childbirth, and the puerperium. Usually combined with the practice of gynecology
pediatrics pē-dē-AT-riks	The branch of medicine that treats children and diseases of children (root ped/o means "child")
pelvimetry pel-VIM-e-trē	Measurement of the pelvis by manual examination or radiographic study to determine whether delivery of a fetus through the vagina will be possible
Pitocin pi-TŌ-sin	Trade name for oxytocin; used to induce and hasten labor
presentation	Term describing the part of the fetus that can be felt by vaginal or rectal examination. Normally the head presents first (vertex presentation), but sometimes the buttocks (breech presentation), face, or other part presents first
Rho-GAM RŌ-gam	Trade name for a preparation of antibody to the Rh(D) antigen; used to prevent hemolytic disease of the newborn in cases of Rh incompatibility

PASSport to Success®

Go to the pronunciation glossary on the Student Resources to hear these words pronounced.

Terminology | Abbreviations

Pregnancy and Birth

AB	Abortion		GIFT	Gamete intrafallopian transfer
AFP	Alpha-fetoprotein		hCG	Human chorionic gonadotropin
AGA	Appropriate for gestational age		HDN	Hemolytic disease of the newborn
AI	Artificial insemination		IVF	In vitro fertilization
ART	Assisted reproductive technology		LMP	Last menstrual period
C-section	Cesarean section		NB	Newborn
CPD	Cephalopelvic disproportion		NICU	Neonatal intensive care unit
CVS	Chorionic villus sampling		OB	Obstetrics
D&E	Dilatation and evacuation		PDA	Patent ductus arteriosus
ECMO	Extracorporeal membrane oxygenation		PIH	Pregnancy-induced hypertension
EDC	Estimated date of confinement		PKU	Phenylketonuria
FHR	Fetal heart rate		SVD	Spontaneous vaginal delivery
FHT	Fetal heart tone		UC	Uterine contractions
FTND	Full-term normal delivery		UTP	Uterine term pregnancy
FTP	Full-term pregnancy		VBAC	Vaginal birth after cesarean section
GA	Gestational age		ZIFT	Zygote intrafallopian transfer

Chapter Review

LABELING EXERCISE

Female Reproductive System > Write the name of each numbered part on the corresponding line of the answer sheet.

Anus   Oviduct (fallopian tube)
Cervix   Peritoneal cavity
Clitoris   Posterior fornix
Cul-de-sac   Rectum
Fimbriae   Urethra
Labium majus   Urinary bladder
Labium minus   Uterus
Ovary   Vagina

1. _____   9. _____

2. _____   10. _____

3. _____   11. _____

4. _____   12. _____

5. _____   13. _____

6. _____   14. _____

7. _____   15. _____

8. _____   16. _____

Ovulation and Fertilization > Write the name of each numbered part on the corresponding line of the answer sheet.

Cervix
Body of uterus
Fimbriae
Greater vestibular
    (Bartholin) gland
Implanted embryo

Ovary
Oviduct (fallopian tube)
Ovum
Sperm cells (spermatozoa)
Vagina

1. _____

2. _____

3. _____

4. _____

5. _____

6. _____

7. _____

8. _____

9. _____

10. _____

TERMINOLOGY

Matching> Match the following terms and write the appropriate letter to the left of each number:

_____ **1.** clitoris
_____ **2.** gestation
_____ **3.** oxytocin
_____ **4.** zygote
_____ **5.** vulva

a. fertilized egg
b. female erectile tissue
c. external female genitalia
d. period of development in the uterus
e. hormone that stimulates labor

_____ **6.** menostasis
_____ **7.** metrorrhagia
_____ **8.** menarche
_____ **9.** gynecogenic
_____ **10.** metratrophia

a. producing female characteristics
b. wasting of uterine tissue
c. excess uterine bleeding
d. suppression of menstruation
e. first menstrual period

_____ **11.** congenital
_____ **12.** leiomyoma
_____ **13.** atresia
_____ **14.** rubella
_____ **15.** mutation

a. fibroid
b. absence of a normal body opening
c. present at birth
d. genetic change
e. German measles

Supplementary Terms

_____ **16.** puerperium
_____ **17.** areola
_____ **18.** meconium
_____ **19.** hymen
_____ **20.** lochia

a. uterine discharge after childbirth
b. period after childbirth
c. first feces of the newborn
d. a pigmented ring
e. membrane that covers the vaginal opening

_____ **21.** hirsutism
_____ **22.** dyspareunia
_____ **23.** vernix caseosa

a. whitish vaginal discharge
b. excess hair growth
c. pain during intercourse

——— **24.** leukorrhea
——— **25.** fontanel

d. soft spot between cranial bones
e. fetal protective covering

Fill in the blanks:

26. The female gonad is the _____ .

27. The ovarian follicle encloses a developing _____ .

28. The tissue that nourishes and maintains the developing fetus is the _____ .

29. The secretion of milk from the mammary glands is called _____ .

30. Loss of an embryo or fetus before 20 weeks or 500 g is termed a(n) _____ .

31. Parametritis (*par-a-mē-TRĪ-tis*) means inflammation of the tissue near the _____ .

32. Polymastia (*pol-ē-MAS-tē-a*) means the presence of more than one pair of _____ .

True–False > Examine the following statements. If the statement is true, write T in the first blank. If the statement is false, write F in the first blank and correct the statement by replacing the underlined word in the second blank.

33. Parturition is <u>childbirth</u>.   ———   _____

34. The fallopian tube is the <u>oviduct</u>.   ———   _____

35. The lining of the uterus is the <u>myometrium</u>.   ———   _____

36. After ovulation, the ovarian follicle becomes a <u>fimbriae</u>.   ———   _____

37. Fertilization of an ovum occurs in the <u>uterus</u>.   ———   _____

38. The Pap smear is a test for <u>cervical</u> cancer.   ———   _____

39. Agalactia is the lack of <u>milk</u> production.   ———   _____

40. For the first 2 months, the developing offspring is called a <u>fetus</u>.   ———   _____

Define the following terms:

41. retrouterine (*re-trō-Ū-ter-in*)_____

42. hysteropathy (*his-te-ROP-a-thē*) _____

43. metromalacia (*mē-trō-ma-LĀ-shē-a*) _____

44. pyosalpinx (*pī-ō-SAL-pinx*) _____

45. colpostenosis (*kol-pō-ste-NŌ-sis*) _____

46. postnatal (*pōst-NĀ-tal*) _____

47. inframammary (*in-fra-MAM-a-rē*) _____

48. extraembryonic (*eks-tra-em-brē-ON-ik*) _____

49. nulligravida (*nul-i-GRAV-i-da*) _____

50. tripara (*TRIP-a-ra*) _____

51. teratogenic (*TER-at-ō-jen-ik*) _____

Write words for the following:

52. hernia of an oviduct   _____

53. suture of the vulva (episi/o-)   _____

54. narrowing of the uterus (metr/o) _____

55. surgical removal of the uterus   _____
(hyster/o) and oviducts

56. radiograph of the breast   _____
(mamm/o)

57. abnormal or difficult labor   _____

58. rupture of the amniotic sac   _____

59. study of the embryo   _____

60. measurement of a fetus   _____

Synonyms > Write one word that means the same as the following:

61. neonate   _____

62. para 1   _____

63. gravida 0   _____

Opposites > Write a word that means the opposite of the following:

64. antepartum   _____

65. postnatal   _____

66. dystocia   _____

67. ovulatory   _____

Adjectives > Write the adjective form of the following:

68. cervix   _____

69. uterus   _____

70. perineum   _____

71. vagina   _____

72. embryo   _____

73. amnion   _____

Plurals > Write the plural form of the following:

74. ovum   _____

75. cervix   _____

76. fimbria   _____

77. labium   _____

Chapter Review *(continued)*

Eliminations > In each of the sets below, underline the word that does not fit in with the rest and explain the reason for your choice:

78. umbilical cord — labia majora — amniotic fluid — chorion — placenta

_____

79. colostrum — progesterone — LH — estrogen — FSH

_____

80. hemophilia — albinism — measles — PKU — cystic fibrosis

_____

81. amniocentesis — chorionic villus sampling — karyotype — ultrasonography — candidiasis

_____

82. placental abruption — spina bifida — pregnancy-induced hypertension — placenta previa — eclampsia

_____

Word Building > Write a word for the following definitions using the word parts provided.

-graphy   episi/o   -plasty   intra-   cervic/o   mamm/o   -itis   -al   -tomy   trans-

83. plastic repair of the vulva _____

84. inflammation of the cervix _____

85. radiographic study of the breast _____

86. plastic repair of the breast _____

87. radiographic study of the cervix _____

88. incision of the vulva _____

89. within the cervix _____

90. plastic repair of the cervix _____

91. incision of the cervix _____

92. through the cervix _____

Write the meaning of the following abbreviations:

93. hCG _____

94. TSS _____

95. IUD _____

96. DUB _____

97. LMP _____

98. ZIFT _____

99. GA _____

100. FHR _____

101. VBAC _____

Word Analysis ➤ Define the following words and give the meaning of the word parts in each. Use a dictionary if necessary.

102. antiangiogenesis (*an-tē-an-jē-ō-JEN-e-sis*) _____

    a. anti _____

    b. angi/o _____

    c. gen _____

    d. e/sis _____

103. gynecomastia (*jin-e-kō-MAS-tē-a*) _____

    a. gynec/o _____

    b. mast/o _____

    c. -ia _____

104. oxytocia (*ok-sē-TŌ-sē-a*) _____

                                                 sharp, acute

    a. oxy _____

    b. toc _____

    c. -ia _____

105. oligohydramnios (*ol-i-gō-hī-DRAM-nē-os*) _____

    a. oligo- _____

    b. hydr/o _____

    c. amnio(s) _____

PASSport to Success®   Go to the word exercises on the Student Resources for additional review exercises.

Case Studies

➤ Case Study 15-1: Total Abdominal Hysterectomy with Bilateral Salpingo-Oophorectomy

M.T., a 60-year-old gravida 2, para 2, had spent 3 months under the care of her gynecologist for treatment of postmenopausal bleeding and cervical dysplasia. She had had several vaginal examinations with Pap smears, a uterine ultrasound, colposcopy with endocervical biopsies, and a D&C with cone biopsy. She wanted to take hormone therapy, but her doctor thought she was at too much risk with the abnormal cells on her cervix and the excessive bleeding.

She had a TAH & BSO under general anesthesia with no complications and an uneventful recovery. Her uterus had been prolapsed on abdominal examination, but there was no sign of malignancy or PID. The pathology report revealed several uterine leiomyomas and stenosis of the right oviduct. She was discharged on the second postoperative day with few activity restrictions.

➤ Case Study 15-2: In Vitro Fertilization

C.A. had worked as a technologist in the IVF lab at University Medical Center for 4 years. Her department was

(continued)

Case Studies (continued)

the Advanced Reproductive Technology Program. Although her work was primarily in the laboratory, she followed each patient through all five phases of the IVF and embryo transfer treatment cycle: follicular development, aspiration of the preovulatory follicles, sperm preparation, IVF, and embryo transfer. Her department does both GIFT and ZIFT.

While the female patient is in surgery having an ultrasound-guided transvaginal oocyte retrieval, C.A. examines the recently donated sperm for motility and quantity. She prepares to inoculate the sample into the cytoplasm of the ova as soon as she receives the cells from the OR. After inoculation, she places the sterile Petri dish with the fertilized oocytes into an incubator until they are ready to be introduced into the female patient.

➤ Case Study 15-3: Cesarean Section Birth

A.Y., a gravida 2, para 1 at 39 weeks' gestation, had been in active labor for several hours, fully effaced and dilated, yet unable to progress. She had had an uneventful pregnancy with good health, moderate weight gain, good fetal heart sounds, and no signs or symptoms of pregnancy-induced hypertension. X-ray pelvimetry revealed CPD with the fetus in the right occiput posterior position. Changes in fetal heart rate indicated fetal distress. A.Y. was transported to the OR for emergency C-section under spinal anesthesia.

After being placed in the supine position, A.Y. had a urethral catheter inserted and her abdomen was prepped with antimicrobial solution. After draping, a transverse suprapubic incision was made. Dissection was continued through the muscle layers to the uterus, with care not to nick the bladder. The uterus was incised through the lower segment, 2 cm from the bladder. The fetal head was gently elevated through the incision while the assistant put gentle pressure on the fundus. The baby's mouth and nose were suctioned with a bulb syringe, and the umbilical cord was clamped and cut. The baby was handed off to an attending pediatrician and OB nurse and placed in a radiant neonate warmer bed. The Apgar score was 9/9. The placenta was gently delivered from the uterus, and the scrub nurse checked for three vessels and filled two sterile test tubes with cord blood for lab analysis. A.Y. was given an injection of Pitocin to stimulate uterine contraction. The uterus and abdomen were closed, and A.Y. was transported to the PACU (postanesthesia care unit).

CASE STUDY QUESTIONS

Multiple choice. Select the best answer and write the letter of your choice to the left of each number:

_____ 1. M.T. is a gravida 2, para 2. This means:
   a. she has four children from two pregnancies
   b. she has had two pregnancies and two births
   c. she has had four pregnancies and two births
   d. she has had two pregnancies and two sets of twins
   e. she has one set of twins

_____ 2. An endocervical biopsy is:
   a. a tissue sample from the cul-de-sac
   b. a cone-shaped tissue sample from the uterine fundus
   c. a tissue sample from within the neck
   d. a tissue sample from the lining of the cervix
   e. a scraping of tissue cells from the vaginal wall

_____ 3. A curettage is a(n):
   a. suturing
   b. scraping
   c. cutting
   d. examination
   e. incision

_____ 4. A colposcopy is an endoscopic examination of the:
   a. vagina
   b. fundus
   c. intraperitoneal pelvic floor
   d. pouch of Douglas
   e. uterus and fallopian tubes

_____ 5. Another name for a leiomyoma is a(n):
   a. ectopic pregnancy
   b. uterine fibroid
   c. myoma
   d. a and b
   e. b and c

_____ 6. Pregnancy-induced hypertension is also called:
   a. tubal pregnancy
   b. congenital mutation
   c. ectopic pregnancy
   d. preeclampsia
   e. placenta previa

_____ 7. The occiput of the fetus is the:
   a. forehead
   b. foot
   c. back of the head
   d. chin
   e. shoulder

_____ 8. Pitocin is the trade name for:
   a. progesterone
   b. estrogen
   c. chorionic gonadotropin
   d. FSH
   e. oxytocin

Write a term from the case studies with each of the following meanings:

9. displaced downward _____

10. cell produced by fertilization _____

11. measurement of the pelvis _____

12. upper rounded portion of the uterus _____

(continued)

Case Studies *(continued)*

13. method for rating a newborn's physical condition

_____

14. afterbirth _____

Define each of the following abbreviations:

15. D&C _____

16. BSO _____

17. PID _____

18. HRT _____

19. IVF _____

20. CPD _____

21. OB _____

22. GYN _____

23. GU _____

PASSport to Success®   Go to the word exercises on the Student Resources for additional review exercises.

The Endocrine System

CHAPTER CONTENTS

OBJECTIVES

After study of this chapter you should be able to:

1. Define hormones.
2. Compare steroid and amino acid hormones.
3. Label a diagram of the endocrine system.
4. Name the hormones produced by the endocrine glands and briefly describe the function of each.
5. Identify and use roots pertaining to the endocrine system.
6. Describe the main disorders of the endocrine system.
7. Interpret abbreviations used in endocrinology.
8. Analyze several case studies concerning disorders of the endocrine system.

PRETEST

Multiple choice. Select the best answer and write the letter of your choice to the left of each number.

___ 1. The secretions of the endocrine glands are called:

    a. enzymes   c. lymph
    b. sera   d. hormones

___ 2. The small gland in the brain that controls other glands is the:

    a. pituitary   c. appendix
    b. thymus   d. corpus luteum

___ 3. The glands that are located above the kidneys are the:

    a. thyroids   c. adrenals
    b. follicles   d. fimbriae

___ 4. Gigantism results from overproduction of:

    a. growth hormone   c. erythropoietin
    b. oxytocin   d. prolactin

___ 5. Diabetes mellitus involves the
hormone insulin, which is made by the:

    a. thymus   c. kidney
    b. seminal vesicle   d. pancreas

___ 6. A goiter involves the:

    a. adrenal   c. calyx
    b. zygote   d. thyroid

The body's main controlling systems are the endocrine system and the nervous system (discussed in Chapters 17 and 18). The endocrine system consists of a widely distributed group of glands that secrete regulatory substances called **hormones**. Because hormones are released into the blood, the **endocrine** glands are known as the *ductless glands*, as compared to glands that secrete through ducts, such as sweat glands and digestive glands. Despite the fact that hormones circulating in the blood reach all parts of the body, only certain tissues respond to a specific hormone. The tissue that is influenced by a specific hormone is called the **target tissue**. The cells in a target tissue have specific **receptors** on their membranes or within the cell to which the hormone attaches, enabling it to act.

Hormones

Hormones are produced in extremely small amounts and are highly potent. By means of their actions on various target tissues, they affect growth, metabolism, reproductive activity, and behavior. (Box 16-1 describes some old ideas about the effects of substances circulating in the blood.)

Chemically, hormones fall into two categories:

- **Steroid hormones**, which are made from lipids. Steroids are produced by the sex glands (gonads) and the outer region (cortex) of the **adrenal glands**.

- Hormones made of amino acids, which include proteins and protein-like compounds. All of the endocrine glands aside from the gonads and adrenal cortex produce amino acid hormones.

The production of hormones is controlled mainly by negative feedback—that is, the hormone itself, or some product of hormone activity, acts as a control over further manufacture of the hormone—a self-regulating system. Hormone production may also be controlled by the nervous system or by other hormones.

The Endocrine Glands

Refer to Figure 16-1 to locate the endocrine glands described below. Box 16-2 lists the endocrine glands, along with the hormones they secrete and their functions.

Pituitary

The **pituitary gland**, or **hypophysis**, is a small gland beneath the brain. It is divided into an anterior lobe (adenohypophysis) and a posterior lobe (neurohypophysis). Both lobes are connected to and controlled by the **hypothalamus**, a part of the brain.

The anterior pituitary produces six hormones. One of these is growth hormone (somatotropin), which stimulates bone growth and acts on other tissues as well (see Box 16-3). The remainder of the pituitary hormones

Box 16-1   Focus on Words

Are You in a Good Humor?

In ancient times, people accepted the theory that a person's state of health depended on the balance of four body fluids. These fluids, called "humors," were yellow bile, black bile, phlegm, and blood. A predominance of any one of these humors would determine a person's mood or temperament. Yellow bile caused anger; black bile caused depression; phlegm (mucus) made a person sluggish; blood resulted in cheerfulness and optimism.

Although we no longer believe in humoralism, we still have adjectives in our vocabulary that reflect these early

beliefs. Choleric describes a person under the influence of yellow bile; melancholic describes the effects of black bile (melano- means black or dark); a phlegmatic person is slow to respond; a sanguine individual "goes with the flow." (*Sanguine* is derived from the Greek word for blood.)

The humors persist today in the adjective *humoral*, which describes substances carried in the blood or other body fluids. The term applies to hormones and other circulating materials that influence body responses. Humoral immunity is immunity based on antibodies carried in the bloodstream.

16

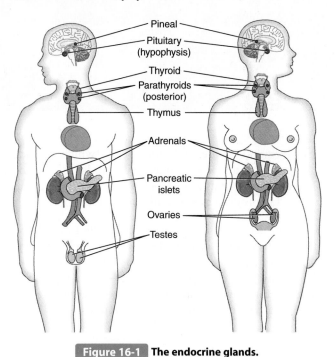

Pineal
Pituitary
(hypophysis)
Thyroid
Parathyroids
(posterior)
Thymus
Adrenals
Pancreatic
islets
Ovaries
Testes

Figure 16-1 **The endocrine glands.**

regulate other glands, including the thyroid, adrenals, gonads, and mammary glands (see Box 16-2). The ending -tropin, as in *gonadotropin*, indicates a hormone that acts on another gland. The adjective ending is -tropic, as in *adrenocorticotropic*.

The posterior pituitary releases two hormones that are actually produced in the hypothalamus. These hormones are stored in the posterior pituitary until they are needed:

- Antidiuretic hormone (ADH) acts on the kidneys to conserve water and also promotes constriction of blood vessels. Both of these actions increase blood pressure.
- Oxytocin stimulates uterine contractions and promotes milk "letdown" in the breasts during lactation.

Thyroid and Parathyroids

The **thyroid gland** consists of two lobes on either side of the larynx and upper trachea. The lobes are connected

Box 16-2   For Your Reference

The Endocrine Glands and Their Hormones

GLAND	HORMONE	PRINCIPAL FUNCTIONS
anterior pituitary *pi-TŪ-i-tar-ē*	GH (growth hormone), also called somatotropin (*sō-ma-tō-TRŌ-pin*)	Promotes growth of all body tissues
	TSH (thyroid-stimulating hormone)	Stimulates thyroid gland to produce thyroid hormones
	ACTH (adrenocorticotropic hormone) (*a-drē-nō-kor-ti-kō-TRŌ-pik*)	Stimulates adrenal cortex to produce cortical hormones; aids in protecting body in stress situations (injury, pain)
	FSH (follicle-stimulating hormone)	Stimulates growth and hormonal activity of ovarian follicles; stimulates growth of testes; promotes sperm cell development
	LH (luteinizing hormone) (*LŪ-tē-in-ī-zing*)	Causes development of corpus luteum at site of ruptured ovarian follicle in female; stimulates testosterone secretion in male
	PRL (prolactin) (*prō-LAK-tin*)	Stimulates milk secretion by mammary glands
posterior pituitary	ADH (antidiuretic hormone; vasopressin) (*an-tē-dī-ū-RET-ik; vā-sō-PRES-in*)	Promotes water reabsorption in kidney tubules; causes blood vessels to constrict
	oxytocin (*ok-sē-TŌ-sin*)	Causes uterine contraction; causes milk ejection from mammary glands
thyroid	thyroxine or tetraiodothyronine (T₄) and triiodothyronine (T₃) (*thī-ROK-sēn; trī-ī-ō-dō-THĪ-rō-nēn*)	Increase metabolic rate and heat production, influencing both physical and mental activities; required for normal growth
	calcitonin (*kal-si-TŌ-nin*)	Decreases blood calcium level

Box 16-2   For Your Reference (Continued)

The Endocrine Glands and Their Hormones

GLAND	HORMONE	PRINCIPAL FUNCTIONS
parathyroids	parathyroid hormone (PTH) (*par-a-THĪ-royd*)	Regulates calcium exchange between blood and bones; increases blood calcium level
adrenal cortex	cortisol (hydrocortisone) (*KOR-ti-sol*)	Aids in metabolism of carbohydrates, proteins, and fats; active during stress
	aldosterone (*al-DOS-ter-ōn*)	Aids in regulating electrolytes and water balance
	sex hormones	May influence secondary sexual characteristics
adrenal medulla	epinephrine (adrenaline) and norepinephrine (noradrenaline) (*ep-i-NEF-rin; a-DREN-a-lin*)	Respond to stress; increase respiration, blood pressure, and heart rate
pancreatic islets	insulin (*IN-sū-lin*)	Aids glucose transport into cells; required for cellular metabolism of nutrients, especially glucose; decreases blood sugar levels
	glucagon (*GLŪ-ka-gon*)	Stimulates liver to release glucose, thereby increasing blood sugar levels
pineal	melatonin (*mel-a-TŌN-in*)	Regulates mood, sexual development, and daily cycles in response to environmental light
thymus	thymosin (*THĪ-mō-sin*)	Important in development of T cells needed for immunity and in early development of lymphoid tissue
testes	testosterone (*tes-TOS-te-rōn*)	Stimulates growth and development of sexual organs plus development of secondary sexual characteristics; stimulates maturation of sperm cells
ovaries	estrogens (*ES-trō-jenz*)	Stimulate growth of primary sexual organs and development of secondary sexual characteristics
	progesterone (*prō-JES-ter-ōn*)	Prepares uterine lining for implantation of fertilized ovum; aids in maintaining pregnancy; stimulates development of mammary glands' secretory tissue

Box 16-3   Clinical Perspectives

Growth Hormone: Its Clinical Use Is Growing

Growth hormone (GH) is produced by the anterior pituitary. It is released mainly at the beginning of deep sleep, so the old belief that you grow while you sleep has some basis in fact. Although GH affects primarily bone and muscle development during early growth, it has a general stimulating effect on most other tissues throughout life. Its alternative name, soma-totropin, comes from *soma* meaning "body" and *tropin* meaning "acting on." GH is released during times of stress to boost the liver's output of energy-rich fatty acids when blood glucose levels drop. A lack of GH in childhood results in dwarfism, and the hormone was initially prescribed only for children with a GH deficiency. Now it has also been approved for children who are in the lowest percentile of height for their age. If a child is still growing, as shown by x-rays of the hand and wrist, GH will lead to some ultimate increase in height. Because GH increases lean muscle mass, it is also touted as a body-building and anti-aging medication. However, it may have some side effects, and its long-term effects are not known. GH for clinical use was initially obtained from cadaver pituitaries, but it is now made by genetic engineering.

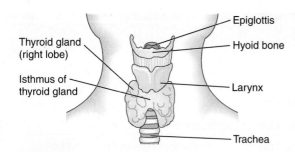

Figure 16-2 **Thyroid gland.** This anterior view shows the gland in relation to the larynx and trachea.

by a narrow band (isthmus) (Fig. 16-2). The thyroid secretes a mixture of hormones, mainly thyroxine (T_4) and triiodothyronine (T_3). Because thyroid hormones contain iodine, laboratories can measure these hormones and study thyroid gland activity by following iodine levels. Most thyroid hormone in the blood is bound to protein, primarily thyroxine-binding globulin (TBG).

On the posterior surface of the thyroid are four to six tiny **parathyroid glands** that affect calcium metabolism (Fig. 16-3). Parathyroid hormone (PTH) increases the blood level of calcium. It works with the thyroid hormone calcitonin, which lowers blood calcium, to regulate calcium balance.

Adrenals

The **adrenal glands**, located atop the kidneys, are divided into two distinct regions: an outer cortex and an inner

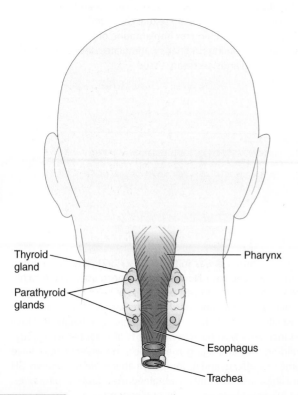

Figure 16-3 **Parathyroid glands.** A posterior view of the thyroid gland shows the parathyroid glands embedded in its surface.

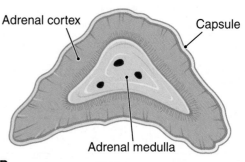

Figure 16-4 **Adrenal glands.** (*A*) The adrenal glands shown on top of each kidney. (*B*) The adrenal gland is divided into a medulla and cortex, each secreting different hormones.

medulla (Fig. 16-4). The hormones produced by this gland are involved in the body's response to stress. The cortex produces steroid hormones:

- Cortisol (hydrocortisone) mobilizes fat and carbohydrate reserves to increase these nutrients in the blood. It also reduces inflammation and is used clinically for this purpose.

- Aldosterone causes the kidneys to conserve sodium and water while eliminating potassium.

- Sex hormones, mainly testosterone, are also produced in small amounts, but their importance is not well understood. Some athletes, illegally and dangerously, take testosterone-like steroids to increase muscle size, strength, and endurance (see Box 20-1).

The medulla of the adrenal gland produces two similar hormones that are released in response to stress. Epinephrine (adrenaline) and norepinephrine (noradrenaline) work with the nervous system to help the body meet challenges.

Pancreatic islet   Digestive cells

Blood vessels

Figure 16-5 Pancreatic cells, microscopic view. Light-staining islet cells are seen among the cell clusters that produce digestive juices.

Pancreas

The endocrine portions of the pancreas are the **pancreatic islets**, small cell clusters within the pancreatic tissue. The term *islet*, meaning "small island," is used because these cells look like little islands in the midst of the many pancreatic cells that secrete digestive juices (Fig. 16-5). The islet cells produce two hormones, insulin and glucagon, that regulate glucose metabolism. Insulin increases cellular use of glucose, thus decreasing blood sugar levels. Glucagon has the opposite effect, increasing blood sugar levels.

Other Endocrine Tissues

There are three additional types of endocrine glands:

- The **pineal gland** is a small gland in the brain (see Fig. 16-1). It regulates mood, daily rhythms, and sexual development in response to environmental light. Its hormone is melatonin, which some people take to help regulate sleep-wake cycles when they travel between time zones.

- The thymus, described in Chapter 9, is considered an endocrine gland because it secretes a hormone, thymosin, that stimulates the immune system's T lymphocytes.

- The gonads, the testes and ovaries described in Chapters 14 and 15, are also included because they secrete hormones in addition to producing the sex cells.

Other organs, including the stomach, kidney, heart, and small intestine, also produce hormones. However, they have other major functions and are discussed with the systems to which they belong.

Finally, **prostaglandins** are a group of hormones produced by many cells. They have a variety of effects, including stimulation of uterine contractions, promotion of inflammation, and vasomotor activities. They are called prostaglandins because they were first discovered in the prostate gland.

Terminology   Key Terms

Normal Structure and Function

Term	Definition
adrenal gland *a-DRĒ-nal*	A gland on the superior surface of the kidney. The outer region (cortex) secretes steroid hormones; the inner region (medulla) secretes epinephrine (adrenaline) and norepinephrine (noradrenaline) (root: *adren/o*)
endocrine *EN-dō-krin*	Pertaining to a ductless gland that secretes hormones into the blood
hormone *HOR-mōn*	A secretion of an endocrine gland. A substance that travels in the blood and has a regulatory effect on tissues, organs, or glands
hypophysis *hī-POF-i-sis*	The pituitary gland (root: *hypophys*); named from *hypo*, meaning "below," and *physis*, meaning "growing," because the gland develops below the hypothalamus
hypothalamus *hī-pō-THAL-a-mus*	A portion of the brain that controls the pituitary gland and is active in maintaining homeostasis
pancreatic islets *Ī-lets*	Clusters of endocrine cells in the pancreas that secrete hormones to regulate glucose metabolism; also called islets of Langerhans or islet cells (root *insul/o* means "island")
parathyroid glands *par-a-THĪ-royd*	Small endocrine glands on the posterior thyroid that act to increase blood calcium levels; there are usually four to six parathyroid glands (roots: *parathyr/o*, *parathyroid/o*); the name literally means "near the thyroid"

(continued)

Terminology   Key Terms (continued)

pineal gland PIN-ē-al	A small gland in the brain (see Fig. 16-1). Appears to regulate mood, daily rhythms, and sexual development in response to environmental light. Secretes the hormone melatonin
pituitary gland pi-TŪ-i-tar-ē	A small endocrine gland at the base of the brain. The anterior lobe secretes growth hormone and hormones that stimulate other glands; the posterior lobe releases ADH and oxytocin manufactured in the hypothalamus
prostaglandins pros-ta-GLAN-dinz	A group of hormones produced throughout the body that have a variety of effects, including stimulation of uterine contractions and regulation of blood pressure, blood clotting, and inflammation
receptor	A site on the cell membrane or within the cell to which a substance, such as a hormone, attaches
steroid hormone STER-oyd	A hormone made from lipids and including the sex hormones and the hormones of the adrenal cortex
target tissue	The specific tissue on which a hormone acts; may also be called the target organ
thyroid gland THĪ-royd	An endocrine gland on either side of the larynx and upper trachea. It secretes hormones that affect metabolism and growth and a hormone (calcitonin) that regulates calcium balance (roots: *thyr/o*, *thyroid/o*)

PASSport to Success®   Go to the pronunciation glossary on the Student Resources to hear these words pronounced.

Roots Pertaining to the Endocrine System

See Table 16-1.

Table 16-1   Roots Pertaining to the Endocrine System

Root	Meaning	Example	Definition of Example
endocrin/o	endocrine glands or system	endocrinopathy en-dō-kri-NOP-a-thē	any disease of the endocrine glands
pituitar	pituitary gland, hypophysis	pituitarism pi-TŪ-i-ta-rizm	condition caused by any disorder of pituitary function
hypophys	pituitary gland, hypophysis	hypophysial hī-pō-FIZ-ē-al (also spelled hypophyseal)	pertaining to the pituitary gland
thyr/o, thyroid/o	thyroid gland	thyrolytic thī-rō-LIT-ik	destroying the thyroid gland
parathyr/o, parathyroid/o	parathyroid gland	hyperparathyroidism hī-per-par-a-THĪ-royd-izm	overactivity of a parathyroid gland
adren/o, adrenal/o	adrenal gland, epinephrine	adrenergic ad-ren-ER-jik	activated (erg) by or related to epinephrine (adrenaline)
adrenocortic/o	adrenal cortex	adrenocorticotropic a-drē-nō-kor-ti-kō-TRŌ-pik	acting on the adrenal cortex
insul/o	pancreatic islets	insular IN-sū-lar	pertaining to islet cells

EXERCISE 16-1

Define the following words:

1. endocrinology (*en-dō-krin-OL-ō-jē*) _____

2. hypophysectomy (*hī-pof-i-SEK-tō-mē*) _____

3. thyrotropic (*thī-rō-TROP-ik*) _____

4. hypoadrenalism (*hī-pō-a-DRĒ-nal-izm*) _____

5. insulitis (*in-sū-LĪ-tis*) _____

Words for conditions resulting from endocrine dysfunctions are formed by adding the suffix *-ism* to the name of the gland or its root and adding the prefix *hyper-* or *hypo-* for overactivity or underactivity of the gland. Use the full name of the gland to form words with the following definitions:

6. condition of underactivity of the thyroid gland _____

7. condition of underactivity of the parathyroid gland _____

8. condition of overactivity of the adrenal gland _____

Use the word root for the gland to form words with the following definitions:

9. condition of overactivity of the adrenal cortex _____

10. condition of underactivity of the pituitary gland (use pituitar) _____

Write a word for the following definitions:

11. physician who specializes in study of the endocrine system _____

12. incision into the thyroid gland _____

13. any disease of the adrenal gland _____

14. inflammation of the adrenal gland _____

15. tumor of the pancreatic islets _____

Clinical Aspects of the Endocrine System

Endocrine diseases usually result from the overproduction (hypersecretion) or underproduction (hyposecretion) of hormones. They may also result from secretion at the wrong time or from failure of the target tissue to respond. The causes of abnormal secretion may originate in the gland itself or may result from failure of the hypothalamus or the pituitary to release the proper amount of stimulating hormones. Some of the common endocrine disorders are described below. Conditions resulting from hypersecretion or hyposecretion of hormones are summarized in Box 16-4.

Pituitary

A pituitary **adenoma** (glandular tumor) usually increases secretion of growth hormone or adrenocorticotropic hormone (ACTH). Less commonly, a tumor affects the secretion of prolactin. An excess of growth hormone in children causes **gigantism**. In adults it causes **acromegaly**, characterized by enlargement of the hands, feet, jaw, and facial features. Treatment is by surgery to remove the tumor (adenomectomy) or by drugs to reduce the blood levels of growth hormone. Excess ACTH overstimulates the adrenal cortex, resulting in **Cushing disease**. Increased prolactin causes milk secretion (galactorrhea) in both males and females. Radiographic studies in cases of pituitary adenoma usually show enlargement of the bony socket (sella turcica) that contains the pituitary.

Pituitary hypofunction, as caused by tumor or interruption of blood supply to the gland, may involve a single hormone but usually affects all functions and is referred to as **panhypopituitarism**. This condition's widespread effects include dwarfism (from lack of growth hormone), lack of sexual development and sexual function, fatigue, and weakness.

A specific lack of ADH from the posterior pituitary results in **diabetes insipidus** in which the kidneys have a decreased ability to conserve water. Symptoms are polyuria (excessive urination) and polydipsia (excessive thirst).

Box 16-4   For Your Reference

Disorders Associated with Endocrine Dysfunction*

HORMONE	HYPERSECRETION	HYPOSECRETION
growth hormone	gigantism (children), acromegaly (adults)	dwarfism (children)
antidiuretic hormone	syndrome of inappropriate ADH (SIADH)	diabetes insipidus
aldosterone	aldosteronism	Addison disease
cortisol	Cushing syndrome	Addison disease
thyroid hormone	Graves disease, thyrotoxicosis	congenital hypothyroidism (children), myxedema (adults)
insulin	hypoglycemia	diabetes mellitus
parathyroid hormone	bone degeneration	tetany (muscle spasms)

*Refer to key terms for pronunciations and descriptions.

Diabetes insipidus should not be confused with **diabetes mellitus (DM)**, a disorder of glucose metabolism described below. The two diseases share the symptoms of polyuria and polydipsia but have entirely different causes. DM is the more common disorder, and when the term *diabetes* is used alone, it generally refers to DM. The word *diabetes* is from the Greek meaning "siphon," referring to the large urinary output in both forms of diabetes.

Thyroid

Because thyroid hormone affects the growth and function of many tissues, a deficiency of this hormone in infancy causes physical and mental retardation as well as other symptoms that together constitute **congenital hypothyroidism**, formerly called *cretinism*. The United States and other developed countries now require testing of newborns for hypothyroidism. If not diagnosed at birth and treated, hypothyroidism will lead to mental retardation within 6 months.

In adults, thyroid deficiency causes **myxedema** in which there is weight gain; lethargy; rough, dry skin; hair loss; and facial swelling. There may be reproductive problems and muscular weakness, pain, and stiffness. A common cause of hypothyroidism in adults is autoimmune destruction of the thyroid. Hypothyroidism in both children and adults is easily treated with thyroid hormone.

The most common form of hyperthyroidism is **Graves disease**, also called *diffuse toxic goiter*. This is an autoimmune disorder in which antibodies stimulate an increased production of thyroid hormone. There is weight loss, irritability, hand tremor, and rapid heart rate (tachycardia). A most distinctive sign is a bulging of the eyeballs, termed **exophthalmos**, caused by swelling of the tissues behind the eyes (Fig. 16-6). Treatment for Graves disease may include antithyroid drugs, surgical removal of all or part of the thyroid, or radiation delivered in the form of radioactive iodine.

A common sign in thyroid disease is an enlarged thyroid, or **goiter**. However, a goiter is not necessarily accompanied by thyroid malfunction. A simple or nontoxic goiter is caused by a dietary iodine deficiency. Such cases are rare in industrialized countries because of iodine addition to salt and other commercial foods.

Figure 16-6 **Graves disease.** A young woman with hyperthyroidism showing a mass in the neck and exophthalmos.

Thyroid function is commonly tested by measuring the gland's radioactive iodine uptake (RAIU). Laboratories use radioimmunoassays to measure blood levels of pituitary thyroid-stimulating hormone (TSH), which varies with changing levels of thyroid hormones. Total and free thyroxine (T_4) and triiodothyronine (T_3) are also measured, as are the levels of TBG, a blood protein that binds to thyroid hormones. Thyroid scans following administration of radioactive iodine are also used to study the activity of this gland.

Parathyroids

Overactivity of the parathyroid glands, usually from a tumor, causes a high level of calcium in the blood. Because this calcium is obtained from the bones, there is also skeletal degeneration and bone pain. A common side effect is the development of kidney stones from the high levels of circulating calcium.

Damage to the parathyroids or their surgical removal, as during thyroid surgery, results in a decrease in blood calcium levels. This causes numbness and tingling in the arms and legs and around the mouth (perioral), as well as **tetany** (muscle spasms). Treatment consists of supplying calcium.

Adrenals

Hypofunction of the adrenal cortex, or **Addison disease,** is usually caused by autoimmune destruction of the gland. It may also result from a deficiency of pituitary ACTH. The lack of aldosterone results in water loss, low blood pressure, and electrolyte imbalance. There is also weakness and nausea and an increase in brown pigmentation. This last symptom is caused by release of a pituitary hormone that stimulates the skin's pigment cells (melanocytes). Once diagnosed, Addison disease is treated with replacement cortical hormones.

An excess of adrenal cortical hormones results in **Cushing syndrome.** Patients with this syndrome have a moon-shaped face, obesity localized in the torso, weakness, excess hair growth (hirsutism), and fluid retention (Fig. 16-7). The most common cause of Cushing syndrome is the therapeutic administration of steroid hormones. An adrenal tumor is another possible cause. If the disorder is caused by a pituitary tumor that increases ACTH production, it is referred to as **Cushing disease.**

The Pancreas and Diabetes

The most common endocrine disorder, and a serious public health problem, is diabetes mellitus (DM), a failure of the body cells to use glucose effectively. The excess glucose accumulates in the blood, causing **hyperglycemia.** Increased urination (polyuria) marks the effort to eliminate the excess glucose in the urine, a condition termed **glycosuria.** The result is dehydration and excessive thirst (polydipsia). There is also weakness, weight loss, and extreme hunger (polyphagia). Unable to use carbohydrates, the body burns

Figure 16-7 **Cushing syndrome.** The woman has a moon face, buffalo hump, increased facial hair, and thinning of the scalp hair.

more fat. This leads to accumulation of ketone bodies in the blood and a shift toward acidosis, a condition termed **ketoacidosis.** If untreated, diabetes will lead to starvation of the central nervous system and coma. Diabetic patients are prone to cardiovascular, neurologic, and visual problems, infections, and renal failure.

TYPES OF DIABETES MELLITUS
There are two main types of DM:

- Type 1 diabetes mellitus (T1DM) is caused by autoimmune destruction of pancreatic islet cells and failure of the pancreas to produce insulin. It has an abrupt onset and usually appears in children and teenagers. Because insulin levels are very low or absent, patients need careful monitoring and regular administration of this hormone. The former names for T1DM, juvenile-onset and insulin-dependent diabetes mellitus (IDDM), are not accurate, because this form of the disease may develop past early youth and also because many people with type 2 diabetes require insulin.

- Type 2 diabetes mellitus (T2DM) accounts for about 90% of diabetes cases. Heredity plays a much greater role in this form of diabetes than in type 1. Type 2 diabetes is initiated by cellular resistance to insulin. Feedback stimulation of the pancreatic islets leads to insulin overproduction followed by a failure of the overworked cells to produce enough insulin. Most cases of type 2 diabetes are linked to obesity, especially upper-body obesity. Although seen mostly in older people, the incidence of type 2 diabetes is increasing among younger generations, presumably because of increased obesity, poor diet, and sedentary habits. For this reason and also because of possible insulin need, the former names, adult-onset DM and non–insulin-dependent DM (NIDDM), have been dropped.

Metabolic syndrome (also called *syndrome X* or *insulin resistance syndrome*) is related to T2DM and describes a state of hyperglycemia caused by insulin resistance in association with some metabolic disorders, including high levels of plasma triglycerides (fats), low levels of high-density lipoproteins (HDLs), hypertension, and coronary heart disease.

Gestational diabetes mellitus (GDM) refers to glucose intolerance during pregnancy. This imbalance usually appears in women with a family history of diabetes and in those who are obese. Women, especially those with predisposing factors, must be monitored during pregnancy for signs of DM because this condition can cause complications for both the mother and the fetus. Gestational diabetes usually disappears after childbirth, but it may be a sign that diabetes will develop later in life. As with other forms of diabetes, a proper diet is the first step to management, with insulin treatment if needed.

DM may also follow other endocrine disorders or treatment with corticosteroids and may be caused by a genetic disorder of the pancreatic islets.

DIAGNOSIS

Diabetes is diagnosed by measuring glucose levels in blood plasma with or without fasting. The standard for diagnosis of diabetes in a random test is >200 mg/dL and for a fasting plasma glucose (FPG) >126 mg/dL. Measuring blood glucose levels after oral administration of glucose is an oral glucose tolerance test (OGTT). Categories of impaired fasting blood glucose (IFG) and impaired glucose tolerance (IGT) are stages between a normal response to glucose and diabetes.

TREATMENT

People with T1DM must monitor blood glucose levels four to eight times a day. Traditionally, this is done with blood obtained by a finger stick, but new methods of monitoring glucose through the skin are available. Systems for continuous monitoring are also available, and these can alert patients to high and low blood glucose levels. Insulin may be given in divided doses by injection or by means of an insulin pump that delivers the hormone around the clock (continuous subcutaneous insulin infusion [CSII]). Newer computerized pumps monitor glucose levels and adjust insulin dosage automatically. Diet must be carefully regulated to keep glucose levels steady.

While managing diabetes, patients monitor their own glucose levels on a daily basis. Every few months, physicians obtain more precise indications of long-term glucose control with a **glycated hemoglobin (HbA1c) test**. This test is based on glucose uptake by red blood cells and reflects the average blood glucose levels for 2 to 3 months before the test.

Exercise and weight loss for those who are overweight are the first approaches to treating type 2 diabetes, and these measures often lead to management of the disorder. Drugs for increasing insulin production or improving cellular responses to insulin may also be prescribed, with insulin treatment given if necessary.

Insulin is now made by genetic engineering. There are various forms with different action times that can be alternated to achieve glucose regulation. Excess insulin may result from a pancreatic tumor, but more often it occurs after administration of too much hormone to a diabetic patient. The resultant **hypoglycemia** leads to **insulin shock,** which is treated by the administration of glucose.

Methods of administering insulin in pills or capsules, inhaler spray, or skin patches are still experimental. Researchers are also studying the possibility of transplanting a healthy pancreas or islet cells to compensate for failed cells. Another area of research is the use of immunosuppression to halt T1DM.

Also used to diagnose endocrine disorders are imaging techniques, other measurements of hormones or their metabolites in plasma and urine, and studies involving hormone stimulation or suppression.

Box 16-5 has information on dieticians and nutritionists, who help people, including those with metabolic disorders, to plan healthful diets.

Box 16-5   Health Professions

Dietitians and Nutritionists

Dietitians and nutritionists specialize in planning and supervising food programs for institutions such as hospitals, schools, and nursing-care facilities. They assess their clients' nutritional needs and design individualized meal plans. Dietitians and nutritionists also work in community settings, educating the public about disease prevention through healthy eating. Increased public awareness about food and nutrition has also led to new opportunities in the food manufacturing industry. To perform their duties, dietitians and nutritionists need a thorough scientific and clinical background. Most dietitians and nutritionists in the United States receive their training from a college or university and take a licensing exam.

Job prospects for dietitians and nutritionists are good. As the American population continues to age, the need for nutritional planning in hospital and nursing-care settings is expected to rise. In addition, many people now place an emphasis on healthy eating and may consult nutritionists privately. The American Dietetic Association at www.eatright.org has information about these careers.

Terminology	Key Terms

Disorders

acromegaly *ak-rō-MEG-a-lē*	Overgrowth of bone and soft tissue, especially in the hands, feet, and face, caused by excess growth hormone in an adult. The name comes from *acro* meaning "extremity" and *megal/o* meaning "enlargement"
Addison disease	A disease resulting from deficiency of adrenocortical hormones. It is marked by darkening of the skin, weakness, and alterations in salt and water balance
adenoma *ad-e-NŌ-ma*	A neoplasm of a gland
congenital hypothyroidism	A condition caused by congenital lack of thyroid secretion and marked by arrested physical and mental development; formerly called cretinism (KRĒ-tin-izm)
Cushing disease	Overactivity of the adrenal cortex resulting from excess production of ACTH by the pituitary
Cushing syndrome	A condition resulting from an excess of hormones from the adrenal cortex. It is associated with obesity, weakness, hyperglycemia, hypertension, and hirsutism (excess hair growth)
diabetes insipidus *dī-a-BĒ-tēz in-SIP-i-dus*	A disorder caused by insufficient release of ADH from the posterior pituitary. It results in excessive thirst and production of large amounts of very dilute urine. The word insipidus means "tasteless," referring to the dilution of the urine
diabetes mellitus *MEL-i-tus*	A disorder of glucose metabolism caused by deficiency of insulin production or failure of the tissues to respond to insulin. Type 1 results from autoimmune destruction of pancreatic islet cells; it generally appears in children and requires insulin administration. Type 2 generally occurs in obese adults; it is treated with diet, exercise, and drugs to improve insulin production or activity, and sometimes insulin. The word *mellitus* comes from the Latin root for honey, referring to the urine's sugar content
exophthalmos *ek-sof-THAL-mos*	Protrusion of the eyeballs, as seen in Graves disease
gigantism *JĪ-gan-tizm*	Overgrowth caused by excess growth hormone from the pituitary during childhood; also called gigantism
glycated hemoglobin (HbA1c) test *GLĪ-kā-ted*	A test that measures the binding of glucose to hemoglobin during the lifespan of a red blood cell. It reflects the average blood glucose level over 2 to 3 months and is useful in evaluating long-term therapy for diabetes mellitus. Also called A1c test
glycosuria *glī-kō-SŪ-rē-a*	Excess sugar in the urine
goiter *GOY-ter*	Enlargement of the thyroid gland. May be toxic or nontoxic. Simple (nontoxic) goiter is caused by iodine deficiency
Graves disease	An autoimmune disease resulting in hyperthyroidism. A prominent symptom is exophthalmos (protrusion of the eyeballs). Also called diffuse toxic goiter
hyperglycemia *hī-per-glī-SĒ-mē-a*	Excess glucose in the blood
hypoglycemia *hī-pō-glī-SĒ-mē-a*	Abnormally low level of glucose in the blood
insulin shock	A condition resulting from an overdose of insulin, causing hypoglycemia
ketoacidosis *kē-tō-as-i-DŌ-sis*	Acidosis (increased acidity of body fluids) caused by excess ketone bodies, as in diabetes mellitus; diabetic acidosis
metabolic syndrome	A state of hyperglycemia caused by cellular resistance to insulin, as seen in type 2 diabetes, in association with other metabolic disorders; syndrome X or insulin resistance syndrome
myxedema *miks-e-DĒ-ma*	A condition caused by hypothyroidism in an adult. There is dry, waxy swelling most notable in the face

(continued)

Terminology	**Key Terms** (continued)

panhypopituitarism *pan-hī-pō-pi-TŪ-i-ta-rism*	Underactivity of the entire pituitary gland
tetany *TET-a-nē*	Irritability and spasms of muscles; may be caused by low blood calcium and other factors

 Go to the pronunciation glossary on the Student Resources to hear these words pronounced.

Terminology	**Supplementary Terms**

Normal Structure and Function

sella turcica *SEL-a TUR-si-ka*	A saddle-shaped depression in the sphenoid bone that contains the pituitary gland (literally means "Turkish saddle")
sphenoid bone *SFĒ-noyd*	A bone at the base of the skull that houses the pituitary gland

Symptoms and Conditions

adrenogenital syndrome *ad-rē-nō-JEN-i-tal*	Condition caused by overproduction of androgens from the adrenal cortex, resulting in masculinization; may be congenital or acquired, usually as a result of an adrenal tumor
Conn syndrome	Hyperaldosteronism caused by an adrenal tumor
craniopharyngioma *krā-nē-ō-far-in-jē-Ō-ma*	A benign tumor of the pituitary gland
Hashimoto disease *ha-shē-MŌ-tō*	A chronic thyroiditis of autoimmune origin
impaired glucose tolerance (IGT)	High blood glucose levels after glucose intake that may signal borderline diabetes mellitus
ketosis *kē-TŌ-sis*	Accumulation of ketone bodies, such as acetone, in the body. Usually results from deficiency or faulty metabolism of carbohydrates, as in cases of diabetes mellitus and starvation
multiple endocrine neoplasia (MEN)	A hereditary disorder that causes tumors in several endocrine glands; classified according to the combination of glands involved
pheochromocytoma *fē-ō-krō-mō-sī-TŌ-ma*	A usually benign tumor of the adrenal medulla or other structures containing chromaffin cells (cells that stain with chromium salts); *phe/o* means "brown" or "dusky." The adrenal tumor causes increased production of epinephrine and norepinephrine
pituitary apoplexy *AP-ō-plek-sē*	Sudden massive hemorrhage and degeneration of the pituitary gland associated with a pituitary tumor. Common symptoms include severe headache, visual problems, and loss of consciousness
seasonal affective disorder (SAD)	A mood disorder with lethargy, depression, excessive need for sleep, and overeating that generally occurs in winter. Thought to be related to melatonin levels as influenced by environmental light. See Box 16-6
Simmonds disease	Hypofunction of the anterior pituitary (panhypopituitarism), usually because of an infarction; pituitary cachexia (*ka-KEK-sē-a*)

(continued)

Terminology | Supplementary Terms (continued)

thyroid storm	A sudden onset of thyrotoxicosis symptoms occurring in patients with hyperthyroidism who are untreated or poorly treated. May be brought on by illness or trauma. Also called thyroid crisis
thyrotoxicosis thī-rō-tok-si-KŌ-sis	Condition resulting from overactivity of the thyroid gland. Symptoms include anxiety, irritability, weight loss, and sweating. The main example of thyrotoxicosis is Graves disease
von Recklinghausen disease	Bone degeneration caused by excess production of parathyroid hormone. Also called Recklinghausen disease of bone

Diagnosis and Treatment

fasting plasma glucose (FPG)	Measurement of blood glucose after a fast of at least 8 hours. A reading ≥126 mg/dL indicates diabetes. Also called fasting blood glucose (FBG) or fasting blood sugar (FBS)
free thyroxine index (FTI, T_7)	Calculation based on the amount of T_4 present and T_3 uptake, used to diagnose thyroid dysfunction
oral glucose tolerance test (OGTT)	Measurement of glucose levels in blood plasma after administration of a challenge dose of glucose to a fasting patient. Used to measure patient's ability to metabolize glucose. A value ≥200 mg/dL in the 2-hour sample indicates diabetes
radioactive iodine uptake test (RAIU)	A test that measures thyroid uptake of radioactive iodine as an evaluation of thyroid function
radioimmunoassay (RIA)	A method of measuring very small amounts of a substance, especially hormones, in blood plasma using radioactively labeled hormones and specific antibodies
thyroid scan	Visualization of the thyroid gland after administration of radioactive iodine
thyroxine-binding globulin (TBG) test	Test that measures the main protein that binds T_4 in the blood
transsphenoidal adenomectomy trans-sfē-NOY-dal ad-e-nō-MEK-tō-mē	Removal of a pituitary tumor through the sphenoid sinus (space in the sphenoid bone)

PASSport to Success® Go to the pronunciation glossary on the Student Resources to hear these words pronounced.

Box 16-6 Clinical Perspectives

Seasonal Affective Disorder: Some Light on the Subject

We all sense that long dark days make us blue and sap our motivation. Are these learned responses, or is there a physical basis for them? Studies have shown that the amount of light in the environment does have a physical effect on behavior. Evidence that light alters mood comes from people who are intensely affected by the dark days of winter—people who suffer from **seasonal affective disorder**, aptly abbreviated SAD. When days shorten, these people feel sleepy, depressed, and anxious. They tend to overeat, especially carbohydrates.

As light strikes the retina of the eye, it starts nerve impulses that decrease the amount of melatonin produced by the pineal gland in the brain. Because melatonin depresses mood, the final effect of light is to elevate mood. Daily exposure to bright lights has been found to improve the mood of most people with SAD. Exposure for 15 minutes after rising in the morning may be enough, but some people require longer sessions both morning and evening. Other aids include aerobic exercise, stress-management techniques, and antidepressant medications.

Terminology   Abbreviations

A1c	Glycated hemoglobin (test)	**LH**	Luteinizing hormone
ACTH	Adrenocorticotropic hormone	**MEN**	Multiple endocrine neoplasia
ADH	Antidiuretic hormone	**NPH**	Neutral protamine Hagedorn (insulin)
BS	Blood sugar	**OGTT**	Oral glucose tolerance test
CSII	Continuous subcutaneous insulin infusion	**PRL**	Prolactin
DM	Diabetes mellitus	**PTH**	Parathyroid hormone
FBG	Fasting blood glucose	**RAIU**	Radioactive iodine uptake
FBS	Fasting blood sugar	**RIA**	Radioimmunoassay
FPG	Fasting plasma glucose	**SIADH**	Syndrome of inappropriate antidiuretic hormone (secretion)
FSH	Follicle-stimulating hormone		
FTI	Free thyroxine index	**T1DM**	Type 1 diabetes mellitus
GDM	Gestational diabetes mellitus	**T2DM**	Type 2 diabetes mellitus
GH	Growth hormone	**T$_3$**	Triiodothyronine
HbA1c	Hemoglobin A1c; glycated hemoglobin	**T$_4$**	Thyroxine; tetraiodothyronine
^{131}I	Iodine-131 (radioactive iodine)	**T$_7$**	Free thyroxine index
IFG	Impaired fasting blood glucose	**TBG**	Thyroxine-binding globulin
IGT	Impaired glucose tolerance	**TSH**	Thyroid-stimulating hormone

Chapter Review

LABELING EXERCISE

Glands of the Endocrine System > Write the name of each numbered part on the corresponding line of the answer sheet.

Adrenals   Pituitary (hypophysis)
Ovaries   Testes
Pancreatic islets Thymus
Parathyroids   Thyroid
Pineal

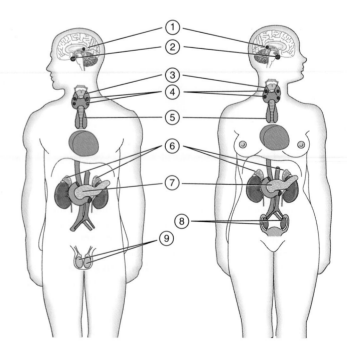

1. _____

2. _____

3. _____

4. _____

5. _____

6. _____

7. _____

8. _____

9. _____

Chapter Review (continued)

Terminology > Match the following terms and write the appropriate letter to the left of each number:

_____ **1.** thymus
_____ **2.** posterior pituitary
_____ **3.** hypothalamus
_____ **4.** islets
_____ **5.** pineal

a. gland that is regulated by light
b. pancreatic endocrine cells
c. part of the brain that controls the pituitary
d. gland important in immunity
e. gland that releases oxytocin

_____ **6.** epinephrine
_____ **7.** growth hormone
_____ **8.** cortisol
_____ **9.** glucagon
_____ **10.** melatonin

a. pancreatic hormone that regulates glucose metabolism
b. hormone produced by the adrenal medulla
c. hormone from the pineal gland
d. somatotropin
e. hormone produced by the adrenal cortex

_____ **11.** ADH
_____ **12.** T$_4$
_____ **13.** ACTH
_____ **14.** T2DM
_____ **15.** HbA1c

a. substance used to monitor blood glucose levels
b. pituitary hormone that regulates water balance
c. a form of diabetes
d. thyroxine
e. hormone that stimulates the adrenal cortex

_____ **16.** ketoacidosis
_____ **17.** myxedema
_____ **18.** Cushing syndrome
_____ **19.** acromegaly
_____ **20.** Addison disease

a. disorder that results from excess growth hormone
b. disorder caused by underactivity of the adrenal cortex
c. a result of uncontrolled diabetes
d. disorder caused by overactivity of the adrenal cortex
e. disorder caused by lack of thyroid hormone

Supplementary Terms

_____ **21.** sella turcica
_____ **22.** Hashimoto disease
_____ **23.** pheochromocytoma
_____ **24.** Simmonds disease
_____ **25.** craniopharyngioma

a. panhypopituitarism
b. tumor of the pituitary gland
c. chronic thyroiditis
d. bony depression that holds the pituitary
e. tumor of the adrenal medulla

Fill in the blanks:

26. The gland under the brain that controls other glands is the _____.

27. The gland in the neck that affects metabolic rate is the _____.

28. The endocrine glands located above the kidneys are the _____.

29. The most common endocrine disorder is _____.

30. Excess glucose in the blood is called _____.

Define the following words:

31. adrenomegaly (*a-drē-nō-MEG-a-lē*) _____.

32. hypopituitarism (*hī-pō-pi-TŪ-i-ta-rizm*) _____.

33. hypophysial (*hī-pō-FIZ-ē-al*) _____.

34. adrenopathy (*a-drē-NOP-a-thē*) _____.

35. thyroidectomy (*thī-roy-DEK-tō-mē*) _____.

36. endocrinologist (*en-dō-kri-NOL-ō-jist*) _____.

Chapter Review (continued)

Write words for the following definitions:

37. tumor of the pancreatic islets _____

38. inflammation of the hypophysis _____

39. pertaining to the adrenal cortex _____

Use the full name of the gland as the root to write words for the following definitions:

40. surgical removal of parathyroid _____
gland

41. removal of one half (hemi-) _____
of the thyroid gland

42. inflammation of the thyroid _____
gland

43. overactivity of the adrenal _____
gland

Use the root *thyr/o* to write words for the following definitions:

44. acting on the thyroid gland _____

45. destructive of (-lytic) thyroid _____
tissue

46. any disease of the thyroid gland _____

True–False > Examine the following statements. If the statement is true, write T in the first blank. If the statement is false, write F in the first blank and correct the statement by replacing the underlined word in the second blank.

47. Diabetes insipidus is caused by a lack of <u>thymosin.</u>   _____   _____

48. The hypophysis is the <u>pituitary</u> gland.   _____   _____

49. The inner region of an organ is the <u>cortex.</u>   _____   _____

50. The thyroid and parathyroids regulate the element <u>sodium.</u>   _____   _____

51. Goiter is an enlargement of the <u>pineal</u> gland.   _____   _____

52. <u>Type 1</u> diabetes mellitus always requires insulin.   _____   _____

53. Thyroid hormones contain the element <u>iodine.</u>   _____   _____

54. The adrenal cortex produces <u>steroid</u> hormones.   _____   _____

Eliminations > In each of the sets below, underline the term that does not fit in with the rest and explain the reason for your choice:

55. GH — TSH — FSH — PTH — ACTH

_____

56. Cushing syndrome — gigantism — dwarfism — acromegaly — thyrotoxicosis

_____

57. TBG — GDM — FPG — IGT — IFG

_____

58. testis — spleen — adrenals — parathyroids — pituitary

_____

Word Building > Write words for the following definitions using the word parts provided.

-ar   adren/o   -megal/o   -oma   thyr/o   -ic   -al   trop   -y   insul/o   path/o   -lytic

59. pertaining to pancreatic islet cells   _____

60. acting on the thyroid gland   _____

61. any disease of the adrenal gland   _____

62. destructive of thyroid tissue   _____

63. tumor of islet cells   _____

64. enlargement of the adrenal gland   _____

65. pertaining to the gland above the kidney   _____

66. enlargement of the thyroid gland   _____

67. acting on the adrenal gland   _____

68. any disease of the thyroid gland   _____

Word Analysis > Define each of the following words, and give the meaning of the word parts in each. Use a dictionary if necessary.

69. craniopharyngioma _____

   a. crani/o _____

   b. pharyng/i _____

   c. -oma _____

70. panhypopituitarism _____

   a. pan- _____

   b. hypo- _____

   c. pituitar _____

   d. -ism _____

71. pheochromocytoma _____

   a. phe/o _____

   b. chrom/o _____

   c. cyt/o _____

   d. -oma _____

Chapter Review (continued)

72. thyrotoxicosis _____

   a. thyr/o _____

   b. toxic/o _____

   c. -sis _____

PASSport
to Success®

Go to the word exercises on the Student Resources for additional review exercises.

Case Studies

▶ Case Study 16-1: Acute Pancreatitis

Two weeks after his emergency cardiac bypass surgery, R.B. was admitted to the hospital with acute pancreatitis, probably triggered by the trauma of the heart surgery. As a nurse, R.B. knew that the mild form of the disease was self-limiting, whereas severe pancreatitis has a mortality rate near 50%. Having survived heart surgery, he was now terrified of developing multisystem organ failure. He had once cared for a patient who died of necrotizing hemorrhagic pancreatitis.

On admission, R.B. had severe stabbing midepigastric pain that radiated to his back, nausea, vomiting, abdominal distention and rigidity, and jaundice. He also had a low-grade fever, hypotension, tachycardia, and decreased breath sounds over all lung fields. His cardiac enzymes were normal, but he showed an increase in serum leukocytes, amylase, and lipase. An abdominal CT scan showed pancreatic inflammation with edema. His chest radiograph showed bilateral pleural effusion and atelectasis.

R.B.'s treatments included NPO, an NG tube, medications to decrease his pain and gastric secretions, and supplemental oxygen. He was monitored for all physiologic parameters, with close attention paid to his fluid and electrolyte balance and intravascular volume. He recovered and was discharged after 6 days.

▶ Case Study 16-2: Hyperparathyroidism

B.E., a 58-year-old woman with a history of hypertension, had a partial nephrectomy 4 years ago for renal calculi. During a routine physical examination, her total serum calcium level was 10.8 mg/dL. Her parathyroid hormone level was WNL; she was in no apparent distress, and the remainder of her physical examination and laboratory data were noncontributory.

B.E. underwent exploratory surgery for an enlarged right superior parathyroid gland. The remaining three glands appeared normal. The enlarged gland was excised, and a biopsy was performed on the remaining glands. The pathology report showed an adenoma of the abnormal gland. On her first postoperative day, she reported perioral numbness and tingling. She had no other symptoms, but her serum calcium level was subnormal. She was given one ampule of calcium gluconate. Within 2 days, her calcium level had improved and she was discharged.

▶ Case Study 16-3: Diabetes Treatment With an Insulin Pump

M.G., a 32-year-old marketing executive, was diagnosed with type 1 diabetes at the age of 3 years. She vividly remembers her mother taking her to the doctor because she had an illness that caused her to feel extremely tired and very thirsty and hungry. She also had begun to wet her bed and had a cut on her knee that would not heal. Her mother had had gestational diabetes during her pregnancy with M.G., and at birth M.G. was described as having "macrosomia" because she weighed 10 lb.

M.G. has managed her disease with meticulous attention to her diet, exercise, preventive health care, regular blood glucose monitoring, and twice-daily injections of regular and NPH insulin, which she rotates among her upper arms, thighs, and abdomen. She continues in a smoking-cessation program supported by weekly acupuncture treatments. She maintains good control of her disease in spite of the inconvenience and time it consumes each day. She will be married next summer and would like to start a family. M.G.'s doctor suggested she try an insulin pump to give her more freedom and enhance her quality of life. After intensive training, she has received her pump. It is about the size of a beeper with a thin catheter that she introduces through a needle into her abdominal subcutaneous tissue. She can administer her insulin in a continuous subcutaneous insulin infusion (CSII) and in calculated meal bolus doses. She still has to test her

(continued)

Case Studies (continued)

blood for hyperglycemia and hypoglycemia and her urine for ketones when her blood sugar is too high. She hopes one day to have an islet transplantation.

CASE STUDY QUESTIONS

Multiple choice. Select the best answer and write the letter of your choice to the left of each number:

_____ 1. Necrotizing hemorrhagic pancreatitis can be described as:
   a. enlargement of the pancreas with anemia
   b. inflammation of the pancreas with tissue death and bleeding
   c. inflammation of the pancreas with overgrowth of tissue
   d. marsupialization of a pancreatic pseudocyst
   e. none of the above

_____ 2. R.B.'s midepigastric pain was located:
   a. inferior to the sternum
   b. periumbilical
   c. cephalad to the clavicle
   d. lateral to the anterior costal margins
   e. anterolateral

_____ 3. Intravascular volume and hemodynamic stability refer to:
   a. measured amount of urine in the drainage bag
   b. speed with which pancreatic fluid moves
   c. movement of cells through a flow cytometer
   d. body fluids and blood pressure
   e. blood count and clotting factors

_____ 4. Renal calculi are:
   a. kidney stones
   b. gallstones
   c. stomach ulcers
   d. bile obstructions
   e. muscle spasms

_____ 5. B.E.'s serum calcium was 10.8 mg/dL, which is:
   a. 5.4 micrograms of calcium in her serous fluid
   b. 10.8 grams of electrolytes in parathyroid hormone
   c. 10.8 milligrams of calcium in 100 mL of blood
   d. 21.6 liters of calcium in 100 g of serum
   e. 10.8 micrograms of calcium in 100 mL of serous parathyroid fluid

_____ 6. B.E. had perioral numbness and tingling. Perioral is:
   a. peripheral to any orifice
   b. lateral to the eye
   c. within the buccal mucosa
   d. around the mouth
   e. circumferential to the perineum

_____ 7. Gestational diabetes occurs:
   a. in a pregnant woman
   b. to any large fetus
   c. during menopause
   d. at the time of puberty
   e. in a large baby with high blood sugar

_____ 8. The term *macrosomia* describes:
   a. excessive weight gain during pregnancy
   b. a large body
   c. an excessive amount of sleep
   d. inability to sleep during pregnancy
   e. too much sugar in the amniotic fluid

_____ 9. M.G. injected the insulin into the subcutaneous tissue, which is:
   a. present only in the abdomen, thighs, and upper arms
   b. a topical application
   c. below the skin
   d. in a large artery
   e. above the pubic bone

_____ 10. An islet transplantation refers to:
   a. transfer of parathyroid cells to the liver
   b. excision of bovine pancreatic cells
   c. surgical insertion of an insulin pump into the abdomen
   d. a total pancreas and kidney transplantation
   e. transfer of insulin-secreting cells into a pancreas

Write the terms from the case studies with the following meanings:

11. yellowish color of the skin

_____

12. enzyme that digests fats

_____

13. surgical excision of a kidney

_____

14. tumor of a gland

_____

15. single-use glass injectable medication container

_____

16. high serum glucose

_____

Abbreviations. Define the following abbreviations:

17. NPO _____

18. NG _____

19. BUN _____

20. WNL _____

21. NPH _____

22. CSII _____

16

CHAPTER

17

The Nervous System and Behavioral Disorders

OBJECTIVES

After study of this chapter you should be able to:

1. Label diagrams showing components of the nervous system.
2. Briefly describe the functions of the regions of the brain.
3. Describe how the central nervous system is protected.
4. Compare the sympathetic and parasympathetic systems.
5. Identify and use word parts pertaining to the nervous system.
6. Describe the major disorders of the nervous system.
7. Describe the major behavioral disorders.
8. List some common symptoms of neurologic disorders.
9. Define abbreviations used in neurology.
10. Interpret case studies involving the nervous system.

PRETEST

Multiple choice. Select the best answer and write the letter of your choice to the left of each number.

___ 1. The basic cell of the nervous system is a(n):

   a. myofiber
   b. neuron
   c. osteoblast
   d. chondrocyte

___ 2. The largest part of the brain is the:

   a. cortex
   b. adrenal
   c. cerebrum
   d. pituitary

___ 3. The midbrain, pons, and medulla oblongata make up the:

   a. brainstem   c. cerebellum
   b. spinal cord   d. thymus

___ 4. Involuntary responses are controlled by the:

   a. voluntary nervous system
   b. somatic nervous system
   c. autonomic nervous system
   d. diaphragm

___ 5. A simple response that requires few cells is a:

   a. reflex   c. sensation
   b. mutation   d. stimulus

___ 6. A disorder, often of unknown cause, characterized by seizures is called:

   a. cystic fibrosis   c. epilepsy
   b. spina bifida   d. thyrotoxicosis

___ 7. An instrument used to study the electric activity of the brain is the:

   a. electrocardiograph
   b. electroencephalograph
   c. CT scanner
   d. sonograph

___ 8. An extreme, persistent fear is a(n):

   a. palliative   c. phobia
   b. prognosis   d. analgesic

17

The nervous system and the endocrine system coordinate and control the body. Together they regulate our responses to the environment and maintain homeostasis. Whereas the endocrine system functions by means of circulating hormones, the nervous system functions by means of electric impulses and locally released chemicals called **neurotransmitters**.

Organization of the Nervous System

For study purposes, the nervous system may be divided into two parts:

- the **central nervous system (CNS)**, consisting of the **brain** and **spinal cord** (Fig. 17-1)

- the **peripheral nervous system (PNS)**, consisting of all nervous tissue outside the brain and spinal cord.

Functionally, the nervous system can be divided into the:

- **somatic nervous system**, which controls skeletal muscles

- **visceral** or **autonomic nervous system (ANS)**, which controls smooth muscle, cardiac muscle, and glands. The ANS regulates responses to stress and helps to maintain homeostasis.

Two types of cells are found in the nervous system. **Neurons**, or nerve cells, make up the conducting tissue of the nervous system. **Neuroglia** are the cells that support and protect nervous tissue.

The Neuron

The neuron is the nervous system's basic functional unit (Fig. 17-2). Each neuron has two types of fibers extending from the cell body:

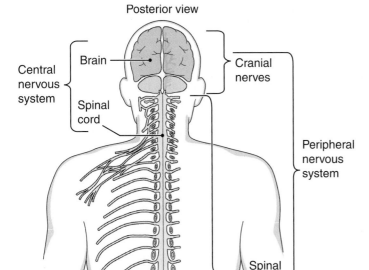

Posterior view

Central nervous system

Brain

Spinal cord

Cranial nerves

Peripheral nervous system

Spinal nerves

Figure 17-1 **Anatomic divisions of the nervous system.**

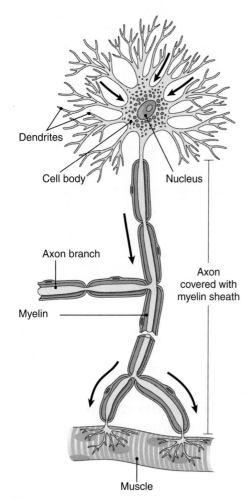

Figure 17-2 **A motor neuron.** The break in the axon denotes length. The *arrows* show the direction of the nerve impulse.

- The **dendrite** carries impulses toward the cell body.
- The **axon** carries impulses away from the cell body.

Some axons are covered with **myelin**, a whitish, fatty material that insulates and protects the axon and speeds electric conduction. Axons so covered are described as *myelinated*, and they make up the **white matter** of the nervous system. Unmyelinated tissue makes up the nervous system's **gray matter**.

Each neuron is part of a pathway that carries information through the nervous system. A neuron that transmits impulses toward the CNS is a **sensory**, or **afferent**, neuron; a neuron that transmits impulses away from the CNS is a **motor**, or **efferent**, neuron. There are also connecting cells within the CNS called **interneurons**.

A **synapse** is the point of contact between two neurons. At the synapse, energy is passed from one cell to another, usually by means of a neurotransmitter, and sometimes by direct transfer of electric current.

See the Student Resources for the animation *The Synapse and the Nerve Impulse*, which illustrates nerve impulse conduction.

Nerves

Individual neuron fibers are held together in bundles like wires in a cable. If this bundle is part of the PNS, it is called a **nerve**. A collection of cell bodies along the pathway of a nerve is a **ganglion**. A few nerves (sensory nerves) contain only sensory neurons, and a few (motor nerves) contain only motor neurons, but most contain both types of fibers and are described as *mixed nerves*.

The Brain

The brain is nervous tissue contained within the cranium. It consists of the **cerebrum, diencephalon, brainstem,** and **cerebellum.** The cerebrum is the largest part of the brain (Fig. 17-3); it is composed largely of white matter with a thin outer layer of gray matter, the **cerebral cortex.** It is within the cortex that the higher brain functions of memory, reasoning, and abstract thought occur. The cerebrum's distinct surface is formed by grooves, or **sulci** (singular: sulcus), and raised areas, or **gyri** (singular: gyrus) that provide additional surface area (Fig. 17-4). The cerebrum is divided into two hemispheres by a deep groove, the longitudinal fissure. Each hemisphere is further divided into lobes with specialized functions (see Fig. 17-4). The lobes are named for the skull bones under which they lie.

The remaining parts of the brain are as follows:

- The diencephalon contains the **thalamus**, the **hypothalamus**, and the pituitary gland (see Fig. 17-3). The thalamus receives sensory information and directs it to the proper portion of the cortex. The hypothalamus controls the pituitary and forms a link between the endocrine and nervous systems.

- The brainstem (see Fig. 17-3) consists of the:
  - **midbrain**, which contains reflex centers for improved vision and hearing
  - **pons**, which forms a bulge on the anterior surface of the brainstem. It contains fibers that connect the brain's different regions.
  - **medulla oblongata**, which connects the brain with the spinal cord. All impulses passing to and from the brain travel through this region. The medulla also has vital centers for control of heart rate, respiration, and blood pressure.

- The cerebellum is under the cerebrum and dorsal to the pons and medulla (see Fig. 17-3). Like the cerebrum, it is divided into two hemispheres. The cerebellum helps to control voluntary muscle movements and to maintain posture, coordination, and balance.

Protecting the Brain

Within the brain are four **ventricles** (cavities) in which **cerebrospinal fluid (CSF)** is formed. This fluid circulates

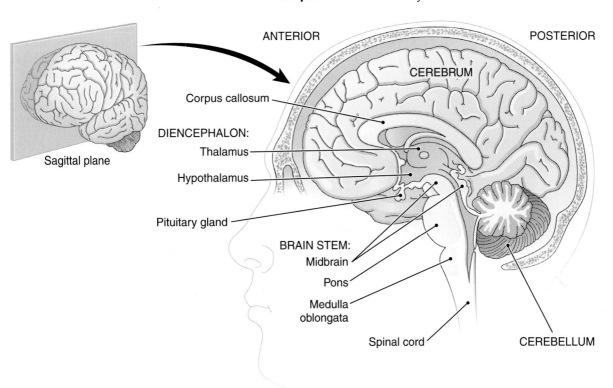

ANTERIOR   POSTERIOR

CEREBRUM

Corpus callosum

DIENCEPHALON:
  Thalamus
  Hypothalamus

Pituitary gland

BRAIN STEM:
  Midbrain
  Pons
  Medulla
  oblongata

Spinal cord   CEREBELLUM

Sagittal plane

Figure 17-3 **Brain, sagittal section.** The main divisions are shown.

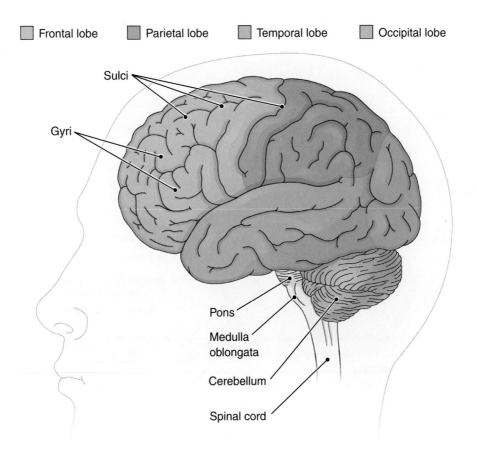

☐ Frontal lobe   ☐ Parietal lobe   ☐ Temporal lobe   ☐ Occipital lobe

Sulci

Gyri

Pons

Medulla
oblongata

Cerebellum

Spinal cord

Figure 17-4 **External surface of the brain, lateral view.** The lobes and surface features of the cerebrum are shown as well as other divisions of the brain and the spinal cord.

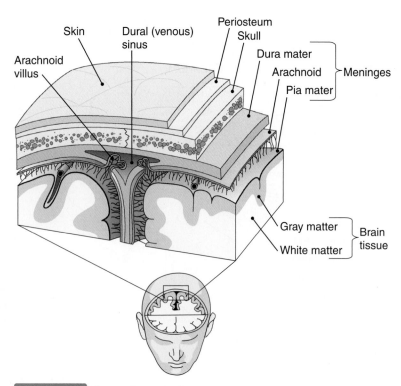

around the brain and spinal cord, acting as a protective cushion for these tissues.

Covering the brain and the spinal cord are three protective layers, together called the **meninges** (Fig. 17-5). All are named with the Latin word *mater*, meaning "mother," to indicate their protective function. They are the:

- **dura mater**, the outermost and toughest of the three. *Dura* means "hard."

- **arachnoid mater**, the thin, weblike middle layer. It is named for the Latin word for spider, because it resembles a spider web.

- **pia mater**, the thin, vascular inner layer, attached directly to the tissue of the brain and spinal cord. *Pia* means "tender."

Twelve pairs of **cranial nerves** connect with the brain (Fig. 17-6). These nerves are identified by Roman numerals and also by name. Box 17-1 is a summary chart of the cranial nerves.

Figure 17-5 **The meninges.** The three protective layers and adjacent tissue are shown in a frontal section of the head.

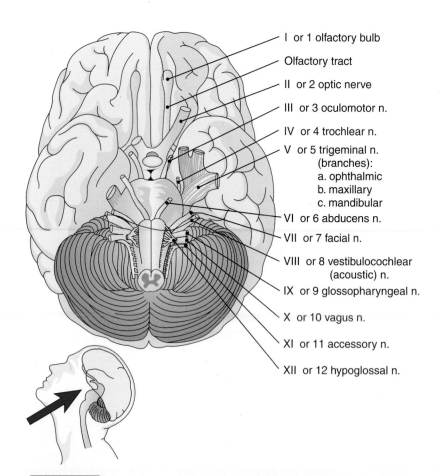

Figure 17-6 **Cranial nerves.** The 12 nerves are shown on one side in an inferior view.

Box 17-1 For Your Reference

The Cranial Nerves

NUMBER	NAME	FUNCTION
I	**olfactory** *ol-FAK-tō-rē*	carries impulses for the sense of smell
II	**optic** *OP-tik*	carries impulses for the sense of vision
III	**oculomotor** *ok-ū-lō-MŌ-tor*	controls movement of eye muscles
IV	**trochlear** *TROK-lē-ar*	controls a muscle of the eyeball
V	**trigeminal** *trī-JEM-i-nal*	carries sensory impulses from the face; controls chewing muscles
VI	**abducens** *ab-DŪ-sens*	controls a muscle of the eyeball
VII	**facial** *FĀ-shal*	controls muscles of facial expression, salivary glands, and tear glands; conducts some impulses for taste
VIII	**vestibulocochlear** *ves-tib-ū-lō-KOK-lē-ar*	conducts impulses for hearing and equilibrium; also called auditory or acoustic nerve
IX	**glossopharyngeal** *glos-ō-fa-RIN-jē-al*	conducts sensory impulses from tongue and pharynx; stimulates parotid salivary gland and partly controls swallowing
X	**vagus** *VĀ-gus*	supplies most organs of thorax and abdomen; controls digestive secretions
XI	**spinal accessory** *ak-SES-ō-rē*	controls muscles of the neck
XII	**hypoglossal** *hī-pō-GLOS-al*	controls muscles of the tongue

The Spinal Cord

The spinal cord begins at the medulla oblongata and tapers to an end between the first and second lumbar vertebrae (Fig. 17-7). It has enlargements in the cervical and lumbar regions, where nerves for the arms and legs join the cord. Seen in cross section (Fig. 17-8), the spinal cord has a central area of gray matter surrounded by white matter. The gray matter projects toward the posterior and the anterior as the dorsal and ventral horns. The white matter contains the ascending and descending **tracts** (fiber bundles) that carry impulses to and from the brain. A central canal contains CSF.

The Spinal Nerves

Thirty-one pairs of **spinal nerves** connect with the spinal cord (see Fig. 17-7). These nerves are grouped in the segments of the cord as follows:

- Cervical: 8
- Thoracic: 12
- Lumbar: 5
- Sacral: 5
- Coccygeal: 1

Each nerve joins the cord by two **roots** (see Fig. 17-8). The dorsal, or posterior, root carries sensory impulses into the cord; the ventral, or anterior, root carries motor impulses away from the cord and out toward a muscle or gland. An enlargement on the dorsal root, the dorsal root ganglion, has the cell bodies of sensory neurons carrying impulses toward the CNS (see Fig. 17-8).

Reflexes

A simple response that requires few neurons is a **reflex** (Fig. 17-9). In a spinal reflex, impulses travel through

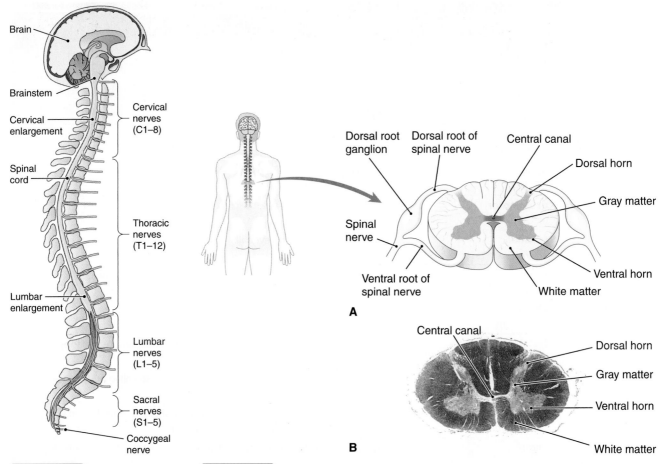

Dorsal root
ganglion

Dorsal root of
spinal nerve

Central canal

Dorsal horn

Gray matter

Spinal
nerve

Ventral root of
spinal nerve

Ventral horn

White matter

A

Central canal

Dorsal horn

Gray matter

Ventral horn

White matter

B

Figure 17-7 **Spinal cord, lateral view.** The divisions of the spinal nerves are shown.

Figure 17-8 **Spinal cord, cross section.** (*A*) Diagram shows the organization of gray and white matter and the roots of the spinal nerves. (*B*) Microscopic view of the spinal cord in cross section (magnification 5×).

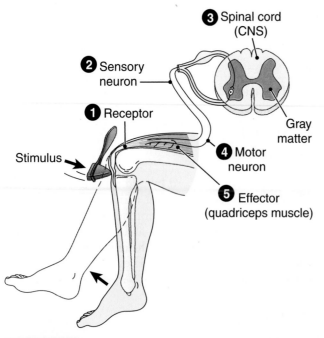

Figure 17-9 **A reflex pathway.** The patellar (knee-jerk) reflex is shown, with numbers indicating the sequence of impulses.

the spinal cord only and do not reach the brain. An example of this type of response is the knee-jerk reflex used in physical examinations. Most neurologic responses, however, involve complex interactions among multiple neurons in the CNS.

The Autonomic Nervous System

The ANS is the division of the nervous system that controls the involuntary actions of muscles and glands (Fig. 17-10). The ANS itself has two divisions:

- The **sympathetic nervous system** motivates our response to stress, the so-called fight-or-flight response. It increases heart rate and respiration rate, stimulates the adrenal gland, and delivers more blood to skeletal muscles.

- The **parasympathetic nervous system** returns the body to a steady state and stimulates maintenance activities, such as digestion of food. Most organs are controlled by both systems and, in general, the two systems have opposite effects on a given organ.

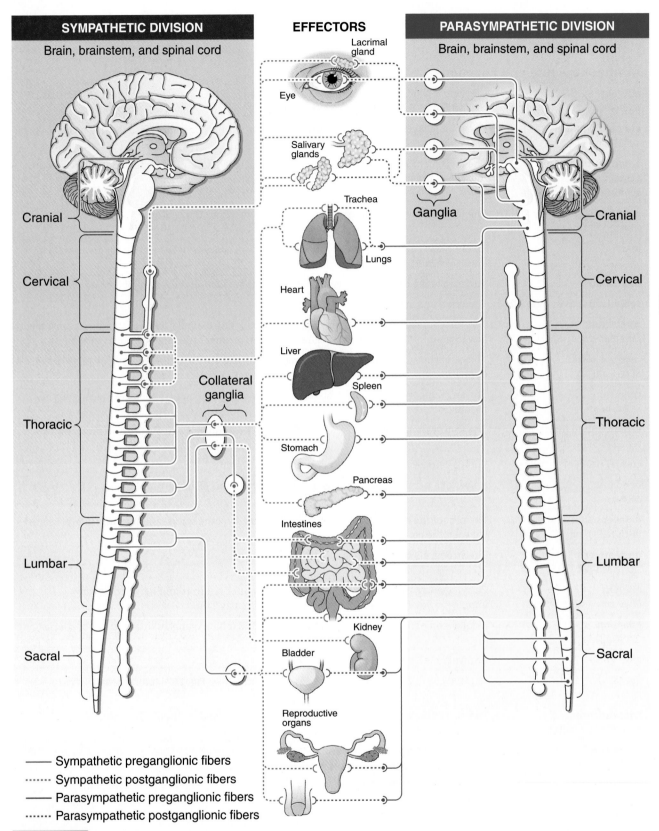

SYMPATHETIC DIVISION	EFFECTORS	PARASYMPATHETIC DIVISION
Brain, brainstem, and spinal cord		Brain, brainstem, and spinal cord

Lacrimal gland
Eye
Salivary glands
Ganglia
Trachea
Lungs
Heart
Liver
Spleen
Stomach
Pancreas
Intestines
Kidney
Bladder
Reproductive organs

Cranial
Cervical
Thoracic
Lumbar
Sacral

Collateral ganglia

—— Sympathetic preganglionic fibers
······ Sympathetic postganglionic fibers
—— Parasympathetic preganglionic fibers
······ Parasympathetic postganglionic fibers

Figure 17-10 **Autonomic nervous system.** Each ANS pathway has two neurons, as shown by the solid and dashed lines. The diagram shows only one side of the body for each division (sympathetic and parasympathetic).

17

Terminology Key Terms

Normal Structure and Function

afferent AF-er-ent	Carrying toward a given point, such as the sensory neurons and nerves that carry impulses toward the CNS (root *fer* means "to carry")
arachnoid mater a-RAK-noyd	The middle layer of the meninges (from the Greek word for spider, because this tissue resembles a spider web)
autonomic nervous system (ANS) aw-tō-NOM-ik	The division of the nervous system that regulates involuntary activities, controlling smooth muscles, cardiac muscle, and glands; the visceral nervous system
axon AK-son	The fiber of a neuron that conducts impulses away from the cell body
brain	The nervous tissue contained within the cranium; consists of the cerebrum, diencephalon, brainstem, and cerebellum (root: *encephal/o*)
brainstem	The part of the brain that consists of the midbrain, pons, and medulla oblongata
central nervous system (CNS)	The brain and spinal cord
cerebellum ser-e-BEL-um	The posterior portion of the brain dorsal to the pons and medulla; helps to coordinate movement and to maintain balance and posture (*cerebellum* means "little brain") (root: *cerebell/o*)
cerebral cortex SER-e-bral	The cerebrum's thin surface layer of gray matter (the cortex is the outer region of an organ) (root: *cortic/o*)
cerebrum SER-e-brum	The large upper portion of the brain; it is divided into two hemispheres by the longitudinal fissure (root: *cerebr/o*)
cerebrospinal fluid (CSF) ser-e-brō-SPĪ-nal	The watery fluid that circulates in and around the brain and spinal cord as a protection
cranial nerves	The 12 pairs of nerves that are connected to the brain
dendrite DEN-drī-t	A fiber of a neuron that conducts impulses toward the cell body
diencephalon dī-en-SEF-a-lon	The part of the brain that contains the thalamus, hypothalamus, and pituitary gland; located between the cerebrum and the brainstem
dura mater DŬ-ra MĀ-ter	The strong, fibrous outermost layer of the meninges
efferent EF-er-ent	Carrying away from a given point, such as the motor neurons and nerves that carry impulses away from the CNS (root *fer* means "to carry")
ganglion GANG-glē-on	A collection of neuron cell bodies outside the CNS (plural: ganglia) (roots: *gangli/o*, *ganglion/o*)
gray matter	Unmyelinated tissue of the nervous system
gyrus JĪ-rus	A raised convolution of the surface of the cerebrum (see Fig. 17-4) (plural: gyri)
hypothalamus hī-pō-THAL-a-mus	The part of the brain that controls the pituitary gland and maintains homeostasis
interneuron in-ter-NŪR-on	Any neuron located between a sensory and a motor neuron in a neural pathway, such as the neurons that transmit impulses within the CNS
medulla oblongata me-DUL-la ob-long-GA-ta	The portion of the brain that connects with the spinal cord. It has vital centers for control of respiration, heart rate, and blood pressure (root: *medull/o*). Often called simply medulla
meninges men-IN-jēz	The three membranes that cover the brain and spinal cord (see Fig. 17-5) (singular: meninx) (roots: *mening/o*, *meninge/o*)
midbrain	The part of the brainstem between the diencephalon and the pons; contains centers for coordination of reflexes for vision and hearing
motor	Producing movement; describes neurons and nerves that carry impulses away from the CNS

(continued)

Terminology	**Key Terms** (continued)
myelin MĪ-e-lin	A whitish, fatty substance that surrounds certain axons of the nervous system
neuroglia nū-ROG-lē-a	The support cells of the nervous system; also called glial cells (from *glia* meaning "glue") (root: *gli/o*)
neuron NŪ-ron	The basic unit of the nervous system; a nerve cell
neurotransmitter nū-rō-TRANS-mit-er	A chemical that transmits energy across a synapse. Examples are epinephrine, acetylcholine (a-sē-til-KŌ-lēn), serotonin (ser-ō-TŌ-nin), and dopamine (DŌ-pa-mēn)
nerve	A bundle of neuron fibers outside the CNS (root: *neur/o*)
parasympathetic nervous system	The part of the automatic nervous system that reverses the response to stress and restores homeostasis. It slows heart rate and respiration rate and stimulates digestive, urinary, and reproductive activities
peripheral nervous system (PNS) per-IF-er-al	The portion of the nervous system outside the CNS
pia mater PĒ-a MĀ-ter	The innermost layer of the meninges
pons ponz	A rounded area on the ventral surface of the brainstem; contains fibers that connect brain regions; adjective: pontine (PON-tēn)
reflex RĒ-fleks	A simple, rapid, and automatic response to a stimulus
root	A branch of a spinal nerve that connects with the spinal cord; the dorsal (posterior) root joins the spinal cord's dorsal gray horn; the ventral (anterior) root joins the spinal cord's ventral gray horn (root: *radicul/o*)
sensory SEN-so-rē	Describing neurons and nerves that carry impulses toward the CNS
somatic nervous system	The division of the nervous system that controls skeletal (voluntary) muscles
spinal cord	The nervous tissue contained within the spinal column; extends from the medulla oblongata to the second lumbar vertebra (root: *myel/o*)
spinal nerves	The 31 pairs of nerves that connect with the spinal cord
sulcus SUL-kus	A shallow furrow or groove, as on the surface of the cerebrum (see Fig. 17-4) (plural: sulci)
sympathetic nervous system	The part of the autonomic nervous system that mobilizes a response to stress; increases heart rate and respiration rate and delivers more blood to skeletal muscles
synapse SIN-aps	The junction between two neurons; also the junction between a motor neuron and a muscle or gland
thalamus THAL-a-mus	The part of the brain that receives all sensory impulses, except those for the sense of smell, and directs them to the proper portion of the cerebral cortex (root: *thalam/o*)
tract trakt	A bundle of neuron fibers within the CNS
ventricle VEN-trik-l	A small cavity, such as one of the cavities in the brain in which CSF is formed (root: *ventricul/o*)
visceral nervous system	The autonomic nervous system
white matter	Myelinated tissue of the nervous system

17

PASSport to Success®

Go to the pronunciation glossary on the Student Resources to hear these words pronounced.

Word Parts Pertaining to the Nervous System

See Tables 17-1 to 17-3.

Table 17-1	Roots for the Nervous System and the Spinal Cord		
Root	**Meaning**	**Example**	**Definition of Example**
neur/o, neur/i	nervous system, nervous tissue, nerve	neurotrophin nū-rō-TRŌ-fin	factor that promotes nerve growth (*troph/o* means "nourish")
gli/o	neuroglia	glial GLĪ-al	pertaining to neuroglia
gangli/o, ganglion/o	ganglion	ganglioma gang-glē-Ō-ma	tumor of a ganglion
mening/o, meninge/o	meninges	meningocele me-NING-gō-sēl	hernia of the meninges
myel/o	spinal cord (also bone marrow)	hematomyelia hē-ma-tō-mī-Ē-lē-a	hemorrhage into the spinal cord
radicul/o	spinal nerve root	radiculopathy ra-dik-ū-LOP-a-thē	any disease of a spinal nerve root

EXERCISE 17-1

Define the following adjectives:

1. neural (NŪ-ral) _____ pertaining to a nerve or the nervous system _____

2. neuroglial (nū-ROG-lē-al) _____

3. radicular (ra-DIK-ū-lar) _____

4. meningeal (me-NIN-jē-al) _____

5. ganglionic (gang-glē-ON-ik) _____

Fill in the blanks:

6. Myelodysplasia (mī-e-lō-dis-PLĀ-sē-a) is abnormal development of the _____ .

7. A neurotropic (nū-rō-TROP-ik) dye has an affinity for the _____ .

8. Meningococci (me-ning-gō-KOK-sī) are bacteria (cocci) that infect the _____ .

9. Radiculalgia (ra-dik-ū-LAL-jē-a) is pain caused by irritation of a(n) _____ .

Define the following terms:

10. ganglionectomy (gang-glē-o-NEK-tō-mē) _____

11. polyradiculitis (pol-ē-ra-dik-ū-LĪ-tis) _____

12. neurolysis (nū-ROL-i-sis) _____

13. meningioma (me-nin-jē-Ō-ma) (combining vowel is i) _____

14. myelography (mī-e-LOG-ra-fē) _____

Write words for the following definitions:

15. tumor of glial cells _____

16. any disease of the nervous system _____

17. inflammation of the spinal cord _____

18. pain in a nerve _____

19. x-ray image of the spinal cord _____

Table 17-2	Roots for the Brain		
Root	**Meaning**	**Example**	**Definition of Example**
encephal/o	brain	anencephaly *an-en-SEF-a-lē*	absence of a brain
cerebr/o	cerebrum (loosely, brain)	infracerebral *in-fra-SER-e-bral*	below the cerebrum
cortic/o	cerebral cortex, outer portion	corticospinal *kor-ti-kō-SPĪ-nal*	pertaining to the cerebral cortex and spinal cord
cerebell/o	cerebellum	supracerebellar *sū-pra-ser-e-BEL-ar*	above the cerebellum
thalam/o	thalamus	thalamotomy *thal-a-MOT-ō-mē*	incision of the thalamus
ventricul/o	cavity, ventricle	intraventricular *in-tra-ven-TRIK-ū-lar*	within a ventricle
medull/o	medulla oblongata (also spinal cord)	medullary *MED-ū-lar-ē*	pertaining to the medulla
psych/o	mind	psychogenic *sī-kō-JEN-ik*	originating in the mind
narc/o	stupor, unconsciousness	narcosis *nar-KŌ-sis*	state of stupor induced by drugs
somn/o, somn/i	sleep	somnolence *SOM-nō-lens*	sleepiness

17

EXERCISE **17-2**

Fill in the blanks:

1. An electroencephalogram (*ē-lek-trō-en-SEF-a-lō-gram*) (EEG) is a record of the electric activity of the _____.

2. The term decerebrate (*dē-SER-e-brāt*) refers to functional loss in the _____.

3. The hypothalamus (*hī-pō-THAL-a-mus*) is below the _____.

4. A psychoactive (*sī-kō-AK-tiv*) drug has an effect on the _____.

5. A narcotic (*nar-KOT-ik*) is a drug that causes _____.

6. Somnambulism (*som-NAM-bū-lizm*) means walking during _____.

7. The term cerebrovascular (*ser-ē-brō-VAS-kū-lar*) refers to blood vessels in the _____.

Write an adjective for the following definitions. Note the endings.

8. pertaining to (-al) the cerebrum _____

9. pertaining to (-al) the cerebral cortex _____

10. pertaining to (-ic) the thalamus _____

11. pertaining to (-ar) the cerebellum _____

12. pertaining to (-ar) a ventricle _____

Define the following words:

13. psychology (*sī-KOL-ō-jē*) _____

14. cerebrospinal (*ser-e-brō-SPĪ-nal*) _____

15. encephalopathy (*en-sef-a-LOP-a-thē*) _____

16. insomnia (*in-SOM-nē-a*) _____

17. extramedullary (*eks-tra-MED-ū-lar-ē*) _____

18. ventriculotomy (*ven-trik-ū-LOT-ō-mē*) _____

Write words for the following definitions:

19. above the cerebrum _____

20. inflammation of the brain _____

21. within the cerebellum _____

22. pertaining to the cerebral cortex and the thalamus _____

23. radiograph of a ventricle _____

Table 17-3	**Suffixes for the Nervous System**		
Suffix	**Meaning**	**Example**	**Definition of Example**
-phasia	speech	heterophasia *het-er-ō-FĀ-zē-a*	uttering words that are different from those intended
-lalia	speech, babble	coprolalia *kop-rō-LĀ-lē-a*	compulsive use of obscene words (*copro-* means "feces")
-lexia	reading	bradylexia *brad-ē-LEK-sē-a*	slowness in reading
-plegia	paralysis	tetraplegia *tet-ra-PLĒ-jē-a*	paralysis of all four limbs
-paresis*	partial paralysis, weakness	hemiparesis *hem-i-pa-RĒ-sis*	partial paralysis of one side of the body
-lepsy	seizure	narcolepsy *NAR-kō-lep-sē*	condition marked by sudden episodes of sleep
-phobia*	persistent, irrational fear	agoraphobia *ag-o-ra-FŌ-bē-a*	fear of being in a public place (from Greek *agora*, meaning "marketplace")
-mania*	excited state, obsession	megalomania *meg-a-lō-MĀ-nē-a*	exaggerated self-importance; "delusions of grandeur"

*May be used alone as a word.

EXERCISE **17-3**

Fill in the blanks:

1. Another term for quadriplegia (*kwa-dri-PLĒ-jē-a*) is _____.

2. Echolalia (*ek-ō-LĀ-lē-a*) refers to repetitive _____.

3. A person with alexia (*a-LEK-sē-a*) lacks the ability to _____.

4. Epilepsy (*EP-i-lep-sē*) is a disease characterized by _____.

5. In myoparesis (*mī-ō-pa-RĒ-sis*), a muscle shows _____.

Define the following words:

6. cardioplegia (*kar-dē-ō-PLĒ-jē-a*) _____.

7. aphasia (*a-FĀ-zē-a*) _____.

8. dyslexia (*dis-LEK-sē-a*) _____.

9. pyromania (*pī-rō-MĀ-nē-a*) _____.

10. gynephobia (*jin-e-FŌ-bē-a*) _____.

11. quadriparesis (*kwa-dri-pa-RĒ-sis*) _____.

Write words for the following definitions:

12. slowness in speech (-lalia)   _____

13. paralysis of one side (hemi-) of the body   _____

14. fear of night and darkness   _____

15. fear of (or abnormal sensitivity to) light   _____

17

Clinical Aspects of the Nervous System

Vascular Disorders

The term **cerebrovascular accident (CVA)**, or **stroke**, applies to any occurrence that deprives brain tissue of oxygen. These events include blockage in a vessel that supplies the brain, a ruptured blood vessel, or some other damage that leads to hemorrhage within the brain. Stroke is the third leading cause of death in developed countries, after cancer and heart attack (myocardial infarction), and is a leading cause of **paralysis** and other neurologic disabilities. Risk factors for a stroke include hypertension, atherosclerosis, heart disease, diabetes mellitus, and cigarette smoking. Heredity is also a factor.

PASSport to Success See the animation *Stroke* on the Student Resources.

THROMBOSIS

Thrombosis is the formation of a blood clot in a vessel. Often, in cases of CVA, thrombosis occurs in the carotid artery, the large vessel in the neck that supplies the brain. Sudden blockage by an obstruction traveling from another part of the body is described as an **embolism**. In cases of stroke, the embolus usually originates in the heart.

These obstructions can be diagnosed by **cerebral angiography** with radiopaque dye, computed tomographic (CT) scans, and other radiographic techniques. In cases of thrombosis, surgeons can remove the blocked section of a vessel and insert a graft. If the carotid artery leading to the brain is involved, a **carotid endarterec-tomy** may be performed to open the vessel. Thrombolytic drugs for dissolving ("busting") such clots are also available.

ANEURYSM

An **aneurysm** (Fig. 17-11) is a localized dilation of a vessel that may rupture and cause hemorrhage. An aneurysm may be congenital or may arise from other causes, especially atherosclerosis, which weakens the vessel wall. Hypertension then contributes to its rupture.

The effects of cerebral hemorrhage vary from massive functional loss to mild sensory or motor impairment, depending on the degree of damage. **Aphasia**, loss or impairment of speech communication, is a common aftereffect. **Hemiplegia** (paralysis of one side of the body) on the side opposite the damage is also seen. It has been found that in cases of hemorrhage, as in other forms of brain injury, that immediate retraining therapy may help to restore lost function.

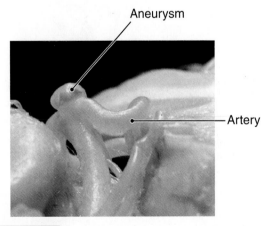

Figure 17-11 **Aneurysm.** A thin-walled aneurysm protrudes from an artery.

Trauma

A **cerebral contusion** is a bruise to the brain's surface, usually caused by a blow to the head. Blood escapes from local vessels, but the injury is not deep.

A more serious injury may cause bleeding into or around the meninges, resulting in a hematoma, a localized collection of clotted blood. Damage to an artery from a skull fracture, usually on the side of the head, may be the cause of an **epidural hematoma** (Fig. 17-12), which appears between the dura mater and the skull bone. The rapidly accumulating blood puts pressure on local vessels and interrupts blood flow to the brain. There may be headache, loss of consciousness, or **hemiparesis** (partial paralysis) on the side opposite the blow. Diagnosis is made by CT scan or magnetic resonance imaging (MRI). If pressure is not relieved within 1 or 2 days, death results.

A **subdural hematoma** (see Fig. 17-12) often results from a blow to the front or back of the head, as when the moving head hits a stationary object. The force of the blow separates the dura from the underlying arachnoid. Blood from a damaged vessel, usually a vein, slowly enters this space. The gradual blood accumulation puts pressure on the brain, causing headache, weakness, and **dementia**. If there is continued bleeding, death results. Figure 17-12

also shows a site of bleeding into the brain tissue itself, forming an intracerebral hematoma.

A cerebral **concussion** results from a blow to the head or from a fall and is usually followed by temporary loss of consciousness and a short period of amnesia. Aftereffects of a concussion may include headache, dizziness, vomiting, fatigue, and even paralysis, among other symptoms. Damage that occurs on the side of the brain opposite a blow as the brain is thrown against the skull is described as a **contrecoup** (*kon-tre-KŪ*) **injury** (from French, meaning "counterblow").

Other injuries may damage the brain directly. Injury to the base of the brain may involve vital centers in the medulla and interfere with respiration and cardiac functions.

Confusion and Coma

Confusion is a state of reduced comprehension, coherence, and reasoning ability resulting in inappropriate responses to environmental stimuli. Confusion may worsen to include loss of language ability, memory loss, reduced alertness, and emotional changes. This condition may accompany a head injury, drug toxicity, extensive surgery, organ failure, infection, or degenerative disease.

Coma is a state of unconsciousness from which one cannot be aroused. Causes of coma include brain injury, **epilepsy**, toxins, metabolic imbalance (such as the ketoacidosis or glucose imbalances associated with diabetes mellitus), and respiratory, hepatic, or renal failure.

Health care professionals use various responses to evaluate coma, for example, reflex behavior and responses to touch, pressure, and mild pain, as from a light pin prick. Laboratory tests, **electroencephalography** (**EEG**), and sometimes CT and MRI scans help to identify the causes of coma.

Infection

Inflammation of the meninges, or **meningitis**, is usually caused by bacteria that enter through the ear, nose, or throat or are carried by the blood. One of these organisms, the meningococcus (*Neisseria meningitidis*), is responsible for meningitis epidemics among individuals living in close quarters. Other bacteria implicated in cases of meningitis include *Haemophilus influenzae*, *Streptococcus pneumoniae*, and *Escherichia coli*. A stiff neck is a common symptom. The presence of pus or lymphocytes in spinal fluid is also characteristic.

Physicians can withdraw fluid for diagnosis by a **lumbar puncture** (Fig. 17-13), using a needle to remove CSF from the meninges in the lumbar region of the spine. This fluid can be examined for white blood cells and bacteria in the case of meningitis, for red blood cells in the case of brain injury, or for tumor cells. The fluid can also be analyzed chemically. Normally, spinal fluid is clear, with glucose and chlorides present but no protein and very few cells.

Figure 17-12   Cranial hematomas. Location of epidural, subdural, and intracerebral hematomas are shown.

A

Third lumbar vertebra

Dura mater

Subarachnoid
space

B

Figure 17-13 **Lumbar puncture.** (*A*) Position of the patient for a lumbar puncture. (*B*) CSF is withdrawn from the subarachnoid space between the third and fourth or fourth and fifth lumbar vertebrae.

Other conditions that can cause meningitis and **encephalitis** (inflammation of the brain) include viral infections, tuberculosis, and syphilis. Viruses that can involve the CNS include the poliovirus, rabies virus, herpesvirus, HIV (human immunodeficiency virus), tick- and mosquito-borne viruses, such as West Nile virus, and rarely, viruses that ordinarily cause relatively mild diseases, such as measles and chickenpox. Aseptic meningitis is a benign, nonbacterial form of the disease caused by a virus.

Varicella–zoster virus, which causes chickenpox, is also responsible for **shingles**, a nerve infection. If someone had chickenpox as a child, the latent virus can become reactivated later in life and spread along peripheral nerves, causing an itching, blistering rash. The name *shingles* comes from the Latin word for belt, as the shingles rash is often near or around the waist. A vaccine is now available for people over 60, and childhood chickenpox vaccinations will prevent shingles in the future.

Neoplasms

Almost all tumors that originate in the nervous system are tumors of nonconducting support cells, the neuroglia. These growths are termed **gliomas** and may be named for the specific cell type involved, such as **astrocytoma**, oligo-dendroglioma, or **neurilemoma** (schwannoma). Because they tend not to metastasize, these tumors may be described as benign. However, they do harm by compressing brain tissue (Fig. 17-14). The symptoms they cause depend on their size and location. There may be **seizures**, headache, vomiting, muscle weakness, or interference with a special sense, such as vision or hearing. If present, edema and **hydrocephalus**, accumulation of excess CSF in the ventricles, add to the tumor's effects (Fig. 17-15).

A **meningioma** is a tumor of the meninges. Because a meningioma does not spread and is localized at the surface, a surgeon can usually remove it completely.

Tumors of nervous tissue generally occur in childhood, and may even originate before birth, when this tissue is actively multiplying. Also, cancer may metastasize to the brain from elsewhere in the body. For unknown reasons, certain forms of cancer, especially melanoma, breast cancer, and lung cancer, tend to spread to the brain.

Degenerative Diseases

Multiple sclerosis (**MS**) commonly attacks people in their 20s or 30s and progresses at intervals and at varying rates. It involves patchy loss of myelin with hardening (sclerosis) of tissue in the CNS. The symptoms include vision problems, tingling or numbness in the arms and legs, urinary incontinence, **tremor** (shaking), and stiff gait. MS is thought to be an autoimmune disorder, but the exact cause is not known.

17

Figure 17-14 **Brain tumor.** MRI shows a large tumor that arises from the cerebellum and pushes the brainstem forward.

Figure 17-15 **Hydrocephalus.** Coronal section of the brain showing marked enlargement of the ventricles caused by a tumor that obstructed the flow of CSF.

A

B

Figure 17-16 **Effects of Alzheimer disease.** (*A*) Normal brain. (*B*) Brain of a patient with Alzheimer disease, showing atrophy of the cortex with narrow gyri and enlarged sulci.

Parkinsonism occurs when, for unknown reasons, certain neurons in the midbrain fail to secrete the neurotransmitter dopamine. This leads to tremors, muscle rigidity, flexion at the joints, akinesia (loss of movement), and emotional problems. Parkinsonism is treated with daily administration of the drug L-**dopa** (levodopa), a form of dopamine that can be carried by the circulation into the brain.

Alzheimer disease (AD) results from unexplained degeneration of neurons and atrophy of the cerebral cortex (Fig. 17-16). These changes cause progressive loss of recent memory, confusion, and mood changes. Dangers associated with AD are injury, infection, malnutrition, and aspiration of food or fluids into the lungs. Originally called presenile dementia and used only to describe cases in patients about 50 years of age, the term is now applied to these same changes when they occur in elderly patients.

AD is diagnosed by CT or MRI scans and confirmed at autopsy. Histologic (tissue) studies show deposits of a substance called **amyloid** in the tissues. The disease may be hereditary. AD commonly develops in people with Down syndrome after age 40, indicating that AD is associated with abnormality on chromosome 21, the same chromosome that is involved in Down syndrome.

Multi-infarct dementia (MID) resembles AD in that it is a progressive cognitive impairment associated with loss of memory, loss of judgment, aphasia, altered motor and sensory function, repetitive behavior, and loss of social skills. The disorder is caused by multiple small strokes that interrupt blood flow to brain tissue and deprive areas of oxygen.

Epilepsy

A prime characteristic of epilepsy is recurrent seizures brought on by abnormal electric activity of the brain. These attacks may vary from brief and mild episodes known as absence (petit mal) seizures to major tonic–clonic (grand mal) seizures with loss of consciousness, **convulsion** (intervals of violent involuntary muscle contractions), and sensory disturbances. In other cases (psychomotor seizures), there is a 1- to 2-minute period of disorientation. Epilepsy may be the result of a tumor, injury, or neurologic disease, but in most cases the cause is unknown.

EEG reveals abnormalities in brain activity and can be used in the diagnosis and treatment of epilepsy. The disorder is treated with antiepileptic and anticonvulsive drugs to control seizures, and sometimes surgery is of help. If seizures cannot be controlled, the individual with epilepsy may have to avoid certain activities that can lead to harm.

Sleep Disturbances

The general term *dyssomnia* includes a variety of possible disorders that result in excessive sleepiness or difficulty in beginning or maintaining sleep. Simple causes for such disorders include schedule changes or travel to different time zones (jet lag). **Insomnia** refers to insufficient or nonrestorative sleep despite ample opportunity to sleep. There may be physical causes for insomnia, but often it is related to emotional upset caused by stressful events. **Narcolepsy** is characterized by brief, uncontrollable attacks of sleep during the day. The disorder is treated with stimulants, regulation of sleep habits, and short daytime naps.

Sleep apnea refers to failure to breathe for brief periods during sleep. It usually results from upper airway obstruction, often associated with obesity, alcohol consumption, or weakened throat muscles, and is usually accompanied by loud snoring with brief periods of silence. Dental appliances that move the tongue and jaw forward may help to prevent sleep apnea. Other options are surgery to correct an obstruction or positive air pressure delivered through a mask.

Sleep disorders are diagnosed by physical examination, a sleep history, and a log of sleep habits, including details of the sleep environment and note of any substances consumed that may interfere with sleep. Study in a sleep laboratory with a variety of electric and other studies, constituting **polysomnography**, may also be needed.

Sleep studies identify two components of normal sleep, each showing a specific EEG pattern. Non–rapid eye movement (NREM) sleep has four stages, which take a person progressively into the deepest level of sleep. If sleepwalking (somnambulism) occurs, it occurs during this stage. NREM sleep is interrupted about every 1.5 hours by episodes of rapid eye movement (REM) sleep, during which the eyes move rapidly, although they are closed. Dreaming occurs during REM sleep and muscles lose tone, while heart rate, blood pressure, and brain activity increase.

Others

Many hereditary diseases affect the nervous system. Some of these are described in Chapter 15. Hormonal imbalances that involve the nervous system are described in Chapter 16. Finally, drugs, alcohol, toxins, and nutritional deficiencies may act on the nervous system in a variety of ways.

Box 17-2 has information on occupational therapists, who are often involved in treating people with neurologic disturbances.

17

Box 17-2   Health Professions

Careers in Occupational Therapy

Occupational therapy (OT) helps people with physical or mental disability achieve independence at home and at work by teaching them "skills for living." Many people can benefit, including those:

- Recovering from traumas such as fractures, amputations, burns, spinal cord injury, stroke, and heart attack.
- With chronic conditions such as arthritis, multiple sclerosis, Alzheimer disease, and schizophrenia.
- With developmental disabilities such as Down syndrome, cerebral palsy, spina bifida, muscular dystrophy, and autism.

OTs work as part of multidisciplinary teams, which include physicians, nurses, physical therapists, speech pathologists, and social workers. They assess their clients' capabilities and develop individualized treatment programs that help them

recover from injury or compensate for permanent disability. Treatment may include teaching activities ranging from work tasks to dressing, cooking, and eating, and using adaptive equipment such as wheelchairs and computers. OT assistants implement treatment plans and report results to a therapist. To perform these duties, OTs and assistants need a thorough scientific and clinical background. Most OTs in the United States have bachelor's or master's degrees and must pass a national licensing exam. Assistants typically train in a 2-year program and also take a licensing exam.

OTs and their assistants work in hospitals, clinics, and nursing care facilities, and also visit homes and schools. As the population continues to age and the need for rehabilitative therapy increases, job prospects remain good. The American Occupational Therapy Association at www.aota.org has more information on OT careers.

Behavioral Disorders

This section is an introduction to some of the behavioral disorders that involve the nervous system. Criteria for clinical diagnosis of these and other behavioral and mental disorders are set forth in the *Diagnostic and Statistical Manual of Mental Disorders* (DSM) of the American Psychiatric Association.

Anxiety Disorders

Anxiety is a feeling of fear, worry, uneasiness, or dread. It may be associated with physical problems or drugs and is often prompted by feelings of helplessness or loss of self-esteem. Generalized anxiety disorder (GAD) is characterized by chronic excessive and uncontrollable worry about various life circumstances, often with no basis. It may be accompanied by muscle tensing, restlessness, dyspnea, palpitations, insomnia, irritability, or fatigue.

Panic disorder is a form of anxiety disorder marked by episodes of intense fear. A person with panic disorder may isolate himself or herself or avoid social situations for fear of having a panic attack or in response to attacks.

A **phobia** is an extreme, persistent fear of a specific object or situation (Box 17-3). It may center on social situations, particular objects, such as animals or blood, or activities, such as flying or driving through tunnels.

Obsessive–compulsive disorder (OCD) is a condition marked by disturbing thoughts or images that are persistent and intrusive. To relieve anxiety about these thoughts or images, the person with OCD engages in repetitive behavior that interferes with normal daily activities, although he or she knows that such behavior is unreasonable. These patterns include repeated washing; performing rituals; arranging, touching, or counting objects; and repeating words or phrases. OCD is associated with perfectionism and rigidity in behavior. Some specialists believe that OCD is related to low levels of the neurotransmitter serotonin in the brain. Treatment is with behavioral therapy and antidepressant drugs that increase the brain's serotonin levels (Box 17-4).

When a highly stressful, catastrophic event results in persistent emotional difficulties, the condition is described as **posttraumatic stress disorder (PTSD)**. People who are abused, whose lives are threatened, who witness a crime, who experience a natural disaster, and especially those who are combat veterans are subject to PTSD. Responses include anger, fear, sleep disturbances, and physical symptoms, including changes in brain chemistry and hormone imbalances. PTSD is often associated with other emotional problems such as **depression**, withdrawal, substance abuse, and impaired social and family relationships. Patients need early treatment with emotional support, protection, psychotherapy, and drugs to treat depression and anxiety.

Mood Disorders

Depression is a mental state characterized by profound feelings of sadness, emptiness, hopelessness, inability to concentrate, and lack of interest or pleasure in activities. Depression is often accompanied by insomnia, loss of appetite, and suicidal tendencies. Depression frequently coexists with other physical or emotional conditions.

Dysthymia is a chronic mood disorder that lasts for several months to years and is often triggered by a serious event. Depression is a common symptom, as well as eating disorders, sleep disturbances, fatigue, lack of concentration, indecision, and feelings of hopelessness.

In **bipolar disorder** (formerly called manic depressive illness), normal moods alternate with episodes of depression and **mania**, a state of elation, which may include agitation, hyperexcitability, or hyperactivity. Treatment for bipolar disorder may differ from therapy

---

Box 17-3   Focus on Words

Phobias and Manias

Some of the terms for phobias and manias are just as strange and interesting as the behaviors themselves.

Agoraphobia is fear of being in a public place. The agora in ancient Greece was the marketplace. Xenophobia is an irrational fear of strangers, taken from the Greek root *xen/o*, which means strange or foreign. Acrophobia, a fear of heights, is taken from the root *acro-*, meaning terminal, highest, or topmost. In most medical terms, this root is used to mean extremity, as in *acrocyanosis*. Hydrophobia is a fear of or aversion to water (*hydr/o*). The term was used as an alternative name for rabies, because people infected with this paralytic disease had difficulty swallowing water and other liquids.

Trichotillomania is the odd practice of compulsively pulling out one's hair in response to stress. The word comes from the root for hair (*trich/o*) plus a Greek word that means "to pull." Kleptomania, also spelled cleptomania, is from the Greek word for thief, and describes an irresistible urge to steal in the absence of need.

Terminology	**Key Terms** (continued)
phobia *FŌ-bē-a*	An extreme, persistent fear of a specific object or situation
posttraumatic stress disorder (PTSD)	Persistent emotional disturbances that follow exposure to life-threatening, catastrophic events, such as trauma, abuse, natural disasters, and warfare
psychosis *sī-KŌ-sis*	A mental disorder extreme enough to cause gross misperception of reality with delusions and hallucinations
schizophrenia *skiz-ō-FRĔ-nē-a*	A poorly understood group of severe mental disorders with features of psychosis, delusions, hallucinations, and withdrawn or bizarre behavior (*schizo* means "split" and *phren* means "mind")

PASSport to Success® Go to the pronunciation glossary on the Student Resources to hear these words pronounced.

17

Terminology	**Supplementary Terms**

Normal Structure and Function

acetylcholine (Ach) *as-ē-til-KŌ-lēn*	A neurotransmitter; activity involving acetylcholine is described as cholinergic
basal ganglia	Four masses of gray matter in the cerebrum and upper brainstem that are involved in movement and coordination
blood–brain barrier	A special membrane between circulating blood and the brain that prevents certain damaging substances from reaching brain tissue
Broca area *BRŌ-ka*	An area in the left frontal lobe of the cerebrum that controls speech production
circle of Willis	An interconnection (anastomosis) of several arteries supplying the brain; located at the base of the cerebrum
contralateral *kon-tra-LAT-er-al*	Affecting the opposite side of the body
corpus callosum *KOR-pus ka-LŌ-sum*	A large band of connecting fibers between the cerebral hemispheres
dermatome *DER-ma-tōm*	The area of the skin supplied by a spinal nerve; term also refers to an instrument used to cut skin for grafting (see Chapter 21)
epinephrine *ep-i-NEF-rin*	A neurotransmitter; also called adrenaline; activity involving epinephrine is described as adrenergic
ipsilateral *ip-si-LAT-er-al*	On the same side; unilateral
leptomeninges *lep-to-men-IN-jēz*	The pia mater and arachnoid together
nucleus *NŪ-klē-us*	A collection of nerve cells within the central nervous system
plexus *PLEKS-us*	A network, as of nerves or blood vessels

(continued)

Terminology	**Supplementary Terms** (continued)

pyramidal tracts pi-RAM-i-dal	A group of motor tracts involved in fine coordination. Most of the fibers in these tracts cross in the medulla to the opposite side of the spinal cord and affect the opposite side of the body. Fibers not included in the pyramidal tracts are described as extrapyramidal
reticular activating system (RAS) re-TIK-ū-lar	A widespread system in the brain that maintains wakefulness
Schwann cells shvon	Cells that produce the myelin sheath around peripheral axons
Wernicke area VER-ni-kē	An area in the temporal lobe concerned with speech comprehension

Symptoms and Conditions

amyotrophic lateral sclerosis (ALS) a-mī-ō-TROF-ik	A disorder marked by muscular weakness, spasticity, and exaggerated reflexes caused by degeneration of motor neurons; Lou Gehrig disease
amnesia am-NĒ-zē-a	Loss of memory
apraxia a-PRAK-sē-a	Inability to move with purpose or to use objects properly
ataxia a-TAK-sē-a	Lack of muscle coordination; dyssynergia
athetosis ath-e-TŌ-sis	Involuntary, slow, twisting movements in the arms, especially the hands and fingers
Bell palsy PAWL-zē	Paralysis of the facial nerve
berry aneurysm AN-ū-rizm	A small saclike aneurysm of a cerebral artery
catatonia kat-a-TŌ-nē-a	A phase of schizophrenia in which the patient is unresponsive; there is a tendency to remain in a fixed position without moving or talking
cerebral palsy SER-e-bral PAWL-zē	A nonprogressive neuromuscular disorder usually caused by damage to the CNS near the time of birth. May include spasticity, involuntary movements, or ataxia
chorea KOR-ē-a	A nervous condition marked by involuntary twitching of the limbs or facial muscles
claustrophobia claws-trō-FŌ-bē-a	Fear of being shut in or enclosed (from Latin claudere, "to shut")
compulsion kom-PUL-shun	A repetitive, stereotyped act performed to relieve tension
Creutzfeldt–Jakob disease (CJD) KROITS-felt YA-kob	A slow-growing degenerative brain disease caused by a prion (PRĪ-on), an infectious protein. Related to bovine spongiform encephalopathy (BSE, "mad cow disease") in cattle
delirium de-LIR-ē-um	A sudden and temporary state of confusion marked by excitement, physical restlessness, and incoherence
dysarthria dis-AR-thrē-a	Defect in speech articulation caused by lack of control over the required muscles
dysmetria dis-MĒ-trē-a	Disturbance in the path or placement of a limb during active movement. In hypometria, the limb falls short; in hypermetria, the limb extends beyond the target
euphoria ū-FOR-ē-a	An exaggerated feeling of well-being; elation

(continued)

Terminology	Supplementary Terms (continued)
glioblastoma *glī-ō-blas-TŌ-ma*	A malignant astrocytoma
Guillain–Barré syndrome *gē-YAN-bar-RĀ*	An acute polyneuritis with progressive muscular weakness that usually occurs after a viral infection; in most cases recovery is complete, but may take several months to years
hematomyelia *hē-ma-tō-mī-Ē-lē-a*	Hemorrhage of blood into the spinal cord, as from an injury
hemiballism *hem-ē-BAL-izm*	Jerking, twitching movements of one side of the body
Huntington disease	A hereditary disease of the CNS that usually appears between ages 30 and 50. The patient shows progressive dementia and chorea, and death occurs within 10 to 15 years
hypochondriasis *hī-pō-kon-DRĪ-a-sis*	Abnormal anxiety about one's health
ictus *IK-tus*	A blow or sudden attack, such as an epileptic seizure
lethargy *LETH-ar-jē*	A state of sluggishness or stupor
migraine *MĪ-grān*	Chronic intense, throbbing headache that may result from vascular changes in cerebral arteries. Possible causes include genetic factors, stress, trauma, and hormonal fluctuations. Headache might be signaled by visual disturbances, nausea, photophobia, and tingling sensations
neurofibromatosis *nū-rō-fī-brō-ma-TŌ-sis*	A condition involving multiple tumors of peripheral nerves
neurosis *nū-RŌ-sis*	An emotional disorder caused by unresolved conflicts, with anxiety as a main characteristic
paraplegia *par-a-PLĒ-jē-a*	Paralysis of the legs and lower part of the body
parasomnia *par-a-SOM-nē-a*	Condition of having undesirable phenomena, such as nightmares, occur during sleep or become worse during sleep
quadriplegia *kwa-dri-PLĒ-jē-a*	Paralysis of all four limbs; tetraplegia
Reye syndrome *rī*	A rare acute encephalopathy occurring in children after viral infections. The liver, kidney, and heart may be involved. Linked to administration of aspirin during a viral illness
sciatica *sī-AT-i-ka*	Neuritis characterized by severe pain along the sciatic nerve and its branches
somatoform disorders *sō-MA-tō-form*	Conditions associated with symptoms of physical disease, such as pain, hypertension, or chronic fatigue, with no physical basis
somnambulism *som-NAM-bū-lizm*	Walking or performing other motor functions while asleep and out of bed; sleepwalking
stupor *STŪ-por*	A state of unconsciousness or lethargy with loss of responsiveness
syringomyelia *sir-in-gō-mī-Ē-lē-a*	A progressive disease marked by formation of fluid-filled cavities in the spinal cord
tic	Involuntary, spasmodic, recurrent, and purposeless motor movements or vocalizations
tic douloureux *tik dū-lū-RŪ*	Episodes of extreme pain in the area supplied by the trigeminal nerve; also called trigeminal neuralgia
tabes dorsalis *TĀ-bēz dor-SAL-is*	Destruction of the dorsal (posterior) portion of the spinal cord with loss of sensation and awareness of body position, as seen in advanced cases of syphilis
Tourette syndrome *tū-RET*	A tic disorder with intermittent motor and vocal manifestations that begins in childhood. There also may be obsessive and compulsive behavior, hyperactivity, and distractibility

17

(continued)

Terminology — Supplementary Terms (continued)

transient ischemic attack (TIA) *is-KĒ-mik*	A sudden, brief, and temporary cerebral dysfunction usually caused by interruption of blood flow to the brain
Wallerian degeneration *wahl-LĒ-rē-an*	Degeneration of a nerve distal to an injury
whiplash	Cervical injury caused by rapid acceleration and deceleration resulting in damage to muscles, ligaments, disks, and nerves

Additional terms related to neurologic symptoms can be found in Chapters 18 (on the senses) and 20 (on the muscular system).

Diagnosis and Treatment

Babinski reflex *ba-BIN-skē*	A spreading of the outer toes and extension of the big toe over the others when the sole of the foot is stroked. This response is normal in infants but indicates a lesion of specific motor tracts in adults
evoked potentials	Record of the brain's electric activity after sensory stimulation. Included are visual evoked potentials (VEPs), brainstem auditory evoked potentials (BAEPs), and somatosensory evoked potentials (SSEPs), obtained by stimulating the hand or leg. These tests are used to evaluate CNS function
Glasgow coma scale	A system for assessing level of consciousness by assigning a score to each of three responses: eye opening, motor responses, and verbal responses
Positron emission tomography (PET)	Use of radioactive glucose or other metabolically active substance to produce images of biochemical activity in tissues. Used for study of the living brain, both healthy and diseased, and also in cardiology. Figure 17-17 compares CT, MRI, and PET scans
Romberg sign	Inability to maintain balance when the eyes are shut and the feet are close together
sympathectomy *sim-pa-THEK-tō-mē*	Interruption of sympathetic nerve transmission either surgically or chemically
trephination *tref-i-NĀ-shun*	Cutting a piece of bone out of the skull; the instrument used is a trepan (*tre-PAN*) or trephine (*tre-FĪN*)

Psychoactive Drugs

antianxiety agents *an-tē-ang-ZĪ-e-tē*	Relieve anxiety by means of a calming, sedative effect on the CNS, for example, chlordiazepoxide (Librium), diazepam (Valium), alprazolam (Xanax); anxiolytic
antidepressants (other than those listed in separate categories below)	Block the reuptake of neurotransmitters such as serotonin, norepinephrine, dopamine, alone or in combination, for example, bupropion (Wellbutrin, Zyban), mirtazapine (Remeron), nefazodone (Serzone), venlafaxine (Effexor XR), atomoxetine (Strattera)
monoamine oxidase inhibitors (MAOI) *mō-nō-A-mēn OK-si-dās*	Block an enzyme that breaks down norepinephrine and serotonin, thus prolonging their action, for example, phenelzine (Nardil), tranylcypromine (Parnate), isocarboxazid (Marplan)
neuroleptics *nū-rō-LEP-tiks*	Drugs used to treat psychosis, including schizophrenia, for example, clozapine (Clozaril), haloperidol (Haldol), risperidone (Risperdal), olanzapine (Zyprexa); antipsychotic. Action mechanism unknown, but may interfere with neurotransmitters
selective serotonin reuptake inhibitors (SSRIs) *ser-ō-TŌ-nin*	Block the reuptake of serotonin in the brain, thus increasing levels, for example, fluoxetine (Prozac), citalopram (Celexa), paroxetine (Paxil), sertraline (Zoloft)
stimulants *STIM-ū-lantz*	Promote activity and a sense of well-being, for example, methylphenidate (Ritalin), dextroamphetamine (Dexedrine), amphetamine + dextroamphetamine (Adderall)
tricyclic antidepressants (TCAs) *trī-SĪ-klik*	Block the reuptake of norepinephrine, serotonin, or both, for example, amitriptyline (Elavil), clomipramine (Anafranil), imipramine (Tofranil), doxepin (Sinequan), trimipramine (Surmontil)

PASSport to Success® Go to the pronunciation glossary on the Student Resources to hear these words pronounced.

Figure 17-17 **Brain images.** (*A*) CT scan of a normal adult brain. (*B*) MRI of the brain showing a subdural hematoma (*arrows*). (*C*) PET scan showing regions of different metabolic activity.

17

Terminology | Abbreviations

ACh	Acetylcholine	**LP**	Lumbar puncture
AD	Alzheimer disease	**MAOI**	Monoamine oxidase inhibitor
ADHD	Attention-deficit/hyperactivity disorder	**MID**	Multi-infarct dementia
ALS	Amyotrophic lateral sclerosis	**MS**	Multiple sclerosis
ANS	Autonomic nervous system	**NICU**	Neurological intensive care unit
BAEP	Brainstem auditory evoked potentials	**NPH**	Normal pressure hydrocephalus
CBF	Cerebral blood flow	**NREM**	Non–rapid eye movement (sleep)
CJD	Creutzfeldt–Jakob disease	**OCD**	Obsessive–compulsive disorder
CNS	Central nervous system	**PDD**	Pervasive developmental disorder
CP	Cerebral palsy	**PET**	Positron emission tomography
CSF	Cerebrospinal fluid	**PNS**	Peripheral nervous system
CVA	Cerebrovascular accident	**PTSD**	Posttraumatic stress disorder
CVD	Cerebrovascular disease	**RAS**	Reticular activating system
DSM	*Diagnostic and Statistical Manual of Mental Disorders*	**REM**	Rapid eye movement (sleep)
DTR	Deep tendon reflexes	**SSEP**	Somatosensory evoked potentials
EEG	Electroencephalogram; electroencephalograph(y)	**SSRI**	Selective serotonin reuptake inhibitor
GAD	Generalized anxiety disorder	**TCA**	Tricyclic antidepressant
ICP	Intracranial pressure	**TIA**	Transient ischemic attack
LMN	Lower motor neuron	**UMN**	Upper motor neuron
LOC	Level of consciousness	**VEP**	Visual evoked potentials

Chapter Review

LABELING EXERCISE

Anatomic Divisions of the Nervous System > Write the name of each numbered part on the corresponding line of the answer sheet.

Brain   Peripheral nervous system
Central nervous system   Spinal cord
Cranial nerves   Spinal nerves

1. _____

2. _____

3. _____

4. _____

5. _____

6. _____

Chapter Review (continued)

Motor Neuron > Write the name of each numbered part on the corresponding line of the answer sheet.

Axon branch   Dendrites
Axon covered with   Muscle
   myelin sheath   Myelin
Cell body   Nucleus

1. _____

2. _____

3. _____

4. _____

5. _____

6. _____

7. _____

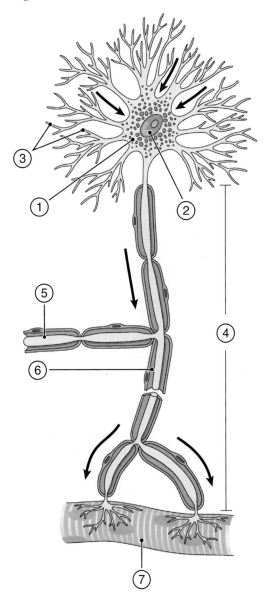

Chapter Review (continued)

External Surface of the Brain > Write the name of each numbered part on the corresponding line of the answer sheet.

Cerebellum   Parietal lobe
Frontal lobe   Pons
Gyri   Spinal cord
Medulla oblongata   Sulci
Occipital lobe   Temporal lobe

1. _____

2. _____

3. _____

4. _____

5. _____

6. _____

7. _____

8. _____

9. _____

10. _____

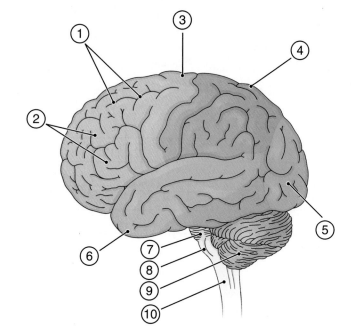

Spinal Cord, Lateral View > Write the name of each numbered part on the corresponding line of the answer sheet.

Brain   Lumbar enlargement
Brainstem   Lumbar nerves
Cervical enlargement Sacral nerves
Cervical nerves   Spinal cord
Coccygeal nerve   Thoracic nerves

1. _____

2. _____

3. _____

4. _____

5. _____

6. _____

7. _____

8. _____

9. _____

10. _____

Spinal Cord, Cross Section > Write the name of each numbered part on the corresponding line of the answer sheet.

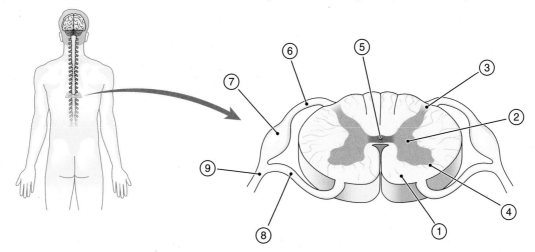

Central canal   Spinal nerve
Dorsal horn   Ventral horn
Dorsal root ganglion   Ventral root of
Dorsal root of spinal nerve   spinal nerve
Gray matter   White matter

1. _____   6. _____

2. _____   7. _____

3. _____   8. _____

4. _____   9. _____

5. _____

Reflex Pathway > Write the name of each numbered part on the corresponding line of the answer sheet.

Effector   Sensory neuron
Motor neuron   Spinal cord (CNS)
Receptor

Stimulus

1. _____

2. _____

3. _____

4. _____

5. _____

Chapter Review *(continued)*

TERMINOLOGY

Matching > Match the following terms and write the appropriate letter to the left of each number:

_____	**1.** myelin	**a.**	region that connects the brain and spinal cord
_____	**2.** diencephalon	**b.**	part of the brain that contains the thalamus and pituitary
_____	**3.** ganglion	**c.**	whitish material that covers some axons
_____	**4.** medulla oblongata	**d.**	rounded area on the ventral surface of the brain
_____	**5.** pons	**e.**	collection of neuron cell bodies
_____	**6.** amyloid	**a.**	accumulation of CSF in the brain
_____	**7.** aphasia	**b.**	excessive fear of pain
_____	**8.** hydrocephalus	**c.**	substance associated with Alzheimer disease
_____	**9.** paranoia	**d.**	mental disorder associated with delusions of persecution
_____	**10.** odynophobia	**e.**	loss of speech communication
_____	**11.** aneurysm	**a.**	partial paralysis or weakness
_____	**12.** convulsion	**b.**	paralysis of the bladder
_____	**13.** meningomyelocele	**c.**	series of violent, involuntary muscle contractions
_____	**14.** paresis	**d.**	localized dilation of a blood vessel
_____	**15.** cystoplegia	**e.**	hernia of the meninges and spinal cord

Supplementary Terms

_____	**16.** plexus	**a.**	network
_____	**17.** corpus callosum	**b.**	area of skin supplied by a spinal nerve
_____	**18.** dermatome	**c.**	a neurotransmitter
_____	**19.** acetylcholine	**d.**	a band of connecting fibers in the brain
_____	**20.** ictus	**e.**	a sudden blow or attack
_____	**21.** lethargy	**a.**	fear of being enclosed
_____	**22.** ataxia	**b.**	state of sluggishness
_____	**23.** claustrophobia	**c.**	loss of memory
_____	**24.** euphoria	**d.**	lack of muscle coordination
_____	**25.** amnesia	**e.**	sense of elation
_____	**26.** PTSD	**a.**	type of psychoactive drug
_____	**27.** SSRI	**b.**	system that maintains wakefulness
_____	**28.** DSM	**c.**	mental disturbances that follow trauma
_____	**29.** RAS	**d.**	degenerative brain disease
_____	**30.** CJD	**e.**	reference for diagnosis of mental disorders

Fill in the blanks:

31. The largest part of the brain is the _____.

32. The scientific name for a nerve cell is _____.

33. The junction between two nerve cells is a(n) _____.

34. The support cells of the nervous system are the _____.

35. The fluid that circulates around the central nervous system is _____.

36. The membranes that cover the brain and spinal cord are the _____.

37. A simple, rapid, automatic response to a stimulus is a(n) _____.

38. The sympathetic and parasympathetic systems make up the _____.

39. A chemical that acts at a synapse is a(n) _____.

40. The posterior portion of the brain that coordinates muscle movement is the _____.

Define the following words:

41. radicular (*ra-DIK-ū-lar*) _____

42. hemiparesis (*hem-i-pa-RĒ-sis*) _____

43. anencephaly (*an-en-SEF-a-lē*) _____

44. polyneuritis (*pol-ē-nū-RĪ-tis*) _____

45. corticothalamic (*kor-ti-kō-tha-LAM-ik*) _____

46. psychotherapy (*sī-kō-THER-a-pē*) _____

47. panplegia (*pan-PLĒ-jē-a*) _____

48. encephalomalacia (*en-sef-a-lō-ma-LĀ-shē-a*) _____

49. dyssomnia (*dis-SOM-nē-a*) _____

17

Write words for the following definitions:

50. study of the nervous system   _____

51. inflammation of the spinal cord and meninges   _____

52. excision of a ganglion   _____

53. any disease of the nervous system   _____

54. creation of an opening into a brain ventricle   _____

55. paralysis of one side of the body   _____

56. within the cerebellum   _____

57. difficulty in reading   _____

58. fear of water   _____

59. paralysis of one limb   _____

True–False > Examine the following statements. If the statement is true, write T in the first blank. If the statement is false, write F in the first blank and correct the statement by replacing the underlined word in the second blank.

60. <u>Sensory</u> fibers conduct impulses toward the CNS.   _____   _____

61. CSF forms in the <u>ventricles</u> of the brain.   _____   _____

62. The cervical nerves are in the region of the <u>neck</u>.   _____   _____

63. Myelinated neurons make up the <u>gray</u> matter of the CNS.   _____   _____

64. The spinal nerves are part of the <u>central</u> nervous system.   _____   _____

65. The fiber that carries impulses toward the neuron cell body
is the <u>axon</u>.   _____   _____

66. There are <u>twelve</u> pairs of cranial nerves.   _____   _____

67. The outermost layer of the meninges is the <u>pia</u> mater.   _____   _____

Opposites > Write a word that means the opposite of the following words:

68. extramedullary _____

69. ipsilateral _____

70. postganglionic _____

71. tachylalia _____

72. motor _____

73. dorsal _____

74. afferent _____

Adjectives > Write the adjective form of the following words:

75. ganglion _____

76. cortex _____

77. dura _____

78. meninges _____

79. psychosis _____

Plurals > Write the plural form of the following words:

80. ganglion _____

81. ventricle _____

82. meninx _____

83. gyrus _____

Eliminations > In each of the sets below, underline the word that does not fit in with the rest and explain the reason for your choice:

84. CVA — lumbar puncture — embolism — thrombus — TIA

_____

85. glioma — astrocytoma — meningioma — hematoma — neurilemmoma

_____

86. gyri — sulci — mania — ventricles — lobes

_____

87. MID — CNS — ADHD — OCD — GAD

_____

Word Building > Write a word for the following definitions using the word parts provided.

-plegia   myel/o   -a-   -itis   dys-   brady-   my/o   tetra-   -paresis   -phasia   gangli/o   hemi-

88. paralysis of the spinal cord _____

89. lack of speech _____

90. partial paralysis of one side of the body _____

Chapter Review (continued)

91. muscle weakness _____

92. abnormal or difficult speech production _____

93. paralysis of a ganglion _____

94. paralysis of all four limbs _____

95. inflammation of the spinal cord _____

96. slowness of speech _____

97. paralysis of one side of the body _____

98. inflammation of a ganglion _____

Word Analysis > Define each of the following words, and give the meaning of the word parts in each. Use a dictionary if necessary.

99. hematomyelia (*hē-ma-tō-mī-Ē-lē-a*) _____

    a. hemat/o _____

    b. myel/o _____

    c. -ia _____

100. myelodysplasia (*mī-e-lō-dis-PLĀ-sē-a*) _____

    a. myel/o _____

    b. dys- _____

    c. plas _____

    d. -ia _____

101. polyneuroradiculitis (*pol-ē-nū-rō-ra-dik-ū-LĪ-tis*) _____

    a. poly- _____

    b. neur/o _____

    c. radicul/o _____

    d. -itis _____

102. dyssynergia (*dis-sin-ER-jē-a*) _____

    a. dys- _____

    b. syn- _____

    c. erg _____

    d. -ia _____

PASSport to **Success**® Go to the word exercises on the Student Resources for additional review exercises.

Case Studies

➤ Case Study 17-1: Pediatric Brain Tumor

B.C., a 6-year-old first-grade student, was referred to a pediatric neurologist by his primary pediatrician for a neuro consult. He had presented with an acute onset of headaches, vomiting on waking in the morning, and progressive ataxia. The neurologist conducted a thorough neuro exam and ordered a CT scan, MRI, and lumbar puncture (LP) to look for possible tumor cells. When the LP revealed suspicious cells and the scans showed a tissue density, he was referred to a neurosurgeon for treatment of a suspected infratentorial astrocytoma (neuroglial tumor) of the posterior fossa.

B.C. had a craniotomy with tumor resection 5 days later. The cerebellar tumor was found to be noninfiltrating and was enclosed within a cyst, which was totally removed. B.C. spent 2 days in the neurological intensive care unit (NICU) because he was on seizure precautions and monitoring for increased intracranial pressure (ICP). A regimen of focal radiation followed after recovery from surgery. His spine was also treated because of the potential spread of tumor cells in the CSF. B.C. did not have chemotherapy because of the danger that hydrocephalus might develop, which generally requires a ventriculoperitoneal (VP) shunt.

B.C. was discharged 6 days after his surgery with a mild hemiparesis, which was expected to resolve within the next few weeks. He was scheduled for 6 weeks of outpatient rehabilitation, and his prognosis was good.

➤ Case Study 17-2: Cerebrovascular Accident (CVA)

A.R., a 62-year-old man, was admitted to the ER with right hemiplegia and aphasia. He had a history of hypertension and recent transient ischemic attacks (TIAs), yet was in good health when he experienced a sudden onset of right-sided weakness. He arrived in the ER via ambulance within 15 minutes of onset and was received by a member of the hospital's stroke team. He had a rapid general assessment and neuro exam, including a Glasgow Coma Scale (GCS) rating, to determine his candidacy for fibrinolytic (clot-dissolving) therapy.

He was sent for a noncontrast CT scan to look for evidence of hemorrhagic or ischemic stroke, postcardiac arrest ischemia, hypertensive encephalopathy, craniocerebral or cervical trauma, meningitis, encephalitis, brain abscess, tumor, and subdural or epidural hematoma. The CT scan, read by the radiologist, did not show intracerebral or subarachnoid hemorrhage. A.R. was diagnosed with probable acute ischemic stroke within 1 hour of the onset of symptoms and cleared as a candidate for immediate fibrinolytic treatment.

He was admitted to the NICU for 48-hour observation to monitor his neuro status and vital signs. He was discharged after 3 days with a prognosis of full recovery.

➤ Case Study 17-3: Neuroleptic Malignant Syndrome

J.N., a 21-year-old woman with chronic paranoid schizophrenia, was admitted to the hospital with a diagnosis of pneumonia. She was brought to the ER by her mother, who said J.N. had been very lethargic, had a temperature of 104°F, and had had muscular rigidity for 3 days. She took Haldol (haloperidol) and Cogentin (benztropine mesylate). Her mother stated that J.N.'s psychiatrist had changed her neuroleptic medication the week before. Her secondary diagnosis was stated as neuroleptic malignant syndrome, a rare and life-threatening disorder associated with the use of antipsychotic medications. This drug-induced condition is usually characterized by alterations in mental status, temperature regulation, and autonomic and extrapyramidal functions.

J.N. was monitored for potential hypotension, tachycardia, diaphoresis, dyspnea, dysphagia, and changes in her level of consciousness (LOC). Her medications were discontinued, she was hydrated with IV fluids, and her body temperature was monitored for fluctuations. She was treated with bromocriptine, a dopamine antagonist, and dantrolene, a muscle relaxant and antispasmodic.

After 5 days, J.N. was transferred to a mental health facility and restarted on low-dose neuroleptics. She was monitored to prevent a recurrence. Both J.N. and her family were educated about neuroleptic malignant syndrome in preparation for her discharge back home in 2 weeks.

CASE STUDY QUESTIONS

Multiple choice. Select the best answer and write the letter of your choice to the left of each number:

_____ 1. A neurologist is a physician who:
   a. performs brain surgery
   b. practices psychiatry
   c. practices psychology
   d. treats with natural and herbal medicine
   e. treats disorders of the nervous system

_____ 2. A diagnostic procedure in which fluid is withdrawn from the spinal subarachnoid space is a(n):
   a. thoracentesis
   b. lumbar puncture
   c. ventriculogram
   d. intracranial window
   e. trephine

_____ 3. B.C.'s tumor was in the cerebellum, which controls voluntary movement, balance, and coordination. His motor dysfunction is called:
   a. ataxia
   b. neurolepsis
   c. dysphagia
   d. dyspnea
   e. seizure

(continued)

Case Studies *(continued)*

_____ 4. A VP shunt is a surgical treatment for hydro-cephalus. Excess CSF is shunted (drained) from the _____ by way of tubing tunneled to the _____ cavity.
   a. vortex, ventricular
   b. ventricles, peritoneal
   c. peritoneum, ventricular
   d. ventricles, thoracic
   e. midbrain, stomach

_____ 5. Ischemic stroke is generally caused by:
   a. hemorrhage
   b. hematoma
   c. thrombosis
   d. hemiparesis
   e. hemangioma

_____ 6. Thrombolytic therapy is directed toward:
   a. stabilizing blood cells
   b. destroying RBCs
   c. triggering blood clotting
   d. decreasing CSF
   e. dissolving a blood clot

_____ 7. A general term for any disorder or alteration of brain tissue is:
   a. cerebrocyst
   b. encephalopathy
   c. neurocytoma
   d. dysencephaloma
   e. psychosomatic

_____ 8. J.N. had disease manifestations related to involuntary functions and to movement controlled by motor fibers outside the pyramidal tracts. These functions are:
   a. antispasmodic and voluntary
   b. autonomic and neuroleptic
   c. autonomic and voluntary
   d. extrapyramidal and pyramidal
   e. autonomic and extrapyramidal

Write terms from the case studies with the following meanings:

 9. tumor of astrocytes

   _____

10. surgical opening into the skull

   _____

11. sudden attack typical of epilepsy

   _____

12. partial paralysis on one side

   _____

13. inability to speak or understand speech

   _____

14. inflammation of the meninges

   _____

15. collection of blood below the dura mater

   _____

16. perceived feeling of threat or harm

   _____

17. drug that relieves muscle spasms

   _____

18. antipsychotic medications

   _____

19. a physician who treats psychiatric disorders

   _____

Define the following abbreviations:

20. CT _____

21. LP _____

22. NICU _____

23. ICP _____

24. CSF _____

25. CVA _____

26. TIA _____

27. LOC _____

17

CHAPTER

18

The Senses

CHAPTER CONTENTS

OBJECTIVES

After study of this chapter you should be able to:

1. Explain the role of the sensory system.
2. Label diagrams of the ear and the eye, and briefly describe the function of each part.
3. Describe the pathway of nerve impulses from the ear to the brain.
4. Describe the roles of the retina and the optic nerve in vision.
5. Identify and use word parts pertaining to the senses.
6. Describe the main disorders pertaining to the ear and the eye.
7. Interpret abbreviations used in the study of the ear and the eye.
8. Analyze several case studies pertaining to vision or hearing.

PRETEST

Multiple choice. Select the best answer and write the letter of your choice to the left of each number.

___ 1. The scientific name for the sense of smell is:

   a. osmosis   c. olfaction
   b. dialysis   d. gustation

___ 2. The term *tactile* refers to the sense of:

   a. pain   c. taste
   b. touch   d. temperature

___ 3. The two senses located in the ear are:

   a. hearing and equilibrium
   b. hearing and vision
   c. balance and taste
   d. equilibrium and pressure

___ 4. Inflammation of the ear is called:

    a. parotitis   c. otitis
    b. mastitis   d. orchitis

___ 5. The receptor layer of the eye is the:

    a. lens   c. retina
    b. cornea   d. pinna

___ 6. The scientific name for the white of the eye is:

    a. sclera   c. pupil
    b. vitreous body d. conjunctiva

___ 7. Clouding of the lens is termed:

    a. vertigo   c. cataract
    b. tinnitus   d. glaucoma

The sensory system is our network for detecting stimuli from the internal and external environments. It is needed to maintain homeostasis, provide us with pleasure, and protect us from harm. Pain, for example, is an important warning sign of tissue damage. The signals generated in the various **receptors** of the sensory system must be transmitted to the central nervous system for interpretation.

The Senses

The senses are divided according to whether they are widely distributed or localized in special sense organs. The receptors for the general senses are found throughout the body. Many are located in the skin (Fig. 18-1). These senses include:

- Pain. These receptors are found in the skin and also in muscles, joints, and internal organs.

- Touch, the **tactile** sense, located in the skin. Sensitivity to touch depends on the concentration of these receptors in different areas, high on the fingers, lips, and tongue, for example, but low at the back of the neck or back of the hand.

- Pressure, or deep touch, located beneath the skin and in deeper tissues.

- Temperature. Receptors for heat and cold are located in the skin and also in the hypothalamus, which regulates body temperature.

    - **Proprioception,** the awareness of body position. Receptors in muscles, tendons, and joints help to judge body position and coordinate muscle activity. They also help to maintain muscle tone.

The special senses are localized within complex sense organs in the head. These include:

- **Gustation** (taste) is located in receptors in taste buds on the tongue. These receptors basically detect only sweet, sour, bitter, and salty, although researchers have recently identified receptors for alkali (bases), metallic taste, and the amino acid glutamate, as found in the flavor enhancer MSG. The senses of smell and taste are chemical senses, that is, they respond to chemicals in solution.

- **Olfaction** (smell) is located in receptors in the nose. Many more chemicals can be discriminated by smell than by taste. Both senses are important in stimulating appetite and warning of harmful substances.

- **Hearing** receptors are located in the ear. These receptors respond to movement created by sound waves as they travel through the ear.

Figure 18-1 **Receptors for general senses in the skin.** Synapses for these pathways are in the spinal cord.

- **Equilibrium** receptors are also located in the ear. These receptors are activated by changes in the position of cells as we move.

- **Vision** receptors are light sensitive and located deep within the **eye**, protected by surrounding bone and other support structures. The coordinated actions of external and internal eye muscles help in the formation of a clear image.

Suffixes pertaining to the senses are listed in Table 18-1. The remainder of this chapter concentrates on hearing and vision, the senses that have received the most clinical attention.

Terminology   Key Terms

SENSES

Normal Structure and Function

equilibrium ē-kwi-LIB-rē-um	The sense of balance
gustation gus-TĀ-shun	The sense of taste; Latin *geusis* means "taste"
hearing HĒR-ing	The sense or perception of sound
olfaction ol-FAK-shun	The sense of smell; root *osm/o* means "smell"
proprioception prō-prē-ō-SEP-shun	The awareness of posture, movement, and changes in equilibrium; receptors are located in muscles, tendons, and joints
receptor rē-SEP-tor	A sensory nerve ending or a specialized structure associated with a sensory nerve that responds to a stimulus
tactile TAK-til	Pertaining to the sense of touch
vision VIZH-un	The sense by which the shape, size, and color of objects are perceived by means of the light they give off

PASSport to Success® — Go to the pronunciation glossary on the Student Resources to hear these words pronounced.

Table 18-1   Suffixes Pertaining to the Senses

Suffix	Meaning	Example	Definition of Example
-esthesia	sensation	cryesthesia krī-es-THĒ-zē-a	sensitivity to cold
-algesia	pain	hypalgesia* hī-pal-JĒ-zē-a	decreased sensitivity to pain
-osmia	sense of smell	pseudosmia sū-DOS-mē-a	false sense of smell
-geusia	sense of taste	parageusia par-a-GŪ-zē-a	abnormal (para-) sense of taste

*Prefix hyp/o.

EXERCISE **18-1**

Define the following words:

1. dysesthesia (*dis-es-thē-zē-a*)   _____

2. parosmia (*par-OZ-mē-a*)   _____

3. ageusia (*a-GŪ-zē-a*)   _____

Write words for the following definitions:

4. lack (an-) of sensation   _____

5. false sense of taste   _____

6. sensitivity to temperature   _____

7. excess sensitivity to pain   _____

8. abnormal (dys-) sense of taste   _____

9. muscular (my/o-) sensation   _____

The Ear

The ear has the receptors for both hearing and equilibrium. For study purposes, it may be divided into three parts: the outer, middle, and inner ear (Fig. 18-2).

The outer ear consists of the projecting **pinna** (auricle) and the **external auditory canal** (meatus). This canal ends at the **tympanic membrane**, or eardrum, which transmits sound waves to the middle ear. Glands in the external canal produce a waxy material, **cerumen**, which protects the ear and helps to prevent infection.

18

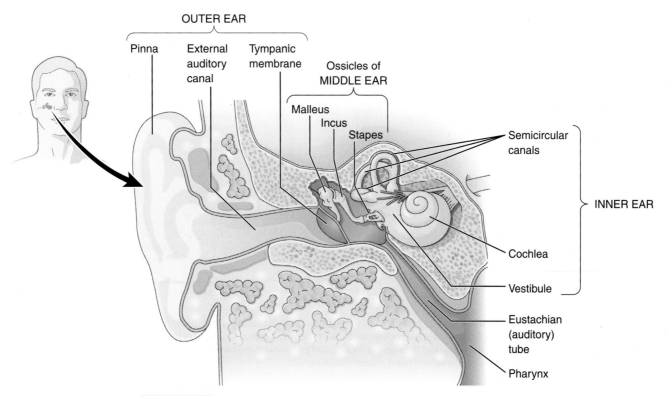

Figure 18-2 **The ear.** Structures in the outer, middle, and inner divisions are shown.

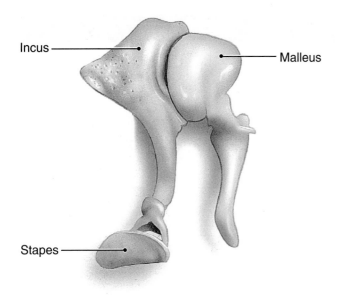

Incus

Malleus

Stapes

Figure 18-3 **The ossicles of the middle ear.** The malleus is in contact with the tympanic membrane. The base of the stapes is in contact with the oval window of the inner ear.

Spanning the middle ear cavity are three **ossicles** (small bones), each named for its shape: the **malleus** (hammer), **incus** (anvil), and **stapes** (stirrup) (Fig. 18-3). Sound waves traveling over the ossicles are transmitted from the footplate of the stapes to the inner ear. The

eustachian (auditory) **tube** connects the middle ear with the nasopharynx and serves to equalize pressure between the outer ear and the middle ear.

The inner ear, because of its complex shape, is described as a **labyrinth**, which means "maze" (Fig. 18-4). It consists of an outer bony framework containing a similarly shaped membranous channel. The entire labyrinth is filled with fluid.

The **cochlea**, shaped like a snail's shell, has the specialized **organ of Corti**, which is concerned with hearing. Cells in this receptor organ respond to sound waves traveling through the cochlea's fluid-filled ducts. Sound waves enter the cochlea from the base of the stapes through an opening, the oval window, and leave through another opening, the round window (see Fig. 18-4).

The sense of equilibrium is localized in the **vestibular apparatus**. This structure consists of the chamberlike **vestibule** and three projecting **semicircular canals**. Special cells within the vestibular apparatus respond to movement. (The senses of vision and proprioception are also important in maintaining balance.)

Nerve impulses are transmitted from the ear to the brain by way of the **vestibulocochlear nerve**, the eighth cranial nerve, also called the acoustic or auditory nerve. The cochlear branch of this nerve transmits impulses for hearing from the cochlea; the vestibular branch transmits impulses concerned with equilibrium from the vestibular apparatus (see Fig. 18-4). Roots pertaining to the ear and hearing are in Table 18-2.

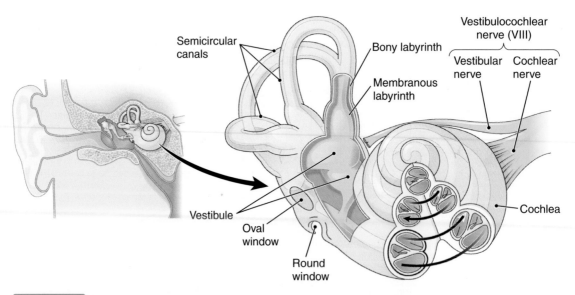

Semicircular canals

Bony labyrinth

Membranous labyrinth

Vestibulocochlear nerve (VIII)

Vestibular nerve   Cochlear nerve

Cochlea

Vestibule

Oval window

Round window

Figure 18-4 **The inner ear.** The outer bony labyrinth contains the membranous labyrinth. Receptors for equilibrium are in the vestibule and the semicircular canals. The cochlea contains the hearing receptor, the organ of Corti. Sound waves enter the cochlea through the oval window, travel through the cochlea, and exit through the round window. The inner ear transmits impulses to the brain in the vestibulocochlear nerve (eighth cranial nerve).

Terminology   Key Terms

THE EAR

Normal Structure and Function

cerumen *se-RŪ-men*	The brownish, waxlike secretion formed in the external ear canal to protect the ear and prevent infection; adjective: ceruminous (*se-RŪ-mi-nus*)
cochlea *KOK-lē-a*	The coiled portion of the inner ear that contains the receptors for hearing (root: *cochle/o*)
eustachian tube *ū-STĀ-shen*	The tube that connects the middle ear with the nasopharynx and serves to equalize pressure between the outer and middle ear (root: *salping/o*); auditory tube
external auditory canal	Tube that extends from the pinna of the ear to the tympanic membrane; external auditory meatus
incus *ING-kus*	The middle ossicle of the ear
labyrinth *LAB-i-rinth*	The inner ear, named for its complex structure, which resembles a maze
malleus *MAL-ē-us*	The ossicle of the middle ear that is in contact with the tympanic membrane and the incus
ossicles *OS-i-klz*	The small bones of the middle ear, the malleus, incus, and stapes
organ of Corti *KOR-tē*	The hearing receptor, which is located in the cochlea
pinna *PIN-a*	The projecting part of the outer ear; auricle (AW-ri-kl)
semicircular canals	The three curved channels of the inner ear that hold receptors for equilibrium
stapes *STĀ-pēz*	The ossicle that is in contact with the inner ear (roots: *staped/o*, *stapedi/o*)
tympanic membrane *tim-PAN-ik*	The membrane between the external auditory canal and the middle ear (tympanic cavity); the eardrum. It serves to transmit sound waves to the ossicles of the middle ear (roots: *myring/o*, *tympan/o*)
vestibular apparatus *ves-TIB-ū-lar*	The portion of the inner ear that is concerned with the sense of equilibrium; consists of the vestibule and the semicircular canals (root: *vestibul/o*)
vestibule *VES-ti-būl*	The chamber in the inner ear that holds some of the receptors for equilibrium
vestibulocochlear nerve *ves-tib-ū-lō-KOK-lē-ar*	The nerve that transmits impulses for hearing and equilibrium from the ear to the brain; eighth cranial nerve; auditory or acoustic nerve

PASSport to Success®

Go to the pronunciation glossary on the Student Resources to hear these words pronounced.

Table 18-2	Roots Pertaining to the Ear and Hearing		
Root	**Meaning**	**Example**	**Definition of Example**
audi/o	hearing	audiology aw-ē-OL-ō-jē	the study of hearing
acous, acus, cus	sound, hearing	acoustic a-KŪ-stik	pertaining to sound or hearing
ot/o	ear	ototoxic ō-tō-TOKS-ik	poisonous or harmful to the ear
myring/o	tympanic membrane	myringotome mi-RING-gō-tōm	knife used for surgery on the eardrum
tympan/o	tympanic cavity (middle ear), tympanic membrane	tympanometry tim-pa-NOM-e-trē	measurement of transmission through the tympanic membrane and middle ear
salping/o	tube, eustachian tube	salpingoscopy sal-ping-GOS-kō-pē	endoscopic examination of the eustachian tube
staped/o, stapedi/o	stapes	stapedoplasty stā-pē-dō-PLAS-tē	plastic repair of the stapes
labyrinth/o	labyrinth (inner ear)	labyrinthitis lab-i-rin-THĬ-tis	inflammation of the inner ear (labyrinth)
vestibul/o	vestibule, vestibular apparatus	vestibulotomy ves-tib-ū-LOT-ō-mē	incision of the vestibule of the inner ear
cochle/o	cochlea of inner ear	retrocochlear ret-rō-KOK-lē-ar	behind the cochlea

EXERCISE 18-2

Fill in the blanks:

1. Audition (*aw-DISH-un*) is the act of _____ .

2. Hyperacusis (*hī-per-a-KŪ-sis*) is abnormally high sensitivity to _____ .

3. Otogenic (*ō-tō-JEN-ik*) means originating in the _____ .

Define the following adjectives:

4. auditory (*AW-di-tor-ē*) _____

5. otic (*Ō-tik*) _____

6. labyrinthine (*lab-i-RIN-thēn*) _____

7. stapedial (*stā-PĒ-dē-al*) _____

8. vestibular (*ves-TIB-ū-lar*) _____

9. cochlear (*KOK-lē-ar*) _____

Write words for the following definitions:

10. pain in the ear _____

11. measurement of hearing (audi/o-) _____

12. plastic repair of the middle ear _____

13. incision of the tympanic membrane _____

14. within the cochlea _____

15. pertaining to the vestibular apparatus and cochlea _____

16. incision of the labyrinth _____

17. endoscope for examining the eustachian tube _____

18. excision of the stapes _____

Define the following words:

19. otitis (ō-TĪ-tis) _____

20. audiometer (aw-dē-OM-e-ter) _____

21. vestibulopathy (ves-tib-ū-LOP-a-thē) _____

22. salpingopharyngeal (sal-ping-gō-fa-RIN-jē-al) _____

23. myringoscope (mi-RING-gō-skōp) _____

Clinical Aspects of Hearing

Hearing Loss

Hearing impairment may result from disease, injury, or developmental problems that affect the ear itself or any nervous pathways concerned with the sense of hearing.

Sensorineural hearing loss results from damage to the inner ear, the eighth cranial nerve, or central auditory pathways. Heredity, toxins, exposure to loud noises, and the aging process are possible causes for this type of hearing loss. It may range from inability to hear certain sound frequencies to a complete loss of hearing (deafness). People with extreme hearing loss that originates in the inner ear may benefit from a cochlear implant. This prosthesis stimulates the cochlear nerve directly, bypassing the receptor cells of the inner ear, and may allow the recipient to hear medium to loud sounds.

Conductive hearing loss results from blockage in sound transmission to the inner ear. Causes include obstruction, severe infection, or fixation of the middle ear ossicles. Often, physicians can successfully treat the conditions that cause conductive hearing loss.

Box 18-1 has information on careers in audiology, the study and treatment of hearing disorders.

Otitis

Otitis is any inflammation of the ear. **Otitis media** refers to an infection that leads to fluid accumulation in the middle ear cavity. One cause is malfunction or obstruction of the eustachian tube, as by allergy, enlarged adenoids, injury, or congenital abnormalities. Another cause is infection that spreads to the middle ear, most commonly from the upper respiratory tract. Continued infection may lead to accumulation of pus and perforation of the eardrum. Otitis media usually affects children under 5 years of age and may result in hearing loss. If not treated with antibiotics, the infection may spread to other regions of the ear and head. An incision, a **myringotomy**, and placement of a tube in the tympanic membrane helps to ventilate and drain the middle ear cavity in cases of otitis media.

Otitis externa is the inflammation of the external auditory canal. Infections in this region may be caused by a fungus or bacterium and are most common among those living in hot climates and among swimmers, leading to the alternative name, "swimmer's ear."

Otosclerosis

In **otosclerosis**, the bony structure of the inner ear deteriorates and then reforms into spongy bone tissue that

18

Box 18-1 **Health Professions**

Audiologists

Audiologists specialize in preventing, diagnosing, and treating hearing disorders that may be caused by injury, infection, birth defects, noise, or aging. They take a complete patient history to diagnose hearing disorders and use specialized equipment to measure hearing acuity. Audiologists design and implement individualized treatment plans, which may include fitting clients with assistive listening devices, such as hearing aids, or teaching alternative communication skills, such as lip reading. Audiologists also measure workplace and community noise levels and teach the public how to prevent hearing loss. Most audiologists in the United States have master's degrees or the equivalent from an accredited college or university and must pass a national licensing exam.

Audiologists work in a variety of settings, such as hospitals, nursing care facilities, schools, and clinics. Job prospects are good, as the need for audiologists' specialized skills will increase as populations age. The American Academy of Audiology at www.audiology.org has more information on this career.

may eventually harden. Most commonly, the stapes becomes fixed against the inner ear and is unable to vibrate, resulting in conductive hearing loss. The cause of otosclerosis is unknown, but some cases are hereditary. Surgeons usually can remove the damaged bone. In a **stapedectomy**, the stapes is removed and a prosthetic bone is inserted.

Ménière Disease

Ménière disease is a disorder that affects the inner ear. It seems to involve production and circulation of the fluid that fills the inner ear, but the cause is unknown. The symptoms are **vertigo** (dizziness), hearing loss, pronounced **tinnitus** (ringing in the ears), and a feeling of pressure in the ear. The course of the disease is uneven,

and symptoms may become less severe with time. Ménière disease is treated with drugs to control nausea and dizziness, such as those used to treat motion sickness. In severe cases, the inner ear or part of the eighth cranial nerve may be destroyed surgically.

Acoustic Neuroma

An **acoustic neuroma** (also schwannoma or neurilemoma) is a tumor that arises from the neurilemma (sheath) of the eighth cranial nerve. As the tumor enlarges, it presses on surrounding nerves and interferes with blood supply. This leads to tinnitus, dizziness, and progressive hearing loss. Other symptoms develop as the tumor presses on the brainstem and other cranial nerves. Usually, it is necessary to remove the tumor surgically.

Terminology   Key Terms

THE EAR

Disorders

acoustic neuroma *a-KŪ-stik nū-RŌ-ma*	A tumor of the eighth cranial nerve sheath; although benign, it can press on surrounding tissue and produce symptoms; also called an acoustic or vestibular schwannoma or acoustic neurilemoma
conductive hearing loss	Hearing impairment that results from blockage of sound transmission to the inner ear
Ménière disease *men-NYĀR*	A disease associated with increased fluid pressure in the inner ear and characterized by hearing loss, vertigo, and tinnitus
otitis externa *ō-TĪ-tis ex-TER-na*	Inflammation of the external auditory canal; swimmer's ear
otitis media *ō-TĪ-tis MĔ-dē-a*	Inflammation of the middle ear with accumulation of serous (watery) or mucoid fluid
otosclerosis *ō-tō-skle-RŌ-sis*	Formation of abnormal and sometimes hardened bony tissue in the ear. It usually occurs around the oval window and the footplate (base) of the stapes, causing immobilization of the stapes and progressive loss of hearing
sensorineural hearing loss *sen-sō-rē-NŪ-ral*	Hearing impairment that results from damage to the inner ear, eighth cranial nerve, or auditory pathways in the brain
tinnitus *tin-Ī-tus*	A sensation of noises, such as ringing or tinkling, in the ear
vertigo *VER-ti-gō*	An illusion of movement, as of the body moving in space or the environment moving about the body; usually caused by disturbances in the vestibular apparatus. Used loosely to mean dizziness or lightheadedness

Treatment

myringotomy *mir-in-GOT-ō-mē*	Surgical incision of the tympanic membrane; performed to drain the middle ear cavity or to insert a tube into the tympanic membrane for drainage
stapedectomy *stā-pē-DEK-tō-mē*	Surgical removal of the stapes; it may be combined with insertion of a prosthesis to correct otosclerosis

Go to the pronunciation glossary on the Student Resources to hear these words pronounced.

Terminology   Supplementary Terms

Normal Structure and Function

aural *AW-ral*	Pertaining to or perceived by the ear
decibel (dB) *DES-i-bel*	A unit for measuring the relative intensity of sound
hertz (Hz)	A unit for measuring the frequency (pitch) of sound
mastoid process	A small projection of the temporal bone behind the external auditory canal; it consists of loosely arranged bony material and small, air-filled cavities
stapedius *stā-PĒ-dē-us*	A small muscle attached to the stapes. It contracts in the presence of a loud sound, producing the acoustic reflex

Symptoms and Conditions

cholesteatoma *kō-lē-stē-a-TŌ-ma*	A cystlike mass containing cholesterol that is most common in the middle ear and mastoid region; a possible complication of chronic middle ear infection
labyrinthitis *lab-i-rin-THĪ-tis*	Inflammation of the ear's labyrinth (inner ear); otitis interna
mastoiditis *mas-toyd-Ī-tis*	Inflammation of the air cells of the mastoid process
presbycusis *prez-bē-KŪ-sis*	Loss of hearing caused by aging; also presbyacusis

Diagnosis and Treatment

audiometry *aw-de-OM-e-trē*	Measurement of hearing
electronystagmography (ENG) *ē-lek-trō-nis-tag-MOG-ra-fē*	A method for recording eye movements by means of electrical responses; such movements may reflect vestibular dysfunction
otorhinolaryngology (ORL) *ō-tō-rī-nō-lar-in-GOL-ō-jē*	The branch of medicine that deals with diseases of the ear(s), nose, and throat (ENT); also called otolaryngology (OL)
otoscope *Ō-tō-skōp*	Instrument for examining the ear (see Fig. 7-6)
Rinne test *RIN-ne*	Test that measures hearing by comparing results of bone conduction and air conduction (Fig. 18-5)
spondee *spon-dē*	A two-syllable word with equal stress on each syllable; used in hearing tests; examples are toothbrush, baseball, cowboy, pancake
Weber test	Test for hearing loss that uses a vibrating tuning fork placed at the center of the head (Fig. 18-6)

PASSport to Success®   Go to the pronunciation glossary on the Student Resources to hear these words pronounced.

Figure 18-5 **The Rinne test.** This test assesses both air and bone conduction of sound.

Figure 18-6 **The Weber test.** This test assesses bone conduction of sound.

Terminology Abbreviations

The Ear

ABR	Auditory brainstem response
AC	Air conduction
AD	Right ear (Latin, *auris dexter*)
AS	Left ear (Latin, *auris sinistra*)
BAEP	Brainstem auditory evoked potentials
BC	Bone conduction
dB	Decibel
ENG	Electronystagmography
ENT	Ear(s), nose, and throat
HL	Hearing level
Hz	Hertz
OL	Otolaryngology
OM	Otitis media
ORL	Otorhinolaryngology
ST	Speech threshold
TM	Tympanic membrane
TTS	Temporary threshold shift

The Eye and Vision

The eye is protected by its position within a bony socket or **orbit**. It is also protected by the eyelids, or **palpebrae**, eyebrows, and eyelashes (Fig. 18-7). The **lacrimal (tear) glands** (Fig. 18-8) constantly bathe and cleanse the eyes with a lubricating fluid that drains into the nose. The protective **conjunctiva** is a thin membrane that lines the eyelids and covers the anterior portion of the eye. This membrane folds back to form a narrow space between

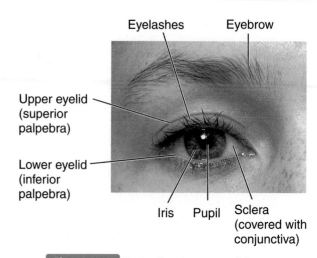

Figure 18-7 **Protective structures of the eye.**

Figure 18-8 **Lacrimal apparatus.** The right lacrimal (tear) gland and its associated ducts are shown.

the eyeball and the eyelids. Medications can be instilled into this conjunctival sac.

The wall of the eye is composed of three layers (Fig. 18-9). Named from outermost to innermost, they are as follows:

1. The **sclera**, commonly called the *white of the eye*, is the tough surface protective layer. The sclera extends over the eye's anterior portion as the transparent **cornea**.

2. The **uvea** is the middle layer, which consists of the:

   - **choroid**, a vascular and pigmented layer located in the posterior portion of the eyeball. The choroid provides nourishment for the **retina**.

   - **ciliary body**, which contains a muscle that controls the shape of the **lens** to allow for near and far vision, a process known as **accommodation** (Fig. 18-10). The lens must become more rounded for viewing close objects.

   - **iris**, a muscular ring that controls the size of the **pupil**, thus regulating the amount of light that enters the eye (Fig. 18-11). The genetically controlled pigments of the iris determine eye color.

3. The retina is the innermost layer and the actual visual receptor. It consists of two types of specialized cells that respond to light:

   - The **rods** function in dim light, provide low **visual acuity** (sharpness), and do not respond to color.

   - The **cones** are active in bright light, have high visual acuity, and respond to color.

Proper vision requires the **refraction** (bending) of light rays as they pass through the eye to focus on a specific point on the retina. The impulses generated within the rods and cones are transmitted to the brain by way of the optic nerve (second cranial nerve). Where the optic nerve connects to the retina, there are no rods or cones. This point, at which there is no visual perception, is called the **optic disk**, or blind spot (Fig. 18-12). The **fovea** is a tiny depression in the retina near the optic nerve that has a high concentration of cones and

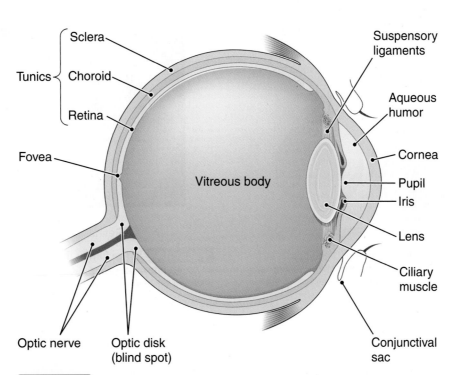

Figure 18-9 **The eye.** The three layers of the eyeball are shown along with other structures involved in vision.

Figure 18-10 **Accommodation for near vision.** When viewing a close object, the lens must become more rounded to focus light rays on the retina.

is the point of greatest visual acuity. The fovea is surrounded by a yellowish spot called the **macula** (see Fig. 18-12).

The eyeball is filled with a jellylike **vitreous body** (see Fig. 18-9), which helps maintain the shape of the eye and also refracts light. The **aqueous humor** is the fluid that fills the eye anterior to the lens, maintaining the cornea's shape and refracting light. This fluid is constantly produced and drained from the eye.

Six muscles attached to the outside of each eye coordinate eye movements to achieve **convergence**, that is, coordinated movement of the eyes so that they both are fixed on the same point.

Box 18-2 explores the Greek origins of some medical words, including some pertaining to the eye.

> **PASSport to Success®** The animation *The Retina* on the Student Resources illustrates in motion the structure and function of this light-sensitive layer of the eye.

Figure 18-11 **Function of the iris.** In bright light, muscles in the iris constrict the pupil, limiting the light that enters the eye. In dim light, the iris dilates the pupil to allow more light to enter the eye.

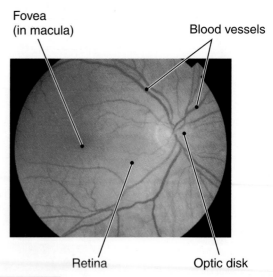

Figure 18-12 **The fundus (back) of the eye as seen through an ophthalmoscope.** The optic disk (blind spot) is shown as well as the fovea, the point of sharpest vision, in the retina.

Box 18-2 Focus on Words

The Greek Influence

Some of our most beautiful (and difficult to spell and pronounce) words come from Greek. *Esthesi/o* means "sensation". It appears in the word *anesthesia*, a state in which there is lack of sensation, particularly pain. It is found in the word *esthetics* (also spelled aesthetics), which pertains to beauty, artistry, and appearance. The prefix *presby*, in the terms *presbycusis* and *presbyopia*, means "old," and these conditions appear with aging. The root *cycl/o*, pertaining to the ringlike ciliary body of the eye, is from the Greek word for circle or wheel. The same root appears in the words *bicycle* and *tricycle*. Also pertaining to the eye, the term *iris* means "rainbow" in Greek, and the iris is the colored part of the eye.

The root *-sthen/o* means "strength," and occurs in the words *asthenia*, meaning lack of strength, or weakness, and *neurasthenia*, an old term for vague "nervous exhaustion," now applied to conditions involving chronic symptoms of generalized fatigue, anxiety, and pain. The root also appears in the word *calisthenics* in combination with the root *cali-*, meaning "beauty." So the rhythmic strengthening and conditioning exercises that are done in calisthenics literally give us beauty through strength.

The Greek root *steth/o* means "chest," although a stethoscope is used to listen to sounds in other parts of the body as well as the chest.

Asphyxia is derived from the Greek root *sphygm/o* meaning "pulse." The word is literally "stoppage of the pulse," which is exactly what happens when one suffocates. This same root is found in *sphygmomanometer*, the apparatus used to measure blood pressure. One look at the word and one attempt to pronounce it make clear why most people call the device a blood pressure cuff!

Terminology Key Terms

THE EYE

Normal Structure and Function

Term	Definition
accommodation a-kom-ō-DĀ-shun	Adjustment of the lens' curvature to allow for vision at various distances
aqueous humor AK-wē-us	Fluid that fills the eye anterior to the lens
choroid KOR-oyd	The dark, vascular, middle layer of the eye (roots: *chori/o, choroid/o*); part of the uvea (see below)
ciliary body SIL-ē-ar-ē	The muscular portion of the uvea that surrounds the lens and adjusts its shape for near and far vision (root: *cycl/o*)
cone	A specialized cell in the retina that responds to light; cones have high visual acuity, function in bright light, and respond to colors
conjunctiva kon-junk-TĪ-va	The mucous membrane that lines the eyelids and covers the eyeball's anterior surface
convergence kon-VER-jens	Coordinated movement of the eyes toward fixation on the same point
cornea KOR-nē-a	The clear, anterior portion of the sclera (roots: *corne/o, kerat/o*)
eye	The organ of vision (roots: *opt/o, ocul/o, ophthalm/o*); Latin *ops* means "eye"

(continued)

Terminology	**Key Terms** (continued)
fovea FŌ-vē-a	The tiny depression in the retina that is the point of sharpest vision; fovea centralis, central fovea
iris Ī-ris	The muscular colored ring between the lens and the cornea; regulates the amount of light that enters the eye by altering the size of the pupil at its center (roots: *ir, irid/o, irit/o*); plural: irides (IR-i-dēz)
lacrimal glands LAK-ri-mal	Pertaining to tears (roots: *lacrim/o, dacry/o*)
lens lenz	The transparent, biconvex structure in the anterior portion of the eye that refracts light and functions in accommodation (roots: *lent/i, phak/o*)
macula MAK-ū-la	A small spot or colored area; used alone to mean the yellowish spot in the retina that contains the fovea
optic disk	The point where the optic nerve joins the retina; at this point, there are no rods or cones; also called the blind spot or optic papilla
orbit OR-bit	The bony cavity that contains the eyeball
palpebra PAL-pe-bra	An eyelid; a protective fold (upper or lower) that closes over the anterior surface of the eye (roots: *palpebr/o, blephar/o*); adjective: palpebral; plural: palpebrae (pal-PĒ-brē)
pupil PŪ-pil	The opening at the center of the iris (root: *pupill/o*)
refraction rē-FRAK-shun	The bending of light rays as they pass through the eye to focus on a specific point on the retina; also the determination and correction of ocular refractive errors
retina RET-i-na	The innermost, light-sensitive layer of the eye; contains the rods and cones, the specialized receptor cells for vision (root: *retin/o*)
rod	A specialized cell in the retina that responds to light; rods have low visual acuity, function in dim light, and do not respond to color
sclera SKLĒR-a	The tough, white, fibrous outermost layer of the eye; the white of the eye (root: *scler/o*)
uvea Ū-vē-a	The middle, vascular layer of the eye (root: *uve/o*); consists of the choroid, ciliary body, and iris
visual acuity a-KŪ-i-tē	Sharpness of vision
vitreous body VIT-rē-us	The transparent jellylike mass that fills the eyeball's main cavity; also called vitreous humor

 PASSport to Success®   Go to the pronunciation glossary on the Student Resources to hear these words pronounced.

Word Parts Pertaining to the Eye and Vision

See Tables 18-3 to 18-5.

Table 18-3	Roots for External Eye Structures		
Root	**Meaning**	**Example**	**Definition of Example**
blephar/o	eyelid	symblepharon *sim-BLEF-a-ron*	adhesion of the eyelid to the eyeball (*sym-* means "together")
palpebr/o	eyelid	palpebral *PAL-pe-bral*	pertaining to an eyelid
dacry/o	tear, lacrimal apparatus	dacryorrhea *dak-rē-ō-RĒ-a*	discharge from the lacrimal apparatus
dacryocyst/o	lacrimal sac	dacryocystocele *dak-rē-ō-SIS-tō-sēl*	hernia of the lacrimal sac
lacrim/o	tear, lacrimal apparatus	lacrimation *lak-ri-MA-shun*	secretion of tears

EXERCISE 18-3

Define the following words:

1. nasolacrimal (*nā-zō-LAK-ri-mal*) _____

2. interpalpebral (*in-ter-PAL-pe-bral*) _____

3. blepharoplegia (*BLEF-a-rō-plē-jē-a*) _____

4. dacryocystectomy (*dak-rē-ō-sis-TEK-tō-mē*) _____

Use the roots indicated to write words that mean the following:

5. spasm of the eyelid (blephar/o) _____

6. stone in the lacrimal apparatus (dacry/o) _____

7. inflammation of a lacrimal sac _____

18

Table 18-4	Roots for the Eye and Vision		
Root	**Meaning**	**Example**	**Definition of Example**
opt/o	eye, vision	optometer *op-TOM-e-ter*	instrument for measuring the refractive power of the eye
ocul/o	eye	sinistrocular *si-nis-TROK-ū-lar*	pertaining to the left eye
ophthalm/o	eye	exophthalmos *eks-of-THAL-mos*	protrusion of the eyeball
scler/o	sclera	episcleritis *ep-i-skle-rī-tis*	inflammation of the tissue on the surface of the sclera
corne/o	cornea	circumcorneal *sir-kum-KOR-nē-al*	around the cornea

(continued)

Table 18-4	Continued		

Root	Meaning	Example	Definition of Example
kerat/o	cornea	keratoplasty KER-a-tō-plas-tē	plastic repair of the cornea; corneal transplant
lent/i	lens	lentiform LEN-ti-form	resembling a lens
phak/o, phac/o	lens	aphakia a-FĀ-kē-a	absence of a lens
uve/o	uvea	uveal Ū-vē-al	pertaining to the uvea
chori/o, choroid/o	choroid	subchoroidal sub-kor-OYD-al	below the choroid
cycl/o	ciliary body, ciliary muscle	cycloplegic sī-klō-PLĒ-jik	pertaining to or causing paralysis of the ciliary muscle
ir, irit/o, irid/o	iris	iridoschisis ir-i-DOS-ki-sis	splitting of the iris
pupill/o	pupil	iridopupillary ir-i-dō-PŪ-pi-ler-ē	pertaining to the iris and the pupil
retin/o	retina	retinoscopy ret-in-OS-kō-pē	examination of the retina

EXERCISE 18-4

Fill in the blanks:

1. The oculomotor (ok-ū-lō-MŌ-tor) nerve controls movements of the _____.

2. The science of orthoptics (or-THOP-tiks) deals with correcting defects in _____.

3. The term *phacolysis* (fa-KOL-i-sis) means destruction of the _____.

4. A keratometer (ker-a-TOM-e-ter) is an instrument for measuring the curves of the _____.

5. Lenticonus is conical protrusion of the _____.

Identify and define the roots pertaining to the eye in the following words:

	Root	Meaning of Root
6. optometrist (op-TOM-e-trist)	_____	_____
7. microphthalmos (mī-krof-THAL-mus)	_____	_____
8. interpupillary (in-ter-PŪ-pi-ler-ē)	_____	_____
9. phacotoxic (fak-ō-TOK-sik)	_____	_____
10. uveitis (ū-vē-Ī-tis)	_____	_____
11. iridodilator (ir-id-ō-DĬ-lā-tor)	_____	_____
12. retrolental (ret-rō-LEN-tal)	_____	_____

Write words for the following definitions:

13. inflammation of the uvea and sclera _____

14. softening of the lens (use phac/o) _____

15. pertaining to the pupil _____

16. surgical fixation of the retina _____

17. inflammation of the ciliary body _____

Use the root *ophthalm/o* to write words for the following definitions:

18. an instrument used to examine the eye   _____

19. the medical specialty that deals with the eye and diseases of the eye   _____

Use the root *irid/o* to write words for the following definitions:

20. surgical removal of (part of) the iris   _____

21. paralysis of the iris   _____

Define the following words:

22. dextrocular (*deks-TROK-ū-lar*) _____

23. retinoschisis (*ret-i-NOS-ki-sis*) _____

24. sclerotome (*SKLĒR-ō-tōm*) _____

25. optical (*OP-ti-kal*) _____

26. keratitis (*ker-a-TĪ-tis*) _____

27. cyclotomy (*sī-KLOT-ō-mē*) _____

28. iridocyclitis (*ir-i-dō-sī-KLĪ-tis*) _____

29. chorioretinal (*kor-ē-ō-RET-i-nal*) _____

30. lenticular (*len-TIK-ū-lar*) _____

18

Table 18-5	Suffixes for the Eye and Vision*		
Suffix	**Meaning**	**Example**	**Definition of Example**
-opsia	vision	heteropsia *het-er-OP-sē-a*	unequal vision in the two eyes
-opia	eye, vision	hemianopia *hem-ē-an-Ō-pe-a*	blindness in half the visual field

*Compounds of *-ops* (eye) + *-ia*.

EXERCISE 18-5

Use the suffix *-opsia* to write words for the following definitions:

  1. a visual defect in which objects seem larger (macr/o) than they are _____

  2. lack of (a-) color (chromat/o) vision (complete color blindness) _____

Use the suffix *-opia* to write words for the following definitions:

  3. double vision _____

  4. changes in vision due to old age (use the prefix *presby-* meaning "old") _____

The suffix *-opia* is added to the root *metr/o* (measure) to form words pertaining to the refractive power of the eye. Add a prefix to *-metropia* to form words for the following:

  5. a lack of (perfect) refractive power in the eye _____

  6. unequal refractive powers in the two eyes _____

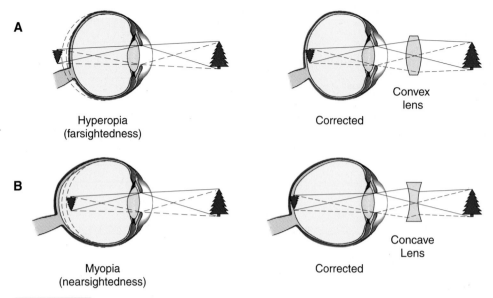

A

Hyperopia
(farsightedness)

Convex
lens

Corrected

B

Myopia
(nearsightedness)

Concave
Lens

Corrected

Figure 18-13 **Errors of refraction.** (*A*) Hyperopia (farsightedness). (*B*) Myopia (nearsightedness). A convex (outwardly curved) lens corrects for hyperopia; a concave (inwardly curved) lens corrects for myopia.

Clinical Aspects of Vision

Errors of Refraction

If the eyeball is too long, images will form in front of the retina. To focus clearly, one must bring an object closer to the eye. This condition of nearsightedness is technically called **myopia** (Fig. 18-13). The opposite condition is **hyperopia**, or farsightedness, in which the eyeball is too short and images form behind the retina. One must move an object away from the eye for clear focus. The same effect is produced by **presbyopia**, which accompanies aging. The lens loses elasticity and can no longer accommodate for near vision, so a person becomes increasingly farsighted.

An **astigmatism** is an irregularity in the curve of the cornea or lens that distorts light entering the eye and blurs vision.

Glasses can compensate for most of these refractive impairments, as shown for nearsightedness and farsightedness in Figure 18-13. See also Box 18-3 for information on a surgical technique to correct refractive errors.

Infection

Several microorganisms can cause **conjunctivitis** (inflammation of the conjunctiva). This is a highly infectious disease commonly called "pinkeye."

The bacterium *Chlamydia trachomatis* causes **trachoma**, inflammation of the cornea and conjunctiva that results in scarring. This disease is rare in the United States and other industrialized countries, but is a common cause of blindness in underdeveloped countries, although it is easily cured with sulfa drugs and antibiotics.

Gonorrhea is the usual cause of an acute conjunctivitis in newborns called **ophthalmia neonatorum**. An antibiotic ointment is routinely used to prevent such eye infections in newborns.

Disorders of the Retina

Retinal detachment, separation of the retina from the underlying layer of the eye (the choroid), may be caused by a tumor, hemorrhage, or injury to the eye (Fig. 18-14). This condition interferes with vision and is commonly repaired with laser surgery.

Degeneration of the macula, the point of sharpest vision, is a common cause of visual problems in the elderly. When associated with aging, this deterioration is described as **age-related macular degeneration (AMD)**. In one form of macular degeneration ("dry"), material accumulates on the retina. Vitamins C and E, beta carotene, and zinc supplements may delay this process. In another form, neovascular ("wet") AMD, abnormal blood vessels grow under the retina, causing it to detach. Laser surgery may stop the growth of these vessels and delay vision loss. More recently, ophthalmologists have had success in delaying the progress of wet AMD with regular intraocular injections of a drug (Lucentis) that inhibits blood vessel formation. Macular degeneration typically affects central vision but not peripheral vision (Fig. 18-15). Other causes of macular degeneration are drug toxicity and hereditary diseases.

Circulatory problems associated with diabetes mellitus eventually cause changes in the retina referred to as **diabetic retinopathy**. In addition to vascular damage, there is a yellowish, waxy exudate high in lipoproteins.

Vitreous body

Detached retina

Fluid

Retinal tear

Figure 18-14 **Retinal detachment.**

Figure 18-15 **Visual loss associated with macular degeneration.** The center of the visual field is affected, but peripheral vision is usually unaffected.

Figure 18-16 **Cataract.** The white appearance of the pupil in this eye is due to complete opacity of the lens.

With time, new blood vessels form and penetrate the vitreous humor, causing hemorrhage, detachment of the retina, and blindness.

Cataract

A **cataract** is an opacity (cloudiness) of the lens (Fig. 18-16). Causes of cataract include disease, injury, chemicals, and exposure to physical forces, especially the ultraviolet radiation in sunlight. The cataracts that frequently appear with age may result from exposure to environmental factors in combination with degeneration attributable to aging.

To prevent blindness, an ophthalmologist must remove the cloudy lens surgically. Commonly, the lens' anterior capsule is removed along with the cataract, leaving the posterior capsule in place (Fig. 18-17). In **phacoemulsification**, the lens is fragmented with high-frequency ultrasound and extracted through a small incision (see Box 18-3). After cataract removal, an artificial intraocular lens (IOL) is usually implanted to compensate for the missing lens. The original type of implant provides vision only within a fixed distance; newer implants are designed to allow for near and far accommodation. Alternatively, a person can wear a contact lens or special glasses.

18

Box 18-3   Clinical Perspectives

Eye Surgery: A Glimpse of the Cutting Edge

Cataracts, glaucoma, and refractive errors are common eye disorders. In the past, cataract and glaucoma treatments concentrated on managing the diseases. Refractive errors were corrected using eyeglasses and, more recently, contact lenses. Today, laser and microsurgical techniques can remove cataracts, reduce glaucoma, and allow people with refractive errors to put their eyeglasses and contacts away. These cutting-edge procedures include:

■ LASIK (laser in situ keratomileusis) to correct refractive errors. During this procedure, a surgeon uses a laser to reshape the cornea so that it refracts light directly onto the retina, rather than in front of or behind it. A microkeratome (surgical knife) is used to cut a flap in the cornea's outer layer. A computer-controlled laser sculpts the middle layer of the cornea and then the flap is replaced. The procedure takes only a few minutes and patients recover their vision quickly and usually with little postoperative pain.

■ Phacoemulsification to remove cataracts. During this procedure, a surgeon makes a very small incision (approximately 3 mm long) through the sclera near the cornea's outer edge. An ultrasonic probe is inserted through this opening and into the center of the lens. The probe uses sound waves to emulsify the lens' central core, which is then suctioned out. An artificial lens is then permanently implanted in the lens capsule (see Fig. 18-17). The procedure is typically painless, although the patient may feel some discomfort for 1 to 2 days afterward.

■ Laser trabeculoplasty to treat glaucoma. This procedure uses a laser to help drain fluid from the eye and lower intraocular pressure. The laser is aimed at drainage canals located between the cornea and iris and makes several burns that are believed to open the canals and allow better fluid drainage. The procedure is typically painless and takes only a few minutes.

Figure 18-17 **Cataract extraction surgeries.** (*A*) Cross section of normal eye anatomy. (*B*) Extracapsular lens extraction involves removing the lens but leaving the posterior capsule intact to receive a synthetic intraocular lens. (*C*) Intracapsular lens extraction involves removing the lens and lens capsule and implanting a synthetic intraocular lens in the anterior chamber.

Glaucoma

Glaucoma is an abnormal increase in pressure within the eyeball. It occurs when more aqueous humor is produced than can be drained away from the eye. There is pressure on blood vessels in the eye and on the optic nerve, leading to blindness. There are many causes of glaucoma, and screening for this disorder should be a part of every routine eye examination. Fetal infection with German measles (rubella) early in pregnancy can cause glaucoma, as well as cataracts and hearing impairment. Glaucoma is usually treated with medication to reduce pressure in the eye and occasionally is treated with surgery (see Box 18-3).

Terminology   Key Terms

THE EYE

Disorders

age-related macular degeneration (AMD)	Deterioration of the macula associated with aging; macular degeneration impairs central vision
astigmatism a-STIG-ma-tizm	An error of refraction caused by irregularity in the curvature of the cornea or lens
cataract KAT-a-rakt	Opacity of the lens of the eye
conjunctivitis kon-junk-ti-VĪ-tis	Inflammation of the conjunctiva; pinkeye
diabetic retinopathy ret-i-NOP-a-thē	Degenerative changes in the retina associated with diabetes mellitus
glaucoma glaw-KŌ-ma	An eye disease caused by increased intraocular pressure that damages the optic disk and causes vision loss. Usually results from faulty fluid drainage from the anterior eye
hyperopia hī-per-Ō-pē-a	A refractive error in which light rays focus behind the retina and objects can be seen clearly only when far from the eye; farsightedness; also called hypermetropia
myopia mī-Ō-pē-a	A refractive error in which light rays focus in front of the retina and objects can be seen clearly only when very close to the eye; nearsightedness
ophthalmia neonatorum of-THAL-mē-a nē-ō-nā-TOR-um	Severe conjunctivitis usually caused by infection with gonococcus during birth

(continued)

Terminology Key Terms (continued)

phacoemulsification *fak-ō-ē-MUL-si-fi-kā-shun*	Removal of a cataract by ultrasonic destruction and extraction of the lens
presbyopia *prez-bē-Ō-pē-a*	Changes in the eye that occur with age; the lens loses elasticity and the ability to accommodate for near vision
retinal detachment	Separation of the retina from its underlying layer
trachoma *tra-KŌ-ma*	An infection caused by *Chlamydia trachomatis* leading to inflammation and scarring of the cornea and conjunctiva; a common cause of blindness in underdeveloped countries

PASSport to Success® Go to the pronunciation glossary on the Student Resources to hear these words pronounced.

Terminology Supplementary Terms

THE EYE

Normal Structure and Function

canthus *KAN-thus*	The angle at either end of the slit between the eyelids
diopter *DĪ-op-ter*	A measurement unit for the refractive power of a lens
emmetropia *em-e-TRŌ-pē-a*	The normal condition of the eye in refraction, in which parallel light rays focus exactly on the retina
fundus *FUN-dus*	A bottom or base; the region farthest from the opening of a structure. The eye's fundus is the posterior portion of the interior eyeball as seen with an ophthalmoscope
meibomian gland *mī-BŌ-mē-an*	A sebaceous gland in the eyelid
tarsus *TAR-sus*	The framework of dense connective tissue that gives shape to the eyelid; tarsal plate
zonule *ZON-ūl*	A system of fibers that holds the lens in place; also called suspensory ligaments

Symptoms and Conditions

amblyopia *am-blē-Ō-pē-a*	A condition that occurs when visual acuity is not the same in the two eyes in children (prefix *ambly* means "dim"). Disuse of the poorer eye will result in blindness if not corrected. Also called "lazy eye"
anisocoria *an-ī-sō-KŌ-rē-a*	Condition in which the two pupils (root: *cor/o*) are not of equal size
blepharoptosis *blef-a-rop-TŌ-sis*	Drooping of the eyelid
chalazion *ka-LĀ-zē-on*	A small mass on the eyelid resulting from inflammation and blockage of a meibomian gland
druzen *DRŪ-zen*	Small growths that appear as tiny yellowish spots beneath the retina of the eye; typically occur with age but also occur in certain abnormal conditions

(continued)

18

Terminology	**Supplementary Terms** (continued)
floater FLŌ-ter	A small moving object in the field of vision that originates in the vitreous body. Floaters appear as spots or threads and are caused by benign degenerative or embryonic deposits in the vitreous body that cast a shadow on the retina
hordeolum hor-DĒ-ō-lum	Inflammation of a sebaceous gland of the eyelid; a sty
keratoconus ker-a-tō-KŌ-nus	Conical protrusion of the corneal center
miosis mī-Ō-sis	Abnormal contraction of the pupils (from Greek, meaning "diminution")
mydriasis mi-DRĬ-a-sis	Pronounced or abnormal dilation of the pupil
nyctalopia nik-ta-LŌ-pē-a	Night blindness. Inability to see well in dim light or at night (root: *nyct/o*); often due to lack of vitamin A, which is used to make the pigment needed for vision in dim light
nystagmus nis-TAG-mus	Rapid, involuntary, rhythmic movements of the eyeball; may occur in neurologic diseases or disorders of the inner ear's vestibular apparatus
papilledema pap-il-e-DĒ-ma	Swelling of the optic disk (papilla); choked disk
phlyctenule FLIK-ten-ūl	A small blister or nodule on the cornea or conjunctiva
pseudophakia sū-dō-FĀ-kē-a	A condition in which a cataractous lens has been removed and replaced with a plastic lens implant
retinitis ret-in-Ī-tis	Inflammation of the retina; causes include systemic disease, infection, hemorrhage, exposure to light
retinitis pigmentosa ret-in-Ī-tis pig-men-TŌ-sa	A hereditary chronic degenerative disease of the retina that begins in early childhood. There is atrophy of the optic nerve and clumping of pigment in the retina
retinoblastoma ret-in-ō-blas-TŌ-ma	A malignant glioma of the retina; usually appears in early childhood and is sometimes hereditary; fatal if untreated, but current cure rates are high
scotoma skō-TŌ-ma	An area of diminished vision within the visual field
strabismus stra-BIZ-mus	A deviation of the eye in which the visual lines of each eye are not directed to the same object at the same time. Also called heterotropia or squint. The various forms are referred to as -*tropias*, with the direction of turning (trop/o) indicated by a prefix, such as esotropia (inward), exotropia (outward), hypertropia (upward), and hypotropia (downward). The suffix -*phoria* is also used, as in esophoria
synechia sin-EK-ē-a	Adhesion of parts, especially adhesion of the iris to the lens and cornea (plural: synechiae)
xanthoma zan-THŌ-ma	A soft, slightly raised, yellowish patch or nodule usually on the eyelids; occurs in the elderly; also called xanthelasma

Diagnosis and Treatment

canthotomy kan-THOT-ō-mē	Surgical division of a canthus
cystitome SIS-ti-tōm	Instrument for incising the lens capsule
electroretinography (ERG) ē-lek-trō-ret-i-NOG-ra-fē	Study of the retina's electrical response to light stimulation

(continued)

Terminology   Supplementary Terms (continued)

enucleation ē-nū-klē-Ā-shun	Surgical removal of the eyeball
gonioscopy gō-nē-OS-kō-pē	Examination of the angle between the cornea and the iris (anterior chamber angle) in which fluids drain out of the eye (root *goni/o* means "angle")
keratometer ker-a-TOM-e-ter	An instrument for measuring the curvature of the cornea
mydriatic mid-rē-AT-ik	A drug that causes dilation of the pupil
phorometer fo-ROM-e-ter	An instrument for determining the degree and kind of strabismus
retinoscope RET-in-ō-skōp	An instrument used to determine refractive errors of the eye; also called a skiascope (SKĪ-a-skōp)
slit-lamp biomicroscope	An instrument for examining the eye under magnification
Snellen chart SNEL-en	A chart printed with letters of decreasing size used to test visual acuity when viewed from a set distance; results reported as a fraction giving a subject's vision compared with normal vision at a distance of 20 feet
tarsorrhaphy tar-SOR-a-fē	Suturing together of all or part of the upper and lower eyelids
tonometer tō-NOM-e-ter	An instrument used to measure fluid pressure in the eye

 PASSport to Success® Go to the pronunciation glossary on the Student Resources to hear these words pronounced.

18

Terminology   Abbreviations

THE EYE

A, Acc	Accommodation
AMD	Age-related macular degeneration
ARC	Abnormal retinal correspondence
As, AST	Astigmatism
cc	With correction
Em	Emmetropia
EOM	Extraocular movement, muscles
ERG	Electroretinography
ET	Esotropia
FC	Finger counting
HM	Hand movements

IOL	Intraocular lens
IOP	Intraocular pressure
NRC	Normal retinal correspondence
NV	Near vision
OD	Right eye (Latin, *oculus dexter*)
OS	Left eye (Latin, *oculus sinister*)
OU	Both eyes (Latin, *oculi unitas*); also each eye (Latin, *oculus uterque*)
sc	Without correction
VA	Visual acuity
VF	Visual field
XT	Exotropia

Chapter Review

LABELING EXERCISE

The Ear > Write the name of each numbered part on the corresponding line of the answer sheet.

Cochlea   Outer ear
Eustachian (auditory) tube   Pinna
External auditory canal   Semicircular canals
Incus   Stapes
Inner ear   Tympanic membrane
Malleus   Vestibule
Ossicles of middle ear

1. _____   8. _____

2. _____   9. _____

3. _____   10. _____

4. _____   11. _____

5. _____   12. _____

6. _____   13. _____

7. _____

Chapter Review (continued)

The Eye > Write the name of each numbered part on the corresponding line of the answer sheet.

Aqueous humor
Choroid
Ciliary muscle
Conjunctival sac
Cornea
Fovea
Iris

Lens
Optic disk (blind spot)
Optic nerve
Pupil
Retina
Sclera
Vitreous body

1. _____
2. _____
3. _____
4. _____
5. _____
6. _____
7. _____
8. _____
9. _____
10. _____
11. _____

12. _____
13. _____
14. _____

Suspensory ligaments

TERMINOLOGY

Matching > Match the following terms and write the appropriate letter to the left of each number:

_____ **1.** lens
_____ **2.** ossicle
_____ **3.** rods and cones
_____ **4.** vestibular apparatus
_____ **5.** iris

a. small bone
b. structure that changes shape for near and far vision
c. muscular ring that regulates light entering the eye
d. location of equilibrium receptors
e. vision receptors

_____ **6.** tactile
_____ **7.** tinnitus
_____ **8.** hyperesthesia
_____ **9.** fovea
_____ **10.** hemianopia

a. increased sensation
b. blindness in half the visual field
c. point of sharpest vision
d. pertaining to touch
e. sensation of noises in the ear

_____ **11.** phacosclerosis
_____ **12.** ophthalmoplegia
_____ **13.** anacusis
_____ **14.** parosmia
_____ **15.** keratoplasty

a. corneal transplant
b. abnormal smell perception
c. paralysis of an eye muscle
d. hardening of the lens
e. total loss of hearing

Supplementary Terms

_____ **16.** diopter
_____ **17.** mastoid process
_____ **18.** stapedius
_____ **19.** canthus
_____ **20.** decibel

a. angle between the eyelids
b. small muscle attached to an ear ossicle
c. projection of the temporal bone
d. unit of sound intensity
e. unit for measuring the refractive power of the lens

Chapter Review (continued)

_____	**21.** emmetropia	**a.**	rapid, involuntary eye movements
_____	**22.** nystagmus	**b.**	normal refraction of the eye
_____	**23.** mydriasis	**c.**	commonly called "lazy eye"
_____	**24.** druzen	**d.**	abnormal dilation of the pupil
_____	**25.** amblyopia	**e.**	small growths beneath the retina

_____	**26.** AMD	**a.**	irregularity in the curve of the eye
_____	**27.** AS	**b.**	left ear
_____	**28.** AST	**c.**	otorhinolaryngology
_____	**29.** ENT	**d.**	eye disorder associated with aging
_____	**30.** OU	**e.**	both eyes

Fill in the blanks:

31. The scientific name for the eardrum is _____.

32. The term _ceruminous_ applies to _____.

33. The ossicle that is in contact with the inner ear is the _____.

34. The outermost layer of the eye wall is the _____.

35. The bending of light rays as they pass through the eye is _____.

36. The innermost layer of the eye that contains the receptors for vision is the _____.

37. The transparent extension of the sclera that covers the front of the eye is the _____.

38. The sense of awareness of body position is _____.

Define the following words:

39. audiologist _____

40. ophthalmometer _____

41. aphakia _____

42. subscleral _____

43. iridotomy _____

44. myringotomy _____

45. perilental _____

46. dacryorrhea _____

47. chorioretinal _____

48. keratoiritis _____

Write words for the following definitions:

49. any disease of the retina _____

50. absence of pain _____

51. surgical removal of the stapes _____

52. drooping of the eyelid _____

53. plastic repair of the ear _____

54. pertaining to the vestibular apparatus
and cochlea _____

55. hardening of the tympanic membrane _____

56. measurement of the pupil _____

57. pertaining to tears _____

58. excision of (part of) the ciliary body _____

59. endoscopic examination of the
auditory tube _____

Adjectives > Write the adjective form of the following words:

60. cochlea _____

61. palpebra _____

62. vestibule _____

63. uvea _____

64. cornea _____

65. sclera _____

66. pupil _____

Opposites > Write words that mean the opposite of the following:

67. mydriasis _____

68. esotropia _____

69. cc _____

70. myopia _____

71. hyperesthesia _____

72. OD _____

73. hypalgesia _____

18

Chapter Review *(continued)*

Word Building > Write words for the following definitions using the word parts provided.

-pexy   -ia   osm/o   kerat/o   -al   -schisis   -scopy   pseud/o-   retin/o   an-   -plasty   salping/o   sub-   myring/o

74. false sense of smell _____

75. plastic repair of the tympanic membrane _____

76. examination of the retina _____

77. examination of the eustachian tube _____

78. absence of the sense of smell _____

79. splitting of the retina _____

80. examination of the tympanic membrane _____

81. beneath the retina _____

82. surgical fixation of the retina _____

83. examination of the cornea _____

True–False > Examine the following statements. If the statement is true, write T in the first blank. If the statement is false, write F in the first blank and correct the statement by replacing the underlined word in the second blank.

84. In bright light the pupils <u>dilate</u>. _____   _____

85. Gustation is the sense of <u>taste</u>. _____   _____

86. The malleus is located in the <u>middle ear</u>. _____   _____

87. An osmoceptor is a receptor for the sense of <u>balance</u>. _____   _____

88. Hypergeusia is an abnormal increase in the sense of <u>touch</u>. _____   _____

89. The eustachian tube is also called the <u>auditory tube</u>. _____   _____

90. The organ of Corti is located in the <u>cochlea</u>. _____   _____

91. A myringotomy is incision of the <u>vestibule</u>. _____   _____

92. The lacrimal gland produces <u>aqueous humor</u>. _____   _____

Eliminations > In each of the sets below, underline the word that does not fit in with the rest and explain the reason for your choice:

93. pressure — temperature — smell — touch — pain

_____

94. cochlea — pinna — vestibule — oval window — semicircular canals

_____

95. malleus — lacrimal gland — eyelash — conjunctiva — palpebra

_____

96. glaucoma — myopia — cataract — macular degeneration — presbycusis

_____

Word Analysis > Define the following words and give the meaning of the word parts in each. Use a dictionary if necessary.

97. asthenopia (*as-the-NŌ-pē-a*) _____

    a. a- _____

    b. sthen/o _____

    c. -op(s) _____

    d. -ia _____

98. pseudophakia (*sū-dō-FĀ-kē-a*) _____

    a. pseudo _____

    b. phak/o _____

    c. -ia _____

99. cholesteatoma (*kō-lē-stē-a-TŌ-ma*) _____

    a. chol/e _____

    b. steat/o _____

    c. -oma _____

100. exotropia (*ek-sō-trō-pē-a*) _____

    a. ex/o- _____

    b. trop/o _____

    c. -ia _____

101. anisometropia (*an-ī-sō-me-TRŌ-pē-a*) _____

    a. an- _____

    b. iso- _____

    c. metr/o _____

    d. op(s) _____

    e. -ia _____

PASSport to Success®   Go to the word exercises on the Student Resources for additional review exercises.

Case Studies

➤ Case Study 18-1: Medical Records

An electrical fire in the physicians' dictation room left a charred mass of burned and water-damaged medical records. Discharge charts had been stacked awaiting physician sign-off before they could be returned to Medical Records for storage. Several medical transcriptionists spent 3 days sorting through the remains to reassemble the charts, all of which were from the patients of the large otorhinolaryngology practice. In addition to patient identification information, the transcriptionists matched word cues to create piles of similar documents. Patients treated for middle and inner ear problems were identified with words such as stapedectomy, tympanoplasty, myringotomy, cochlear, cholesteatoma, otosclerosis, labyrinth, otitis media, and acoustic neuroma. Patients treated for external ear conditions were grouped using terms such as otoplasty, pinna, postauricular, and otitis externa. Mastoid, laryngeal, and nasal surgery patients were grouped separately. Restoring the charts was an impossible task, and the records were determined to be either incomplete or a total loss. The only document to survive the fire was an audiology report.

➤ Case Study 18-2: Audiology Report

S.R., a 55-year-old man, reported decreased hearing sensitivity in his left ear for the past 3 years. In addition to hearing loss, he was experiencing tinnitus and aural fullness. Pure-tone test results revealed normal hearing sensitivity for the right ear and a moderate sensorineural hearing loss in the left ear. Speech thresholds were appropriate for the degree of hearing loss noted. Word recognition was excellent for the right ear and poor for the left ear when the signal was present at a suprathreshold level. Tympanograms were characterized by normal shape, amplitude, and peak pressure points bilaterally. The contralateral acoustic reflex was normal for the right ear but absent for the left ear at the frequencies tested (500 to 4000 Hz). The ipsilateral acoustic reflex was present with the probe in the right ear and absent with the probe in the left ear. Brainstem auditory evoked potentials (BAEPs) were within normal range for the right ear. No repeatable response was observed from the left ear. A subsequent MRI showed a 1 cm acoustic neuroma.

➤ Case Study 18-3: Phacoemulsification with Intraocular Lens Implant

W.S., a 68-year-old woman, was scheduled for surgery for a cataract and relief from "floaters," which she had noticed in her visual field since her surgery for a retinal detachment the previous year. She reported to the ambulatory surgery center an hour before her scheduled procedure. Before transfer to the operating room, she spoke with her ophthalmologist and reviewed the surgical plan. Her right eye was identified as the operative eye and it was marked with a "yes" and the surgeon's initials on the lid. She was given anesthetic drops in the right eye and an intravenous bolus of 2.0 mg of midazolam (Versed).

In the OR, W.S. and her operative eye were again identified by the surgeon, anesthetist, and nurses. After anesthesia and akinesia were achieved, the eye area was prepped and draped in sterile sheets. An operating microscope with video system was positioned over her eye. A 5-0 silk suture was placed through the superior rectus muscle to retract the eye. A lid speculum was placed to open the eye. A minimal conjunctival peritomy was performed, and hemostasis was achieved with wet-field cautery. The anterior chamber was entered at the 10:30 o'clock position. A capsulotomy was performed after Healon was placed in the anterior chamber. Phacoemulsification was carried out without difficulty. The remaining cortex was removed by irrigation and aspiration.

An intraocular lens (IOL) was placed into the posterior chamber. Miochol was injected to achieve papillary miosis, and the wound was closed with one 10-0 suture. Subconjunctival Celestone and Garamycin were injected. The lid speculum and retraction suture were removed. After application of Eserine and Bacitracin ointments, the eye was patched and a shield was applied. W.S. left the OR in good condition and was discharged to home 4 hours later.

CASE STUDY QUESTIONS

Multiple choice. Select the best answer and write the letter of your choice to the left of each number:

_____ 1. The medical specialty of otorhinolaryngology is most often referred to as:

    a. ENT, or ear, nose, and throat
    b. optometry
    c. PERLA
    d. oral surgery
    e. EENT/dental

_____ 2. The surgery to remove one of the microscopic bones of the middle ear is a(n):

    a. stapedectomy
    b. mastoidectomy
    c. myringotomy
    d. tympanoplasty
    e. otoplasty

_____ 3. The procedure in question 2 may require construction of a new eardrum, a procedure called a(n):

    a. otoplasty
    b. myringotomy
    c. stapes transfer
    d. tympanoplasty
    e. otoscope

(continued)

Case Studies (continued)

____ 4. Mastoid surgery incisions are made postauricularly, which is:

    a. anterior to the ear drum
    b. over the left ear
    c. behind the ear
    d. inferior to the tympanic membrane
    e. between the ears

____ 5. The study of hearing is termed:

    a. acousticology
    b. radio frequency
    c. light spectrum
    d. otology
    e. audiology

____ 6. Sensorineural hearing loss may result from:

    a. damage to the second cranial nerve
    b. otitis media
    c. otosclerosis
    d. damage to the eighth cranial nerve
    e. stapedectomy

____ 7. Ultrasound destruction and aspiration of the
lens is called:

    a. catarectomy
    b. phacoemulsification
    c. stapedectomy
    d. radial keratotomy
    e. refraction

____ 8. The term *akinesia* means:

    a. movement
    b. lack of sensation
    c. washing
    d. lack of movement
    e. incision

____ 9. The term that means "on the same side" is:

    a. contralateral
    b. bilateral
    c. distal
    d. ventral
    e. ipsilateral

____ 10. Another name for an acoustic neuroma is:

    a. macular degeneration
    b. acoustic neurilemoma
    c. auditory otosclerosis
    d. 8th cranial labyrinthitis
    e. acoustic glaucoma

Write terms from the case studies with the following
meanings:

11. record obtained by tympanometry

    _____

12. pertaining to or perceived by the ear

    _____

13. inflammation of the middle ear

    _____

14. inflammation of the external ear

    _____

15. physician who specializes in conditions of the eye

    _____

16. within the eye

    _____

17. abnormal contraction of the pupil

    _____

18. generic drug name for Versed

    _____

Abbreviations. Define the following abbreviations:

19. Hz _____

20. BAEP _____

21. OD _____

22. IOL _____

18

CHAPTER 19

The Skeleton

CHAPTER CONTENTS

OBJECTIVES

After study of this chapter you should be able to:

1. Compare the axial skeleton and the appendicular skeleton.
2. Briefly describe the formation of bone tissue.
3. Describe the structure of a long bone.
4. Compare a suture, a symphysis, and a synovial joint.
5. Identify and use roots pertaining to the skeleton.
6. Describe the main disorders that affect the skeleton and joints.
7. Describe the common methods used to diagnose and treat disorders of the skeleton.
8. Interpret abbreviations used in relation to the skeleton.
9. Label diagrams of the skeleton.

PRETEST

Multiple choice. Select the best answer and write the letter of your choice to the left of each number.

____ 1. The root oste/o means:

    a. cartilage   c. bone
    b. fat   d. heart

____ 2. The root myel/o refers to the spinal cord. Used in reference to bones it means:

    a. bone marrow   c. bone shaft
    b. joint   d. membrane

___ 3. A bone of the spinal column is a(n):

    a. cortex   c. labyrinth
    b. ventricle   d. vertebra

___ 4. The large, flared superior bone of the pelvis is the:

    a. duodenum   c. thorax
    b. ilium   d. phalange

___ 5. The bones of the wrist are the:

    a. ribs   c. carpals
    b. cervices   d. digits

___ 6. The bone of the thigh is the:

    a. patella   c. cranium
    b. umbilicus   d. femur

___ 7. A general term for inflammation of a joint is:

    a. arthritis   c. epididymitis
    b. conjunctivitis d. myocarditis

___ 8. Chondrosarcoma is a tumor that originates in:

    a. adipose tissue c. cartilage
    b. bone   d. muscle

The **skeleton** forms the framework of the body, protects vital organs, and works with the muscular system to produce movement at the **joints**. The human adult skeleton is composed of 206 **bones**, which are organized for study into two divisions.

Divisions of the Skeleton

The axial skeleton forms the central core or "axis" of the body's bony framework (Fig. 19-1). It consists of:

- the skull, made up of 8 cranial bones and 14 bones of the face (Fig. 19-2). The skull bones are joined by immovable joints (sutures), except for the joint between the lower jaw (mandible) and the temporal bone of the cranium, the temporomandibular joint (TMJ).

- the spinal column (Fig. 19-3) consisting of 26 vertebrae. Between the vertebrae are disks of **cartilage** that add strength and flexibility to the spine. The five groups of vertebrae, listed from superior to inferior with the number of bones in each group are:

  1. cervical (7), designated C1 to C7. The first and second cervical vertebrae also have specific names, the **atlas** and the **axis**, respectively (see Fig. 19-3).

  2. thoracic (12), designated T1 to T12.

  3. lumbar (5), designated L1 to L5.

  4. the sacrum (S), composed of five fused bones.

  5. the coccyx (Co), composed of four to five fused bones.

- the **thorax**, consisting of 12 pairs of ribs joined by cartilage to the sternum (breast bone). The rib cage encloses and protects the thoracic organs.

The appendicular skeleton is attached or "appended" to the axial skeleton (see Fig. 19-1). The upper division includes:

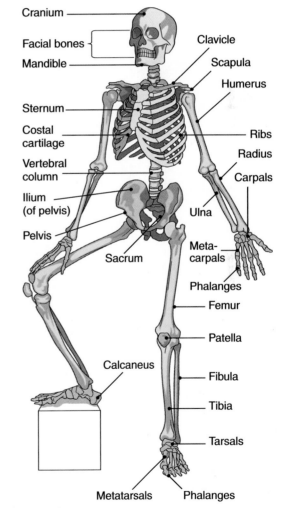

Figure 19-1 **The skeleton.** The axial skeleton is shown in yellow; the appendicular in blue.

- the bones of the shoulder girdle, the clavicle (collar bone) and scapula (shoulder blade)

- the bones of the upper extremities (arms), the humerus, radius, ulna, carpals (wrist bones), metacarpals (bones of the palm), and phalanges (finger bones)

19

447

The lower division includes:

- the **pelvic bones**, two large bones that join the sacrum and coccyx to form the bony **pelvis**. Each pelvic or hip bone (os coxae) is formed by three fused bones, the large, flared **ilium**, the ischium, and the pubis (Fig. 19-4). The deep socket in the hip bone that holds the head of the femur is the **acetabulum**.

- the bones of the lower extremities (legs), the femur, patella (kneecap), tibia, fibula, tarsals (ankle bones), metatarsals (bones of the instep), and phalanges (toe bones). The large tarsal bone that forms the heel is the calcaneus (*kal-KĀ-nē-us*), shown in Figure 19-1.

All of these bone groups, and also the hyoid under the jaw and the ear ossicles, are listed with phonetic pronunciations and described in Reference Box 19-1.

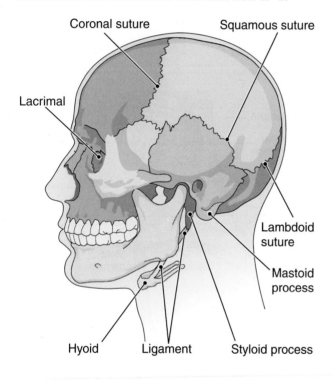

Bones of the skull:

- Frontal
- Parietal
- Sphenoid
- Temporal
- Nasal
- Maxilla
- Occiptial
- Zygomatic
- Mandible

Figure 19-2 **The skull from the left.** An additional cranial bone, the ethmoid (*ETH-moyd*), is visible mainly from the interior of the skull. The hyoid is considered part of the axial skeleton but is not attached to any other bones. The tongue and other muscles are attached to the hyoid.

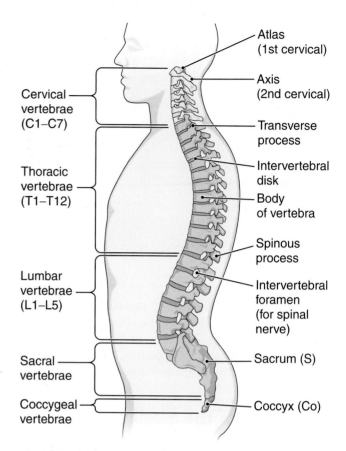

Figure 19-3 **Vertebral column, left lateral view.** The number of vertebrae in each group and the abbreviations for each are shown. The sacrum and coccyx are formed from fused bones.

Bone Formation

Bone is formed by the gradual addition of calcium and phosphorus salts to cartilage, a type of dense connective tissue. This process of **ossification** begins before birth and continues to adulthood. Although bone appears to be inert, it is actually living tissue that is constantly being replaced and remodeled throughout life. Three types of cells are involved in these changes:

- **osteoblasts,** the cells that produce bone,

- **osteocytes,** mature bone cells that help to maintain bone tissue,

- **osteoclasts,** involved in the breakdown of bone tissue to release needed minerals or to allow for reshaping and repair.

The process of destroying bone so that its components can be taken into the circulation is called **resorption**. This activity occurs continuously and is normally in balance with bone formation. In disease states, resorption may occur more rapidly or more slowly than bone production.

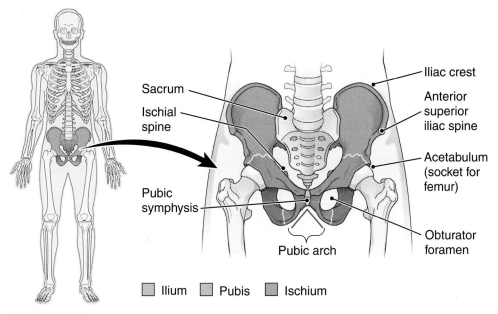

Figure 19-4 **The pelvic bones.** Each pelvic, or hip, bone is formed from three fused bones, the ilium, ischium, and pubis. Together with the sacrum and coccyx, they form the bony pelvis. The acetabulum is the socket for the femur.

Box 19-1   For Your Reference

Bones of the Skeleton

REGION	BONES	DESCRIPTION
Axial Skeleton (*AK-sē-al*)		
SKULL		
Cranium (*KRĀ-nē-um*)	Cranial bones (8)	Chamber enclosing the brain; houses the ear and forms part of the eye socket
Facial portion (*FĀ-shal*)	Facial bones (14)	Form the face and chambers for sensory organs
Hyoid (*HĪ-oyd*)		U-shaped bone under mandible (lower jaw); used for muscle attachments
Ossicles (*OS-i-klz*)	Ear bones (3)	Transmit sound waves through middle ear
TRUNK		
Vertebral column (*VER-te-bral*)	Vertebrae (26) (*VER-te-brē*)	Encloses the spinal cord
Thorax (*THŌ-raks*)	Sternum (*STER-num*)	Anterior bone of the thorax
	Ribs (12 pair)	Enclose the organs of the thorax
Appendicular Skeleton (*ap-en-DIK-ū-lar*)		

(continued)

Box 19-1 For Your Reference (Continued)

Bones of the Skeleton

REGION	BONES	DESCRIPTION
UPPER DIVISION		
Shoulder girdle	Clavicle (KLAV-i-kel)	Anterior; between sternum and scapula
	Scapula (SKAP-ū-la)	Posterior, anchors muscles that move arm
Upper extremity	Humerus (HŪ-mer-us)	Proximal arm bone
	Ulna (UL-na)	Medial bone of forearm
	Radius (RĀ-dē-us)	Lateral bone of forearm
	Carpals (8) (KAR-palz)	Wrist bones
	Metacarpals (5) (met-a-KAR-palz)	Bones of palm
	Phalanges (14) (fa-LAN-jēz)	Bones of fingers
LOWER DIVISION		
Pelvic bones (PEL-vic)	Os coxae (2) (os KOK-sē)	Join sacrum and coccyx of vertebral column to form the bony pelvis
Lower extremity	Femur (FĒ-mur)	Thigh bone
	Patella (pa-TEL-a)	Kneecap
	Tibia (TIB-ē-a)	Medial bone of leg
	Fibula (FIB-ū-la)	Lateral bone of leg
	Tarsal bones (7) (TAR-sal)	Ankle bones. The large heel bone is the calcaneus (kal-KĀ-nē-us)
	Metatarsals (5) (met-a-TAR-salz)	Bones of instep
	Phalanges (14) (fa-LAN-jēz)	Bones of toes

PASSport to Success® The animation *Bone Growth* on the Student Resources shows the growth process in a long bone.

Structure of a Long Bone

A typical long bone (Fig. 19-5) has a shaft or **diaphysis** composed of compact bone tissue. Within the shaft is a medullary cavity containing the yellow form of **bone marrow**, which is high in fat. The irregular **epiphysis** at either end is made of a less dense, spongy (cancellous) bone tissue (Fig. 19-6). The spaces in spongy bone contain the blood-forming red bone marrow. A layer of cartilage covers the epiphysis to protect the bone surface at a joint. The thin layer of fibrous tissue, or **periosteum**, that covers the bone's outer surface nourishes and protects the bone and also generates new bone cells for growth and repair.

Between the diaphysis and the epiphysis at each end, in a region called the **metaphysis**, is the growth region or **epiphyseal plate**. Long bones continue to grow in length at these regions throughout childhood and into early adulthood. When the bone stops elongating, this area becomes fully calcified but remains visible as the epiphyseal line (see Fig. 19-5).

Long bones are found in the arms, legs, hands, and feet. Other bones are described as:

■ flat (e.g., cranial bones, ribs, scapulae),

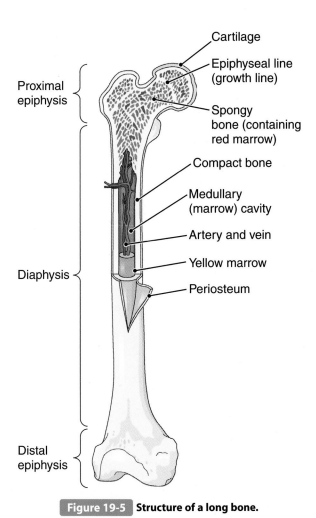

Figure 19-5 **Structure of a long bone.**

(Labels in figure: Cartilage; Epiphyseal line (growth line); Proximal epiphysis; Spongy bone (containing red marrow); Compact bone; Medullary (marrow) cavity; Diaphysis; Artery and vein; Yellow marrow; Periosteum; Distal epiphysis)

- short (e.g., wrist and ankle bones),
- irregular (e.g., facial bones, vertebrae).

Joints

The joints, or **articulations**, are classified according to the degree of movement they allow:

- A **suture** is an immovable joint held together by fibrous connective tissue, as is found between the bones of the skull (see Fig. 19-2).
- A **symphysis** is a slightly movable joint connected by fibrous cartilage. Examples are the joints between the bodies of the vertebrae (see Fig. 19-3) and the joint between the pubic bones (see Fig. 19-4).
- A **synovial joint**, or **diarthrosis**, is a freely movable joint. Such joints allow for a wide range of movements, as described in Chapter 20. **Tendons** attach muscles to bones to produce movement at the joints.

Freely movable joints are subject to wear and tear, and they therefore have some protective features (Fig. 19-7). The cavity of a diarthrotic joint contains **synovial fluid**, which cushions and lubricates the joint. This fluid is produced by the synovial membrane that lines the joint cavity. The ends of the articulating bones are cushioned and protected by cartilage. A fibrous capsule, continuous with the periosteum, encloses the joint. Synovial joints are stabilized and strengthened by **ligaments**, which connect the articulating bones. A **bursa** is a small sac of synovial fluid that cushions the area around a joint. Bursae are found at stress points between tendons, ligaments, and bones (see Fig. 19-7).

19

Figure 19-6 **Bone tissue, longitudinal section.** The epiphysis (end) of this long bone has an outer layer of compact bone. The remainder of the tissue is spongy (cancellous) bone, shown by the arrows. Transverse growth lines are also visible.

Figure 19-7 **The knee joint, sagittal section.** The knee joint is an example of a freely movable, synovial joint, also called a diarthrosis. Synovial fluid fills the joint cavity. Other protective structures such as cartilage, joint capsule, ligaments, and bursae are also shown.

(Labels in figure: Suprapatellar bursa; Synovial membrane; Femur; Quadriceps tendon; Articular cartilage; Patella; Joint capsule; Prepatellar bursa; Meniscus (cartilage); Fat pad; Joint cavity; Infrapatellar bursae; Tibia; Patellar ligament)

Terminology | Key Terms

Normal Structure and Function

acetabulum as-e-TAB-ū-lum	The bony socket in the hip bone that holds the head of the femur (from the Latin word for vinegar because it resembles the base of a vinegar cruet)
articulation ar-tik-ū-LĀ-shun	A joint (adjective: articular)
atlas AT-las	The first cervical vertebra (see Fig. 19-3) (root: atlant/o)
axis AK-sis	The second cervical vertebra (see Fig. 19-3)
bone bōn	A calcified form of dense connective tissue; osseous tissue; also an individual unit of the skeleton made of such tissue (root: oste/o)
bone marrow	The soft material that fills bone cavities. Yellow marrow fills the central cavity of the long bones; blood cells are formed in red bone marrow, which is located in spongy bone tissue (root: myel/o)
bursa BUR-sa	A fluid-filled sac that reduces friction near a joint (root: burs/o)
cartilage KAR-ti-lij	A type of dense connective tissue that is found in the skeleton, larynx, trachea, and bronchi. It is the precursor to most bone tissue (root: chondr/o)
diarthrosis di-ar-THRŌ-sis	A freely movable joint; also called a synovial joint (adjective: diarthrotic)
diaphysis dī-AF-i-sis	The shaft of a long bone
epiphyseal plate ep-i-FIZ-ē-al	The growth region of a long bone; located in the metaphysis, between the diaphysis and epiphysis. When bone growth ceases, this area appears as the epiphyseal line
epiphysis e-PIF-i-sis	The irregularly shaped end of a long bone
ilium IL-ē-um	The large, flared, superior portion of the pelvic bone (root: ili/o) (adjective: iliac)
joint	The junction between two bones; articulation (root: arthr/o)
ligament LIG-a-ment	A strong band of connective tissue that joins one bone to another
metaphysis me-TAF-i-sis	The region of a long bone between the diaphysis (shaft) and epiphysis (end); during development, the growing region of a long bone
ossification os-i-fi-KĀ-shun	The formation of bone tissue (from Latin os, meaning "bone")
osteoblast OS-tē-ō-blast	A cell that produces bone tissue
osteoclast OS-tē-ō-clast	A cell that destroys bone tissue
osteocyte OS-tē-ō-sīt	A mature bone cell that nourishes and maintains bone tissue
pelvis	The large ring of bone at the inferior trunk. Formed of the two hip bones (os coxae) joined to the sacrum and coccyx (plural: pelves). Each os coxae is formed of three bones, the superior, flared ilium (IL-ē-um), ischium (IS-kē-um), and pubis (PŪ-bis)
periosteum per-ē-OS-tē-um	The fibrous membrane that covers a bone's surface

(continued)

Terminology Key Terms (continued)

resorption rē-SORP-shun	Removal of bone by breakdown and absorption into the circulation
skeleton SKEL-e-ton	The body's bony framework, consisting of 206 bones. The axial portion (80 bones) is composed of the skull, spinal column, ribs, and sternum. The appendicular skeleton (126 bones) contains the bones of the arms and legs, shoulder girdle, and pelvis
suture SŪ-chur	An immovable joint, such as the joints between the skull bones
symphysis SIM-fi-sis	A slightly movable joint
synovial fluid sin-O-vē-al	The fluid contained in a freely movable (diarthrotic) joint; synovia (root: synov/i)
synovial joint	A freely movable joint; has a joint cavity containing synovial fluid; a diarthrosis
tendon TEN-don	A fibrous band of connective tissue that attaches a muscle to a bone
thorax THŌ-raks	The upper part of the trunk between the neck and the abdomen; formed by the 12 pairs of ribs and sternum

PASSport to Success® Go to the pronunciation glossary on the Student Resources to hear these words pronounced.

Roots Pertaining to the Skeleton, Bones, and Joints

See Tables 19-1 and 19-2.

Table 19-1 Roots for Bones and Joints

Root	Meaning	Example	Definition of Example
oste/o	bone	osteopenia os-tē-ō-PĒ-nē-a	deficiency of bone tissue
myel/o	bone marrow; also, spinal cord	myeloid MĪ-e-loyd	pertaining to or resembling bone marrow
chondr/o	cartilage	chondroblast KON-drō-blast	a cartilage-forming cell
arthr/o	joint	arthrosis ar-THRŌ-sis	joint; condition affecting a joint
synov/i	synovial fluid, joint, or membrane	asynovia a-sin-Ō-vē-a	lack of synovial fluid
burs/o	bursa	peribursal per-i-BER-sal	around a bursa

EXERCISE **19-1**

Fill in the blanks:

1. Osteolysis (*os-tē-OL-i-sis*) is destruction of _____.

2. Myelogenous (*mī-e-LOJ-e-nus*) means originating in _____.

3. Arthrodesis (*ar-THROD-e-sis*) is fusion of a(n) _____.

4. A chondroma (*kon-DRŌ-ma*) is a tumor of _____.

5. A bursolith (*BUR-sō-lith*) is a stone in a(n) _____.

Define the following words:

6. osteoid (*OS-tē-oyd*) _____

7. myelopoiesis (*mī-e-lō-poy-Ē-sis*) _____

8. chondromalacia (*kon-drō-ma-LĀ-shē-a*) _____

9. arthrocentesis (*ar-thrō-sen-TĒ-sis*) _____

10. bursitis (*bur-SĪ-tis*) _____

11. synovial (*sin-Ō-vē-al*) _____

Write words for the following definitions:

12. inflammation of bone and bone marrow   _____

13. a bone-forming cell   _____

14. tumor of bone marrow   _____

15. incision of a bursa   _____

16. inflammation of a synovial membrane   _____

17. plastic repair of a joint   _____

18. any disease of a joint   _____

19. pertaining to or resembling cartilage   _____

20. instrument for examining the interior of a joint   _____

The word ostosis means "bone growth." Use this as a suffix for the following two words:

21. excess growth of bone   _____

22. abnormal growth of bone   _____

Table 19-2   Roots for the Skeleton

Root	Meaning	Example	Definition of Example
crani/o	skull, cranium	craniometry *krā-ne-OM-e-trē*	measurement of the cranium
spondyl/o	vertebra	spondylolysis *spon-di-LOL-i-sis*	destruction and separation of a vertebra
vertebr/o	vertebra, spinal column	paravertebral *pa-ra-VER-te-bral*	near the vertebrae or spinal column
rachi/o	spine	rachischisis *rā-KIS-ki-sis*	fissure (-schisis) of the spine; spina bifida

Table 19-2	Continued		
Root	**Meaning**	**Example**	**Definition of Example**
cost/o	rib	costochondral *kos-tō-KON-dral*	pertaining to a rib and its cartilage
sacr/o	sacrum	presacral *prē-SĀ-kral*	in front of the sacrum
coccy, coccyg/o	coccyx	coccygeal* *kok-SIJ-ē-al*	pertaining to the coccyx
pelvi/o	pelvis	pelviscope *PEL-vi-skōp*	endoscope for examining the pelvis
ili/o	ilium	iliopelvic *il-ē-ō-PEL-vik*	pertaining to the ilium and pelvis

*Note spelling.

EXERCISE 19-2

Adjectives. Write adjectives for the following definitions:

1. pertaining to (-al) the skull _____

2. pertaining to (-al) a rib _____

3. pertaining to (-ic) the pelvis _____

4. pertaining to (-ac) the ilium _____

5. pertaining to (-al) the spinal column _____

6. pertaining to (-al) the sacrum _____

Define the following terms:

7. craniotomy (*krā-nē-OT-ō-mē*) _____

8. prevertebral (*prē-VER-te-bral*) _____

9. spondylodynia (*spon-di-lō-DIN-ē-a*) _____

10. suprapelvic (*sū-pra-PEL-vik*) _____

Write words for the following definitions:

11. fissure of the skull _____

12. inflammation of the vertebrae (use spondyl/o) _____

13. plastic repair of a vertebra (use vertebr/o) _____

14. surgical excision of a rib _____

15. surgical puncture of the spine; spinal tap _____

16. pertaining to the sacrum and ilium _____

17. pertaining to the cranium and sacrum _____

18. measurement of the pelvis _____

19. around the sacrum _____

20. excision of the coccyx _____

21. pertaining to the ilium and coccyx _____

22. below the ribs _____

19

Clinical Aspects of the Skeleton

Disorders of the skeleton often involve surrounding tissues—ligaments, tendons, and muscles—and may be studied together as diseases of the musculoskeletal system. (The muscular system is described in Chapter 20.) The medical specialty that concentrates on diseases of the skeletal and muscular systems is **orthopedics**. Physical therapists and occupational therapists must also understand these systems (see Box 19-2). (Some colorful terms used to describe musculoskeletal abnormalities are given in Box 19-3.)

Most abnormalities of the bones and joints appear on simple radiographs (see Fig. 19-8 for a radiograph of a normal joint). Radioactive bone scans, computed tomography (CT), and magnetic resonance imaging (MRI) scans are used as well. Also indicative of disorders are changes in blood levels of calcium and **alkaline phosphatase**, an enzyme needed for bone calcification.

Infection

Osteomyelitis is an inflammation of bone caused by pus-forming bacteria that enter through a wound or are carried by the blood. Often the blood-rich ends of the long

---

Box 19-2   Health Professions

Careers in Physical Therapy

Physical therapy restores mobility and relieves pain in cases of arthritis or musculoskeletal injuries. Individuals with heart disease and brain injury, or those who are recovering from burns or major surgery, may benefit as well from physical therapy.

Physical therapists (PTs) work closely with physicians, nurses, occupational therapists, speech pathologists, and audiologists. Some treat a wide range of ailments, whereas others specialize in pediatrics, geriatrics, orthopedics, sports medicine, neurology, or cardiology. Regardless of specialty, physical therapists are responsible for examining their patients and developing individualized treatment programs. The examination includes a medical history and tests measuring strength, mobility, balance, coordination, and endurance. The treatment plan may include stretching and exercise to improve mobility;

hot packs, cold compresses, and massage to reduce pain; and the use of crutches, prostheses, and wheelchairs. Physical therapy assistants are responsible for implementing a treatment plan, teaching patients exercises and equipment use, and reporting results back to the physical therapist. Most physical therapists in the United States have bachelor's or master's degrees and must pass a national licensing exam. Assistants typically train in a 2-year program.

Physical therapists and physical therapist assistants practice in hospitals and clinics and may also visit homes and schools. As the American population continues to age and the need for rehabilitative therapy increases, job prospects are good. For more information about careers in physical therapy, contact the American Physical Therapy Association at www.apta.org.

Box 19-3   Focus on **Words**

Names That Are Like Pictures

Some conditions are named by terms that are very descriptive. In orthopedics, several names for types of bursitis are based on the repetitive stress that leads to the irritation. For example, "tailor's bottom" involves the ischial ("sit") bones of the pelvis, as might be irritated by sitting tailor-fashion to sew. "Housemaid's knee" comes from the days of scrubbing floors on hands and knees, and "tennis elbow" is named for the sport that is its most common cause. "Student's elbow" results from leaning to pore over books while studying, although today a student is more likely to have neck and wrist problems from working at a computer.

The term *knock-knee* describes genu valgum, in which the knees are abnormally close and the space between the ankles

is wide. The opposite is genu varum, in which the knees are far apart and the bottom of the legs are close together, giving rise to the term *bowleg*. A dowager's hump appears dorsally between the shoulders as a result of osteoporosis and is most commonly seen in elderly women.

Injury to the roots of nerves that supply the arm may cause the arm to abduct slightly and rotate medially with the wrist flexed and the fingers pointing backward, a condition colorfully named "waiter's tip position." "Popeye's shoulder" is sign of a separation or tear at the head of the biceps tendon. The affected arm, when abducted with the elbow flexed, reveals a bulge on the upper arm—just like Popeye's!

Humerus

Fat pad
Radius shaft
Radius head
Radius neck
Ulna

Joint space

Ulnar olecranon
(elbow)

Figure 19-8   Radiograph of a normal left elbow joint, lateral view. The olecranon
(ō-LEK-ra-non) is the proximal ulnar enlargement that forms the prominent bone of the elbow.

bones are invaded, and the infection then spreads to other regions, such as the bone marrow and even the joints. The use of antibiotics has greatly reduced the threat of osteomyelitis.

Tuberculosis may spread to bone, especially the long bones of the arms and legs and the bones of the wrist and

ankle. Tuberculosis of the spine is **Pott disease**. Infected vertebrae are weakened and may collapse, causing pain, deformity, and pressure on the spinal cord. Antibiotics can control tuberculosis as long as the strains are not resistant to these drugs and the host is not weakened by other diseases.

Fractures

A **fracture** is a break in a bone, usually caused by trauma. The effects of a fracture depend on the break's location and severity; the amount of associated injury; possible complications, such as infections; and success of healing, which may take months. In a closed or simple fracture, the skin is not broken. If the fracture is accompanied by a wound in the skin, it is described as an open fracture. Various types of fractures are listed in Reference Box 19-4 and illustrated in Figure 19-9.

Reduction of a fracture refers to realignment of the broken bone. If no surgery is required, the reduction is described as closed; an open reduction is one that requires surgery to place the bone in proper position. Rods, plates, or screws might be needed to ensure proper healing. A splint or cast is often needed during the healing phase to immobilize the bone. **Traction** refers to using pulleys and weights to maintain

Box 19-4   For Your Reference

19

Types of Fractures

FRACTURE	DESCRIPTION
closed	a simple fracture with no open wound
Colles KOL-ēz	fracture of the distal end of the radius with backward displacement of the hand
comminuted COM-i-nū-ted	fracture in which the bone is splintered or crushed
compression	fracture caused by force from both ends, as to a vertebra
greenstick	one side of the bone is broken and the other side is bent
impacted	one fragment is driven into the other
oblique	break occurs at an angle across the bone; usually one fragment slips by the other
open	fracture is associated with an open wound, or broken bone protrudes through the skin
Pott	fracture of the distal end of the fibula with injury to the tibial joint
spiral	fracture is in a spiral or S shape; usually caused by twisting injuries
transverse	a break at right angles to the long axis of a bone

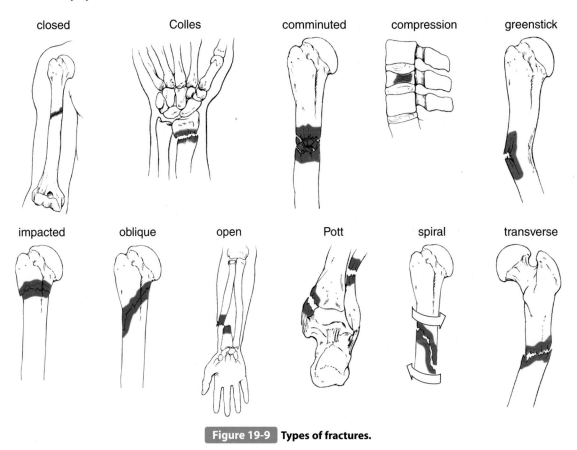

closed   Colles   comminuted   compression   greenstick

impacted   oblique   open   Pott   spiral   transverse

Figure 19-9   **Types of fractures.**

alignment of a fractured bone during healing. A traction device may be attached to the skin or attached to the bone itself by means of a pin or wire.

Metabolic Bone Diseases

Osteoporosis is a loss of bone mass that results in bone weakening (Fig. 19-10). A decrease in estrogens after menopause makes women over age 50 most susceptible to the effects of this disorder. Efforts to prevent osteoporosis include a healthful diet, adequate intake of calcium and vitamin D, and engaging in regular weight-bearing exercises, such as walking, running, aerobics,

Figure 19-10   **Osteoporosis.** Femoral head showing osteoporosis (*right*) compared with a normal control (*left*).

and weight training. These exercises stimulate bone growth and also contribute to the balance and muscle strength needed to prevent falls. Perimenopausal hormone replacement therapy (HRT) prevents bone loss, but because of safety concerns, this treatment is currently being reevaluated. Some drugs are available for reducing bone resorption and increasing bone density. These include the **bisphosphonates** and **selective estrogen receptor modulators (SERMs)** described in Chapter 15.

Osteoporosis is diagnosed and monitored using a DEXA (dual-energy x-ray absorptiometry) scan, an imaging technique that measures bone mineral density (BMD). The diagnostic term **osteopenia** refers to a lower-than-average bone density, which is not considered to be abnormal. Osteopenia may progress to osteoporosis, but does not necessarily need treatment.

Other conditions that can lead to bone loss include nutritional deficiencies; disuse, as in paralysis or immobilization in a cast; and excess steroids from the adrenal cortex. Overactivity of the parathyroid glands also leads to osteoporosis because parathyroid hormone causes calcium release from bones to raise blood calcium levels. Certain drugs, smoking, lack of exercise, and high intake of alcohol, caffeine, and proteins may also contribute to the development of osteoporosis.

In **osteomalacia** there is a softening of bone tissue because of diminished calcium salt formation. Possible causes include deficiency of vitamin D, needed to absorb regions (see Fig. 19-3). Any exaggeration or deviation of these curves is described as **curvature of the spine.** Three common types of spinal curvatures are shown in Figure 19-18 and described as follows:

- **Kyphosis** is an exaggerated curve in the thoracic region, popularly known as "hunchback."

- **Lordosis** is an exaggerated curve in the lumber region, popularly known as "swayback."

- **Scoliosis** is a sideways curvature of the spine in any region.

Spinal curvatures may be congenital or may result from muscle weakness or paralysis, poor posture, joint problems, disk degeneration, extreme obesity, or disease, such as spinal tuberculosis, rickets, or osteoporosis. Extreme cases may cause pain, breathing problems, or degenerative changes.

Bracing the spine during childhood may help to correct a curvature. If surgery is needed, vertebrae are fused and bone grafts and implants are used to stabilize the spine. It is now sometimes possible for surgeons to make these corrections endoscopically.

Terminology | Key Terms

Disorders

ankylosing spondylitis *ang-ki-LŌ-sing spon-di-LĪ-tis*	A chronic, progressive inflammatory disease involving the spinal joints and surrounding soft tissue, most common in young males; also called rheumatoid spondylitis
ankylosis *ang-ki-LŌ-sis*	Immobility and fixation of a joint
arthritis *ar-THRĪ-tis*	Inflammation of a joint
chondrosarcoma *kon-drō-sar-KŌ-ma*	A malignant tumor of cartilage
curvature of the spine *KER-va-chūr*	An exaggerated spinal curve, such as scoliosis, lordosis, or kyphosis (see Fig. 19-18)
degenerative joint disease (DJD)	Osteoarthritis (see below)
fracture *FRAK-chūr*	A break in a bone. In a closed or simple fracture, the broken bone does not penetrate the skin; in an open fracture, there is an accompanying wound in the skin (see Fig. 19-9)
gout *gowt*	A form of acute arthritis, usually beginning in the knee or foot, caused by deposit of uric acid salts in the joints
herniated disk *HER-nē-āt-ed*	Protrusion of the center (nucleus pulposus) of an intervertebral disk into the spinal canal; ruptured or "slipped" disk
kyphosis *kī-FŌ-sis*	An exaggerated curve of the spine in the thoracic region; hunchback, humpback (see Fig. 19-18)
lordosis *lor-DŌ-sis*	An exaggerated curve of the spine in the lumbar region; swayback (see Fig. 19-18)
osteoarthritis (OA) *os-tē-ō-ar-THRĪ-tis*	Progressive deterioration of joint cartilage with growth of new bone and soft tissue in and around the joint; the most common form of arthritis; results from wear and tear, injury, or disease; also called degenerative joint disease (DJD)
osteogenic sarcoma *os-tē-ō-JEN-ik*	A malignant bone tumor; osteosarcoma
osteomalacia *os-tē-ō-ma-LĀ-shē-a*	A softening and weakening of the bones due to vitamin D deficiency or other disease
osteomyelitis *os-tē-ō-mī-e-LĪ-tis*	Inflammation of bone and bone marrow caused by infection, usually bacterial
osteopenia *os-tē-ō-PĒ-nē-a*	A lower-than-average bone density, which may foreshadow osteoporosis

(continued)

Terminology	Key Terms (continued)

Term	Definition
osteoporosis os-tē-ō-po-RŌ-sis	A condition characterized by reduction in bone density, most common in white women past menopause; predisposing factors include poor diet, inactivity, and low estrogen levels
Paget disease PAJ-et	Skeletal disease of the elderly characterized by bone thickening and distortion with bowing of long bones; osteitis deformans
Pott disease	Inflammation of the vertebrae, usually caused by tuberculosis
rheumatoid arthritis (RA) RŪ-ma-toyd	A chronic autoimmune disease of unknown origin resulting in inflammation of peripheral joints and related structures; more common in women than in men
rheumatoid factor	A group of antibodies found in the blood in cases of rheumatoid arthritis and other systemic diseases
rickets RIK-ets	Faulty bone formation in children, usually caused by a deficiency of vitamin D
sciatica sī-AT-i-ka	Severe pain in the leg along the course of the sciatic nerve, usually related to spinal nerve root irritation
scoliosis skō-lē-Ō-sis	A sideways curvature of the spine in any region (see Fig. 19-18)
spondylolisthesis spon-di-lō-LIS-the-sis	A forward displacement of one vertebra over another (-listhesis means "a slipping")
spondylolysis spon-di-LOL-i-sis	Degeneration of the articulating portions of a vertebra allowing for spinal distortion, specifically in the lumbar region

Treatment

alkaline phosphatase AL-ka-lin FOS-fa-tās	An enzyme needed in the formation of bone; serum activity of this enzyme is useful in diagnosis
arthrocentesis ar-thrō-sen-TĒ-sis	Aspiration of fluid from a joint by needle puncture
arthrodesis ar-THROD-e-sis	Surgical immobilization (fusion) of a joint; artificial ankylosis
arthroplasty AR-thrō-plas-tē	Partial or total replacement of a joint with a prosthesis
arthroscopy ar-THROS-kō-pē	Use of an endoscope to examine the interior of a joint or to perform surgery on the joint (see Fig. 19-14); the instrument used is an arthroscope
diskectomy dis-KEK-tō-mē	Surgical removal of a herniated intervertebral disk; also spelled discectomy
orthopedics or-thō-PĒ-diks	The study and treatment of disorders of the skeleton, muscles, and associated structures; literally "straight" (ortho) "child" (ped); also spelled orthopaedics
reduction of a fracture	Return of a fractured bone to a normal position; may be closed (not requiring surgery) or open (requiring surgery)
traction TRAK-shun	The process of drawing or pulling, such as traction of the head in the treatment of injuries to the cervical vertebrae

Drugs

antiinflammatory agent	Drug that reduces inflammation; includes steroids, such as cortisone, and nonsteroidal anti-inflammatory drugs (NSAIDs)
bisphosphonate bis-FOS-fō-nāt	Agent used to prevent and treat osteoporosis; increases bone mass by decreasing bone turnover. Examples are alendronate (Fosamax), risedronate (Actonel), and ibandronate (Boniva)

(continued)

Terminology	**Key Terms** (continued)
nonsteroidal antiinflammatory drug (NSAID)	Drug that reduces inflammation but is not a steroid; examples include aspirin and ibuprofen and other inhibitors of prostaglandins, naturally produced substances that promote inflammation
selective estrogen receptor modulator (SERM)	Drug that acts on estrogen receptors. Raloxifene (Evista) is used to prevent bone loss after menopause. Other SERMs are used to prevent and treat estrogen-sensitive breast cancer

PASSport to Success® Go to the pronunciation glossary on the Student Resources to hear these words pronounced.

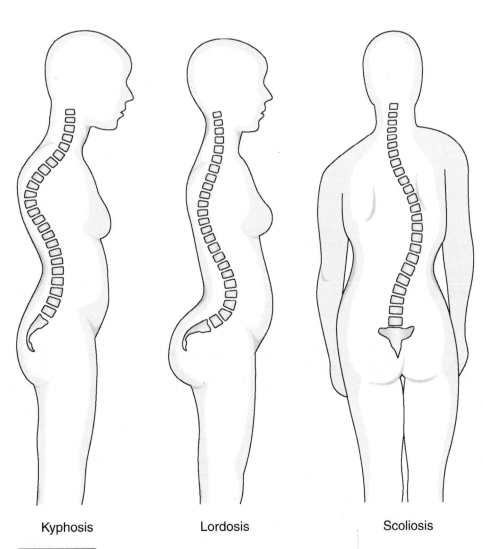

Kyphosis   Lordosis   Scoliosis

Figure 19-18 **Curvatures of the spine.** Kyphosis is an exaggerated thoracic curve; lordosis is an exaggerated lumbar curve; scoliosis is a sideways curve in any region.

19

Terminology Supplementary Terms

Normal Structure and Function*

annulus fibrosus AN-ū-lus fī-BRŌ-sus	The outer ringlike portion of an intervertebral disk
calvaria kal-VAR-ē-a	The domelike upper portion of the skull
coxa KOK-sa	Hip
cruciate ligaments KRŪ-shē-āt	Ligaments that cross in the knee joint to connect the tibia and fibula. They are the anterior cruciate ligament (ACL) and the posterior cruciate ligament (PCL). *Cruciate* means "shaped like a cross"
genu JE-nu	The knee
glenoid cavity GLEN-oyd	The bony socket in the scapula that articulates with the head of the humerus
hallux HAL-uks	The great toe
malleolus ma-LĒ-ō-lus	The projection of the tibia or fibula on either side of the ankle
meniscus me-NIS-kus	Crescent-shaped disk of cartilage found in certain joints, such as the knee joint. In the knee, the medial meniscus and the lateral meniscus separate the tibia and femur; plural: menisci (me-NIS-kī); *meniscus* means "crescent"
olecranon ō-LEK-ra-non	The process of the ulna that forms the elbow
os	Bone (plural: ossa)
osseous OS-ē-us	Pertaining to bone
symphysis pubis SIM-fi-sis	The anterior pelvic joint, formed by the union of the two pubic bones (see Fig. 19-4); also called pubic symphysis

*See Box 19-6 for a list of bone markings.

Symptoms and Conditions

achondroplasia a-kon-drō-PLĀ-zha	Decreased growth of cartilage in the growth plate of long bones resulting in dwarfism; a genetic disorder
Baker cyst	Mass formed at the knee joint by distention of a bursa with excess synovial fluid resulting from chronic irritation
bunion BUN-yun	Inflammation and enlargement of the metatarsal joint of the great toe, usually with displacement of the great toe toward the other toes
bursitis bur-SĪ-tis	Inflammation of a bursa, a small fluid-filled sac near a joint; causes include injury, irritation, and joint disease; the shoulder, hip, elbow, and knee are common sites
carpal tunnel syndrome	Numbness and weakness of the hand caused by pressure on the median nerve as it passes through a tunnel formed by carpal bones
chondroma kon-DRŌ-ma	A benign tumor of cartilage

(continued)

Terminology   Supplementary Terms (continued)

Ewing tumor	A bone tumor that usually appears in children 5 to 15 years of age. It begins in the shaft of a bone and spreads readily to other bones. It may respond to radiation therapy, but then returns. Also called Ewing sarcoma
exostosis *eks-os-TŌ-sis*	A bony outgrowth from the surface of a bone
giant cell tumor	A bone tumor that usually appears in children and young adults. The ends of the bones are destroyed, commonly at the knee, by a large mass that does not metastasize
hammertoe *HAM-er-tō*	Change in position of the toe joints so that the toe takes on a clawlike appearance and the first joint protrudes upward, causing irritation and pain on walking
hallux valgus	Painful condition involving lateral displacement of the great toe at the metatarsal joint. There is also enlargement of the metatarsal head and bunion formation
Heberden nodes *HĒ-ber-den*	Small, hard nodules formed in the cartilage of the distal finger joints in osteoarthritis
hemarthrosis *hē-mar-THRŌ-sis*	Bleeding into a joint cavity
Legg–Calvé–Perthes disease *leg-kahl-vā-PER-tez*	Degeneration (osteochondrosis) of the femur's proximal growth center. The bone is eventually restored, but there may be deformity and weakness. Most common in young boys. Also called coxa plana
multiple myeloma *mī-e-LŌ-ma*	A cancer of blood-forming cells in bone marrow (see Chapter 10)
neurogenic arthropathy *nū-rō-JEN-ik ar-THROP-a-thē*	Degenerative joint disease caused by impaired nervous stimulation; most common cause is diabetes mellitus; Charcot arthropathy
Osgood–Schlatter disease *oz-good-SHLAHT-er*	Degeneration (osteochondrosis) of the tibia's proximal growth center causing pain and tendinitis at the knee
osteochondroma *os-tē-ō-kon-DRŌ-ma*	A benign tumor consisting of cartilage and bone
osteochondrosis *os-tē-ō-kon-DRŌ-sis*	Disease of a bone's growth center in children; tissue degeneration is followed by recalcification
osteodystrophy *os-tē-ō-DIS-trŏ-fē*	Abnormal bone development
osteogenesis imperfecta (OI) *os-tē-ō-JEN-e-sis* *im-per-FEK-ta*	A hereditary disease resulting in the formation of brittle bones that fracture easily. There is faulty synthesis of collagen, the main structural protein in connective tissue
osteoma *os-tē-Ō-ma*	A benign bone tumor that usually remains small and localized
Reiter syndrome *RĪ-ter*	Chronic polyarthritis that usually affects young men; occurs after a bacterial infection and is common in those infected with HIV; may also involve the eyes and genitourinary tract
spondylosis *spon-di-LŌ-sis*	Degeneration and ankylosis of the vertebrae resulting in pressure on the spinal cord and spinal nerve roots; often applied to any degenerative lesion of the spine
sprain	Trauma to a joint involving the ligaments
subluxation *sub-luk-SĀ-shun*	A partial dislocation
talipes *TAL-i-pēz*	A deformity of the foot, especially one occurring congenitally; clubfoot

19

(continued)

Terminology   Supplementary Terms (continued)

valgus *VAL-gus*	Bent outward
varus *VAR-us*	Bent inward
von Recklinghausen disease *fon REK-ling-how-zen*	Loss of bone tissue caused by increased parathyroid hormone; bones become decalcified and deformed, and fracture easily

Diagnosis and Treatment

allograft *AL-ō-graft*	Graft of tissue between individuals of the same species but different genetic makeup; homograft, allogenic graft (see autograft)
arthroclasia *ar-thrō-KLĀ-zha*	Surgical breaking of an ankylosed joint to provide movement
aspiration *as-pi-RĀ-shun*	Removal by suction, as removal of fluid from a body cavity; also inhalation, such as accidental inhalation of material into the respiratory tract
autograft *AW-tō-graft*	Graft of tissue taken from a site on or in the body of the person receiving the graft; autologous graft (see allograft)
calcitonin *kal-si-TŌ-nin*	A thyroid hormone that decreases resorption (loss) of bone tissue; used in the treatment of Paget disease and osteoporosis; also called thyrocalcitonin
chondroitin *kon-DRŌ-i-tin*	A complex polysaccharide found in connective tissue; used as a dietary supplement, usually with glucosamine, for treatment of joint pain
glucosamine *glū-KŌS-a-mēn*	A dietary supplement used in the treatment of joint pain
goniometer *gō-nē-OM-e-ter*	A device used to measure joint angles and movements (root *goni/o* means "angle")
iontophoresis *ī-on-tō-for-Ē-sis*	Introduction into the tissue by means of electric current, using the ions of a given drug; used in the treatment of musculoskeletal disorders
laminectomy *lam-i-NEK-tō-mē*	Excision of the posterior arch (lamina) of a vertebra
meniscectomy *men-i-SEK-tō-mē*	Removal of the crescent-shaped cartilage (meniscus) of the knee joint
myelogram *MĪ-e-lō-gram*	Radiograph of the spinal canal after injection of a radiopaque dye; used to evaluate a herniated disk
osteoplasty *OS-tē-ō-plas-tē*	Scraping and removal of damaged bone from a joint
prosthesis *PROS-thē-sis*	An artificial organ or part, such as an artificial limb

 PASSport to Success Go to the pronunciation glossary on the Student Resources to hear these words pronounced.

Box 19-6   For Your Reference

Bone Markings

MARKING	DESCRIPTION
condyle *KON-dīl*	smooth, rounded protuberance at a joint
crest	raised, narrow ridge (see iliac crest in Fig. 19-4)
epicondyle *ep-i-KON-dīl*	projection above a condyle
facet *FAS-et*	small, flattened surface
foramen *for-Ā-men*	rounded opening (see foramen for spinal nerve in Fig. 19-3)
fossa *FOS-a*	hollow cavity
meatus *mē-Ā-tus*	long channel within a bone
process	projection (see mastoid process and styloid process in Fig. 19-2)
sinus *SĪ-nus*	air-filled space or channel
spine	sharp projection (see ischial spine in Fig. 19-4)
trochanter *trō-KAN-ter*	large, blunt projection as at the top of the femur
tubercle *TŪ-ber-kl*	small, rounded projection
tuberosity *tū-ber-OS-i-tē*	large, rounded projection

19

Terminology   Abbreviations

ACL	Anterior cruciate ligament		**HNP**	Herniated nucleus pulposus
AE	Above the elbow		**IM**	Intramedullary
AK	Above the knee		**L**	Lumbar vertebra; numbered L1 to L5
ASF	Anterior spinal fusion		**MCP**	Metacarpophalangeal (joint)
BE	Below the elbow		**MTP**	Metatarsophalangeal (joint)
BK	Below the knee		**NSAID(s)**	Nonsteroidal antiinflammatory drug(s)
BMD	Bone mineral density		**OA**	Osteoarthritis
C	Cervical vertebra; numbered C1 to C7		**OI**	Osteogenesis imperfecta
Co	Coccyx; coccygeal		**ORIF**	Open reduction internal fixation
DEXA	Dual-energy x-ray absorptiometry (scan)		**ortho, ORTH**	Orthopedics
DIP	Distal interphalangeal (joint)		**PCL**	Posterior cruciate ligament
DJD	Degenerative joint disease		**PIP**	Proximal interphalangeal (joint)
Fx	Fracture		**PSF**	Posterior spinal fusion

(continued)

Terminology	**Abbreviations** (continued)		
RA	Rheumatoid arthritis	THA	Total hip arthroplasty
S	Sacrum; sacral	TKA	Total knee arthroplasty
SERM	Selective estrogen receptor modulator	TMJ	Temporomandibular joint
T	Thoracic vertebra; numbered T1 to T12	Tx	Traction

Chapter Review

LABELING EXERCISE

The Skeleton > Write the name of each numbered part on the corresponding line of the answer sheet.

Calcaneus
Carpals
Clavicle
Cranium
Facial bones
Femur
Fibula
Humerus
Ilium
Mandible
Metacarpals
Metatarsals
Patella

Pelvis
Phalanges
Phalanges
Radius
Ribs
Sacrum
Scapula
Sternum
Tarsals
Tibia
Ulna
Vertebral column

1. _____
2. _____
3. _____
4. _____
5. _____
6. _____
7. _____
8. _____
9. _____
10. _____
11. _____
12. _____
13. _____
14. _____
15. _____
16. _____
17. _____
18. _____
19. _____
20. _____
21. _____
22. _____
23. _____
24. _____
25. _____

Chapter Review *(continued)*

Skull from the Left > Write the name of each numbered part on the corresponding line of the answer sheet.

Frontal   Occipital
Hyoid   Parietal
Lacrimal   Sphenoid
Mandible   Temporal
Maxilla   Zygomatic
Nasal

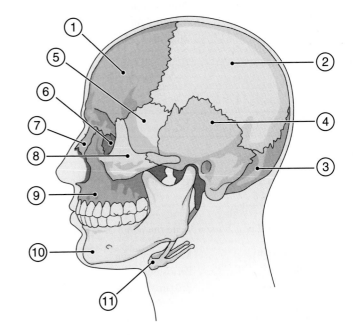

1. _____
2. _____
3. _____
4. _____
5. _____
6. _____
7. _____
8. _____
9. _____
10. _____
11. _____

Vertebral Column > Write the name of each numbered part on the corresponding line of the answer sheet.

Body of vertebra   Lumbar vertebrae
Cervical vertebrae   Sacrum
Coccyx   Thoracic vertebrae
Intervertebral disk

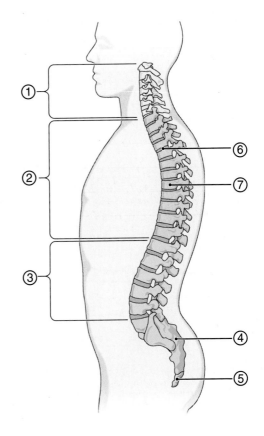

1. _____
2. _____
3. _____
4. _____
5. _____
6. _____
7. _____

19

Chapter Review *(continued)*

The Pelvic Bones > Write the name of each numbered part on the corresponding line of the answer sheet.

Ilium   Pubic symphysis
Ischium   Acetabulum
Pubis   Sacrum

1. _____

2. _____

3. _____

4. _____

5. _____

6. _____

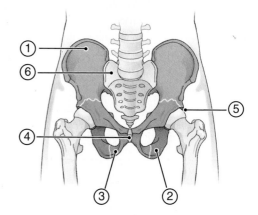

Structure of a Long Bone > Write the name of each numbered part on the corresponding line of the answer sheet.

Artery and vein   Medullary cavity
Cartilage   Periosteum
Compact bone   Proximal epiphysis
Diaphysis   Spongy bone
Distal epiphysis   (containing
Epiphyseal line   red marrow)
   (growth line)   Yellow marrow

1. _____

2. _____

3. _____

4. _____

5. _____

6. _____

7. _____

8. _____

9. _____

10. _____

11. _____

TERMINOLOGY

Matching > Match the following terms and write the appropriate letter to the left of each number:

_____ **1.** periosteum
_____ **2.** epiphysis
_____ **3.** symphysis
_____ **4.** osteoclast
_____ **5.** resorption

a. end of a long bone
b. breakdown and removal of tissue
c. cell that breaks down bone
d. membrane that covers a bone
e. slightly movable joint

_____ **6.** scoliosis
_____ **7.** ankylosis
_____ **8.** osteopenia
_____ **9.** spondylolisthesis
_____ **10.** rachiocentesis

a. immobility of a joint
b. spinal tap
c. displacement of a vertebra
d. sideways curvature of the spine
e. deficiency of bone tissue

Supplementary Terms

_____ **11.** laminectomy
_____ **12.** calvaria
_____ **13.** subluxation
_____ **14.** hallux
_____ **15.** olecranon

a. great toe
b. part of the ulna that forms the elbow
c. excision of part of a vertebra
d. upper portion of the skull
e. partial dislocation

_____ **16.** meniscus
_____ **17.** genu
_____ **18.** prosthesis
_____ **19.** goniometer
_____ **20.** arthroclasia

a. breaking of a joint
b. device used to measure joint angles
c. knee
d. crescent-shaped cartilage
e. artificial part

Fill in the blanks:

21. The study and treatment of disorders of the skeleton, muscles, and associated structures is _____.

22. The type of tissue that covers the ends of the bones at the joints is _____.

23. A band of connective tissue that connects a bone to another bone is a(n) _____.

24. The part of the vertebral column that articulates with the ilium is the _____.

25. A fluid-filled sac near a joint is a(n) _____.

26. The fluid that fills a freely movable joint is _____.

27. The term *costochondral* refers to a rib and its _____.

28. Myelogenesis is the formation of _____.

29. Hemarthrosis is bleeding into a(n) _____.

30. Spondylarthritis (*spon-dil-ar-THRĪ-tis*) is arthritis of the _____.

31. Rachischisis (*rā-KIS-ki-sis*) is fissure of the _____.

19

Define the following words:

32. myelitis (*mī-e-LĪ-tus*) _____

33. osteogenesis (*os-tē-ō-JEN-i-sis*) _____

34. arthrodesis (*ar-THROD-e-sis*) _____

35. synovectomy (*sin-ō-VEK-tō-mē*) _____

36. chondrocyte (*KON-drō-sīt*) _____

37. intraosteal (*in-tra-OS-tē-al*) _____

38. peribursal (*per-i-BER-sal*) _____

39. spondylitis (*spon-di-LĪ-tis*) _____

40. polyarticular (*pol-ē-ar-TIK-ū-lar*) _____

41. subcostal (*sub-KOS-tal*) _____

42. coccydynia (*kok-sē-DIN-ē-a*) _____

Write words for the following definitions:

43. formation of cartilage _____

44. death (-necrosis) of bone tissue _____

45. incision into the cranium _____

46. tumor of bone and cartilage _____

47. narrowing of a joint _____

48. surgical excision of cartilage _____

49. stone in a bursa _____

50. measurement of the pelvis _____

51. endoscopic examination of a joint _____

52. pertaining to the sacrum and ilium _____

53. surgical excision of the coccyx _____

54. near the sacrum _____

Adjectives > Write the adjective form of the following words:

55. cranium _____

56. ilium _____

57. coccyx _____

58. pelvis _____

59. vertebra _____

True–False > Examine each of the following statements. If the statement is true, write T in the first blank. If the statement is false, write F in the first blank and correct the statement by replacing the underlined word in the second blank.

60. The growth region of a long bone is in the <u>metaphysic</u>.   _____   _____

61. The tarsal bones are found in the <u>wrist</u>.   _____   _____

62. An immovable joint is a <u>suture</u>.   _____   _____

63. The femur is part of the <u>axial</u> skeleton.   _____   _____

64. The <u>cervical</u> vertebrae are located in the neck.   _____   _____

65. The cells that produce cartilage are <u>chondroblasts</u>.   _____   _____

66. Blood cells are formed in <u>yellow</u> bone marrow.   _____   _____

67. An exaggerated thoracic curve of the spine is <u>kyphosis</u>.   _____   _____

68. The term *varus* means bent <u>inward</u>.   _____   _____

Eliminations > In each of the sets below, underline the word that does not fit in with the rest and explain the reason for your choice:

69. trochanter — process — hyoid — meatus — condyle

_____

70. lambdoid — occipital — parietal — frontal — sphenoid

_____

71. sacr/o — rachi/o — spondyl/o — vertebr/o — cost/o

_____

72. Pott — sciatic — impacted — comminuted — greenstick

_____

73. T — C — L — Co — OA

_____

19

Word Building > Write words for the following definitions using the word parts provided.

spondyl/o   -plasty   arthr/o   -lysis   -odynia   oste/o   -tome

74. destruction of bone tissue _____

75. instrument for incising a joint _____

76. pain in a vertebra _____

77. loosening or separation of a joint _____

78. instrument for cutting bone tissue _____

79. plastic repair of a joint _____

80. pain in a bone _____

81. destruction of a vertebra _____

82. pain in a joint _____

83. plastic repair of a bone _____

Chapter Review (continued)

Word Analysis > Define the following words and give the meaning of the word parts in each. Use a dictionary if necessary.

84. osteochondrosis (*os-tē-ō-kon-DRŌ-sis*) _____

    a. oste/o _____

    b. chondr/o _____

    c. -sis _____

85. spondylosyndesis (*spon-di-lō-SIN-de-sis*) _____

    a. spondyl/o _____

    b. syn- _____

    c. -desis _____

86. exostosis (*eks-os-TŌ-sis*) _____

    a. ex/o _____

    b. ost(e)/o _____

    c. -sis _____

87. achondroplasia (*a-kon-drō-PLĀ-zha*) _____

    a. a- _____

    b. chondr/o _____

    c. plas _____

    d. -ia _____

PASSport to Success® Go to the word exercises on the Student Resources for additional review exercises.

Case Studies

▸ Case Study 19-1: Arthroplasty of the Right TMJ

S.A., a 38-year-old teacher, was admitted for surgery for degenerative joint disease (DJD) of her right temporomandibular joint (TMJ). She has experienced chronic pain in her right jaw, neck, and ear since her automobile accident the previous year. S.A.'s diagnosis was confirmed by CT scan and was followed up with conservative therapy, which included a bite plate, NSAIDs, and steroid injections. She had also tried hypnosis in an attempt to manage her pain but was not able to gain relief. Her doctor referred her to an oral surgeon who specializes in TMJ disorders. S:A. was scheduled for an arthroplasty of the right TMJ to remove diseased bone

on the articular surface of the right mandibular condyle.

On the following day, she was transported to the OR for surgery. She was given general endotracheal anesthesia, and a vertical incision was made from the superior aspect of the right ear down to the base of the attachment of the right earlobe. After appropriate dissection and retraction, the posterior–superior aspect of the right zygomatic arch was bluntly dissected anteroposteriorly. With a nerve stimulator, the zygomatic branch of the facial nerve was identified and retracted from the surgical field with a vessel loop. The periosteum was then incised along the superior aspect of the arch. An inferior dissection was then made along the capsular ligament and retracted posteriorly. With a Freer elevator, the

(continued)

Case Studies (continued)

meniscus was freed, and a horizontal incision was made to the condyle. With a Hall drill and saline coolant, a high condylectomy of approximately 3 mm of bone was removed while conserving function of the external pterygoid muscle. The stump of the condyle was filed smooth and irrigated copiously with NSS. The lateral capsule, periosteum, subcutaneous tissue, and skin were then closed with sutures. The facial nerve was tested before closing and confirmed to be intact. A pressure pack and Barton bandage were applied. The sponge, needle, and instrument counts were correct. Estimated blood loss (EBL) was approximately 50 mL.

S.A. was discharged on the second postoperative day with instructions for a soft diet, daily mouth-opening exercises, an antibiotic (Keflex 500 mg po q6h), Tylenol no. 3 po q4h prn for pain, and four weekly postoperative appointments.

➤ Case Study 19-2: Osteogenesis Imperfecta

M.H., a 3-year-old boy with osteogenesis imperfecta (OI) type III, was admitted to the pediatric orthopedic hospital for treatment of yet another fracture. Since birth he has had 15 arm and leg fractures as a result of his congenital disease. This latest fracture occurred when he twisted at the hip while standing in his wheeled walker. He has been in a research study and receives a bisphosphonate infusion every 2 months. He is short in stature with short limbs for his age, and has bowing of both legs.

M.H. was transferred to the OR and carefully lifted to the OR table by the staff. After he was anesthetized, he was positioned with gentle manipulation, and his left hip was elevated on a small gel pillow. After skin preparation and sterile draping, a stainless steel rod was inserted into the medullary canal of his left femur to reduce and stabilize the femoral fracture. The muscle, fascia, subcutaneous tissue, and skin were sutured closed. Three nurses gently held M.H. in position on a pediatric spica box while the surgeon applied a hip spica (body cast) to stabilize the fixation, protect the leg, and maintain abduction. M.H. was transferred to the postanesthesia care unit (PACU) for recovery. The surgeon dictated the procedure as an open reduction internal fixation (ORIF) of the left femur with intramedullary (IM) rodding and application of spica cast.

➤ Case Study 19-3: Idiopathic Adolescent Scoliosis

Four years ago, L.R., who is now 15, had a posterior spinal fusion (PSF) for correction of idiopathic adolescent scoliosis in a pediatric orthopedic hospital in another state. Her spinal curvature had been surgically corrected with the insertion of bilateral laminar and pedicle hooks and two 3/16-inch rods. A bone autograft was taken from her right posterior superior ilium and applied along the lateral processes of T4 to L2 to complete the fusion.

During a follow-up visit, she presented with a significant prominence of the right scapula and back pain in the mid and lower back. She denied numbness or tingling of the lower extremities, bowel or bladder problems, chest pain, and shortness of breath. A CT scan of the upper thoracic spine showed a prominent rotatory scoliosis deformity of the right posterior thorax with acute angulation of the ribs. Her deformity is a common consequence of overcorrection of prior spinal fusion surgery, called crankshaft phenomenon.

L.R. was referred to the chief spinal surgeon of a local pediatric orthopedic hospital for removal of the spinal instrumentation, posterior spinal osteotomies from T4 to L2, insertion of replacement hooks and rods, bilateral rib resections, autograft bone from the resected ribs, partial scapulectomy and possible bone allograft, and bilateral chest tube placement. The surgical plan was explained to her and her mother and consent was obtained and signed. The surgical procedure as well as the potential benefits versus risks were discussed. L.R. and her mother stated that they fully understood and provided consent to proceed with the plan for surgery.

CASE STUDY QUESTIONS

Multiple choice. Select the best answer and write the letter of your choice to the left of each number:

_____ 1. A condylectomy is:
   a. removal of a joint capsule
   b. plastic repair of a vertebra
   c. removal of a rounded bone protuberance
   d. enlargement of a cavity
   e. removal of a tumor

_____ 2. The articulating surface of a bone is located:
   a. under the epiphysis
   b. in a joint
   c. around the bone marrow
   d. at a muscle attachment
   e. at a tendon attachment

_____ 3. The dissection directed anteroposteriorly was done:
   a. posterior–superior
   b. circumferential
   c. front to back
   d. top to bottom
   e. perpendicular to the mandible

_____ 4. Another term for bow-legged is:
   a. internal rotation
   b. knock-kneed
   c. adduction
   d. varus
   e. valgus

_____ 5. An IM rod is placed:
   a. inferior to the femoral condyle
   b. into the acetabulum
   c. within the medullary canal
   d. on top of the periosteum
   e. lateral to the epiphyseal growth plates

19

(continued)

Case Studies (continued)

_____ 6. The anatomic area described as thoracic or as the thorax is the:
  a. chest
  b. lower pelvis
  c. between sternum and umbilicus
  d. shoulders
  e. posterior abdomen

_____ 7. L.R.'s spinal fusion will immobilize the spinal levels of T4 to L2. These segments describe the _____ and _____ vertebrae.
  a. cervical, lumbar
  b. sacral, cranial
  c. lamina, disks
  d. thoracic, lumbar
  e. lumbar, thoracic

_____ 8. The grafted bone for L.R.'s fusion came from her own right ilium. The proper name for this is a(n):
  a. allograft
  b. autograft
  c. heterograft
  d. iliograft
  e. homograft

Write terms from the case studies that mean the following:

9. pertaining to the cheekbone

_____

10. the membrane around a bone

_____

11. a crescent-shaped cartilage in a joint

_____

12. on both sides

_____

13. plastic repair of a joint

_____

14. term for a disease of unknown origin

_____

15. removal of the shoulder blade

_____

16. a break in a bone

_____

17. surgical openings into bones

_____

Abbreviations. Define the following abbreviations:

18. DJD _____

19. MRI _____

20. NSAIDs _____

21. CT _____

22. NSS _____

23. TMJ _____

24. OI _____

25. ORIF _____

26. PSF _____

27. EBL _____

The Muscular System

CHAPTER

20

CHAPTER CONTENTS

OBJECTIVES

After study of this chapter you should be able to:

1. Compare the location and function of smooth, cardiac, and skeletal muscles.
2. Describe the typical structure of a skeletal muscle.
3. Briefly describe the mechanism of muscle contraction.
4. Explain how muscles work together to produce movement.
5. Describe the main types of movements produced by muscles.
6. List some of the criteria for naming muscles.
7. Identify and use the roots pertaining to the muscular system.
8. Describe the main disorders that affect muscles.
9. Label diagrams of the superficial anterior and posterior muscles.
10. Interpret abbreviations pertaining to muscles.
11. Analyze several case studies involving muscles.

PRETEST

Multiple choice. Select the best answer and write the letter of your choice to the left of each number.

____ 1. The neuromuscular junction is between a muscle and a:

    a. gland   c. bone
    b. neuron   d. gonad

____ 2. In the muscular system, the opposite of the origin is the:

    a. counterorigin   c. diaphragm
    b. prime mover   d. insertion

___ 3. The quadriceps femoris muscle forms the anterior part of the:

    a. neck   c. thigh
    b. back   d. abdomen

___ 4. The opposite of flexion is:

    a. rotation   c. relaxation
    b. antiflexion   d. extension

___ 5. The opposite of abduction is:

    a. adduction   c. periduction
    b. circumduction   d. pronation

___ 6. The band of connective tissue that attaches a muscle to a bone is a:

    a. cartilage   c. tendon
    b. bursa   d. diaphysis

___ 7. Polymyositis is inflammation of many:

    a. sense organs   c. glands
    b. muscles   d. bones

___ 8. The word *kinesis* means:

    a. movement   c. stretching
    b. bending   d. pain

The main characteristic of **muscle** tissue is its ability to contract. When stimulated, muscles shorten to produce movement of the skeleton, vessel walls, or internal organs. Muscles may also remain partially contracted to maintain posture. In addition, the heat generated by muscle contraction is the main source of body heat.

Types of Muscles

There are three types of muscle tissue in the body (Fig. 20-1):

- **Smooth (visceral) muscle** makes up the walls of the hollow organs, such as the stomach, intestines, and uterus, and the walls of ducts, such as the blood vessels and bronchioles. Smooth muscle operates involuntarily and is responsible for peristalsis, the wavelike movements that propel materials through the systems.

- **Cardiac muscle** makes up the myocardium of the heart wall. It functions involuntarily and is responsible for the heart's pumping action.

- **Skeletal muscle** is attached to bones and is responsible for voluntary movement. It also maintains posture and generates a large proportion of body heat. All of these voluntary muscles together make up the muscular system.

Skeletal Muscle

The discussion that follows describes the characteristics of skeletal muscle, which has been the most extensively studied of the three muscle types.

Muscle Structure

Muscles are composed of individual cells, often referred to as fibers because they are so long and threadlike. These cells are held together in **fascicles** (bundles) by connective tissue (Fig. 20-2). Covering each muscle is a sheath of

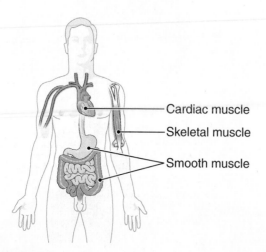

Figure 20-1 **Muscle types.** Smooth muscle makes up the wall of ducts and hollow organs, such as the stomach and intestine; cardiac muscle makes up the heart wall; skeletal muscle is attached to bones.

- Cardiac muscle
- Skeletal muscle
- Smooth muscle

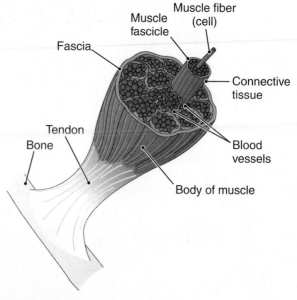

Figure 20-2 **Structure of a skeletal muscle.** Connective tissue coverings are shown as is the tendon that attaches the muscle to a bone.

Muscle fiber (cell)
Muscle fascicle
Fascia
Connective tissue
Tendon
Bone
Blood vessels
Body of muscle

Axon of motor neuron

Synaptic cleft

Synaptic vesicle

Mitochondrion

Neurotransmitter (acetylcholine)

A   Muscle fiber (cell)   Axon branches   Myosin   Actin   Muscle fiber nucleus

B   Muscle cell membrane

Figure 20-3 **Neuromuscular junction (NMJ).** (*A*) The branched end of a motor neuron makes contact with the membrane of a muscle fiber (cell). (*B*) Enlarged view of the NMJ showing release of neurotransmitter (acetylcholine) from a neuron and its attachment to a muscle cell membrane. Mitochondria generate ATP, the cells' energy compound.

connective tissue or **fascia.** These supporting tissues merge to form the **tendons** that attach the muscle to bones.

Muscle Action

Skeletal muscles are stimulated to contract by motor neurons of the nervous system (Fig. 20-3). At the **neuromuscular junction (NMJ),** the synapse (junction) where a branch of a neuron meets a muscle cell, the neurotransmitter **acetylcholine (ACh)** is released from small vesicles

(sacs) in an axon branch. ACh interacts with the muscle cell membrane to prompt cellular contraction. Two special protein filaments in muscle cells, **actin** and **myosin,** interact to produce the contraction. ATP (the cell's energy compound) and calcium are needed for this response. Box 20-1 discusses the use of steroids to increase muscle development and strength.

Most skeletal muscles contract rapidly to produce movement and then relax rapidly unless stimulation continues. Sometimes muscles are kept in a steady partially

---

Box 20-1   **Clinical Perspectives**

Anabolic Steroids: Winning at All Costs?

Anabolic steroids mimic the effects of the male sex hormone testosterone by promoting metabolism and stimulating growth. These drugs are legally prescribed to promote muscle regeneration and prevent atrophy from disuse after surgery. However, athletes also purchase them illegally, using them to increase muscle size and strength and improve endurance.

When steroids are used illegally to enhance athletic performance, the doses needed are large enough to cause serious side effects. They increase blood cholesterol levels, which may lead to atherosclerosis, heart disease, kidney failure, and

stroke. Steroids damage the liver, making it more susceptible to disease and cancer, and they suppress the immune system, increasing the risk of infection and cancer. In men, steroids cause impotence, testicular atrophy, low sperm count, infertility, and the development of female sex characteristics such as breasts (gynecomastia). In women, steroids disrupt ovulation and menstruation and produce male sex characteristics such as breast atrophy, clitoral enlargement, increased body hair, and deepening of the voice. In both sexes, steroids increase the risk for baldness and, especially in men, they cause mood swings, depression, and violence.

20

contracted state, to maintain posture, for example. This state of firmness is called **tonus**, or muscle tone.

The animation *The Neuromuscular Junction and Neurotransmitters* on the Student Resources shows events at the neuromuscular junction and the role of acetylcholine in muscle contraction.

Muscles work in pairs to produce movement at the joints. As one muscle, the **prime mover**, contracts, an opposing muscle, the **antagonist**, must relax. For example, when the biceps brachii on the anterior surface of the upper arm contracts to flex the arm, the triceps brachii on the posterior surface must relax (Fig. 20-4). When the arm is extended, these actions are reversed. In a given movement, the point where the muscle is attached to a stable part of the skeleton is the **origin**; the point where a muscle is attached to a moving part of the skeleton is the **insertion**.

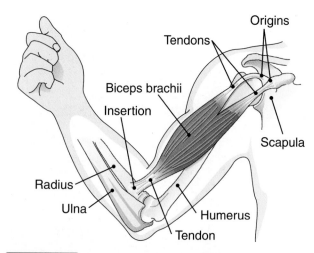

Figure 20-4 Muscle attachments to bones. Three attachments of the biceps brachii are shown, two origins and one insertion.

Box 20-2 describes various types of movements at the joints; these are illustrated in Figure 20-5. See also Box 20-3 for a description of careers in physical fitness.

Box 20-2   For Your Reference

Types of Movement

MOVEMENT	DEFINITION	EXAMPLE
flexion *FLEK-shun*	closing the angle at a joint	bending at the knee or elbow
extension *eks-TEN-shun*	opening the angle at a joint	straightening at the knee or elbow
abduction *ab-DUK-shun*	movement away from the midline of the body	outward movement of the arm at the shoulder
adduction *a-DUK-shun*	movement toward the midline of the body	return of lifted arm to the body
rotation *rō-TĀ-shun*	turning of a body part on its own axis	turning of the forearm from the elbow
circumduction *ser-kum-DUK-shun*	circular movement from a central point	describing a circle with an outstretched arm
pronation *prō-NĀ-shun*	turning downward	turning the palm of the hand downward
supination *sū-pin-Ā-shun*	turning upward	turning the palm of the hand upward
eversion *ē-VER-zhun*	turning outward	turning the sole of the foot outward
inversion *in-VER-zhun*	turning inward	turning the sole of the foot inward
dorsiflexion *dor-si-FLEK-shun*	bending backward	moving the foot so that the toes point upward, away from the sole of the foot
plantar flexion	bending the sole of the foot	pointing the toes downward

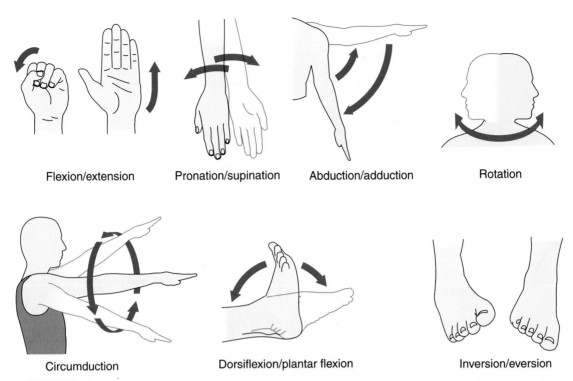

Flexion/extension   Pronation/supination   Abduction/adduction   Rotation

Circumduction   Dorsiflexion/plantar flexion   Inversion/eversion

Figure 20-5 **Types of movement.** Muscle contraction produces movement at the joints. Some muscles are named for the type of movement they produce, such as flexor, extensor, and adductor.

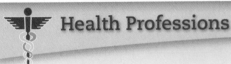

Box 20-3 **Health Professions**

Careers in Exercise and Fitness

Several related careers are concerned with the management of exercise programs for therapy, health maintenance, and recreation. The American College of Sports Medicine (ACSM) at www.acsm.org has information on these fields and some certification programs.

- **Exercise physiologists** study the mechanisms involved in physical exercise and the body's physiologic responses to exercise. They design programs for general health, athletics, and rehabilitation for disability or disease, such as cardiovascular and respiratory diseases. They may work in a clinical setting in cooperation with physicians, in private industry, in health clubs, or in teaching. Most exercise physiologists (EPs) have a master's degree, but some jobs may require only a bachelor's degree. A PhD is needed for teaching or research. EPs may be certified through ACSM or the Center for Exercise Physiology (CEP). The American Society of Exercise Physiologists at www.asep.org has information about this profession.

- **Athletic trainers** specialize in the prevention and treatment of musculoskeletal injuries. They advise clients on the proper use of exercise equipment and devices, such as braces, that help prevent injuries. They work in cooperation with physicians in private establishments, in health care facilities, and with athletes and sports teams. An athletic trainer's job may have a set schedule, but if working for a sports team, may require long and irregular hours. A

majority of athletic trainers have a master's degree or higher. Employment opportunities in health care and teaching are expected to be good, although jobs with sports teams are limited. The National Athletic Trainers' Association at www.nata.org has more information on this career.

- **Fitness workers** is a category that includes a variety of career activities, such as personal trainers and group fitness, yoga, and Pilates instructors. These professionals lead, instruct, and motivate individuals or groups in all types of exercise activities. Traditionally, they have worked in studios, health clubs, or private homes, but they are increasingly found in the workplace, where they organize and direct fitness programs for employees. Their jobs may involve administrative duties as well. Personal trainers must be certified, and certification is encouraged for other fitness professionals. Candidates must have a high school diploma, certification in CPR, and must pass a written exam and sometimes a practical exam as well. Increasingly, a bachelor's degree is required, and those who wish to progress to management jobs may need a higher degree. Instructors who specialize in a particular exercise method, such as Pilates or yoga, have their own training standards. Job opportunities in these fields are expected to increase with an aging population and increasing concern for good health and physical fitness. The National Commission for Certifying Agencies at www.noca.org can help locate accredited fitness certification programs.

20

Figure 20-6 Superficial muscles, anterior view.

Naming of Muscles

A muscle can be named by its location (near a bone, for example), by the direction of its fibers, or by its size, shape, or number of attachment points (heads), as indicated by the suffix -*ceps*. It may also be named for its action, adding the suffix -*or* to the root for the action. For example, a muscle that produces flexion at a joint is a flexor. Examine the muscle diagrams in Figures 20-6 and 20-7. See how many of these criteria you can find in the muscle names. Note that sometimes more than one criterion is used in the name.

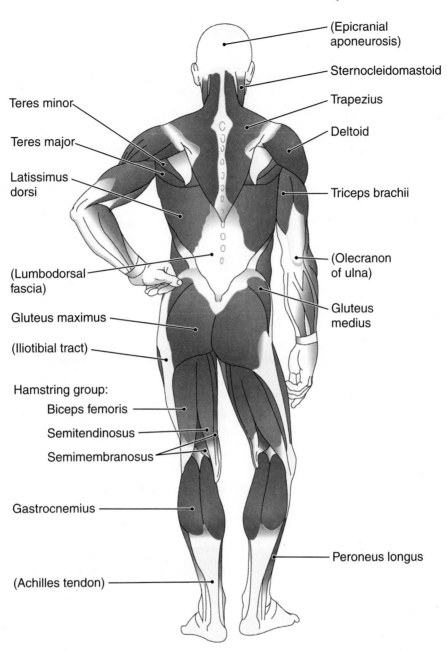

Figure 20-7 **Superficial muscles, posterior view.** Associated structures are labeled in parentheses.

Terminology	Key Terms

Normal Structure and Function

acetylcholine (ACh) *as-e-til-KŌ-lēn*	A neurotransmitter that stimulates contraction of skeletal muscles
actin *AK-tin*	One of the two contractile proteins in muscle cells; the other is myosin
antagonist *an-TAG-ō-nist*	The muscle that opposes a prime mover; it must relax when the prime mover contracts
cardiac muscle *KAR-dē-ak*	Involuntary muscle that makes up the wall of the heart

Terminology	**Key Terms** (continued)
fascia FASH-ē-a	The fibrous sheath of connective tissue that covers a muscle; called *deep fascia* to differentiate it from the superficial fascia that underlies the skin (root: *fasci/o*); plural: fasciae
fascicle FAS-i-kel	A small bundle, as of muscle or nerve fibers
insertion in-SER-shun	In a given movement, the point where a muscle is attached to a moving part of the skeleton
muscle MUS-el	An organ that produces movement by contracting; also the tissue that composes such organs (roots: *my/o, muscul/o*)
myosin MĪ-ō-sin	One of the two contractile proteins in muscle cells; the other is actin
neuromuscular junction (NMJ) nū-rō-MUS-kū-lar JUNK-shun	The point of contact, or synapse, between a branch of a motor neuron and a muscle cell
origin OR-i-jin	In a given movement, the point where a muscle is attached to a stable part of the skeleton
prime mover PRĪM	The muscle that carries out a given movement; agonist (AG-on-ist)
skeletal muscle SKEL-e-tal	Voluntary muscle that moves the skeleton and maintains posture
smooth muscle	Involuntary muscle that makes up the wall of hollow organs, vessels, and ducts; visceral muscle
tendon TEN-dun	A fibrous band of connective tissue that attaches a muscle to a bone (roots: *ten/o, tendin/o*)
tonus TŌ-nus	A state of steady, partial muscle contraction that maintains firmness; muscle tone (root: *ton/o*)

PASSport to Success® Go to the pronunciation glossary on the Student Resources to hear these words pronounced.

Roots Pertaining to Muscles

See Table 20-1.

Table 20-1	**Roots Pertaining to Muscles**

Root	Meaning	Example	Definition of Example
my/o	muscle	myositis* mī-ō-SĪ-tis	inflammation of muscle
muscul/o	muscle	musculature MUS-kyŭ-la-chur	muscle arrangement in a part or the whole body
in/o	fiber	inotropic in-ō-TROP-ik	acting on (muscle) fibers
fasci/o	fascia	fasciodesis fash-ē-OD-e-sis	binding (suture) of a fascia to a tendon or other fascia

Table 20-1	Continued		
Root	**Meaning**	**Example**	**Definition of Example**
ten/o, tendin/o	tendon	tenostosis *ten-os-TŌ-sis*	ossification of a tendon
ton/o	tone	cardiotonic *kar-dē-ō-TON-ik*	having a strengthening action on the heart muscle
erg/o	work	ergonomics	study of the efficient use of energy during work
kin/o-, kine, kinesi/o, kinet/o	movement	kinesis *ki-NĒ-sis*	movement (adjective: kinetic)

*Note addition of s to this root before the suffix -itis.

EXERCISE 20-1

Define the following adjectives:

1. muscular _____

2. fascial _____

3. tendinous _____

4. tonic _____

5. kinetic _____

Fill in the blanks:

6. Myoglobin (*mī-ō-GLŌ-bin*) is a type of protein (globin) found in _____.

7. Inosclerosis (*in-ō-skle-RŌ-sis*) is hardening of tissue from an increase in _____.

8. Fasciitis (*fash-ē-Ī-tis*) is inflammation of _____.

9. Dystonia (*dis-TŌ-nē-a*) is abnormal muscle _____.

10. An ergograph (*ER-gō-graf*) is an instrument for recording muscle _____.

11. Kinesia (*kī-NĒ-sē-a*) is a term for sickness caused by _____.

12. Myofibrils (*mī-ō-FĪ-brils*) are small fibers found in _____.

13. The muscularis layer in the wall of a hollow organ or duct is composed of _____.

Define the following terms:

14. hypermyotonia (*hī-per-mī-ō-TŌ-nē-a*) _____

15. fasciorrhaphy (*fash-ē-OR-a-fē*) _____

16. tendinitis (*ten-di-NĪ-tis*), also tendonitis (*ten-don-Ī-tis*) _____

17. musculotendinous (*mus-kū-lō-TEN-di-nus*) _____

18. tenodesis (*ten-OD-e-sis*) _____

19. myalgia (*mī-AL-jē-a*) _____

20. kinesitherapy (*ki-nē-si-THER-a-pē*) _____

21. myotenositis (*mī-ō-ten-ō-SĪ-tis*) _____

22. myofascial (*mī-ō-FASH-ē-al*) _____

20

23. ergogenic (er-gō-JEN-ik) _____

24. atony (AT-ō-nē) _____

25. dyskinesia (dis-kī-NĒ-zē-a) _____

Write words for the following definitions:

26. any disease of muscle _____

27. excision of fascia _____

28. incision of a tendon (use ten/o) _____

29. inflammation of many (poly-) muscles _____

30. pertaining to muscles and the skeleton _____

31. study of movement (use kinesi/o) _____

32. plastic repair of a tendon and its muscle _____

Clinical Aspects of the Muscular System

Muscle function may be affected by disorders elsewhere, particularly in the nervous system and connective tissue. The conditions described below affect the muscular system directly or involve the muscles and have not been described in other chapters. Any disorder of muscles is described as a myopathy.

Techniques for diagnosing muscle disorders include electrical studies of muscle in action, **electromyography (EMG)**, and serum assay of enzymes released in increased amounts from damaged muscles, mainly **creatine kinase (CK)**.

Muscular Dystrophy

Muscular dystrophy refers to a group of hereditary diseases involving progressive, noninflammatory muscular degeneration. There is weakness and wasting of muscle tissue with its gradual replacement by connective tissue and fat. There may also be cardiomyopathy (cardiac muscle disease) and mental impairment.

The most common form is Duchenne muscular dystrophy, a sex-linked disease passed from mother to son. This appears at 3 to 4 years of age, and patients are incapacitated by age 10 to 15. Death is commonly caused by respiratory failure or infection.

Multiple System Disorders Involving Muscles

POLYMYOSITIS

Polymyositis is inflammation of skeletal muscle leading to weakness, frequently associated with dysphagia (difficulty in swallowing) or cardiac problems. The cause is unknown and may be related to viral infection or autoimmunity. Often the disorder is associated with some other systemic disease such as rheumatoid arthritis or lupus erythematosus.

When the skin is involved, the condition is termed **dermatomyositis**. In this case, there is erythema (redness of the skin), dermatitis (inflammation of the skin), and a typical lilac-colored rash, predominantly on the face. In addition to enzyme studies and EMG, clinicians use muscle biopsy in diagnosis.

FIBROMYALGIA SYNDROME

Fibromyalgia syndrome (FMS) is a difficult-to-diagnose condition involving the muscles. It is associated with widespread muscle aches, tenderness, and stiffness, along with fatigue and sleep disorders in the absence of neurologic abnormalities or any other known cause. The disorder may coexist with other chronic diseases, may follow a viral infection, and may involve immune system dysfunction. A current theory is that FMS results from hormonal or neurotransmitter imbalances that increase sensitivity to pain. Treatments for FMS include a carefully planned exercise program and medication with pain relievers, muscle relaxants, or antidepressants.

CHRONIC FATIGUE SYNDROME

Chronic fatigue syndrome (CFS) involves persistent fatigue of no known cause that may be associated with impaired memory, sore throat, painful lymph nodes, muscle and joint pain, headaches, sleep problems, and immune disorders. The condition often occurs after a viral infection. Epstein–Barr virus (the cause of mononucleosis), herpesvirus, and other viruses have been suggested as possible causes of CFS. No traditional or alternative therapies have been consistently successful in treating CFS.

MYASTHENIA GRAVIS

Myasthenia gravis (MG) is an acquired autoimmune disease in which antibodies interfere with muscle stimulation at the neuromuscular junction. There is a progressive loss of muscle power, especially in the external eye muscles and facial muscles.

Box 20-4   Focus on Words

Some Colorful Musculoskeletal Terms

Some common terms for musculoskeletal disorders have interesting origins. A charley horse describes muscular strain and soreness, especially in the legs. The term comes from common use of the name Charley for old lame horses that were kept around for family use when they could no longer be used for hard work. Wryneck, technically torticollis, uses the word *wry* meaning twisted or turned, as in the word awry (*a-RĪ*), meaning amiss or out of position.

A bunion, technically called hallux valgus, is an enlargement of the first joint of the great toe with bursitis at the joint. It probably comes from the word bony, changed to bunny, and used to mean a bump on the head and then a swelling on a joint. A clavus is commonly called a corn because it is a hardened or horny thickening of the skin in an area of friction or pressure.

AMYOTROPHIC LATERAL SCLEROSIS

Also named Lou Gehrig disease after a famous baseball player who died of the disorder, **amyotrophic lateral sclerosis (ALS)** is a progressive degeneration of motor neurons that leads to muscle atrophy (amyotrophy). Early signs are weakness, cramping, and muscle twitching. The facial or respiratory muscles may be affected early depending on the site of degeneration. Mental function, sensory perception, as well as bowel and bladder function usually remain intact. The disease progresses and eventually leads to death from respiratory muscle paralysis in 3 to 5 years.

Stress Injuries

Not as grave as the above diseases perhaps, but much more common, are musculoskeletal disorders caused by physical stress. These include accidental injuries and work- or sports-related damage caused by overexertion or repetitive motion, so called **repetitive strain injury (RSI)**. Damages to soft tissues include muscle **strain**, inflammation or tearing of ligaments and tendons, and bursitis. **Tenosynovitis**, commonly called **tendinitis**, is inflammation of a tendon, tendon sheath, and the synovial membrane at a joint. The signs of these injuries are pain, fatigue, weakness, stiffness, numbness, and reduced range of motion (ROM). (The origins of some colorful terms for such conditions are given in Box 20-4.)

Stress injuries may involve any muscles or joints, but some common upper extremity conditions are:

- Rotator cuff (RTC) injury—The RTC, which strengthens the shoulder joint, is formed by four muscles, the supraspinatus, infraspinatus, teres minor, and subscapularis, the "SITS" muscles (Fig. 20-8). Inflammation or tearing of the RTC

A   Posterior view

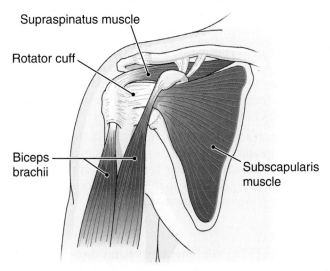

B   Anterior view

Figure 20-8   **Anatomy of the rotator cuff.** Four muscles contribute to the rotator cuff that strengthens the shoulder. They are the supraspinatus, infraspinatus, teres minor, and subscapularis. Two adjacent muscles are also shown, the deltoid and biceps brachii. (*A*) Posterior. (*B*) Anterior.

can occur in people who repeatedly perform over-head activities, such as swimming, painting, or pitching.

■ Epicondylitis—The medial and lateral epicondyles (projections) of the distal humerus are attachment points for muscles that flex and extend the wrist and fingers. Inflammation of these tendons of origin causes pain at the elbow and forearm on lifting, carrying, squeezing, or typing. These stress injuries are often sports related, leading to the terms "golfer's elbow" and "tennis elbow" for medial and lateral epicondylitis, respectively. A brace worn below the elbow to distribute stress on the joint may be helpful.

■ Carpal tunnel syndrome (CTS)—CTS involves the tendons of the finger flexor muscles and the nerves that supply the hand and fingers (Fig. 20-9). Hand numbness and weakness is caused by pressure on the median nerve as it passes through a tunnel formed by the carpal (wrist) bones. CTS commonly appears in people who use their hands and fingers strenuously, such as musicians and keyboarders.

■ Trigger finger—This is a painful snapping, triggering, or locking of a finger as it is moved. It is caused by inflammation and swelling of the flexor tendon sheath at the metacarpophalangeal joint that prevents the tendon from sliding back and forth.

Some stress injuries that involve the lower extremities are:

■ Hamstring strain—The hamstring is a large muscle group in the posterior thigh that extends from the hip to the knee and flexes the knee (see Fig. 20-7). A "pulled hamstring" is common in athletes who stop and start running suddenly. It is treated with stretching and strengthening activities.

■ Shin splint—This is pain in the leg's anterior tibial region from running on hard surfaces or overuse of the foot flexors, as in athletes and dancers. Help comes from good shoes with adequate support and avoidance of hard surfaces for exercise.

■ Achilles tendinitis—The Achilles (a-KIL-ēz) tendon is a large tendon that attaches the calf muscles to the heel and is used to plantar flex the foot at the ankle (see Fig. 20-7). Damage to the Achilles tendon hampers or prevents walking and running.

TREATMENT

Orthopedists diagnose musculoskeletal disorders by MRI and other imaging techniques, ROM measurements, and strength testing. Treatment of stress injuries usually begins conservatively with rest, elevation, ice packs, bracing, and medications, such as

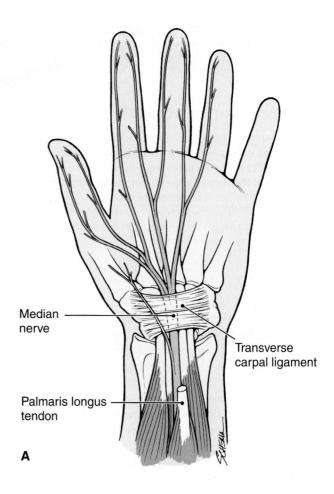

Median nerve

Transverse carpal ligament

Palmaris longus tendon

A

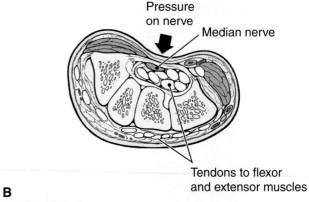

Pressure on nerve

Median nerve

Tendons to flexor and extensor muscles

B

Figure 20-9 **Carpal tunnel syndrome.** (*A*) Pressure on the median nerve as it passes through the carpal (wrist) bones causes numbness and weakness in the areas of the hand supplied by the nerve. (*B*) Cross section of the wrist showing compression of the median nerve.

analgesics, antiinflammatory agents, and muscle relaxants. (The acronym PRICE represents this simple approach—protection, rest, ice, compression, elevation.) Treatment may progress to steroid injections, ultrasound therapy for deep heat, strengthening exercises, or even surgery.

13. _____   19. _____

14. _____   20. _____

15. _____   21. _____

16. _____   22. _____

17. _____   23. _____

18. _____   24. _____

Superficial Muscles, Posterior View > Write the name of each numbered part on the corresponding line of the answer sheet.

Deltoid   Peroneus longus
Gastrocnemius   Sternocleidomastoid
Gluteus maximus   Teres major
Gluteus medius   Teres minor
Hamstring group   Trapezius
Latissimus dorsi   Triceps brachii

1. _____

2. _____

3. _____

4. _____

5. _____

6. _____

7. _____

8. _____

9. _____

10. _____

11. _____

12. _____

Posterior view

TERMINOLOGY

Matching > Match the following terms and write the appropriate letter to the left of each number:

_____ **1.** masseter   **a.** main muscle of the calf
_____ **2.** deltoid   **b.** muscle of the upper back and neck
_____ **3.** pectoralis major **c.** muscle used in chewing; jaw muscle
_____ **4.** gastrocnemius   **d.** large muscle of the upper chest
_____ **5.** trapezius   **e.** triangular muscle that covers the shoulder

_____ **6.** dystonia   **a.** instrument for measuring muscle work
_____ **7.** ergometer   **b.** slowness of movement
_____ **8.** inotropic   **c.** a small bundle of fibers
_____ **9.** bradykinesia   **d.** acting on muscle fibers
_____ **10.** fascicle   **e.** abnormal muscle tone

20

Chapter Review *(continued)*

Supplementary Terms

_____ **11.** glycogen	**a.** substance that stores energy in muscle cells
_____ **12.** tetany	**b.** flat, white, sheetlike tendon
_____ **13.** aponeurosis	**c.** muscular spasms and cramps
_____ **14.** creatine	**d.** complex sugar stored in muscles
_____ **15.** lactic acid	**e.** a byproduct of anaerobic muscle contractions

_____ **16.** asterixis	**a.** wryneck
_____ **17.** ataxia	**b.** lack of muscle coordination
_____ **18.** torticollis	**c.** awareness of movement
_____ **19.** atrophy	**d.** wasting of tissue
_____ **20.** kinesthesia	**e.** rapid, jerky movements, especially of the hands

_____ **21.** clonus	**a.** forcible tearing away of a part
_____ **22.** athetosis	**b.** acute infectious disease that affects muscles
_____ **23.** spasm	**c.** intermittent muscle contractions
_____ **24.** tetanus	**d.** sudden involuntary muscle contraction
_____ **25.** avulsion	**e.** condition marked by slow, twisting movements

Fill in the blanks:

26. The neurotransmitter released at the neuromuscular junction is _____.

27. The sheath of connective tissue that covers a muscle is called _____.

28. The number of origins (heads) in the triceps brachii muscle is _____.

29. A muscle that produces extension at a joint is called a(n) _____.

30. A band of connective tissue that attaches a muscle to a bone is a(n) _____.

31. The strong, cordlike tendon that attaches the calf muscle to the heel is the _____.

32. Movement away from the midline of the body is termed _____.

33. A musculotropic substance acts on _____.

Define the following words:

34. myology (*mī-OL-ō-jē*) _____

35. myofascial (*mī-ō-FASH-ē-al*) _____

36. tendinoplasty (*TEN-din-ō-plas-tē*) _____

37. inositis (*in-ō-SĪ-tis*) _____

38. hypotonia (*hī-pō-TŌ-nē-a*) _____

39. hyperkinesia (*hī-per-ki-NĒ-sē-a*) _____

Write words for the following definitions:

40. inflammation of muscle (use my/o-) _____

41. death of muscle tissue _____

42. suture of fascia _____

43. absence of muscle tone _____

44. excision of fascia   _____

45. study of movement   _____

46. surgical incision of a tendon (use ten/o-)   _____

47. pertaining to a tendon   _____

Opposites > Write a word that means the opposite of the following terms as they pertain to muscles:

48. prime mover   _____

49. origin   _____

50. abduction   _____

51. pronation   _____

52. extension   _____

Adjectives > From the supplementary terms, write the adjective form of the following words:

53. ataxia   _____

54. athetosis   _____

55. spasm   _____

56. clonus   _____

True–False > Examine the following statements. If the statement is true, write T in the first blank. If the statement is false, write F in the first blank and correct the statement by replacing the underlined word in the second blank.

57. The part of a neuron that contacts a muscle cell is the <u>axon</u>.   _____   _____

58. Skeletal muscle is <u>voluntary.</u>   _____   _____

59. The <u>origin</u> of a muscle is attached to a moving part.   _____   _____

60. The hamstring group is in the <u>anterior</u> thigh.   _____   _____

61. <u>Pronation</u> means turning downward.   _____   _____

62. Smooth muscle is also called <u>visceral</u> muscle.   _____   _____

63. The quadriceps muscle has <u>three</u> components.   _____   _____

64. In an <u>isotonic</u> contraction, a muscle shortens.   _____   _____

Eliminations > In each of the sets below, underline the word that does not fit in with the rest and explain the reason for your choice:

65. fascicle — fiber — tendon — osteoblast — fascia

_____

66. soleus — flexor carpi — biceps brachii — brachioradialis — extensor carpi

_____

67. vastus intermedius — intercostals — vastus lateralis — vastus medialis — rectus femoris

_____

20

68. circumduction — inversion — actin — dorsiflexion — rotation

_____

69. EMG — ALS — FMS — CFS — MG

_____

Abbreviations > Write the meaning of each of the following:

70. CTS _____

71. ACh _____

72. RTC _____

73. NMJ _____

74. CK _____

Word Building > Write a word for the following definitions using the word parts provided.

-ia   ten/o   -al   alg/o   -itis   -desis   -blast   -lysis   fasci/o   my/o

75. an immature muscle cell _____

76. binding of a fascia _____

77. pain in a tendon _____

78. destruction of muscle tissue _____

79. binding of a tendon _____

80. inflammation of fascia _____

81. separation of a tendon _____

82. pertaining to fascia _____

83. pain in a muscle _____

Word Analysis > Define each of the following words, and give the meaning of the word parts in each. Use a dictionary if necessary.

84. dermatomyositis (*der-ma-tō-mī-ō-SĪ-tis*) _____

    a. dermat/o _____

    b. my/o(s) _____

    c. -itis _____

85. myasthenia (*mī-as-THĒ-nē-a*) _____

    a. my/o _____

    b. a- _____

    c. sthen/o _____

    d. -ia _____

Chapter Review *(continued)*

86. dyssynergia (*dis-in-ER-jē-a*) _____

   a. dys- _____

   b. syn- _____

   c. erg/o _____

   d. -ia _____

87. amyotrophic (*a-mī-ō-TRŌ-fik*) _____

   a. a- _____

   b. my/o _____

   c. troph/o _____

   d. -ic _____

PASSport to Success® Go to the word exercises on the Student Resources for additional review exercises.

Case Studies

▶ Case Study 20-1: Rotator Cuff Tear

M.L., a 56-year-old business executive and former college football player, was referred to an orthopedic surgeon for recurrent shoulder pain. M.L. was unable to abduct his right arm without pain even after 6 months of physical therapy and NSAIDs. In addition, he had taken supplements of glucosamine, chondroitin, and S-adenosylmethionine for several months in an effort to protect the flexibility of his shoulder joint. M.L. recalled a shoulder dislocation resulting from a football injury 35 years earlier. An MRI scan confirmed a complete rotator cuff tear. The surgeon recommended the Bankart procedure for M.L.'s injury to restore his joint stability, alleviate his pain, and permit him to return to his former normal activities, including golf.

After anesthesia induction and positioning in a semisitting (beach chair) position, the surgeon made an anterosuperior deltoid incision (the standard deltopectoral approach) and divided the coracoacromial ligament at the acromial attachment. The rotator cuff was identified after the deltoid was retracted and the clavipectoral fascia was incised. The subscapularis tendon was incised proximal to its insertion. After capsular incision, inspection showed a large pouch inferiorly in the capsule, consistent with laxity (instability). The capsule's torn edges were anchored to the rim of the glenoid fossa with heavy nonabsorbable sutures. A flap

from the subscapularis tendon was transposed and sutured to the supraspinatus and infraspinatus muscles to bridge the gap. An intraoperative ROM examination showed that the external rotation could be performed past neutral and that the shoulder did not dislocate. The wound was closed, and a shoulder immobilizer sling was applied. M.L. was referred to PT to begin therapy in 3 weeks and was assured he would be able to play golf in 6 months.

▶ Case Study 20-2: Brachial Plexus Injury

T.D., a 16-year-old high school student, had a severe football accident 3 months before his admission. He sustained a right brachial plexus injury, resulting in a flail arm. He had no recovery and was on medication for neurologic pain. He reported that he had no feeling or motion in his right shoulder or arm. He had atrophy over the supraspinatus and infraspinatus muscles and also subluxation of his shoulder and deltoid atrophy. He had no active motion of the right upper extremity and no sensation. The rest of his orthopedic exam showed full ROM of his hips, knees, and ankles with intact sensation and palpable distal pulses as well as normal motor function. He was diagnosed with a possible middle trunk brachial plexus injury from C7. He was scheduled for an EMG, nerve conduction studies, and

20

(continued)

Case Studies (continued)

somatosensory evoked potentials (SSEPs). His diaphragm was examined under fluoroscopy to R/O phrenic nerve injury.

With middle trunk brachial plexus injury, damage to the subscapular nerve will interrupt conduction to the subscapularis and teres major muscles. Damage to the long thoracic nerve prevents conduction to the serratus anterior muscles. Injury to the pectoral nerves affects the pectoralis major and minor muscles.

T.D. was scheduled for a brachial plexus exploration with possible nerve graft, nerve transfer, bilateral sural (calf) nerve harvest, or gracilis muscle graft from his right thigh.

▶ Case Study 20-3: "Wake Up" Test during Spinal Fusion Surgery

L.N.'s somatosensory evoked potentials (SSEPs) were monitored throughout her spinal fusion surgery to provide continuous information on the functional state of her sensory pathways from the median and posterior tibial nerves through the dorsal column to the primary somatosensory cortex. Before surgery, needle electrodes were inserted into L.N.'s right and left quadriceps muscles to determine nerve conduction through L2 to L4, into the anterior tibialis muscles to measure passage through L5, and into the gastrocnemius muscles to measure S1 to S2. Electrodes were placed in her rectus abdominis to monitor S1 to S2. All electrodes were taped in place, and the wires were plugged into a transformer box with feedback to a computer. A neuromonitoring technologist placed the electrodes and attended the computer monitor throughout the case. During the procedure, selected muscle groups were stimulated with 15 to 40 milliamperes (mA) of current to test the nerves and muscles. Data fed back into the computer confirmed the neuromuscular integrity and status of the spinal fixation, the instrumentation, and implants.

After the pedicle screws, hooks, and wires were in place and the spinal rods were cinched down to straighten the spine, L.N. was permitted to emerge temporarily from anesthesia and muscle paralysis medication to a lightly sedated but pain-free state. She was given commands to move her feet, straighten her legs, and wiggle her toes to test all neuromuscular groups that could be affected by misplaced or compressed spinal fixation devices. Her feet were watched, and movement was announced to the team. Dorsiflexion cleared the tibialis anterior muscles; plantar flexion cleared the gastrocnemius muscles. Knee flexion cleared the hamstring muscle group, and knee extension determined function of the quadriceps group. L.N. had a successful "wake-up" test. She was put back into deep anesthesia, and her incision was closed. A postoperative "wake-up" test was repeated after she was moved to her bed. The surgical instruments and tables were kept sterile until after all of the monitored muscle groups were tested and showed voluntary movement. The electrodes were removed, and she was taken to postanesthesia care unit (PACU) for recovery.

CASE STUDY QUESTIONS

Multiple choice. Select the best answer and write the letter of your choice to the left of each number.

_____ 1. The insertion of the muscle is:
    a. the thick middle portion
    b. the point of attachment to the moving bone
    c. the point of attachment to the stable bone
    d. the fibrous sheath
    e. the connective tissue

_____ 2. M.L. was unable to abduct his affected arm. This motion is:
    a. toward the midline
    b. circumferential
    c. in the same direction as the muscle fibers
    d. away from the midline
    e. a position with the palm facing upward

_____ 3. An anterosuperior deltoid incision would be made:
    a. perpendicular to the muscle fibers
    b. below the fascia sheath
    c. behind the glenoid fossa
    d. in the best area
    e. at the top and to the front of the deltoid muscle

_____ 4. The subscapularis tendon arises from the subscapularis:
    a. fascia
    b. nerve
    c. bone
    d. extensor
    e. flexor

_____ 5. The intraoperative ROM examination was performed:
    a. in the OR corridor
    b. during surgery
    c. before surgery
    d. after surgery
    e. in the interventional radiology suite

_____ 6. M.L.'s arm and shoulder were immobilized after surgery to:
    a. encourage movement beyond the point of pain
    b. minimize rapid ROM
    c. maintain adduction and external rotation
    d. prevent movement
    e. stop bleeding

_____ 7. T.D. had atrophy of the supraspinatus and infraspinatus muscles. The term *atrophy* here refers to:
    a. hypercontraction
    b. intermittent contraction and relaxation
    c. muscle tissue wasting
    d. paralysis
    e. painful discoloration

(continued)

Case Studies (continued)

_____ 8. Another term for subluxation is:
   a. dislocation
   b. hyperextension
   c. turning inside out
   d. overlapping
   e. stretched beyond original shape

_____ 9. A palpable distal pulse means that the pulse can be:
   a. heard at the foot
   b. felt at the top of the thigh
   c. felt at the foot
   d. obliterated with light
   e. undetectable

_____ 10. The pectoralis major and pectoralis minor muscles are located:
   a. below the knees
   b. behind the thighs
   c. in the lower back
   d. in the upper chest
   e. on the lateral side of the arms

_____ 11. The quadriceps muscle group is made up of:
   a. smooth and cardiac muscle fibers
   b. four muscles in the thigh
   c. three muscles in the leg and one in the anterior chest
   d. fascia and tendon sheaths
   e. tendons and fascia around the shoulder

_____ 12. The nerve supply for the rectus abdominis muscle runs through S1–S2. This anatomic region is:
   a. the first and second sural sheath
   b. subluxation and suppuration
   c. sacral disk space 1 and 2
   d. sacral disk space 3
   e. somatosensory electrodes 1 and 2

_____ 13. The movement of elevating the toes toward the anterior ankle is:
   a. supination
   b. pronation
   c. dorsiflexion
   d. plantar flexion
   e. external rotation

_____ 14. Knee extension results in:
   a. a bent knee
   b. a ballet position with the toes turned out
   c. bilateral abduction
   d. inversion
   e. a straight leg

Write terms from the case studies with the following meanings:

15. pertaining to the arm

_____

16. pertaining to treatment of skeletal and muscular disorders

_____

17. bending at a joint

_____

18. to point the toes downward

_____

Define the following abbreviations:

19. PT _____

20. ROM _____

21 R/O _____

22. EMG _____

23. SSEP _____

24. PACU _____

20

CHAPTER 21

The Skin

CHAPTER CONTENTS

OBJECTIVES

After study of this chapter you should be able to:

1. Compare the epidermis, dermis, and subcutaneous tissue.
2. Describe the roles of keratin and melanin in the skin.
3. Name and describe the glands in the skin.
4. Describe the structure of hair and nails.
5. Identify and use roots pertaining to the skin.
6. Describe the main disorders that affect the skin.
7. Label a diagram of the skin.
8. Analyze several case studies involving the skin.

PRETEST

Multiple choice. Select the best answer and write the letter of your choice to the left of each number.

___ 1. The uppermost portion of the skin is called the:

   a. fossa
   b. cuticle
   c. epidermis
   d. epiphysis

___ 2. A hair grows within a sheath called the:

   a. follicle
   b. hyaline
   c. fascia
   d. vesicle

___ 3. The glands that secrete an oily substance that lubricates the skin are the:

   a. sweat glands
   b. sebaceous glands
   c. mammary glands
   d. foramina

____ 4. The rule of nines is a system used to evaluate:

    a. burns   c. inflammation
    b. fever   d. immunity

____ 5. A pigmented skin tumor is a(n):

    a. chondrosarcoma c. lymphoma
    b. melanoma   d. adenoma

____ 6. The root *hidr/o* pertains to:

    a. tears   c. blood
    b. saliva   d. sweat

____ 7. Onychomycosis is a fungal infection of a(n):

    a. eyelid   c. hair
    b. nail   d. bone

Like the eyes, the **skin** is a readily visible reflection of one's health. Its color, texture, and resilience reveal much, as does the condition of the **hair** and **nails**. The skin and its associated structures make up the **integumentary system**. This body-covering system protects against infection, dehydration, ultraviolet radiation, and injury. Extensive damage to the skin, such as by burns, can result in a host of dangerous complications.

The skin helps to regulate temperature by evaporation of sweat and by changes in the diameter of surface blood vessels, which control how much heat is lost to the environment. The skin also contains receptors for the sensory perceptions of touch, temperature, pressure, and pain. Medication can be delivered through the skin from patches, as explained in Box 21-1.

The word **derma** (from Greek) means (skin) and is used as an ending in words pertaining to the skin, such as xeroderma (dryness of the skin) and **scleroderma** (hardening of the skin). The adjective **cutaneous** refers to the skin and is from the Latin word *cutis* for skin.

Anatomy of the Skin

The skin's outermost portion is the **epidermis**, consisting of four to five layers (strata) of epithelial cells (Fig. 21-1). The deepest layer, the stratum basale, or basal layer, produces new cells. As these cells gradually rise toward the surface, they die and become filled with **keratin**, a protein that thickens and toughens the skin. The outermost

---

Box 21-1   Clinical Perspectives

Medication Patches: No Bitter Pill to Swallow

For most people, pills are a convenient way to take medication, but for some, they have drawbacks. Pills must be taken at regular intervals to ensure consistent dosing, and they must be digested and absorbed into the bloodstream before they can begin to work. For those who have difficulty swallowing or digesting pills, transdermal (TD) patches offer an effective alternative to oral medications.

TD patches deliver a consistent dose of medication that diffuses at a constant rate through the skin into the bloodstream. There is no daily schedule to follow, nothing to swallow, and no stomach upset. TD patches can also deliver medication to unconscious patients, who would otherwise require intravenous drug delivery. TD patches are used in hormone replacement therapy, to treat heart disease, to manage pain, and to suppress motion sickness. Nicotine patches are also used as part of programs to quit smoking.

TD patches must be used carefully. Drug diffusion through the skin takes time, so it is important to know how long the patch must be in place before it is effective. It is also important to know when the medication's effects disappear after the patch is removed. Because the body continues to absorb what has already diffused into the skin, removing the patch does not entirely remove the medicine. There is also a danger that patches may become unsafe when heated, as by exercise, high fever, or a hot environment, such as a hot tub, heating pad, or sauna. When heat dilates the capillaries in the skin, a dangerous increase in dosage may result as more medication enters the blood.

A recent advance in TD drug delivery is iontophoresis. Based on the principle that like charges repel each other, this method uses a mild electrical current to move ionic drugs through the skin. A small electrical device attached to the patch uses positive current to "push" positively charged drug molecules through the skin, and a negative current to push negatively charged ones. Even though very low levels of electricity are used, people with pacemakers should not use iontophoretic patches. Another disadvantage of these patches is that they can move only ionic drugs through the skin.

21

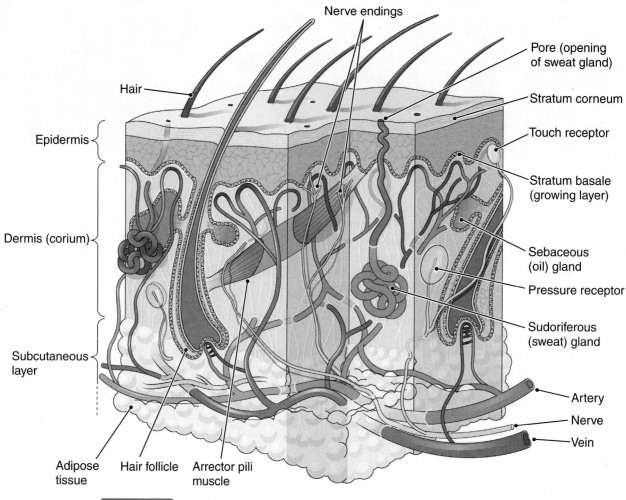

Figure 21-1 **Cross section of the skin.** The skin layers and associated structures are shown.

epidermal layer, the stratum corneum or horny layer, is composed of flat, dead, protective cells that are constantly being shed and replaced. Some of the cells in the epidermis produce **melanin**, a pigment that gives the skin color and protects against sunlight.

The **dermis** is beneath the epidermis. It contains connective tissue, nerves, blood vessels, lymphatics, and sensory receptors. This layer supplies nourishment and support for the skin. The **subcutaneous tissue** beneath the dermis is composed mainly of connective tissue and fat.

Associated Skin Structures

Specialized structures within the skin are part of the integumentary system:

- The **sudoriferous (sweat) glands** act mainly in temperature regulation by releasing a watery fluid that evaporates to cool the body.

- The **sebaceous glands** release an oily fluid, **sebum**, that lubricates the hair and skin and prevents drying.

- **Hair** is widely distributed over the body. Each hair develops within a sheath or **hair follicle** and grows from its base within the skin's deep layers. A small muscle (arrector pili) attached to the follicle raises the hair to produce "goosebumps" when one is frightened or cold. In animals this is a warning sign and a means of insulation.

- **Nails** develop from a growing region at the proximal end (Fig. 21-2). The cuticle, technically named the eponychium (*ep-ō-NIK-ē-um*), is an extension of the epidermis onto the surface of the nail plate. A lighter region distal to the cuticle is called the lunula because it looks like a half moon. Here the underlying skin is thicker and blood does not show as much through the nail.

Hair and nails are composed of nonliving material consisting mainly of keratin. Both function in protection.

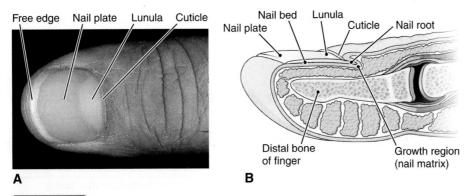

Figure 21-2 **Nail structure.** (*A*) Photograph of a nail, superior view. (*B*) Midsagittal section of a fingertip showing the growth region and tissue surrounding the nail plate.

Terminology | Key Terms

Normal Structure and Function

Term	Definition
cutaneous *kū-TĀ-nē-us*	Pertaining to the skin (from Latin *cutis*, meaning "skin")
derma *DER-ma*	Skin (from Greek)
dermis *DER-mis*	The layer of the skin between the epidermis and the subcutaneous tissue; the true skin or corium
epidermis *ep-i-DER-mis*	The outermost layer of the skin (from *epi-*, meaning "upon or over" and *derm*, meaning "skin")
hair *hār*	A threadlike keratinized outgrowth from the skin (root: *trich/o*)
hair follicle *FOL-i-kel*	The sheath in which a hair develops
integumentary system *in-teg-ū-MEN-ta-rē*	The skin and its associated glands, hair, and nails
keratin *KER-a-tin*	A protein that thickens and toughens the skin and makes up hair and nails (root: *kerat/o*)
melanin *MEL-a-nin*	A dark pigment that gives color to the hair and skin and protects the skin against the sun's radiation (root: *melan/o*)
nail *nāl*	A platelike keratinized outgrowth of the skin that covers the dorsal surface of the terminal phalanges (root: *onych/o*)
sebaceous gland *se-BĀ-shus*	A gland that produces sebum; usually associated with a hair follicle (root: *seb/o*)
sebum *SĒ-bum*	A fatty secretion of the sebaceous glands that lubricates the hair and skin (root: *seb/o*)
skin	The tissue that covers the body; the integument (roots: *derm/o*, *dermat/o*)
subcutaneous tissue *sub-kū-TĀ-nē-us*	The layer of tissue beneath the skin; also called the hypodermis
sudoriferous gland *sū-dor-IF-er-us*	A sweat gland (root: *hidr/o*)

PASSport to Success® Go to the pronunciation glossary on the Student Resources to hear these words pronounced.

21

Roots Pertaining to the Skin

See Table 21-1.

Table 21-1	Roots Pertaining to the Skin		
Root	**Meaning**	**Example**	**Definition of Example**
derm/o, dermat/o	skin	dermabrasion *derm-a-BRĀ-zhun*	surgical procedure used to resurface the skin and remove imperfections
kerat/o	keratin, horny layer of the skin	keratinous *ke-RAT-i-nus*	containing keratin; horny
melan/o	dark, black, melanin	melanosome *MEL-a-nō-sōm*	a small cellular body that produces melanin
hidr/o	sweat, perspiration	anhidrosis *an-hī-DRŌ-sis*	absence of sweating
seb/o	sebum, sebaceous gland	seborrhea *seb-or-Ē-a*	excess flow of sebum (adjective: seborrheic)
trich/o	hair	trichomycosis *trik-ō-mī-KŌ-sis*	fungal infection of the hair
onych/o	nail	onychia *ō-NIK-ē-a*	inflammation of the nail and nail bed (not an -itis ending)

EXERCISE 21-1

Identify and define the roots in the following words:

	Root	**Meaning of Root**
1. hypodermis (*hī-pō-DER-mis*)	_____	_____
2. seborrheic (*seb-ō-RĒ-ik*)	_____	_____
3. hypermelanosis (*hī-per-mel-a-NŌ-sis*)	_____	_____
4. dyskeratosis (*dis-ker-a-TŌ-sis*)	_____	_____
5. hypohidrosis (*hī-pō-hī-DRŌ-sis*)	_____	_____
6. hypertrichosis (*hī-per-tri-KŌ-sis*)	_____	_____
7. eponychium (*ep-ō-NIK-ē-um*)	_____	_____

Fill in the blanks:

8. Dermatopathology (*der-ma-tō-pa-THOL-ō-jē*) is study of diseases of the _____.

9. Keratolysis (*ker-a-TOL-i-sis*) is loosening of the skin's _____.

10. A melanocyte (*MEL-a-nō-sīt*) is a cell that produces _____.

11. Trichoid (*TRIK-oyd*) means resembling a(n) _____.

12. Onychomycosis (*on-i-kō-mī-KŌ-sis*) is a fungal infection of a(n) _____.

13. Hidradenitis (*hī-drad-e-NĪ-tis*) is inflammation of a gland that produces _____.

14. A hypodermic (*hī-pō-DER-mik*) injection is given under the _____.

Write words for the following definitions:

15. loosening or separation of the skin _____

16. a tumor containing melanin _____

17. formation (-genesis) of keratin   _____

18. instrument for cutting the skin   _____

19. study of the hair   _____

20. excess production of sweat   _____

21. softening of a nail   _____

22. study of the skin and skin diseases   _____

Use *-derma* as a suffix meaning "skin" to write words for the following:

23. hardening of the skin   _____

24. presence of pus in the skin   _____

Clinical Aspects of the Skin

Many diseases are manifested by changes in the quality of the skin or by specific lesions. Some types of skin lesions are described and illustrated in Box 21-2 and appear later in photographs of specific skin disorders. The study of the skin and skin diseases is **dermatology**, but careful observation of the skin, hair, and nails should be part of every physical examination. The skin should be examined for color, unusual pigmentation, and

---

Box 21-2   For Your Reference

Types of Skin Lesions

LESION	DESCRIPTION
bulla *BUL-a*	raised, fluid-filled lesion larger than a vesicle (plural: bullae)
fissure *FISH-ūr*	crack or break in the skin
macule *MAK-ūl*	flat, colored spot
nodule *NOD-ūl*	solid, raised lesion larger than a papule; often indicative of systemic disease
papule *PAP-ūl*	small, circular, raised lesion at the surface of the skin
plaque *plak*	superficial, flat, or slightly raised differentiated patch more than 1 cm in diameter
pustule *PUS-tūl*	raised lesion containing pus; often in a hair follicle or sweat pore
ulcer *UL-ser*	lesion resulting from destruction of the skin and perhaps subcutaneous tissue
vesicle *VES-i-kal*	small, fluid-filled, raised lesion; a blister or bleb
wheal *wēl*	smooth, rounded, slightly raised area often associated with itching; seen in urticaria (hives), such as that resulting from allergy

Bulla   Fissure

Macule   Nodule

Papule   Plaque

Pustule   Ulcer

Vesicle   Wheal

21

Nurse Practitioners

A nurse practitioner (NP) is a nurse with an advanced degree, beyond a registered nurse (RN) degree, who provides health care services similar to those of a physician. Most have a master's degree or a doctorate as well as advanced, specialized clinical training. NPs practice in many settings, but most work in collaboration with physicians to help provide individualized care. Their approach focuses not only on treatment of disease but also on disease prevention, patient education, and counseling. Their duties may include routine examinations, testing, diagnosis, treatment, and minor surgeries. They manage a patient's total health care, including treatment of chronic conditions, such as diabetes or high blood pressure. An NP may specialize in an area, including acute care, women's health, oncology, dermatology, and occupational health. A pediatric nurse practitioner can provide most medical services needed by children, referring to physicians when necessary.

NPs are licensed in all states, and in most they are able to dispense and prescribe medications without a physician's co-signature. They may bill insurance agencies for services. NPs can lower health care costs by early intervention and patient education. Their professional organizations include the American Academy of Nurse Practitioners at www.aanp.org and the American College of Nurse Practitioners at www.acnpweb.org.

lesions. It should be palpated to evaluate its texture, temperature, moisture, firmness, and any tenderness. See Box 21-3 on nurse practitioners who, among other health care professionals, observe the skin in diagnosis.

Wounds

Wounds are caused by trauma, as in cases of accidents or attacks, or by surgery and other therapeutic or diagnostic procedures. Wounds may affect not only the injured area but also other body systems. Infection and hemorrhage may complicate wounds, as do **dehiscence**, disruption of the wound layers, and **evisceration**, protrusion of internal organs through the lesion.

As a wound heals, fluid and cells drain from the damaged tissue. This drainage, called **exudate**, may be clear, bloody (sanguinous), or pus-containing (purulent). Tubes may be used to remove exudate from the site of a wound.

 See the animation *Wound Healing* on the Student Resources.

Proper wound healing depends on cleanliness and care of the lesion and also on proper circulation, good general health, and good nutrition. The edges of a deep wound should be joined by sutures, either stitches, or for simple cuts in areas that can be kept dry and immobilized, with a tissue adhesive (glue). Healing is accompanied by scar formation or **cicatrization** (an alternative name for a scar is a cicatrix). Permanent scarring is lessened by appropriate wound care, but some people, especially those of African or Asian descent, may tend to form **keloids** because of excess collagen formation dur-

ing healing (Fig. 21-3). Plastic surgery can often improve keloids and other unsightly scars.

Various types of dressings are used to protect wounded areas and promote healing. Vacuum-assisted closure (VAC) uses negative pressure to close the tissues and begin the healing process. Healing may be promoted by **débridement**, the removal of dead or damaged tissue from a wound. Box 21-4 mentions the origin of the word débridement and gives the meaning of other medical terms taken from French. Débridement may be accomplished by cutting or scrubbing away the dead tissue or by means of enzymes. A thick, dark crust or scab (eschar) may be removed in an **escharotomy**.

Deep wounds may require skin grafting for proper healing. Grafts may be a full-thickness skin graft (FTSG), which consists of the epidermis and dermis, or a split-thickness skin graft (STSG), consisting of the epidermis only. Skin is cut for grafting with a **dermatome**.

Figure 21-3 **Keloid.** Marked overgrowth of scar tissue following earlobe piercing.

Box 21-4	Focus on Words

The French Connection

Many scientific and medical terms are adapted from foreign languages. Most of the roots come from Latin and Greek; others are derived from German or French. Sometimes a foreign word is used "as is." Débridement, removal of dead or damaged tissue from a wound, comes from the French, meaning removal of a restraint, such as the bridle of a harness. Also from French, a contrecoup injury occurs when the head is thrown forward and back, as in a car accident, and the brain is injured by hitting the skull on the side opposite the blow. *Contrecoup* in French means "counterblow." Tic douloureux, a disorder causing pain along the path of the trigeminal nerve in the face, translates literally as "painful spasm." A sound heard while listening to the body with a stethoscope is a bruit, a word in French that literally means "noise." Lavage, which refers to irrigation of a cavity, is a French word meaning "washing."

BURNS

Most burns are caused by hot objects, explosions, or scalding. They may also be caused by electricity, contact with harmful chemicals, or abrasion. Burns are assessed in terms of the depth of damage and the percentage of body surface area (BSA) involved. Depth of tissue destruction is categorized as follows:

1. Superficial partial thickness involves the epidermis and perhaps a portion of the dermis. The tissue is reddened and may blister, as in cases of sunburn.

2. Deep partial thickness involves the epidermis and portions of the dermis. The tissue is blistered and broken and has a weeping surface. Causes include scalding and flash flame.

3. Full thickness involves the full skin and sometimes subcutaneous tissue and underlying tissues as well. The tissue is broken and is dry and pale or charred. These injuries may result in loss of digits or limbs and require skin grafting.

The above classification replaces an older system of ranking burns as first-, second-, and third-degree according to the depth of tissue damage.

The amount of BSA involved in a burn may be estimated by using the **rule of nines**, in which areas of body surface are assigned percentages in multiples of nine (Fig. 21-4). The more accurate Lund and Browder method divides the body into small areas and estimates the proportion of BSA contributed by each.

Infection is a common complication of burns because a major defense against bacterial invasion is damaged. Respiratory complications and shock may also occur.

Treatment of burns includes respiratory care, administration of fluids, wound care, and pain control. Monitoring for cardiovascular complications, infections, and signs of posttraumatic stress are also important.

PRESSURE ULCERS

Pressure ulcers are necrotic skin lesions that appear where the body rests on skin that covers bony projections, such as the sacrum, heel, elbow, ischial bone of the pelvis, or greater trochanter of the femur (see *ulcer*, Box 21-2). The pressure interrupts circulation, leading to thrombosis, ulceration, and tissue death (necrosis). Poor general health, malnutrition, age, obesity, and infection contribute to the development of pressure ulcers.

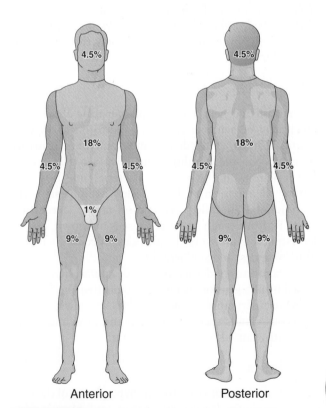

Figure 21-4 **The rule of nines.** Percentage of body surface area (BSA) in the adult is estimated by sectioning the body surface into areas with numerical values related to nine. This method is used to evaluate the extent of skin burns.

Anterior   Posterior

21

Figure 21-5 **Dermatitis.** (*A*) Eczema (atopic dermatitis) on an infant's wrist. (*B*) Contact dermatitis from shoe material. Note several fluid-filled bullae (see Box 21-2).

Pressure ulcer lesions first appear as redness of the skin. If ignored, they may penetrate the skin and underlying muscle, extending even to bone, and may require months to heal.

Pads or mattresses to relieve pressure, regular cleansing and drying of the skin, frequent change in position, and good nutrition help to prevent pressure ulcers. Other terms for pressure ulcers are *decubitus ulcer* and *bedsore*. Both of these terms refer to lying down in bed, although pressure ulcers may appear in anyone with limited movement, not only those who are confined to bed.

Dermatitis

Dermatitis is a general term for inflammation of the skin, which may be acute or chronic. Mild forms show **erythema** (redness) and edema, and sometimes **pruritus** (itching), but the condition may worsen to include deeper lesions and secondary bacterial infections. A chronic allergic form of this disorder that appears early in childhood is called **eczema** or **atopic dermatitis** (Fig. 21-5). Although its exact cause is unknown, atopic dermatitis is made worse by allergies, infection, temperature extremes, and skin irritants.

Other forms of dermatitis include contact dermatitis, caused by allergens or chemical irritants (see Fig. 21-5B); seborrheic dermatitis, which involves areas with many sebaceous glands such as the scalp and face; and stasis dermatitis, caused by poor circulation.

Psoriasis

Psoriasis is a chronic overgrowth (hyperplasia) of the epidermis, producing large, erythematous (red) plaques with silvery scales (Fig. 21-6; see also, *plaques*, Box 21-2). The cause is unknown, but there is sometimes a hereditary pattern, and autoimmunity may be involved.

Dermatologists treat psoriasis in the following ways depending on severity:

1. topical agents, including corticosteroids, immuno-suppressants, vitamins A and D
2. phototherapy—exposure to ultraviolet B (UVB) light; administration of the drug psoralen (P) to increase skin sensitivity to light followed by exposure to ultraviolet A (UVA) light; laser treatment
3. systemic suppression of the immune system.

Autoimmune Disorders

The diseases discussed below are caused, at least in part, by autoimmune reactions. They are diagnosed by biopsy of lesions and by antibody studies.

Figure 21-6 **Psoriasis.** Plaques with scales seen at the front of the knee (see *plaque*, Box 21-2).

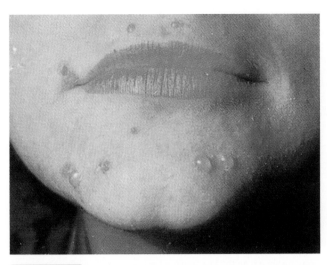

Figure 21-7 **Pemphigus.** Vesicles are shown on the chin (see *vesicle*, Box 21-2).

Pemphigus is characterized by the formation of bullae (blisters) in the skin and mucous membranes caused by a separation of epidermal cells from underlying layers (Fig. 21-7; see also, *bullae*, Box 21-2). Rupture of these lesions leaves deeper skin areas unprotected from infection and fluid loss, much as in cases of burns. The cause is an autoimmune reaction to epithelial cells. Pemphigus is fatal unless treated by suppressing the immune system.

Lupus erythematosus (LE) is a chronic inflammatory autoimmune disease of connective tissue. The more widespread form of the disease, systemic lupus erythematosus (SLE), involves the skin and other organs. SLE is more prevalent in women than in men and has a higher incidence among Asians and blacks than in other populations.

The discoid form (DLE) involves only the skin. It is seen as rough, raised, erythematous papules that are worsened by exposure to the ultraviolet radiation in sunlight (Fig. 21-8). Lupus skin lesions are confined to the face and scalp and may form a typical butterfly-shaped rash across the nose and cheeks.

Scleroderma is a disease of unknown cause that involves thickening and tightening of the skin. There is gradual fibrosis of the dermis because of collagen overproduction. Sweat glands and hair follicles are also involved. A very early sign of scleroderma is Raynaud disease, in which blood vessels in the fingers and toes constrict in the cold, causing numbness, pain, coldness, and tingling. Skin symptoms first appear on the forearms and around the mouth. Internal organs become involved in a diffuse form of scleroderma called progressive systemic sclerosis (PSS).

Skin Cancer

Skin cancer is the most common type of human cancer. Its incidence has been increasing in recent years, mainly because of the mutation-causing effects of sunlight's ultraviolet rays. **Squamous cell carcinoma** and **basal cell carcinoma** are both cancers of epithelial cells. Both appear in areas exposed to sunlight, such as the face and hands. Basal cell carcinoma constitutes more than 75% of all skin cancers. It usually appears as a smooth, pearly papule (Fig. 21-9; see also, *papules*, Box 21-2). Because these cancers are easily seen and do not metastasize, the cure rate after excision is greater than 95%.

Squamous cell carcinoma appears as a painless, firm, red nodule or plaque that may develop surface scales, ulceration, or crusting (Fig. 21-10; see also Box 21-2). This cancer may invade underlying tissue but tends not to metastasize. It is treated by surgical removal and sometimes with x-irradiation or chemotherapy.

Malignant melanoma results from an overgrowth of melanocytes, the pigment-producing cells in the epidermis. It is the most dangerous form of skin cancer because of its tendency to metastasize. This cancer appears as a lesion that is variable in color with an

Figure 21-8 **Discoid (cutaneous) lupus erythematosus.** Erythematous papules and plaques in a typical sun-exposed distribution on the chest.

Figure 21-9 **Basal cell carcinoma.** An initial translucent nodule has spread, leaving a depressed center and a firm, elevated border (see *nodule*, Box 21-2).

21

Figure 21-10 **Squamous cell carcinoma.** Lesions are shown on the face and the back of the hand, sun-exposed areas that are commonly affected.

A   B   C

Figure 21-11 **Malignant melanoma.** Several characteristics are shown. (*A*) Asymmetry. (*B*) Irregular borders. (*C*) Variation in color, a diameter greater than 6 mm, and elevation.

irregular border (Fig. 21-11). It may spread superficially for up to 1 or 2 years before it begins to invade the deeper skin tissues and to metastasize through blood and lymph. The prognosis for cure is good if the lesion is recognized and removed surgically before it enters this invasive stage.

Kaposi sarcoma, once considered rare, is now seen frequently in association with AIDS. It usually appears as distinct brownish areas on the legs. These plaques become raised and firm as the tumor progresses. In those with weakened immune systems, such as patients with AIDS, the cancer can metastasize.

Terminology	Key Terms
atopic dermatitis *a-TOP-ik der-ma-TĪ-tis*	Hereditary, allergic, chronic skin inflammation with pruritus (itching); eczema
basal cell carcinoma *BĀ-sal*	An epithelial tumor that rarely metastasizes and has a high cure rate with surgical removal
cicatrization *sik-a-tri-ZĀ-shun*	The process of scar formation; a scar is a cicatrix (*SIK-a-triks*)
débridement *da-brē-DMON*	Removal of dead or damaged tissue, as from a wound
dehiscence *dē-HIS-ens*	Splitting or bursting, as when the layers of a wound separate

(continued)

Terminology   Key Terms (continued)

dermatitis *der-ma-TĪ-tis*	Inflammation of the skin, often associated with redness and itching; may be caused by allergy, irritants (contact dermatitis), or a variety of diseases
dermatology *der-ma-TOL-ō-jē*	Study of the skin and diseases of the skin
dermatome *DER-ma-tōm*	Instrument for cutting thin skin sections for grafting
eczema *EK-zē-ma*	A general term for skin inflammation with redness, lesions, and itching; atopic dermatitis
erythema *er-i-THĒ-ma*	Diffuse redness of the skin
escharotomy *es-kar-OT-ō-mē*	Removal of scab tissue (eschar) resulting from burns or other skin injuries
evisceration *ē-vis-er-Ā-shun*	Protrusion of internal organs (viscera) through an opening, as through a wound
exudate *EKS-ū-dāt*	Material, which may include fluid, cells, pus, or blood, that escapes from damaged tissue
Kaposi sarcoma *KAP-ō-sē*	Cancerous lesion of the skin and other tissues seen most often in patients with AIDS
keloid *KĒ-loyd*	A raised, thickened scar caused by tissue overgrowth during scar formation
lupus erythematosus (LE) *LŪ-pus er-i-thē-ma-TŌ-sis*	A chronic, inflammatory, autoimmune disease of connective tissue that often involves the skin; types include the more widespread systemic lupus erythematosus (SLE) and a discoid form (DLE) that involves only the skin
malignant melanoma	A metastasizing pigmented skin tumor
pemphigus *PEM-fi-gus*	An autoimmune disease of the skin characterized by sudden, intermittent formation of bullae (blisters); may be fatal if untreated
pressure ulcer	An ulcer caused by pressure to an area of the body, as from a bed or chair; decubitus (*dē-KŪ-bi-tus*) ulcer, bedsore, pressure sore
pruritus *prū-RĪ-tus*	Severe itching
psoriasis *so-RĪ-a-sis*	A chronic hereditary dermatitis with red lesions covered by silvery scales
rule of nines	A method for estimating the extent of body surface area involved in a burn by assigning percentages in multiples of nine to various body regions
scleroderma *sklēr-ō-DER-ma*	A chronic disease that is characterized by thickening and tightening of the skin and that often involves internal organs in a form called progressive systemic sclerosis (PSS)
squamous cell carcinoma	An epidermal cancer that may invade deeper tissues but tends not to metastasize

 PASSport to Success® Go to the pronunciation glossary on the Student Resources to hear these words pronounced.

21

Terminology ⟩ Supplementary Terms

Symptoms and Conditions

acne *AK-nē*	An inflammatory disease of the sebaceous glands and hair follicles usually associated with excess sebum secretion; acne vulgaris
actinic *ak-TIN-ik*	Pertaining to the effects of radiant energy, such as sunlight, ultraviolet light, and x-rays
albinism *AL-bin-izm*	A hereditary lack of pigment in the skin, hair, and eyes
alopecia *al-ō-PĒ-shē-a*	Absence or loss of hair; baldness
Beau lines *bō*	White lines across the fingernails; usually a sign of systemic disease or injury (Fig. 21-12)
bromhidrosis *brō-mi-DRŌ-sis*	Sweat that has a foul odor because of bacterial decomposition; also spelled bromidrosis
carbuncle *CAR-bung-kil*	A localized infection of the skin and subcutaneous tissue, usually caused by staphylococcus, and associated with pain and discharge of pus
comedo *KOM-e-dō*	A plug of sebum, often containing bacteria, in a hair follicle; a blackhead (plural: comedones)
dermatophytosis *der-ma-tō-fi-TŌ-sis*	Fungal infection of the skin, especially between the toes; athlete's foot (root *phyt/o* means "plant")
diaphoresis *dī-a-fō-RĒ-sis*	Profuse sweating
dyskeratosis *dis-ker-a-TŌ-sis*	Any abnormality in keratin formation in epithelial cells
ecchymosis *ek-i-MŌ-sis*	A collection of blood under the skin caused by leakage from small vessels
erysipelas *er-i-SIP-e-las*	An acute infectious skin disease with localized redness and swelling and systemic symptoms
erythema nodosum *nō-DŌ-sum*	Inflammation of subcutaneous tissues resulting in tender, erythematous nodules; may be an abnormal immune response to a systemic disease, an infection, or a drug
exanthem *eks-AN-them*	Any cutaneous eruption that accompanies a disease, such as measles; a rash
excoriation *eks-kō-rē-Ā-shun*	Lesion caused by scratching or abrasion (Fig. 21-13)

(continued)

Figure 21-12 **Beau lines.** These transverse depressions in the nails are associated with acute severe illness.

Figure 21-13 **Skin lesions associated with dermatitis.** (*A*) Excoriation. (*B*) Lichenification.

Terminology **Supplementary Terms** (continued)	
folliculitis *fō-lik-ū-LĪ-tis*	Inflammation of a hair follicle
furuncle *FŪ-rung-kil*	A painful skin nodule caused by staphylococci that enter through a hair follicle; a boil
hemangioma *hē-man-jē-Ō-ma*	A benign tumor of blood vessels; in the skin, called birthmarks or port wine stains
herpes simplex *HER-pēz SIM-pleks*	A group of acute infections caused by herpes simplex virus. Type I herpes simplex virus produces fluid-filled vesicles, usually on the lips, after fever, sun exposure, injury, or stress; cold sore, fever blister. Type II infections usually involve the genital organs
hirsutism *HIR-sū-tizm*	Excessive growth of hair
ichthyosis *ik-thē-Ō-sis*	A dry, scaly condition of the skin (from the root *ichthy/o*, meaning "fish")
impetigo *im-pe-TĪ-gō*	A bacterial skin infection with pustules that rupture and form crusts; most commonly seen in children, usually on the face (Fig. 21-14; see also, *pustules*, Box 21-2)
keratosis *ker-a-TŌ-sis*	Any skin condition marked by thickened or horny growth. Seborrheic keratosis is a benign tumor, yellow or light brown in color, that appears in the elderly. Actinic keratosis is caused by exposure to sunlight and may lead to squamous cell carcinoma
lichenification *lī-ken-i-fi-KĀ-shun*	Thickened marks caused by chronic rubbing, as seen in atopic dermatitis (a lichen is a flat, branching type of plant that grows on rocks and bark) (see Fig. 21-13)
mycosis fungoides *mī-KŌ-sis fun-GOY-dēz*	A rare malignant disease that originates in the skin and involves the internal organs and lymph nodes. There are large, painful, ulcerating tumors
nevus *NĒ-vus*	A defined discoloration of the skin; a congenital vascular skin tumor; a mole, birthmark
paronychia *par-ō-NIK-ē-a*	Infection around a nail (Fig. 21-15). Caused by bacteria or fungi, and may affect multiple nails
pediculosis *pe-dik-ū-LŌ-sis*	Infestation with lice
petechiae *pē-TĒ-kē-e*	Flat, pinpoint, purplish-red spots caused by bleeding within the skin or mucous membrane (singular: petechia)
photosensitization *fō-tō-sen-si-ti-ZĀ-shun*	Sensitization of the skin to light, usually from the action of drugs, plant products, or other substances

(continued)

Figure 21-14 **Impetigo.** This bacterial skin infection, seen here on the nostril, causes pustules that rupture and form crusts (see *pustule*, Box 21-2).

Figure 21-15 **Paronychia.** Infection and inflammation of the proximal and lateral nail folds is shown.

Terminology   Supplementary Terms (continued)

purpura PUR-pū-ra	A condition characterized by hemorrhages into the skin and other tissues
rosacea rō-ZĀ-shē-a	A condition of unknown cause involving redness of the skin, pustules, and overactivity of sebaceous glands, mainly on the face
scabies SKĀ-bēz	A highly contagious skin disease caused by a mite
senile lentigines len-TIJ-i-nēz	Brown macules that appear on sun-exposed skin in adults; liver spots
shingles	An acute eruption of vesicles along the path of a nerve; herpes zoster (HER-pēz ZOS-ter); caused by the same virus that causes chickenpox
tinea TIN-ē-a	A fungal skin infection; ringworm (Fig. 21-16)
tinea versicolor VER-si-kol-or	Superficial chronic fungal infection that causes varied skin pigmentation
urticaria ur-ti-KĀ-rē-a	A skin reaction marked by temporary, smooth, raised areas (wheals) associated with itching; hives (Fig. 21-17; see also, wheals, Box 21-2)
venous stasis ulcer	Ulcer caused by venous insufficiency and stasis of venous blood; usually forms near the ankle (Fig. 21-18; see also, ulcer, Box 21-2)
verruca ver-RŪ-ka	An epidermal tumor; a wart
vitiligo vit-i-LĪ-gō	Patchy disappearance of pigment in the skin; leukoderma (Fig. 21-19)
xeroderma pigmentosum zē-rō-DER-ma pig-men-TŌ-sum	A fatal hereditary disease that begins in childhood with skin discolorations and ulcers and muscle atrophy. There is increased sensitivity to the sun and increased susceptibility to cancer

Diagnosis and Treatment

aloe A-lō	A plant (Aloe vera), the leaves of which contain a gel that is used in treatment of burns and minor skin irritations

(continued)

Figure 21-16 **Tinea corporis (ringworm).** This fungal infection is shown on the face.

Figure 21-17 **Urticaria (hives).** Wheals associated with drug allergy are shown in an infant (see wheal, Box 21-2).

Terminology | Supplementary Terms (continued)

antipruritic *an-ti-prū-RIT-ik*	Agent that prevents or relieves itching
cautery *KAW-ter-ē*	Destruction of tissue by physical or chemical means; cauterization; also the instrument or chemical used for this purpose
dermabrasion *DERM-a-brā-zhun*	A plastic surgical procedure for removing scars or birthmarks by chemical or mechanical destruction of epidermal tissue
dermatoplasty *DER-ma-tō-plas-tē*	Transplantation of human skin; skin grafting
diascopy *dī-AS-kō-pē*	Examination of skin lesions by pressing a glass plate against the skin
fulguration *ful-gū-RĀ-shun*	Destruction of tissue by high-frequency electric sparks
skin turgor *TUR-gor*	Resistance of the skin to deformation. Evidenced by the ability of the skin to return to position when pinched. Skin turgor is a measure of the skin's elasticity and state of hydration. It typically declines with age and may also be a sign of poor nutrition
Wood lamp	An ultraviolet light used to diagnose fungal infections

PASSport to Success®   Go to the pronunciation glossary on the Student Resources to hear these words pronounced.

Figure 21-18 **Venous stasis ulcer.** Lesion on the ankle caused by venous insufficiency and blood stasis (see *ulcer*, Box 21-2).

Figure 21-19 **Vitiligo.** Depigmented macules appear on the skin and may merge into large areas that lack melanin (see *macule*, Box 21-2). The brown pigment seen in the illustration is the person's normal skin color; the pale areas are caused by vitiligo.

21

Terminology   Abbreviations

BSA	Body surface area		SLE	Systemic lupus erythematosus
DLE	Discoid lupus erythematosus		SPF	Sun protection factor
FTSG	Full-thickness skin graft		STSG	Split-thickness skin graft
LE	Lupus erythematosus		UV	Ultraviolet
PSS	Progressive systemic sclerosis		UVA	Ultraviolet A
PUVA	Psoralen ultraviolet A		UVB	Ultraviolet B
SCLE	Subacute cutaneous lupus erythematosus		VAC	Vacuum-assisted closure

Chapter Review

LABELING EXERCISE

Cross Section of the Skin > Write the name of each numbered part on the corresponding line of the answer sheet.

Adipose tissue
Arrector pili muscle
Artery
Dermis (corium)
Epidermis
Hair
Hair follicle
Nerve
Nerve endings

Pore (opening of sweat gland)
Pressure receptor
Sebaceous (oil) gland
Stratum basale (growing layer)
Stratum corneum
Subcutaneous layer
Sudoriferous (sweat) gland
Touch receptor
Vein

1. _____
2. _____
3. _____
4. _____
5. _____
6. _____
7. _____
8. _____
9. _____
10. _____
11. _____
12. _____
13. _____
14. _____
15. _____
16. _____
17. _____
18. _____

TERMINOLOGY

Matching > Multiple choice. Select the best answer and write the letter of your choice to the left of each number:

_____	**1.** follicle	**a.** thickened layer of the epidermis
_____	**2.** stratum corneum	**b.** growing layer of the epidermis
_____	**3.** sebum	**c.** subcutaneous layer
_____	**4.** hypodermis	**d.** sheath that contains a hair
_____	**5.** stratum basale	**e.** oily skin secretion

_____	**6.** débridement	**a.** scar
_____	**7.** pruritus	**b.** atopic dermatitis
_____	**8.** eczema	**c.** removal of dead tissue
_____	**9.** pressure ulcer	**d.** severe itching
_____	**10.** cicatrix	**e.** bedsore

Supplementary Terms

_____	**11.** diaphoresis	**a.** profuse sweating
_____	**12.** nevus	**b.** pertaining to radiant energy
_____	**13.** actinic	**c.** mole or birthmark
_____	**14.** alopecia	**d.** blackhead
_____	**15.** comedo	**e.** baldness

_____	**16.** rosacea	**a.** sweat with a foul odor
_____	**17.** tinea	**b.** infection around a nail
_____	**18.** bromhidrosis	**c.** lack of skin pigmentation
_____	**19.** albinism	**d.** fungal skin infection
_____	**20.** paronychia	**e.** condition causing redness and pustules, mainly on the face

Fill in the blanks:

21. The adjective *cutaneous* refers to the _____.

22. A sudoriferous gland produces _____.

23. The main pigment in skin is _____.

24. The oil-producing glands of the skin are the _____.

25. The protein that thickens the skin and makes up hair and nails is _____.

Define the following words:

26. hypermelanosis (*hī-per-mel a-NŌ-sis*) _____

27. percutaneous (*per-kū-TĀ-nē-us*) _____

28. keratogenic (*ker-a-tō-JEN-ik*) _____

29. seborrhea (*seb-or-Ē-a*) _____

30. pachyderma (*pak-ē-DER-ma*) _____

31. onychia (*ō-NIK-ē-a*) _____

32. xeroderma (*zē-rō-DER-ma*) _____

33. dyskeratosis (*dis-ker-a-TŌ-sis*) _____

21

Chapter Review (continued)

Write words for the following definitions:

34. pertaining to discharge of sebum   _____

35. cell that produces melanin   _____

36. hardening of the skin   _____

37. tumor containing melanin   _____

38. excess production of keratin   _____

39. instrument for cutting the skin   _____

Use the word *hidrosis* (sweating) as an ending for words with the following meanings:

40. absence of sweating   _____

41. excess sweating   _____

42. excretion of colored (chrom/o) sweat   _____

True–False > Examine the following statements. If the statement is true, write T in the first blank. If the statement is false, write F in the first blank and correct the statement by replacing the underlined word in the second blank.

43. The skin and its associated structures
make up the integumentary system.   _____   _____

44. The stratum basale is the outermost layer of the epidermis.   _____   _____

45. The root *trich/o* refers to hair.   _____   _____

46. The dermis is between the epidermis and the
subcutaneous layer.   _____   _____

47. New epidermal cells arise from the stratum corneum.   _____   _____

48. Hirsutism is excess growth of nails.   _____   _____

Word Building > Write a word for the following definitions using the word parts provided.

-lysis   onych/o   -sis   myc/o   path/o   dermat/o   -y   log/o   -oid   trich/o

49. resembling a hair   _____

50. fungal infection of a nail   _____

51. loosening or separation of the skin   _____

52. study of hair   _____

53. loosening of a nail   _____

54. like or resembling skin   _____

55. any disease of a nail   _____

56. fungal infection of the hair   _____

57. any disease of the skin   _____

58. study and treatment of the skin   _____

Chapter Review *(continued)*

Eliminations > In each of the sets below, underline the word that does not fit in with the rest and explain the reason for your choice:

59. nodule — vesicle — keloid — macule — papule

_____

60. impetigo — escharotomy — psoriasis — dermatitis — pemphigus

_____

61. SLE — PSS — SCLE — BSA — DLE

_____

Word Analysis > Define the following words, and give the meaning of the word parts in each. Use a dictionary if necessary.

62. dermatophytosis (*der-ma-tō-fĭ-TŌ-sis*) _____

    a. dermat/o _____

    b. phyt/o _____

    c. -sis _____

63. hidradenoma (*hī-drad-e-NŌ-ma*) _____

    a. hidr/o _____

    b. aden/o _____

    c. -oma _____

64. onychocryptosis (*on-i-kō-krip-TŌ-sis*) _____

    a. onych/o _____

    b. crypt/o _____

    c. -sis _____

65. achromotrichia (*a-krō-mō-TRIK-ē-a*) _____

    a. a- _____

    b. chrom/o _____

    c. trich/o _____

    d. -ia _____

PASSport to **Success**® Go to the word exercises on the Student Resources for additional review exercises.

21

Case Studies

➤ Case Study 21-1: Basal Cell Carcinoma

K.B., a 32-year-old fitness instructor, had noticed a "tiny hard lump" at the base of her left nostril while cleansing her face. The lesion had been present for about 2 months when she consulted a dermatologist. She had recently moved north from Florida, where she had worked as a lifeguard. She thought the lump might have been triggered by the regular tanning salon sessions she had used to retain her tan because it did not resemble the acne pustules, blackheads, or resulting scars of her adolescent years. Although dermabrasion had removed the obvious acne scars and left several areas of dense skin, this lump was brown pigmented and different. K.B. was afraid it might be a malignant melanoma. On examination, the dermatologist noted a small pearly-white nodule at the lower portion of the left ala (outer flared portion of the nostril). There were no other lesions on her face or neck.

A plastic surgeon excised the lesion and was able to reapproximate the wound edges without a full-thickness skin graft. The pathology report identified the lesion as a basal cell carcinoma with clean margins of normal skin and subcutaneous tissue and stated that the entire lesion had been excised. K.B. was advised to wear SPF 30 sun protection on her face at all times and to avoid excessive sun exposure and tanning salons.

➤ Case Study 21-2: Cutaneous Lymphoma

L.C., a 52-year-old female research chemist, has had a history of T cell lymphoma for 8 years. She was initially treated with systemic chemotherapy with methotrexate, until she contracted stomatitis. Continued therapy with topical chemotherapeutic agents brought measurable improvement. She also had a history of hidradenitis.

A recent physical examination showed diffuse erythroderma with scaling and hyperkeratosis, plus alopecia. She had painful leukoplakia and ulcerations of the mouth and tongue. L.C. was hospitalized and given two courses of topical chemotherapy. She was referred to Dental Medicine for treatment of the oral lesions and was discharged in stable condition with an appointment for follow-up in 4 weeks. Her discharge medications included the application of 2% hydrocortisone ointment to the affected lesions q hs, Keralyt gel bid for the hyperkeratosis, and Dyclone and Benadryl for her mouth ulcers prn.

➤ Case Study 21-3: Pressure Ulcer

L.N., an elderly woman in failing health, had recently moved in with her daughter after her hospitalization for a stroke. The daughter reported to the home care nurse that her mother had minimal appetite and was confused and disoriented and that a blister had developed on her lower back since she had been confined to bed. The nurse noted that L.N. had lost weight since her last visit and that her skin was dry, with poor skin turgor. She was wearing an "adult diaper," which was wet. After examining L.N.'s sacrum, the nurse noted a nickel-sized open area, 2 cm in diameter and 1 cm in depth (stage II pressure ulcer), with a 0.5-cm reddened surrounding area with no drainage. L.N. moaned when the nurse palpated the lesion. The nurse also noted reddened areas on L.N.'s elbows and heels.

The nurse provided L.N.'s daughter with instructions for proper skin care, incontinence management, enhanced nutrition, and frequent repositioning to prevent pressure ischemia to the prominent body areas. However, 6 months later, L.N.'s pressure ulcer had deteriorated to class III. She was hospitalized under the care of a plastic surgeon and wound ostomy care nurse. Surgery was scheduled to débride the sacral wound and close it with a full-thickness skin graft taken from her thigh. L.N. was discharged 8 days later to a long-term care facility with orders for an alternating pressure mattress, position change every 2 hours, supplemental nutrition, and meticulous wound care.

CASE STUDY QUESTIONS

Multiple choice. Select the best answer and write the letter of your choice to the left of each number:

_____ 1. K.B.'s basal cell carcinoma may have been caused by chronic exposure to the sun and use of an ultraviolet tanning bed. The scientific explanation for this is the:
   a. autoimmune response
   b. actinic effect
   c. allergic reaction
   d. sun block tanning lotion theory
   e. dermatophytosis

_____ 2. The characteristic pimples of adolescent acne are whiteheads and blackheads. The medical terms for these lesions are:
   a. vesicles and lymphotomes
   b. pustules and blisters
   c. pustules and comedones
   d. vitiligo and macules
   e. furuncles and sebaceous cysts

_____ 3. Which skin cancer is an overgrowth of pigment-producing epidermal cells?
   a. basal cell carcinoma
   b. Kaposi sarcoma
   c. cutaneous lymphoma
   d. melanoma
   e. erythema nodosum

_____ 4. Basal cell carcinoma involves:
   a. subcutaneous tissue
   b. hair follicles
   c. connective tissue
   d. adipose tissue
   e. epithelial cells

(continued)

Case Studies (continued)

____ 5. Hidradenitis is inflammation of a:
   a. sweat gland
   b. salivary gland
   c. sebaceous gland
   d. ceruminous gland
   e. meibomian gland

____ 6. Leukoplakia is:
   a. baldness
   b. ulceration
   c. formation of white patches in the mouth
   d. formation of yellow patches on the skin
   e. formation of scales on the skin

____ 7. Hydrocortisone is a(n):
   a. vitamin
   b. steroid
   c. analgesic
   d. lubricant
   e. diuretic

____ 8. An example of a topical drug is a:
   a. systemic chemotherapeutic agent
   b. drug derived from rain forest plants
   c. subdermal allergy test antigens
   d. skin ointment
   e. Benadryl capsule, 25 mg

____ 9. Stomatitis, a common side effect of systemic chemotherapy, is an inflammatory condition of the:
   a. mouth
   b. colostomy
   c. stomach
   d. teeth and hair
   e. nails

____10. Skin turgor is an indicator of:
   a. elasticity
   b. hydration
   c. aging
   d. nutrition
   e. all of the above

____11. Another name for a pressure ulcer is a:
   a. shearing force
   b. bedsore
   c. decubitus ulcer
   d. a and b
   e. b and c

____12. An FTSG is usually harvested (taken) from another body area with a scalpel, whereas an STSG is harvested with an instrument called a(n) _____, which can cut a thinner graft.
   a. tissue slicer
   b. Keralyt
   c. erythroderm
   d. dermatome
   e. débridement

Write terms from the case studies with the following meanings:

13. skin sanding procedure
_____

14. a solid raised lesion larger than a papule
_____

15. physician who cares for patients with skin diseases
_____

16. connective tissue and fat layer beneath the dermis
_____

17. diffuse redness of the skin
_____

18. increased production of keratin in the skin
_____

19. removal of dead or damaged skin
_____

20. reduced blood flow to tissue
_____

Abbreviations. Define the following abbreviations:

21. FTSG _____
22. STSG _____
23. SPF _____
24. hs _____
25. bid _____

Appendices

Commonly Used Symbols

Appendix 1	Commonly Used Symbols	
Symbol	Meaning	Chapter
1°	primary	7
2°	secondary (to)	7
Δ	change (Greek delta)	7
Ⓛ	left	7
Ⓡ	right	7
↑	increase(d)	7
↓	decrease(d)	7
♂	male	7
♀	female	7
°	degree	7
>	greater than	7
<	less than	7
∧	above	7
∨	below	7
=	equal to	7
≠	not equal to	7
±	doubtful, slight	7
~	approximately	7
×	times	7
#	number, pound	7

Abbreviations and Their Meanings

Appendix 2	Abbreviations and Their Meanings

Abbreviations	Meaning	Chapter	Abbreviations	Meaning	Chapter
ā	before	8	AI	artificial insemination; aromatase inhibitor	15
A, Acc	accommodation	18			
āā	of each	8	AIDS	acquired immunodeficiency syndrome	10, 14
A1c	glycated hemoglobin	16	AK	above the knee	19
Ab	antibody	10	ALL	acute lymphoblastic (lymphocytic) leukemia	10
AB	abortion	15			
ABC	aspiration biopsy cytology	7	ALS	amyotrophic lateral sclerosis	17, 20
ABG(s)	arterial blood gas(es)	11			
ABR	auditory brainstem response	18	AMA	against medical advice	7
			AMB	ambulatory	7
ac	before meals	8	AMD	age-related macular degeneration	18
AC	air conduction	18			
ACE	angiotensin-converting enzyme	9	AMI	acute myocardial infarction	9
			AML	acute myeloblastic (myelogenous) leukemia	10
ACh	acetylcholine	17, 20			
ACL	anterior cruciate ligament	19	ANS	autonomic nervous system	17
ACTH	adrenocorticotropic hormone	16	AP	anteroposterior	7
			APAP	acetaminophen	8
ad lib	as desired	8	APC	atrial premature complex	9
AD	Alzheimer disease; right ear	17, 18	APTT	activated partial thromboplastin time	10
ADH	antidiuretic hormone	13	aq	water, aqueous	8
ADHD	attention-deficit/hyperactivity disorder	17	AR	aortic regurgitation	9
			ARB	angiotensin receptor blocker	9
ADL	activities of daily living	7			
AE	above the elbow	19	ARC	abnormal retinal correspondence	18
AED	automated external defibrillator	9	ARDS	acute respiratory distress syndrome	11
AF	atrial fibrillation	9			
AFB	acid-fast bacillus	11	ARF	acute respiratory failure	11
AFP	alpha-fetoprotein	7, 15	ARF	acute renal failure	13
Ag	antigen	10	ART	assisted reproductive technology	15
AGA	appropriate for gestational age	15	ASA	acetylsalicylic acid (aspirin)	8

(continued)

Appendix 2   Abbreviations and Their Meanings (continued)

Abbreviations	Meaning	Chapter	Abbreviations	Meaning	Chapter
As, Ast	astigmatism	18	C-section	cesarean section	15
AS	atrial stenosis; arteriosclerosis; left ear	9, 18	CA	cancer	6
ASCVD	arteriosclerotic cardiovascular disease	9	CABG	coronary artery bypass graft	9
ASD	atrial septal defect	9	CAD	coronary artery disease	9
ASF	anterior spinal fusion	19	CAM	complementary and alternative medicine	7
ASHD	arteriosclerotic heart disease	9	cap	capsule	8
ASHP	American Society of Health System Pharmacists	8	CAPD	continuous ambulatory peritoneal dialysis	13
AT	atrial tachycardia	9	CBC	complete blood count	10
ATN	acute tubular necrosis	13	CBD	common bile duct	12
AV	atrioventricular	9	CBF	cerebral blood flow	17
BAEP	brainstem auditory evoked potentials	17, 18	CBR	complete bed rest	7
BBB	bundle branch block	9	cc	with correction	18
BC	bone conduction	18	CC	chief complaint	7
BCG	bacille Calmette–Guérin (tuberculosis vaccine)	11	CCPD	continuous cyclic peritoneal dialysis	13
BE	barium enema; below the elbow	12; 19	CCU	coronary care unit, cardiac care unit	9
bid	twice per day	8	CF	cystic fibrosis	11
BK	below the knee	19	CFS	chronic fatigue syndrome	20
BM	bowel movement	12	CHD	coronary heart disease	9
BMD	bone mineral density	19	CHF	congestive heart failure	9
BNO	bladder neck obstruction	14	Ci	Curie	7
BP	blood pressure	7, 9	CIN	cervical intraepithelial neoplasia	15
BPH	benign prostatic hyperplasia (hypertrophy)	14	CIS	carcinoma in situ	6
bpm	beats per minute	7, 9	CJD	Creutzfeldt–Jakob disease	17
BRCA1	breast cancer gene 1	15	CK	creatine kinase	20
BRCA2	breast cancer gene 2	15	CK-MB	creatine kinase MB	9
BRP	bathroom privileges	7	CLL	chronic lymphocytic leukemia	10
BS	bowel sounds; breath sounds; blood sugar	7, 11, 16	cm	centimeter	Appendix 8
BSA	body surface area	21	CMG	cystometrography, cystometrogram	13
BSE	breast self-examination	15	CML	chronic myelogenous leukemia	10
BSO	bilateral salpingo-oophorectomy	15	CNS	central nervous system	17
BT	bleeding time	10	c/o	complains of	7
BUN	blood urea nitrogen	13	Co	coccyx; coccygeal	19
BV	bacterial vaginosis	15	CO_2	carbon dioxide	11
bx	biopsy	7	COLD	chronic obstructive lung disease	11
c̄	with	8	COPD	chronic obstructive pulmonary disease	11
C	Celsius (centigrade); compliance; cervical vertebra	7, 11, 19	CP	cerebral palsy	17

Abbreviations	Meaning	Chapter	Abbreviations	Meaning	Chapter
CPAP	continuous positive airway pressure	11	DRE	digital rectal examination	14
CPD	cephalopelvic disproportion	15	DS	double strength	8
C(P)K	creatine (phospho) kinase	20	DSM	*Diagnostic and Statistical Manual of Mental Disorders*	17
CPR	cardiopulmonary resuscitation	9	DTR	deep tendon reflex(es)	17
CRF	chronic renal failure	13	DUB	dysfunctional uterine bleeding	15
crit	hematocrit	10	DVT	deep vein thrombosis	9
CRP	C-reactive protein	9	Dx	diagnosis	7
C&S	culture and sensitivity	7	EBL	estimated blood loss	7
CSF	cerebrospinal fluid	17	EBV	Epstein–Barr virus	10
CSII	continuous subcutaneous insulin infusion	16	ECG (EKG)	electrocardiogram, electrocardiography	9
CT	computed tomography	7	ECMO	extracorporeal membrane oxygenation	15
CTA	computed tomography angiography	9	ED	erectile dysfunction	14
CTS	carpal tunnel syndrome	20	EDC	estimated date of confinement	15
CVA	cerebrovascular accident	9, 17	EEG	electroencephalogram; electroencephalograph(y)	17
CVD	cardiovascular disease; cerebrovascular disease	9, 17	ELISA	enzyme-linked immunosorbent assay	10
CVI	chronic venous insufficiency	9	elix	elixir	8
CVP	central venous pressure	9	EM	emmetropia	18
CVS	chorionic villus sampling	15	EMG	electromyography, electromyogram	20
CXR	chest x-ray	11	ENG	electronystagmography	18
D&C	dilatation and curettage	15	ENT	ear(s), nose, and throat	18
dB	decibel	18	EOM	extraocular movement, muscles	18
dc, D/C	discontinue; discharge	7, 8	EOMI	extraocular muscles intact	7
DCIS	ductal carcinoma in situ	15	EPO	erythropoietin	10, 13
D&E	dilatation and evacuation	15	ERCP	endoscopic retrograde cholangiopancreatography	12
DES	diethylstilbestrol	15	ERG	electroretinography	18
DEXA	dual-energy x-ray absorptiometry (scan)	19	ERV	expiratory reserve volume	11
DIC	disseminated intravascular coagulation	10	ESR	erythrocyte sedimentation rate	10
DIFF	differential count	10	ESRD	end-stage renal disease	13
DIP	distal interphalangeal	19	ESWL	extracorporeal shock wave lithotripsy	13
DJD	degenerative joint disease	19	ET	esotropia	18
dL	deciliter	Appendix 8	ETOH	alcohol, ethyl alcohol	7
DLE	discoid lupus erythematosus	21	F	Fahrenheit	7
DM	diabetes mellitus	16	FAP	familial adenomatous polyposis	12
DNR	do not resuscitate	7	FBG	fasting blood glucose	16
DOE	dyspnea on exertion	9	FBS	fasting blood sugar	16
DTaP	diphtheria, tetanus, acellular pertussis (vaccine)	11			

Appendix 2   Abbreviations and Their Meanings (continued)

Abbreviations	Meaning	Chapter	Abbreviations	Meaning	Chapter
FC	finger counting	18	HCl	hydrochloric acid	12
FDA	Food and Drug Administration	8	Hct, Ht	hematocrit	10
FEV	forced expiratory volume	11	HCV	hepatitis C virus	12
FFP	fresh frozen plasma	10	HDL	high-density lipoprotein	9
FHR	fetal heart rate	15	HDN	hemolytic disease of the newborn	10, 15
FHT	fetal heart tone	15	HDV	hepatitis D virus	12
FMS	fibromyalgia syndrome	20	HEV	hepatitis E virus	12
FPG	fasting plasma glucose	16	HEENT	head, eyes, ears, nose, and throat	7
FRC	functional residual capacity	11	HIPAA	Health Insurance Portability and Accountability Act	7
FSH	follicle-stimulating hormone	14, 15, 16	HIV	human immunodeficiency virus	10, 14
FTI	free thyroxine index	16	HL	hearing level	18
FTND	full-term normal delivery	15	HM	hand movements	18
FTP	full-term pregnancy	15	HNP	herniated nucleus pulposus	19
FTSG	full-thickness skin graft	21	h/o	history of	7
FUO	fever of unknown origin	6	H&P	history and physical	7
FVC	forced vital capacity	11	HPI	history of present illness	7
Fx	fracture	19	HPS	Hantavirus pulmonary syndrome	11
g	gram	Appendix 8	HPV	human papillomavirus	15
GA	gestational age	15	HR	heart rate	7
GAD	generalized anxiety disorder	17	HRT	hormone replacement therapy	15
GC	gonococcus	14, 15	hs	at bedtime	8
GDM	gestational diabetes mellitus	16	hs-crp	high sensitivity C-reactive protein (test)	9
GERD	gastroesophageal reflux disease	12	HSV	herpes simplex virus	14, 15
GFR	glomerular filtration rate	13	Ht, Hct	hematocrit	10
GH	growth hormone	16	HTN	hypertension	9
GI	gastrointestinal	12	Hx	history	7
GIFT	gamete intrafallopian transfer	15	Hz	Hertz	18
GTT	glucose tolerance test	16	^{131}I	iodine-131	16
gt(t)	drop(s)	8	I&D	incision and drainage	7
GU	genitourinary	13, 14	I&O	intake and output	7
GYN	gynecology	15	IABP	intraaortic balloon pump	9
H&P	history and physical examination	7	IBD	inflammatory bowel disease	12
HAV	hepatitis A virus	12	IBS	irritable bowel syndrome	12
Hb, Hgb	hemoglobin	10	IC	inspiratory capacity	11
HbA1c	hemoglobin A1c; glycated hemoglobin	16	ICD	implantable cardioverter-defibrillator	9
HBV	hepatitis B virus	12, 14	ICP	intracranial pressure	17
hCG	human chorionic gonadotropin	15			

Appendix 2   Abbreviations and Their Meanings *(continued)*

Abbreviations	Meaning	Chapter	Abbreviations	Meaning	Chapter
ICU	intensive care unit	7	LE	lupus erythematosus	21
ID	intradermal	8	LES	lower esophageal sphincter	12
IF	intrinsic factor	10	LH	luteinizing hormone	14, 15, 16
IFG	impaired fasting blood glucose	16	LL	left lateral	7
			LLL	left lower lobe (of lung)	11
Ig	immunoglobulin	10	LLQ	left lower quadrant	5
IGT	impaired glucose tolerance	16	LMN	lower motor neuron	17
			LMP	last menstrual period	15
IM	intramuscular(ly); intramedullary	8, 19	LOC	level of consciousness	17
INH	isoniazid	8, 11	LP	lumbar puncture	17
IOL	intraocular lens	18	LUL	left upper lobe (of lung)	11
IOP	intraocular pressure	18	LUQ	left upper quadrant	5
IPPA	inspection, palpation, percussion, auscultation	7	LV	left ventricle	9
			LVAD	left ventricular assist device	9
IPPB	intermittent positive pressure breathing	11	LVEDP	left ventricular end-diastolic pressure	9
IPPV	intermittent positive pressure ventilation	11	LVH	left ventricular hypertrophy	9
IRV	inspiratory reserve volume	11	lytes	electrolytes	10
ITP	idiopathic thrombocy-topenic purpura	10	μg	microgram	Appendix 8
IU	international unit	8	μL	microliter	10, Appendix 8
IUD	intrauterine device	15	μm	micrometer	Appendix 8
IV	intravenous(ly)	8	m	meter	Appendix 8
IVC	intravenous cholangiogram	12	mcg	microgram	8, Appendix 8
IVCD	intraventricular conduction delay	9			
IVDA	intravenous drug abuse	7	mcL, mcl	microliter	10, Appendix 8
IVF	in vitro fertilization	15	MAOI	monoamine oxidase inhibitor	17
IVP	intravenous pyelography	13			
IVPB	intravenous piggyback	7	MCH	mean corpuscular hemoglobin	10
IVU	intravenous urography	13	MCHC	mean corpuscular hemoglobin concentration	10
JVP	jugular venous pulse	9			
K	potassium	13	MCP	metacarpophalangeal	19
kg	kilogram	Appendix 8	MCV	mean corpuscular volume	10
km	kilometer	Appendix 8	MDS	myelodysplastic syndrome	10
KUB	kidney–ureter–bladder	13	MED(s)	medicine(s), medication(s)	8
KVO	keep vein open	7	MEFR	maximal expiratory flow rate	11
L	lumbar vertebra	19			
L	liter	Appendix 8	MEN	multiple endocrine neoplasia	16
LA	long-acting	8	mEq	milliequivalent	10
LAD	left anterior descending (coronary artery)	9	MET	metastasis	7
LAHB	left anterior hemiblock	9	mg	milligram	8, Appendix 8
LDL	low-density lipoprotein	9			

(continued)

Appendix 2   Abbreviations and Their Meanings (continued)

Abbreviations	Meaning	Chapter	Abbreviations	Meaning	Chapter
MG	myasthenia gravis	20	NSR	normal sinus rhythm	9
MI	myocardial infarction	9	NSS	normal saline solution	7
MID	multi-infarct dementia	17	NV	near vision	18
mL	milliliter	Appendix 8	N/V, N&V, n&v	nausea and vomiting	12
mm	millimeter	Appendix 8	N/V/D	nausea, vomiting, diarrhea	12
MMFR	maximum midexpiratory flow rate	11	O_2	oxygen	11
			OA	osteoarthritis	19
mm Hg	millimeters of mercury	9	OB	obstetrics	15
MMT	manual muscle test(ing)	20	OCD	obsessive–compulsive disorder	17
MN	myoneural	20			
MR	mitral regurgitation, reflux	9	OD	right eye	18
MRI	magnetic resonance imaging	7	ODS	Office of Dietary Supplements	8
MRSA	methicillin-resistant *Staphylococcus aureus*	6	OGTT	oral glucose-tolerance test	16
			OI	osteogenesis imperfecta	19
MS	mitral stenosis; multiple sclerosis	9, 17	OL	otolaryngology	18
			OOB	out of bed	7
MTP	metatarsophalangeal	19	OM	otitis media	18
MUGA	multigated acquisition (scan)	9	ORIF	open reduction internal fixation	19
MVP	mitral valve prolapse	9	ORL	otorhinolaryngology	18
MVR	mitral valve replacement	9	ortho, ORTH	orthopedics	19
Na	sodium	13	OS	left eye	18
NAD	no apparent distress	7	OT	occupational therapy	20
NB	newborn	15	OTC	over-the-counter	8
NCCAM	National Center for Complementary and Alternative Medicine	7	OU	both eyes; each eye	18
			p	after, post	8
NG	nasogastric	12	P	pulse	7, 9
NGU	nongonococcal urethritis	14, 15	PA	posteroanterior; physician assistant	7
NHL	non-Hodgkin lymphoma	10			
NICU	neonatal intensive care unit; neurologic intensive care unit	15, 17	PAC	premature atrial contraction	9
			$Paco_2$	arterial partial pressure of carbon dioxide	11
NKDA	no known drug allergies	7			
NMJ	neuromuscular junction	20	PACU	postanesthesia care unit	19, 20
NPH	neutral protamine Hagedorn (insulin)	16	Pao_2	arterial partial pressure of oxygen	11
NPH	normal pressure hydrocephalus	17	PAP	pulmonary arterial pressure	9
			pc	after meals	8
NPO	nothing by mouth	7	PCA	patient-controlled analgesia	7
NRC	normal retinal correspondence	18			
			PCI	percutaneous coronary intervention	9
NREM	non–rapid eye movement (sleep)	17			
			PCL	posterior cruciate ligament	19
NS, N/S	normal saline	7			
NSAID(s)	nonsteroidal antiinflammatory drug(s)	8, 19	PCOS	polycystic ovarian syndrome	15

Appendix 2 Abbreviations and Their Meanings (continued)

Abbreviations	Meaning	Chapter	Abbreviations	Meaning	Chapter
PCP	*Pneumocystis* pneumonia	10, 11	pp	postprandial (after a meal)	8
PCV	packed cell volume	10	PPD	purified protein derivative (tuberculin)	11
PCWP	pulmonary capillary wedge pressure	9	PPI	proton pump inhibitor	12
PDA	patent ductus arteriosus	15	preop, pre-op	preoperative	7
PDD	pervasive developmental disorder	17	PRICE	protection, rest, ice, compression, and elevation	20
PDR	*Physicians' Desk Reference*	8	PRL	prolactin	16
PE	physical examination	7	prn	as needed	8
PEEP	positive end-expiratory pressure	11	PSA	prostate-specific antigen	14
PEFR	peak expiratory flow rate	11	PSF	posterior spinal fusion	19
PEG	percutaneous endoscopic gastrostomy (tube)	12	PSS	physiologic saline solution; progressive systemic sclerosis	7, 21
PEP	protein electrophoresis	13	PSVT	paroxysmal supraventricular tachycardia	9
PERRLA	pupils equal, (regular) react to light and accommodation	7	pt	patient	7
PET	positron emission tomography	7, 17	PT	physical therapy/therapist	20
PFT	pulmonary function test(s)	11	PT, ProTime	prothrombin time	10
pH	scale for measuring hydrogen ion concentration (acidity or alkalinity)	10	PTCA	percutaneous transluminal coronary angioplasty	9
			PTH	parathyroid hormone	16
Ph	Philadelphia chromosome	10	PTSD	posttraumatic stress disorder	17
PICC	peripherally inserted central catheter	7	PTT	partial thromboplastin time	10
PID	pelvic inflammatory disease	15	PUVA	psoralen ultraviolet A	21
PIH	pregnancy-induced hypertension	15	PVC	premature ventricular contraction	9
PIP	peak inspiratory pressure	11	PVD	peripheral vascular disease	9
PIP	proximal interphalangeal	19	PYP	pyrophosphate	9
PKU	phenylketonuria	15	qam	every morning	8
PMH	past medical history	7	qh	every hour	8
PMI	point of maximal impulse	9	q __ h	every __ hours	8
PMN	polymorphonuclear (neutrophil)	10	qid	four times per day	8
PMS	premenstrual syndrome	15	QNS	quantity not sufficient	7
PND	paroxysmal nocturnal dyspnea	11	QS	quantity sufficient	7
PNS	peripheral nervous system	17	R	respiration	7, 11
po	by mouth, orally	8	RA	rheumatoid arthritis	19
poly, polymorph	neutrophil	10	RAIU	radioactive iodine uptake	16
PONV	postoperative nausea and vomiting	12	RAS	reticular activating system	17
postop, post-op	postoperative	7	RATx	radiation therapy	7
			RBC	red blood cell; red blood (cell) count	10

(continued)

Abbreviations	Meaning	Chapter	Abbreviations	Meaning	Chapter
RDS	respiratory distress syndrome	11	SPECT	single-photon emission-computed tomography	7
REM	rapid eye movement (sleep)	17	SPF	sun protection factor	21
RIA	radioimmunoassay	16	SpO_2	oxygen percent saturation	11
RL	right lateral	7	SR	sustained release	8
RLL	right lower lobe (of lung)	11	$\overline{ss}$	half	8
RLQ	right lower quadrant	5	SSEP	somatosensory evoked potentials	17
RLS	restless legs syndrome	20	SSRI	selective serotonin reuptake inhibitor	17
RML	right middle lobe (of lung)	11	ST	speech threshold	18
R/O	rule out	7	staph	staphylococcus	6
ROM	range of motion	20	STAT	immediately	7
ROS	review of systems	7	STD	sexually transmitted disease	14, 15
RSI	repetitive strain injury	20	STI	sexually transmitted infection	14, 15
RSV	respiratory syncytial virus	11	strep	streptococcus	6
RTC	rotator cuff	20	STSG	split-thickness skin graft	21
RUL	right upper lobe (of lung)	11	supp	suppository	8
RUQ	right upper quadrant	5	susp	suspension	8
RV	residual volume	11	SVD	spontaneous vaginal delivery	15
Rx	drug, prescription, therapy	7, 8	SVT	supraventricular tachycardia	9
$\overline{s}$	without	8	T	temperature; thoracic vertebra	7, 19
S	sacrum; sacral	19	T1DM	type 1 diabetes mellitus	16
S_1	first heart sound	9	T2DM	type 2 diabetes mellitus	16
S_2	second heart sound	9	T_3	triiodothyronine	16
SA	sustained action; sinoatrial	8, 9	T_4	thyroxine, tetraiodothyronine	16
SARS	severe acute respiratory syndrome	11	T_7	free thyroxine index	16
SBE	subacute bacterial endocarditis	9	T&A	tonsils and adenoids, tonsillectomy and adenoidectomy	11
sc	without correction	18	tab	tablet	8
SC, SQ, subcu.	subcutaneous(ly)	8	TAH	total abdominal hysterectomy	15
SCLE	subacute cutaneous lupus erythematosus	21	TB	tuberculosis	11
seg	neutrophil	10	TBG	thyroxine-binding globulin	16
SERM	selective estrogen receptor modulator	15, 19	^{99m}Tc	technetium-99m	9
SG	specific gravity	13	TCA	tricyclic antidepressant	17
SIADH	syndrome of inappropriate antidiuretic hormone	16	TEE	transesophageal echocardiography	9
SIDS	sudden infant death syndrome	11	TGV	thoracic gas volume	11
SITS	supraspinatus, infraspinatus, teres minor, subscapularis (muscles)	20	THA	total hip arthroplasty	19
SK	streptokinase	9	TIA	transient ischemic attack	17
SL	sublingual	8			
SLE	systemic lupus erythematosus	10, 21			

Appendix 2   Abbreviations and Their Meanings *(continued)*

Abbreviations	Meaning	Chapter	Abbreviations	Meaning	Chapter
tid	three times per day	8	URI	upper respiratory infection	11
tinct	tincture	8	USP	*United States Pharmacopeia*	8
TKA	total knee arthroplasty	19	UTI	urinary tract infection	13, 14
TKO	to keep open	7	UTP	uterine term pregnancy	15
TLC	total lung capacity	11	UV	ultraviolet	7, 21
Tm	maximal transport capacity; tubular maximum	13	UVA	ultraviolet A	21
			UVB	ultraviolet B	21
TM	tympanic membrane	18	VA	visual acuity	18
Tn	troponin	9	VAC	vacuum-assisted closure	21
TNM	(primary) tumor, (regional lymph) nodes, (distant) metastases	7	VAD	ventricular assist device	9
TMJ	temporomandibular joint	19	VBAC	vaginal birth after cesarean section	15
tPA	tissue plasminogen activator	9	VC	vital capacity	11
TPN	total parenteral nutrition	12	VD	venereal disease	14, 15
TPR	temperature, pulse, respiration	7	VDRL	Venereal Disease Research Laboratory	14
TPUR	transperineal urethral resection	14	VEP	visual evoked potentials	17
TSE	testicular self-examination	14	VF	ventricular fibrillation; visual field	9, 18
TSH	thyroid-stimulating hormone	16	v fib	ventricular fibrillation	9
TSS	toxic shock syndrome	15	VLDL	very-low-density lipoprotein	9
T(C)T	thrombin (clotting) time	10	VPC	ventricular premature complex	9
TTP	thrombotic thrombocytopenic purpura	10	VRSA	vancomycin-resistant *Staphylococcus aureus*	6
TTS	temporary threshold shift	18	VS	vital signs	7
TUIP	transurethral incision of prostate	14	VSD	ventricular septal defect	9
TURP	transurethral resection of prostate	14	VT	ventricular tachycardia	9
			VTE	venous thromboembolism	9
TV	tidal volume	11	V_{TG}	thoracic gas volume	11
Tx	traction	19	vWF	von Willebrand factor	10
U	units	8	WBC	white blood cell; white blood (cell) count	10
UA	urinalysis	13			
UC	uterine contractions	15	WD	well developed	7
UFE	uterine fibroid embolization	15	WNL	within normal limits	7
			w/o	without	7
UG	urogenital	14	WPW	Wolff–Parkinson–White syndrome	9
UGI	upper gastrointestinal	12	x	times	8
UMN	upper motor neuron	17	XT	exotropia	18
ung	ointment	8	ZIFT	zygote intrafallopian transfer	15

Appendix 3   Word Parts and Their Meanings

Word Part	Meaning	Reference Page	Word Part	Meaning	Reference Page
a-	not, without, lack of, absence	29	-ary	pertaining to	16
ab-	away from	30	-ase	enzyme	53
abdomin/o	abdomen	66	atel/o	imperfect	227
-ac	pertaining to	16	atlant/o	atlas	452
acous, acus	sound, hearing	420	atri/o	atrium	153
acro-	extremity, end	67	audi/o	hearing	420
ad-	toward, near	30	auto-	self	199
aden/o	gland	50	azot/o	nitrogenous compounds	193
adip/o	fat	53	bacill/i, bacill/o	bacillus	90
adren/o	adrenal gland, epinephrine	362	bacteri/o	bacterium	90
adrenal/o	adrenal gland	362	balan/o	glans penis	309
adrenocortic/o	adrenal cortex	362	bar/o	pressure	109
aer/o	air, gas	109	bi-	two, twice	27
-agogue	promotor, stimulator	338	bili	bile	251
-al	pertaining to	16	blast/o, -blast	immature cell, productive cell, embryonic cell	52
alg/o, algi/o, algesi/o	pain	86, 125	blephar/o	eyelid	429
-algesia	pain	88, 416	brachi/o	arm	67
-algia	pain	88	brachy-	short	309
ambly-	dim	435	brady-	slow	87
amnio	amnion	338	bronch/o, bronch/i	bronchus	219
amyl/o	starch	53	bronchiol	bronchiole	219
an-	not, without, lack of, absence	29	bucc/o	cheek	248
			burs/o	bursa	453
andr/o	male	301	calc/i	calcium	193
angi/o	vessel	154	cali/o, calic/o	calyx	277
an/o	anus	250	-capnia	carbon dioxide (level of)	218
ante-	before	34	carcin/o	cancer, carcinoma	86
anti-	against	29, 125	cardi/o	heart	153
aort/o	aorta	154	cec/o	cecum	250
-ar	pertaining to	16	-cele	hernia, localized dilation	88
arter/o, arteri/o	artery	154	celi/o	abdomen	66
arteriol/o	arteriole	154	centesis	puncture, tap	111
arthr/o	joint	453	cephal/o	head	66

Appendix 3   Word Parts and Their Meanings (continued)

Word Part	Meaning	Reference Page	Word Part	Meaning	Reference Page
cerebell/o	cerebellum	387	dent/o, dent/i	tooth, teeth	248
cerebr/o	cerebrum	387	derm/o, dermat/o	skin	506
cervic/o	neck, cervix	66, 325	-desis	binding, fusion	111
chem/o	chemical	125	dextr/o-	right	35
cheil/o	lip	261	di-	two, twice	27
chir/o	hand	108	dia-	through	30
cholangi/o	bile duct	251	dilation, dilatation	expansion, widening	89
chol/e, chol/o	bile, gall	251	dipl/o-	double	27
cholecyst/o	gallbladder	251	dis-	absence, removal, separation	29
choledoch/o	common bile duct	251	duoden/o	duodenum	249
chondr/o	cartilage	453	dys-	abnormal, painful, difficult	87
chori/o, choroid/o	choroid	430			
chrom/o, chromat/o	color, stain	109	ec-	out, outside	35
chron/o	time	109	ectasia, ectasis	dilation, dilatation, distention	89
circum-	around	67	ecto-	out, outside	35
clasis, -clasia	breaking	88	-ectomy	excision, surgical removal	111
clitor/o, clitorid/o	clitoris	326	edema	accumulation of fluid, swelling	89
coccy, coccyg/o	coccyx	455			
cochle/o	cochlea (of inner ear)	420	electr/o	electricity	109
col/o, colon/o	colon	250	embry/o	embryo	338
colp/o	vagina	325	emesis	vomiting	258
contra-	against, opposite	29, 125	-emia	condition of blood	190
copro	feces	388	encephal/o	brain	387
cor/o, cor/e	pupil	435	end/o-	in, within	35
corne/o	cornea	429	endocrin/o	endocrine	362
cortic/o	outer portion, cerebral cortex	387	enter/o	intestine	249
cost/o	rib	455	epi-	on, over	67
counter-	opposite, against	125	epididym/o	epididymis	302
crani/o	skull, cranium	454	episi/o	vulva	326
cry/o	cold	109	equi-	equal, same	32
crypt/o	hidden	306	erg/o	work	109, 487
cus	sound, hearing	420	erythr/o-	red, red blood cell	28, 191
cyan/o-	blue	28	erythrocyt/o	red blood cell	191
cycl/o	ciliary body, ciliary muscle (of eye)	430	esophag/o	esophagus	249
cyst/o	filled sac or pouch, cyst, bladder, urinary bladder	86, 278	-esthesia, -esthesi/o	sensation	416
-cyte, cyt/o	cell	50	eu-	true, good, easy, normal	32
dacry/o	tear, lacrimal apparatus	429	ex/o-	away from, outside	35
dacryocyst/o	lacrimal sac	429	extra-	outside	67
dactyl/o	finger, toe	67	fasci/o	fascia	486
de-	down, without, removal, loss	29	fer	to carry	384
			ferr/i, ferr/o	iron	193
			fet/o	fetus	338

(continued)

Appendix 3   Word Parts and Their Meanings *(continued)*

Word Part	Meaning	Reference Page	Word Part	Meaning	Reference Page
fibr/o	fiber	50	-ic	pertaining to	17
-form	like, resembling	16	-ical	pertaining to	17
galact/o	milk	338	-ics	medical specialty	14
gangli/o, ganglion/o	ganglion	386	-ile	pertaining to	17
			ile/o	ileum	250
gastr/o	stomach	249	ili/o	ilium	455
gen, genesis	origin, formation	52	im-	not	29
ger/e, ger/o	old age	26	immun/o	immunity, immune system	191
-geusia	sense of taste	416			
gingiv/o	gum, gingiva	248	in-	not	29
gli/o	neuroglia	386	infra-	below	67
glomerul/o	glomerulus	277	in/o	fiber, muscle fiber	486
gloss/o	tongue	248	insul/o	pancreatic islets	362
gluc/o	glucose	53	inter-	between	67
glyc/o	sugar, glucose	53	intra-	in, within	67
gnath/o	jaw	248	ir, irit/o, irid/o	iris	430
goni/o	angle	437, 468	-ism	condition of	13
-gram	record of data	110	iso-	equal, same	32
-graph	instrument for recording data	110	-ist	specialist	14
			-itis	inflammation	88
-graphy	act of recording data	110	jejun/o	jejunum	250
gravida	pregnant woman	338	juxta-	near, beside	68
gyn/o, gynec/o	woman	324	kali	potassium	193
hem/o, hemat/o	blood	191	kary/o	nucleus	50
hemi-	half, one side	27	kerat/o	cornea, keratin, horny layer of skin	430, 506
-hemia	condition of blood	190			
hepat/o	liver	251	kin/o, kine, kinesi/o, kinet/o	movement	487
hetero-	other, different, unequal	32			
hidr/o	sweat, perspiration	506	labi/o	lip	248
hist/o, histi/o	tissue	50	labyrinth/o	labyrinth (inner ear)	420
homo-, homeo-	same, unchanging	32	lacrim/o	tear, lacrimal apparatus	429
hydr/o	water, fluid	53	lact/o	milk	338
hyper-	over, excess, increased, abnormally high	31	-lalia	speech, babble	388
			lapar/o	abdominal wall	66
hypn/o	sleep	125	laryng/o	larynx	219
hypo-	under, below, decreased, abnormally low	31	lent/i	lens	430
			-lepsy	seizure	388
hypophys	pituitary, hypophysis	362	leuk/o-	white, colorless, white blood cell	28, 191
hyster/o	uterus	325			
-ia	condition of	13	leukocyt/o	white blood cell	191
-ian	specialist	14	-lexia	reading	388
-ia/sis	condition of	13	lingu/o	tongue	248
-iatrics	medical specialty	14	lip/o	fat, lipid	53
-iatr/o	physician	91	-listhesis	slipping	461
-iatry	medical specialty	14	lith	calculus, stone	86

Appendix 3　Word Parts and Their Meanings *(continued)*

Word Part	Meaning	Reference Page	Word Part	Meaning	Reference Page
-logy	study of	14	nat/i	birth	338
lumb/o	lumbar region, lower back	66	natri	sodium	193
lymphaden/o	lymph node	167	necrosis	death of tissue	89
lymphangi/o	lymphatic vessel	167	neo-	new	32
lymph/o	lymph, lymphatic system, lymphocyte	167, 191	nephr/o	kidney	277
			neur/o, neur/i	nervous system, nerve	386
lymphocyt/o	lymphocyte	191	noct/i	night	112, 287
-lysis	separation, loosening, dissolving, destruction	89	non-	not	29
			normo-	normal	32
-lytic	dissolving, reducing, loosening	125	nucle/o	nucleus	50
			nulli-	never	338
macro-	large, abnormally large	32	nyct/o	night, darkness	112
mal-	bad, poor	87	ocul/o	eye	429
malacia	softening	89	odont/o	tooth, teeth	248
mamm/o	breast, mammary gland	326	-odynia	pain	88
-mania	excited state, obsession	388	-oid	like, resembling	17
mast/o	breast, mammary gland	326	olig/o-	few, scanty, deficiency of	31
medull/o	inner part, medulla oblongata, spinal cord	387	-oma	tumor	88
			onc/o	tumor	86
mega-, megalo-	large, abnormally large	32	onych/o	nail	506
-megaly	enlargement	88	oo	ovum	324
melan/o	black, dark, melanin	28, 506	oophor/o	ovary	324
mening/o, meninge/o	meninges	386	ophthalm/o	eye	429
			-opia	eye, vision	431
men/o, mens	month, menstruation	324	-opsia	vision	431
mes/o-	middle	35	opt/o	eye, vision	429
-meter	instrument for measuring	110	orchid/o, orchi/o	testis	302
metr/o	measure	431	or/o	mouth	248
metr/o, metr/i	uterus	325	ortho-	straight, correct, upright	32
-metry	measurement of	110	-ory	pertaining to	17
micro-	small, one millionth	32	osche/o	scrotum	302
-mimetic	mimicking, simulating	125	-ose	sugar	53
mon/o-	one	27	-o/sis	condition of	13
morph/o	form, structure	50	osm/o	smell	416
muc/o	mucus, mucous membrane	50	-osmia	sense of smell	416
multi-	many	27	oste/o	bone	453
muscul/o	muscle	46	ot/o	ear	420
myc/o	fungus, mold	90	-ous	pertaining to	17
myel/o	bone marrow, spinal cord	191, 386, 453	ovari/o	ovary	324
			ov/o, ovul/o	ovum	324
my/o	muscle	46	-oxia	oxygen (level of)	218
myring/o	tympanic membrane	420	ox/y	oxygen, sharp, acute	193, 353
myx/o	mucus	50			
narc/o	stupor, unconsciousness	125, 387	pachy-	thick	87
nas/o	nose	219			

(continued)

Appendix 3 | Word Parts and Their Meanings *(continued)*

Word Part	Meaning	Reference Page	Word Part	Meaning	Reference Page
palat/o	palate	248	**-poiesis**	formation, production	190
palpebr/o	eyelid	429	**poikilo-**	varied, irregular	32
pan-	all	31	**poly-**	many, much	27
pancreat/o	pancreas	251	**post-**	after, behind	34
papill/o	nipple	50	**pre-**	before, in front of	34
para-	near, beside, abnormal	68, 416	**presby-**	old	431
para	woman who has given birth	338	**prim/i-**	first	27
parathyr/o, parathyroid/o	parathyroid	362	**pro-**	before, in front of	34
-paresis	partial paralysis, weakness	388	**proct/o**	rectum	250
path/o, -pathy	disease, any disease of	86, 88	**prostat/o**	prostate	302
ped/o	foot, child	67, 464	**prote/o**	protein	53
pelvi/o	pelvis	455	**pseudo-**	false	32
-penia	decrease in, deficiency of	190	**psych/o**	mind	387
per-	through	30	**ptosis**	dropping, downward displacement, prolapse	89
peri-	around	67	**ptysis**	spitting	228
perine/o	perineum	326	**puer**	child	345
periton, peritone/o	peritoneum	66	**pulm/o, pulmon/o**	lung	220
-pexy	surgical fixation	111	**pupill/o**	pupil	430
phac/o, phak/o	lens	430	**pyel/o**	renal pelvis	277
phag/o	eat, ingest	52	**pylor/o**	pylorus	249
pharm, pharmac/o	drug, medicine	125	**py/o**	pus	86
pharyng/o	pharynx	219	**pyr/o, pyret/o**	fever, fire	86, 125
-phasia	speech	388	**quadr/i-**	four	27
phil, -philic	attracting, absorbing	52	**rachi/o**	spine	454
phleb/o	vein	154	**radicul/o**	root of spinal nerve	386
-phobia	fear	388	**radi/o**	radiation, x-ray	109
phon/o	sound, voice	109	**re-**	again, back	32
-phonia	voice	218	**rect/o**	rectum	250
phot/o	light	109	**ren/o**	kidney	277
phren/o	diaphragm	220	**reticul/o**	network	50
phrenic/o	phrenic nerve	220	**retin/o**	retina	430
phyt/o	plant	124, 514	**retro-**	behind, backward	68
pituitar	pituitary, hypophysis	362	**rhabd/o**	rod, muscle cell	493
plas, -plasia	formation, molding, development	52	**-rhage, -rhagia**	bursting forth, profuse flow, hemorrhage	88
-plasty	plastic repair, plastic surgery, reconstruction	111	**-rhaphy**	surgical repair, suture	111
-plegia	paralysis	388	**-rhea**	flow, discharge	88
pleur/o	pleura	220	**-rhexis**	rupture	88
-pnea	breathing	218	**rhin/o**	nose	219
pneum/o, pneumat/o	air, gas, lung, respiration	220	**sacchar/o**	sugar	53
			sacr/o	sacrum	455
pneumon/o	lung	220	**salping/o**	tube, oviduct, eustachian (auditory) tube	325, 420
pod/o	foot	67			

Appendix 3 Word Parts and Their Meanings (continued)

Word Part	Meaning	Reference Page	Word Part	Meaning	Reference Page
-schisis	fissure, splitting	88, 454	syn-, sym-	together	35
scler/o	hard, sclera (of eye)	86, 429	synov/i	synovial joint, synovial membrane	453
sclerosis	hardening	90			
-scope	instrument for viewing or examining	110	tachy-	rapid	87
			tax/o	order, arrangement	492
-scopy	examination of	110	tel/e-, tel/o-	end	35
seb/o	sebum, sebaceous gland	506	ten/o, tendin/o	tendon	487
semi-	half, partial	27	terat/o	malformed fetus	344
semin	semen	302	test/o	testis, testicle	302
sept/o	septum, dividing wall, partition	229	tetra-	four	27
			thalam/o	thalamus	387
sial/o	saliva, salivary gland, salivary duct	248	therm/o	heat, temperature	109
sider/o	iron	193	thorac/o	chest, thorax	66
sigmoid/o	sigmoid colon	250	thromb/o	blood clot	191
sinistr/o	left	35	thrombocyt/o	platelet, thrombocyte	191
-sis	condition of	13	thym/o	thymus gland	167
somat/o	body	50	thyr/o, thyroid/o	thyroid	362
-some	body, small body	50	toc/o	labor	338
somn/i, somn/o	sleep	387	-tome	instrument for incising (cutting)	111
son/o	sound, ultrasound	109			
spasm	sudden contraction, cramp	90	-tomy	incision, cutting	111
sperm/i	semen, spermatozoa	302	ton/o	tone	487
spermat/o	semen, spermatozoa	302	tonsill/o	tonsil	167
-spermia	condition of semen	303	tox/o, toxic/o	poison, toxin	86, 125
sphygm/o	pulse	153	toxin	poison	90
spir/o	breathing	220	trache/o	trachea	219
splen/o	spleen	167	trans-	through	30
spondyl/o	vertebra	454	tri-	three	27
staped/o, stapedi/o	stapes	420	trich/o	hair	506
			-tripsy	crushing	111
staphyl/o	grapelike cluster, staphylococcus	90	trop/o	turning	436
			trop, -tropic	act(ing) on, affect(ing)	52, 125
stasis	suppression, stoppage	90	troph/o, -trophy, -trophia	feeding, growth, nourishment	52
steat/o	fatty	53			
stenosis	narrowing, constriction	90	tympan/o	tympanic cavity (middle ear), tympanic membrane	420
steth/o	chest	427			
sthen/o	strength	492			
stoma, stomat/o	mouth	248	un-	not	29
-stomy	surgical creation of an opening	111	uni-	one	27
			-uresis	urination	279
strept/o-	twisted chain, streptococcus	90	ureter/o	ureter	278
			urethr/o	urethra	278
sub-	below, under	67	-uria	condition of urine, urination	279
super-	above, excess	31			
supra-	above	68			

(continued)

Appendix 3   Word Parts and Their Meanings (continued)

Word Part	Meaning	Reference Page	Word Part	Meaning	Reference Page
ur/o	urine, urinary tract	278	**ventricul/o**	cavity, ventricle	153, 387
urin/o	urine	278	**vertebr/o**	vertebra, spinal column	454
uter/o	uterus	325	**vesic/o**	urinary bladder	278
uve/o	uvea (of eye)	430	**vesicul/o**	seminal vesicle	302
uvul/o	uvula	248	**vestibul/o**	vestibule, vestibular apparatus (of ear)	420
vagin/o	sheath, vagina	325			
valv/o, valvul/o	valve	153	**vir/o**	virus	90
varic/o	twisted and swollen vein, varix	163	**vulv/o**	vulva	326
			xanth/o-	yellow	28
vascul/o	vessel	154	**xen/o**	foreign, strange	394
vas/o	vessel, duct, vas deferens	125, 154, 302	**xero-**	dry	87
			-y	condition of	13
ven/o, ven/i	vein	154			

Appendix 4	Meanings and Their Corresponding Word Parts				

Meaning	Word Part(s)	Reference Page	Meaning	Word Part(s)	Reference Page
abdomen	abdomin/o, celi/o	66	artery	arter/o, arteri/o	154
abdominal wall	lapar/o	66	atlas	atlant/o	452
abnormal	dys-, para-	87, 416	atrium	atri/o	153
abnormally high	hyper-	31	attract(ing)	phil, -philic	5t2
abnormally large	macro-, mega-, megalo-	32	auditory (eustachian) tube	salping/o	420
abnormally low	hypo-	31	away from	ab-, ex/o-	30, 35
above	super-, supra-	31, 68	babble	-lalia	388
absence	a-, an-, dis-	29	bacillus	bacill/i, bacill/o	90
absorb(ing)	phil, -philic	52	back	re-	32
accumulation of fluid	edema	89	backward	retro-	68
act of recording data	-graphy	110	bacterium	bacteri/o	90
act(ing) on	trop, -tropic	52, 125	bad	mal-	87
acute	ox/y	353	before	ante-, pre-, pro-	34
adrenal gland	adren/o, adrenal/o	362	behind	post-, retro-	34, 68
adrenaline	adren/o	362	below	hypo-, infra-, sub-	31, 67
adrenal	adren/o	362	beside	para-, juxta-	68
adrenal cortex	adrenocortic/o	362	between	inter-	67
affect(ing)	trop, -tropic	52	bile	bili, chol/e, chol/o	251
after	post-	34	bile duct	cholangi/o	251
again	re-	32	binding	-desis	111
against	anti-, contra-, counter-	29, 125	birth	nat/i	338
air	aer/o, pneumat/o	109, 220	black	melan/o-	28, 506
all	pan-	31	bladder	cyst/o	86, 278
amnion, amniotic sac	amnio	338	bladder (urinary)	cyst/o, vesic/o	86
angle	goni/o	437, 468	blood	hem/o, hemat/o	191
anus	an/o	250	blood (condition of)	-emia, -hemia	190
any disease of	-pathy	88	blood clot	thromb/o	191
aorta	aort/o	154	blue	cyan/o-	28
arm	brachi/o	67	body	somat/o, -some	50
around	circum-, peri-	67	bone	oste/o	453
arrangement	tax/o	492	bone marrow	myel/o	191, 386, 453
arteriole	arteriol/o	154			

(continued)

Appendix 4   Meanings and Their Corresponding Word Parts (continued)

Meaning	Word Part(s)	Reference Page	Meaning	Word Part(s)	Reference Page
brain	encephal/o	387	condition of semen	-spermia	303
breaking	-clasis, -clasia	88	constriction	stenosis	90
breast	mamm/o, mast/o	326	contraction (sudden)	spasm	90
breathing	-pnea, spir/o	218, 220	cornea	corne/o, kerat/o	430
bronchiole	bronchiol	219	correct	ortho-	32
bronchus	bronch/i, bronch/o	219	cramp	spasm	90
bursa	burs/o	453	cranium	crani/o	454
bursting forth	-rhage, -rhagia	88	crushing	-tripsy	111
calcium	calc/i	193	cutting	-tomy	111
calculus	lith	86	cutting instrument	-tome	111
calyx	cali/o, calic/o	277	cyst	cyst/o	86
cancer	carcin/o	86	dark	melan/o-	28, 506
carbon dioxide	-capnia	218	darkness	nyct/o	112
carcinoma	carcin/o	86	data	-gram	110
carry	fer	384	death of tissue	necrosis	89
cartilage	chondr/o	453	decreased, decrease in	hypo-, -penia	31, 190
cavity	ventricul/o	153, 387	deficiency of	oligo-, -penia	31, 190
cecum	cec/o	250	destruction	lysis	89
cell	-cyte, cyt/o	50	development	plas, -plasia	52
cerebellum	cerebell/o	387	diaphragm	phren/o	220
cerebral cortex	cortic/o	387	different	hetero-	32
cerebrum	cerebr/o	387	difficult	dys-	87
cervix	cervic/o	325	dilatation, dilation	ectasia, ectasis	89
chain (twisted)	strept/o	90	distention	ectasia, ectasis	89
cheek	bucc/o	248	dim	ambly-	435
chemical	chem/o	125	discharge	-rhea	88
chest	thorac/o, steth/o	66, 427	disease	path/o, -pathy	86
child	ped/o, puer	345, 464	dissolving	lysis, -lytic	89, 125
choroid	chori/o, choroid/o	430	distention	ectasia, ectasis	89
ciliary body	cycl/o	430	double	dipl/o-	27
ciliary muscle	cycl/o	430	down	de-	29
clitoris	clitor/o, clitorid/o	326	dropping, downward displacement	ptosis	89
clot	thromb/o	191	drug	pharm, pharmac/o	125
coccyx	coccy, coccyg/o	455	dry	xero-	87
cochlea	cochle/o	420	duct	vas/o	154
cold	cry/o	109	ductus deferens	vas/o	302
colon	col/o, colon/o	250	duodenum	duoden/o	249
color	chrom/o, chromat/o	109	ear	ot/o	420
colorless	leuk/o-	28	easy	eu-	32
common bile duct	choledoch/o	251	eat	phag/o	52
condition of	-ia, -ia/sis, -ism, -o/sis, -sis, -y	13	egg cell	oo, ov/o, ovul/o	324
condition of blood	-emia, -hemia	190	electricity	electr/o	109
condition of urine, urination	-uria	279	embryo	embry/o	338

Appendix 4	Meanings and Their Corresponding Word Parts (continued)

Meaning	Word Part(s)	Reference Page	Meaning	Word Part(s)	Reference Page
embryonic cell	-blast, blast/o	52	foreign	xen/o	394
end	tel/e, tel/o, acro	35, 67	form	morph/o	50
endocrine	endocrin/o	362	formation	gen, genesis, plas, -plasia, -poiesis	52, 190
enlargement	-megaly	88			
enzyme	-ase	53	four	quadr/i, tetra-	27
epididymis	epididym/o	302	fungus	myc/o	90
epinephrine	adren/o	362	fusion	-desis	111
equal	iso-, equi-	32	gall	chol/e, chol/o	251
erythrocyte	erythr/o, erythrocyt/o	191	gallbladder	cholecyst/o	251
esophagus	esophag/o	249	ganglion	gangli/o, ganglion/o	386
eustachian (auditory) tube	salping/o	420	gas	aer/o, pneum/o, pneumon/o, pneumat/o	109, 220
examination of	-scopy	110	gingiva (gum)	gingiv/o	248
excess	hyper-, super-	31	gland	aden/o	50
excision	-ectomy	111	glans penis	balan/o	309
excited state	mania	388	glomerulus	glomerul/o	277
expansion	dilation, dilatation, ectasia, ectasis	89	glucose	gluc/o, glyc/o	53
extremity	acro	67	good	eu-	32
eye	ocul/o, ophthalm/o, opt/o, -opia	429, 431	grapelike cluster	staphyl/o	90
			growth	troph/o, -trophy, -trophia	52
eyelid	blephar/o, palpebr/o	427	gum, gingiva	gingiv/o	248
false	pseudo-	32	hair	trich/o	506
fascia	fasci/o	486	half	hemi-, semi-	27
fat	adip/o, lip/o	53	hand	chir/o	108
fatty	steat/o	53	hard	scler/o	86
fear	-phobia	388	hardening	sclerosis	90
feces	copro	388	head	cephal/o	66
feeding	troph/o, -trophy, -trophia	52	hearing	acous, acus, audi/o, cus	420
fetus	fet/o	338	heart	cardi/o	153
fetus (malformed)	terat/o	344	heat	therm/o	109
fever	pyr/o, pyret/o	86, 125	hemorrhage	-rhage, -rhagia	88
few	oligo-	31	hernia	-cele	88
fiber	fibr/o, in/o	50, 486	hidden	crypt/o	306
filled sac or pouch	cyst/o	86	horny layer of skin	kerat/o	506
finger	dactyl/o	67	hypophysis	hypophys, pituitar	362
fire	pyr/o, pyret/o	86	islets (pancreatic)	insul/o	362
first	prim/i-	27	ileum	ile/o	250
fissure	-schisis	88, 454	ilium	ili/o	455
fixation (surgical)	-pexy	111	immature cell	blast/o, -blast	52
flow	-rhea	88	immune system	immun/o	191
fluid	hydr/o	53	immunity	immun/o	191
foot	ped/o, pod/o	67	imperfect	atel/o	227

(continued)

Appendix 4 — Meanings and Their Corresponding Word Parts (continued)

Meaning	Word Part(s)	Reference Page	Meaning	Word Part(s)	Reference Page
in	end/o-, intra-	35, 67	lumbar region, lower back	lumb/o	66
in front of	pre-, pro-	34	lung, lungs	pneum/o, pneumat/o, pneumon/o, pulm/o, pulmon/o	220
incision of	-tomy	111			
increased	hyper-	31			
inflammation	-itis	88	lymph, lymphatic system	lymph/o	167
ingest	phag/o	52			
inner ear	labyrinth/o	420	lymph node	lymphaden/o	167
instrument for incising (cutting)	-tome	111	lymphatic vessel	lymphangi/o	167
			lymphocyte	lympho, lymphocyt/o	191
instrument for measuring	-meter	110	male	andr/o	301
			malformed fetus	terat/o	344
instrument for recording data	-graph	110	mammary gland	mamm/o, mast/o	326
			many	multi-, poly-	27
instrument for viewing or examining	-scope	110	marrow	myel/o	199
			measure	metr/o	431
intestine	enter/o	249	measuring instrument	-meter	110
iris	ir, irid/o, irit/o	430	measurement of	-metry	110
iron	ferr/i, ferr/o, sider/o	193	medical specialty	-ics, -iatrics, iatry	14
irregular	poikilo-	32	medicine	pharm, pharmac/o	125
jaw	gnath/o	248	medulla oblongata	medull/o	387
jejunum	jejun/o	250	melanin	melan/o	506
joint	arthr/o	453	meninges	mening/o, meninge/o	386
keratin	kerat/o	506	menstruation	men/o, mens	324
kidney	nephr/o, ren/o	277	middle	meso-	35
labor	toc/o	338	middle ear	tympan/o	420
labyrinth	labyrinth/o	420	milk	galact/o, lact/o	338
lack of	a-, an-	29	mimicking	-mimetic	125
lacrimal apparatus	dacry/o, lacrim/o	429	mind	psych/o	387
lacrimal sac	dacryocyst/o	429	mold	myc/o	90
large	macro-, mega-, megalo-	32	molding	plas, -plasia	52
			month	men/o, mens	324
larynx	laryng/o	219	mouth	or/o, stoma, stomat/o	248
left	sinistr/o	35	movement	kin/o, kine, -kinesi/o, kinet/o	487
lens	lent/i, phac/o, phak/o	430			
leukocyte	leuk/o, leukocyt/o	291	much	poly-	27
level of carbon dioxide	-capnia	218	mucus	muc/o, myx/o	50
level of oxygen	-oxia	218	mucous membrane	muc/o	50
light	phot/o	109	muscle	my/o, muscul/o	486
like	-form, -oid	16	muscle cell	rhabd/o	493
lip	labi/o, cheil/o	248, 261	muscle fiber	in/o	493
lipid	lip/o	53	nail	onych/o	506
liver	hepat/o	251	narrowing	stenosis	90
localized dilation	-cele	88	near	ad-, juxta-, para-	30, 68
loosening	lysis, -lytic	89, 125	neck	cervic/o	66, 325
loss	de-	29	nerve, nervous system, nervous tissue	neur/o, neur/i	386

Appendix 4   Meanings and Their Corresponding Word Parts *(continued)*

Meaning	Word Part(s)	Reference Page	Meaning	Word Part(s)	Reference Page
network	reticul/o	50	partial paralysis	-paresis	388
neuroglia	gli/o	386	partition	sept/o	229
never	nulli-	338	pelvis	pelvi/o	455
new	neo-	32	perineum	perine/o	326
night	noct/i, nyct/o	112, 287	peritoneum	periton, peritone/o	66
nipple	papill/o	50	perspiration	hidr/o	506
nitrogenous compounds	azot/o	193	pertaining to	-ac, -al, -ar, -ary, -ic, -ical, -ile, -ory, -ous	16
normal	eu-, normo-	32	pharynx	pharyng/o	219
nose	nas/o, rhin/o	219	phrenic nerve	phrenic/o	220
not	a-, an-, in-, im-, non-, un-	29	physician	iatr/o	91
nourishment	troph/o, -trophy, -trophia	52	pituitary	pituitary, hypophys	362
nucleus	kary/o, nucle/o	50	plant	phyt/o	124, 514
obsession	mania	388	plastic repair, plastic surgery	-plasty	111
old	presby-	431	platelet	thrombocyt/o	191
old age	ger/e, ger/o	26	pleura	pleur/o	220
on	epi-	67	poison	tox/o, toxic/o, toxin	86, 90, 125
one	mon/o-, uni-	27	poor	mal-	87
one side	hemi-	27	potassium	kali	193
opening (created surgically)	-stomy	111	pouch (filled)	cyst/o, cyst/i	86
oppose	contra-	29, 125	pregnant woman	gravida	338
opposite	contra-, counter-	29, 125	pressure	bar/o	109
order	tax/o	492	production	-poiesis	190
origin	gen, genesis	52	productive cell	blast/o, -blast	52
other	hetero-	32	profuse flow	-rhage, -rhagia	88
out, outside	ec-, ecto-, ex/o, extra-	35, 67	prolapse	ptosis	89
outer portion	cortic/o	387	promotor	-agogue	338
ovary	ovari/o, oophor/o	324	prostate	prostat/o	302
over	hyper-, epi-	31, 67	protein	prote/o	53
oviduct	salping/o	325	pulse	sphygm/o	153
ovum	oo, ov/o, ovul/o	324	puncture	centesis	111
oxygen	ox/y, -oxia	193, 272	pupil	pupill/o, cor/o, cor/e	430, 435
pain	-algia, -odynia	88	pus	py/o	86
pain	-algesia, alg/o, algi/o, algesi/o	86, 88, 125, 416	pylorus	pylor/o	249
painful	dys-	87	radiation	radi/o	109
palate	palat/o	258	rapid	tachy-	87
pancreas	pancreat/o	251	reading	-lexia	388
pancreatic islets	insul/o	362	reconstruction	-plasty	111
paralysis	-plegia	388	record of data	-gram	110
paralysis (partial)	-paresis	388	recording data (act of)	-graphy	110
parathyroid	parathyr/o, parathyroid/o	362	rectum	rect/o, proct/o	250
partial	semi-	27	red	erythr/o-	28
			red blood cell	erythr/o, erythrocyt/o	191
			reducing	-lytic	125
			removal	de-, dis-	29

(continued)

Appendix 4   Meanings and Their Corresponding Word Parts (continued)

Meaning	Word Part(s)	Reference Page	Meaning	Word Part(s)	Reference Page
removal (surgical)	-ectomy	111	smell (sense of)	-osmia	416
renal pelvis	pyel/o	277	sodium	natri	193
repair (plastic)	-plasty	111	softening	malacia	89
repair (surgical)	-rhaphy	111	sound	phon/o, son/o, acous, acus, cus	109, 420
respiration	pneum/o, pneumat/o	220			
resembling	-form, -oid	16	specialist	-ian, -ist, -logist	14
retina	retin/o	430	specialty	-ics, -iatrics, -iatry	14
rib	cost/o	455	speech	-phasia, -lalia	388
right	dextr/o-	35	sperm, spermatozoa	sperm/i, spermat/o	302
rod	rhabd/o	493	spinal column	vertebr/o	454
root of spinal nerve	radicul/o	386	spinal cord	myel/o, medull/o	386
rupture	-rhexis	88	spinal nerve root	radicul/o	386
sac (filled)	cyst/o, cyst/i	86	spine	rachi/o	454
sacrum	sacr/o	455	spitting	ptysis	228
saliva, salivary gland, salivary duct	sial/o	248	spleen	splen/o	167
			splitting	-schisis	88, 454
same	equi-, homo-, homeo-, iso-	32	stain	chrom/o, chromat/o	109
			stapes	staped/o, stapedi/o	420
sclera (of eye)	scler/o	429	staphylococcus	staphyl/o	90
scanty	oligo-	31	starch	amyl/o	53
scrotum	osche/o	302	stimulator	-agogue	338
sebum, sebaceous gland	seb/o	506	stomach	gastr/o	249
			stone	lith	86
seizure	-lepsy	388	stoppage	stasis	90
self	auto-	199	straight	ortho-	32
semen	semin, sperm/i, spermat/o	302	strange	xen/o	394
			strength	sthen/o	492
semen, condition of	-spermia	303	streptococcus	strept/o	90
seminal vesicle	vesicul/o	302	structure	morph/o	50
sensation	-esthesia, esthesi/o	416	study of	-logy	14
sense of smell	-osmia	416	stupor	narc/o	125, 387
sense of taste	-geusia	416	sugar	glyc/o, sacchar/o, -ose	53
separation	dis-, -lysis	29, 89	sudden contraction	spasm	90
septum	sept/o	229	suppression	stasis	90
sharp	ox/y	353	surgery (plastic)	-plasty	111
short	brachy-	309	surgical creation of an opening	-stomy	111
sigmoid colon	sigmoid/o	250			
simulating	-mimetic	125	surgical fixation	-pexy	111
skin	derm/o, dermat/o	506	surgical removal	-ectomy	111
skull	crani/o	454	surgical repair	-rhaphy	111
sleep	hypn/o, somn/o, somn/i	125, 387	suture	-rhaphy	111
			sweat	hidr/o	506
slipping	-listhesis	461	swelling	edema	89
slow	brady-	87	synovial fluid, joint, membrane	synov/i	453
small	micro-	32			
small body	-some	50			
smell	osm/o	416			

Meaning	Word Part(s)	Reference Page	Meaning	Word Part(s)	Reference Page
tap	centesis	111	upright	ortho-	32
taste (sense of)	-geusia	416	ureter	ureter/o	278
tear	dacry/o, lacrim/o	429	urethra	urethr/o	278
teeth	dent/o, denti, odont/o	248	urinary bladder	cyst/o, vesic/o	278
temperature	therm/o	109	urine, urinary tract, urination	ur/o, -uria	278
tendon	ten/o, tendin/o	487	urination	-uresis	279
testicle	test/o	302	urine	urin/o	278
testis	test/o, orchid/o, orchi/o	302	uterus	hyster/o, metr/o, metr/i, uter/o	325
thalamus	thalam/o	387	uvea	uve/o	430
thick	pachy-	87	uvula	uvul/o	248
thorax	thorac/o	66	vagina	colp/o, vagin/o	325
three	tri-	27	valve	valv/o, valvul/o	153
thrombocyte	thrombocyt/o	191	varicose vein, varix	varic/o	163
through	dia-, per-, trans-	30	varied	poikilo-	32
thymus gland	thym/o	167	vas deferens	vas/o	302
thyroid	thyr/o, thyroid/o	362	vein	ven/o, ven/i, phleb/o	154
time	chron/o	109	vein (twisted, swollen)	varic/o	163
tissue	hist/o, histi/o	50	ventricle	ventricul/o	153, 387
tissue death	necrosis	89	vertebra	spondyl/o, vertebr/o	454
toe	dactyl/o	67	vessel	angi/o, vas/o, vascul/o	125, 154, 302
together	syn-, sym-	35	vestibular apparatus, vestibule	vestibul/o	420
tone	ton/o	487			
tongue	gloss/o, lingu/o	248	virus	vir/o	90
tonsil	tonsill/o	167	vision	opt/o, -opia, -opsia	429, 431
tooth	-dent/o, dent/i, odont/o	248	voice	phon/o, -phonia	109, 218
toward	ad-	30	vomiting	emesis	258
toxin	tox/o, toxic/o	125	vulva	episi/o, vulv/o	326
trachea	trache/o	219	wall, dividing wall	sept/o	229
true	eu-	32	water	hydr/o	53
tube	salping/o	325, 420	weakness	paresis	388
tumor	onc/o, -oma	86, 88	white	leuk/o-	28
turning	trop/o	436	white blood cell	leuk/o, leukocyt/o	191
twice	bi-, di-	27	widening	ectasia, ectasis, dilation, dilatation	89
twisted chain	strept/o	90			
twisted and swollen vein	varic/o	163	within	end/o-, intra-	35, 67
two	bi-, di-, dipl/o-	27	without	a-, an-, de-	29
tympanic cavity	tympan/o	420	woman	gyn/o, gynec/o	324
tympanic membrane	myring/o, tympan/o	420	woman who has given birth	para	338
ultrasound	son/o	109			
unchanging	homo-, homeo-	32	work	erg/o	109, 487
unconsciousness	narc/o	387	x-ray	radi/o	109
under	hypo-, sub-	31, 67	yellow	xanth/o-	28
unequal	hetero-	32			

Word Roots

Appendix 5 — Word Roots

Root	Meaning	Reference Page	Root	Meaning	Reference Page
abdomin/o	abdomen	66	brachi/o	arm	67
acous, acus	sound, hearing	420	bronch/i, bronch/o	bronchus	219
acro	extremity, end	67	bronchiol	bronchiole	219
aden/o	gland	50	bucc/o	cheek	248
adip/o	fat	53	burs/o	bursa	453
adren/o	adrenal gland, epinephrine	362	calc/i	calcium	193
			cali/o, calic/o	calyx	277
adrenal/o	adrenal gland	362	carcin/o	cancer, carcinoma	86
adrenocortic/o	adrenal cortex	362	cardi/o	heart	153
aer/o	air, gas	109	cec/o	cecum	250
alg/o, algi/o, algesi/o	pain	86, 125	celi/o	abdomen	66
			centesis	puncture, tap	111
amnio	amnion	338	cephal/o	head	66
amyl/o	starch	53	cerebell/o	cerebellum	387
andr/o	male	301	cerebr/o	cerebrum	387
angi/o	vessel	154	cervic/o	neck, cervix	66, 325
an/o	anus	250	cheil/o	lip	261
aort/o	aorta	154	chem/o	chemical	125
arter/o, arteri/o	artery	154	chir/o	hand	108
arteriol/o	arteriole	154	cholangi/o	bile duct	251
arthr/o	joint	453	chol/e, chol/o	bile, gall	251
atel/o	incomplete, imperfect	227	cholecyst/o	gallbladder	251
atlant/o	atlas	452	choledoch/o	common bile duct	251
atri/o	atrium	153	chondr/o	cartilage	453
audi/o	hearing	420	chori/o, choroid/o	choroid	430
azot/o	nitrogenous compounds	193	chrom/o, chromat/o	color, stain	109
bacill/i, bacill/o	bacillus	90	chron/o	time	109
bacteri/o	bacterium	90	clasis	breaking	88
balan/o	glans penis	309	clitor/o, clitorid/o	clitoris	326
bar/o	pressure	109	coccy, coccyg/o	coccyx	455
bili	bile	251	cochle/o	cochlea (of inner ear)	420
blast/o	immature cell, productive cell, embryonic cell	52	col/o, colon/o	colon	250
blephar/o	eyelid	429	colp/o	vagina	325

Appendix 5 **Word Roots** *(continued)*

Root	Meaning	Reference Page	Root	Meaning	Reference Page
copro	feces	388	gangli/o, ganglion/o	ganglion	386
cor/o, cor/e	pupil	435	gastr/o	stomach	249
corne/o	cornea	429	gen	origin, formation	52
cortic/o	outer portion, cerebral cortex	387	ger/e, ger/o	old age	26
cost/o	rib	455	gingiv/o	gum, gingiva	248
crani/o	skull, cranium	454	gli/o	neuroglia	386
cry/o	cold	109	glomerul/o	glomerulus	277
crypt/o	hidden	306	gloss/o	tongue	248
cus	sound, hearing	420	gluc/o	glucose	53
cycl/o	ciliary body, ciliary muscle (of eye)	430	glyc/o	sugar, glucose	53
			gnath/o	jaw	248
cyst/o	filled sac or pouch, cyst, bladder, urinary bladder	86, 278	goni/o	angle	437, 468
			gravida	pregnant woman	338
cyt/o	cell	50	gyn/o, gynec/o	woman	324
dacry/o	tear, lacrimal apparatus	429	hem/o, hemat/o	blood	191
dacryocyst/o	lacrimal sac	429	hepat/o	liver	251
dactyl/o	finger, toe	67	hidr/o	sweat, perspiration	506
dent/o, dent/i	tooth, teeth	248	hist/o, histi/o	tissue	50
derm/o, dermat/o	skin	506	hydr/o	water, fluid	53
dilation, dilatation	expansion, widening	89	hypn/o	sleep	125
duoden/o	duodenum	249	hypophys	pituitary, hypophysis	362
ectasia, ectasis	dilation, dilatation, distention	89	hyster/o	uterus	325
			iatr/o	physician	91
edema	accumulation of fluid, swelling	89	ile/o	ileum	250
			ili/o	ilium	455
electr/o	electricity	109	immun/o	immunity, immune system	191
embry/o	embryo	338			
emesis	vomiting	258	in/o	fiber, muscle fiber	486
encephal/o	brain	387	insul/o	pancreatic islets	362
endocrin/o	endocrine	362	ir, irit/o, irid/o	iris	430
enter/o	intestine	249	jejun/o	jejunum	250
epididym/o	epididymis	302	kali	potassium	193
episi/o	vulva	326	kary/o	nucleus	50
erg/o	work	109, 487	kerat/o	cornea, keratin, horny layer of skin	430, 506
erythr/o-	red, red blood cell	28, 191			
erythrocyt/o	red blood cell	191	kin/o, kine, kinesi/o, kinet/o	movement	487
esophag/o	esophagus	249			
fasci/o	fascia	486	labi/o	lip	328
fer	carry	384	labyrinth/o	labyrinth (inner ear)	420
ferr/i, ferr/o	iron	193	lacrim/o	tear, lacrimal apparatus	429
fet/o	fetus	338	lact/o	milk	338
fibr/o	fiber	50	lapar/o	abdominal wall	66
galact/o	milk	338			

(continued)

Appendix 5   Word Roots (continued)

Root	Meaning	Reference Page	Root	Meaning	Reference Page
laryng/o	larynx	219	**neur/o, neur/i**	nervous system, nerve	386
lent/i	lens	430	**noct/i**	night	112
leuk/o	white, colorless, white blood cell	28, 191	**nucle/o**	nucleus	50
			nyct/o	night, darkness	112
leukocyt/o	white blood cell	191	**ocul/o**	eye	429
lingu/o	tongue	248	**odont/o**	tooth, teeth	248
lip/o	fat, lipid	53	**onc/o**	tumor	86
listhesis	slipping	461	**onych/o**	nail	506
lith	calculus, stone	86	**oo**	ovum	324
lumb/o	lumbar region, lower back	66	**oophor/o**	ovary	324
lymphaden/o	lymph node	167	**ophthalm/o**	eye	429
lymphangi/o	lymphatic vessel	167	**opt/o**	eye, vision	429
lymph/o	lymph, lymphatic system, lymphocyte	167, 191	**orchid/o, orchi/o**	testis	302
lymph/o, lymphocyt/o	lymphocyte	191	**or/o**	mouth	248
			osche/o	scrotum	302
lysis	separation, loosening, dissolving, destruction	89	**osm/o**	smell	416
			oste/o	bone	453
malacia	softening	89	**ot/o**	ear	320
mamm/o	breast, mammary gland	326	**ovari/o**	ovary	324
mania	excited state, obsession	388	**ov/o, ovul/o**	ovum	324
mast/o	breast, mammary gland	326	**ox/y**	oxygen, sharp, acute	193, 353
medull/o	inner part, medulla oblongata, spinal cord	387	**palat/o**	palate	248
melan/o	dark, black, melanin	28, 506	**palpebr/o**	eyelid	429
mening/o, meninge/o	meninges	386	**pancreat/o**	pancreas	251
			papill/o	nipple	50
men/o, mens	month, menstruation	324	**para**	woman who has given birth	338
metr/o	measure	431			
metr/o, metr/i	uterus	325	**parathyr/o, parathyroid/o**	parathyroid	362
morph/o	form, structure	50	**paresis**	partial paralysis, weakness	388
muc/o	mucus, mucous membrane	50	**path/o**	disease, any disease of	86
muscul/o	muscle	486	**ped/o**	foot, child	67, 464
myc/o	fungus, mold	90	**pelvi/o**	pelvis	455
myel/o	bone marrow, spinal cord	191, 386, 453	**perine/o**	perineum	326
			periton, peritone/o	peritoneum	66
my/o	muscle	486	**phac/o, phak/o**	lens	430
myring/o	tympanic membrane	420	**phag/o**	eat, ingest	52
myx/o	mucus	50	**pharm, pharmac/o**	drug, medicine	125
narc/o	stupor, unconsciousness	125, 387	**pharyng/o**	pharynx	219
nas/o	nose	219	**phil**	attracting, absorbing	52
nat/i	birth	338	**phleb/o**	vein	154
natri	sodium	193	**phobia**	fear	388
necrosis	death of tissue	89	**phon/o**	sound, voice	109
nephr/o	kidney	277	**phot/o**	light	109

Appendix 5   Word Roots (continued)

Root	Meaning	Reference Page	Root	Meaning	Reference Page
phren/o	diaphragm	220	sial/o	saliva, salivary gland, salivary duct	248
phrenic/o	phrenic nerve	220	sider/o	iron	193
phyt/o	plant	124, 514	sigmoid/o	sigmoid colon	250
pituitar	pituitary, hypophysis	362	somat/o	body	50
plas	formation, molding, development	52	somn/i, somn/o	sleep	387
pleur/o	pleura	220	son/o	sound, ultrasound	109
pneum/o, pneumat/o	air, gas, lung, respiration	220	spasm	sudden contraction, cramp	90
pneumon/o	lung	220	sperm/i	semen, spermatozoa	302
pod/o	foot	67	spermat/o	semen, spermatozoa	302
proct/o	rectum	250	sphygm/o	pulse	153
prostat/o	prostate	302	spir/o	breathing	220
prote/o	protein	53	splen/o	spleen	167
psych/o	mind	387	spondyl/o	vertebra	454
ptosis	dropping, downward displacement, prolapse	89	staped/o, stapedi/o	stapes	420
ptysis	spitting	228	staphyl/o	grapelike cluster, staphylococcus	90
puer	child	345	stasis	suppression, stoppage	90
pulm/o, pulmon/o	lung	220	steat/o	fatty	53
pupill/o	pupil	430	stenosis	narrowing, constriction	90
pyel/o	renal pelvis	277	steth/o	chest	427
pylor/o	pylorus	249	sthen/o	strength	492
py/o	pus	86	stoma, stomat/o	mouth	248
pyr/o, pyret/o	fever, fire	86, 125	synov/i	synovial joint, synovial membrane	453
rachi/o	spine	454			
radicul/o	root of spinal nerve	386	tax/o	order, arrangement	492
radi/o	radiation, x-ray	109	ten/o, tendin/o	tendon	487
rect/o	rectum	250	terat/o	malformed fetus	344
ren/o	kidney	277	test/o	testis, testicle	302
reticul/o	network	50	thalam/o	thalamus	387
retin/o	retina	430	therm/o	heat, temperature	109
rhabd/o	rod, muscle cell	493	thorac/o	chest, thorax	66
rhin/o	nose	219	thromb/o	blood clot	191
sacchar/o	sugar	53	thrombocyt/o	platelet, thrombocyte	191
sacr/o	sacrum	455	thym/o	thymus gland	167
salping/o	tube, oviduct, eustachian (auditory) tube	325, 420	thyr/o, thyroid/o	thyroid	362
			toc/o	labor	338
schisis	fissure	454	ton/o	tone	487
scler/o	hard, sclera (of eye)	86, 429	tonsill/o	tonsil	167
sclerosis	hardening	90	tox/o, toxic/o	poison, toxin	86, 125
seb/o	sebum, sebaceous gland	506	trache/o	trachea	219
semin	semen	302	trich/o	hair	506
sept/o	septum, partition, dividing wall	229	trop/o	turning	436

(continued)

Appendix 5 — Word Roots *(continued)*

Root	Meaning	Reference Page	Root	Meaning	Reference Page
trop	act(ing) on, affect(ing)	52, 125	**varic/o**	twisted and swollen vein, varix	163
troph/o	feeding, growth, nourishment	52	**vascul/o**	vessel	154
tympan/o	tympanic cavity (middle ear), tympanic membrane	420	**vas/o**	vessel, duct, vas deferens	125, 154, 302
ureter/o	ureter	278	**ven/o, ven/i**	vein	154
urethr/o	urethra	278	**ventricul/o**	cavity, ventricle	153, 387
ur/o	urine, urinary tract	278	**vertebr/o**	vertebra, spinal column	454
urin/o	urine	278	**vesic/o**	urinary bladder	278
uter/o	uterus	325	**vesicul/o**	seminal vesicle	302
uve/o	uvea (of eye)	430	**vestibul/o**	vestibule, vestibular apparatus (of ear)	420
uvul/o	uvula	248	**vir/o**	virus	90
vagin/o	sheath, vagina	325	**vulv/o**	vulva	326
valv/o, valvul/o	valve	153	**xen/o**	foreign, strange	394

Metric Measurements

Appendix 8-1 Metric Measurements

Unit	Abbreviation	Metric Equivalent	U.S. Equivalent
Units of Length			
kilometer	km	1000 m	0.62 miles; 1.6 km/mile
meter*	m	100 cm; 1000 mm	39.4 inches; 1.1 yards
centimeter	cm	1/100 m; 0.01 m	0.39 inches; 2.5 cm/inch
millimeter	mm	1/1000 m; 0.001 m	0.039 inches; 25 mm/inch
micrometer	μm	1/1000 mm; 0.001 mm	
Units of Weight			
kilogram	kg	1000 g	2.2 lb
gram*	g	1000 mg	0.035 oz; 28.5 g/oz
milligram	mg	1/1000 g; 0.001 g	
microgram	mcg, μg	1/1000 mg; 0.001 mg	
Units of Volume			
liter*	L	1000 mL	1.06 qt
deciliter	dL	1/10 L; 0.1 L	
milliliter	mL	1/1000 L; 0.001 L	0.034 oz; 29.4 mL/oz
microliter	mcL, mcl, μL	1/1000 mL; 0.001 mL	

*Basic unit.

Appendix 8-2 Metric Prefixes

Prefix	Meaning of Prefix
kilo-	1000
deci-	1/10; one tenth
centi-	1/100; one hundredth
milli-	1/1000; one thousandth
micro-	1/1,000,000; one millionth

Stedman's Medical Dictionary at a Glance

an·ti·bod·y (an′tē-bod′e) *Avoid the jargonsitic use of the plural antibodies when the reference is to a single antibody species.* An immunoglobulin molecule produced by B-lymphoid cells that combine specifically with an immunogen or antigen. A.'s may be present naturally, their specificity is determined through gene rearrangement or somatic replacement or may be synthesized in response to stimulus provided by the introduction of an antigen; a.'s are found in the blood and body fluids, although the basic structure of the molecule consists of two light and two heavy chains, a.'s may also be found as dimers, trimers, or pentamers. After binding antigen, some a.'s may fix, complement, bind to surface receptors on immune cells, and in some cases may neutralize microorganisms. SEE ALSO immunoglobulin. SYN immune protein, protective protein, sensitizer (2).

Usage notes appear in italics before definition

ANTIGEN

Large header for entries with numerous subentries

Indicates term is illustrated

an·ti·gen (Ag) (an′ti-jen). Any substance that, as a result of coming in contact with appropriate cells, induces a state of sensitivity or immune responsiveness and that reacts in a demonstrable way with antibodies or immune cells of the sensitized subject in vivo or in vitro. Modern usage tends to retain the broad meaning of a., employing the terms "antigenic determinant" or "determinant group" for the particular chemical group of a molecule that confers antigenic specificity. SEE ALSO hapten. SYN immunogen. [anti-body) + G, -gen, producing.]

Pronunciation

Main entry

Subentry

Etymologies appear in brackets

Australia a. [MIM*209800], an a. so called because first recognized in an Australian aborigine, but now known to be a subunit of the hepatitis B virus surface antigen. SYN Au a. (2), Aus a.

Abbreviation

Cross references in blue indicate where to find the defined / preferred term. In multi-word terms, the italicized term indicates the main entry under which the term can be found.

carcinoembryonic a. (CEA), a glycoprotein constituent of the glycocalyx of embryonic endodermal epithelium, which may be elevated in the serum of some patients with colon cancer and certain other cancers and in serum of long-term tobacco smokers.

Main word is abbreviated in subentries

conjugated a., SYN conjugated *hapten.*

prostate-specific a. (PSA), a single-chain, 31-kD glycoprotein with 240 amino acid residues and 4 carbohydrate side-chains; a kallikrein protease produced by prostatic epithelial cells and normally found in seminal fluid and circulating blood. Elevations of serum PSA are highly organ-specific but occur in both cancer (adenocarcinoma) and benign disease (e.g. benign prostatic hyperplasia, prostatitis). A significant number of patients with organ-confined cancer have normal PSA values. SEE carcinoma of the prostate. SYN human glandular kallikrein 3.

High profile terms (entries) with broad significance to the practice of medicine and to the world appear in blue boxes

Cross references

KEY

♻	Combining Forms
🅸	Indicates term is illustrated, *see Illustration Index*
SYN	Synonym
Cf.	Compare
[NA]	Nomina Anatomica
[TA]	Terminologia Anatomica
☆	Official alternate Terminologia Anatomica term
[MIM]	Mendelian Inheritance in Man
C.I.	*Color Index*

Answer Key

Chapter 1

Pretest

1. c
2. a
3. d
4. b
5. a
6. c
7. b
8. d
9. a

Chapter Review

1. suffix
2. combining form
3. diarrhea
4. cardiology
5. c
6. b
7. c
8. d
9. *dis-LEK-sē-a*
10. *RŪ-ma-tizm*
11. *nū-MAT-ik*
12. *KEM-ist*
13. *FAR-ma-sē*
14. cardiac
15. hydrogen
16. ocular
17. interface
18. rheumatic
19. gastritis (*gas-TRĪ-tis*)
20. neurology (*nū-ROL-ō-jē*)
21. nephroptosis (*nef-rop-TŌ-sis*)
22. nephrology (*nef-ROL-ō-jē*)
23. neuritis (*nū-RĪ-tis*)
24. cardioptosis (*kar-dē-op-TŌ-sis*)
25. difficult or painful menstruation
    a. abnormal, painful, difficult
    b. menses, menstruation
    c. flow, discharge
26. physician who specializes in study of the heart
    a. heart
    b. study of
    c. specialist in a field of study
27. inflammation of the kidney
    a. kidney
    b. inflammation
28. pertaining to the kidney and stomach
    a. kidney
    b. stomach
    c. pertaining to

Case Study Questions

1. c
2. d
3. b
4. d
5. a
6. hem/o, hemat/o
7. Chapter 7
8. in; within
9. intra-
10. ear; nose; larynx
11. g
12. computed tomography

Chapter 2

Pretest

1. c
2. d
3. a
4. c
5. b
6. a
7. d
8. c
9. a

Chapter Exercises

EXERCISE 2-1

1. -ia
2. -sis
3. -ism
4. -y
5. -ia
6. -ism
7. -sis, -osis
8. -y
9. -sis, -esis

EXERCISE 2-2

1. -ist
2. -logy
3. -iatrics
4. -logy
5. -ian
6. -ist
7. anatomist
8. pediatrician
9. radiologist
10. psychologist
11. technologist; also, technician
12. obstetrician

EXERCISE 2-3

1. -ary
2. -al
3. -ic
4. -ous
5. -form
6. -oid
7. -al, -ical
8. -ile
9. -ic
10. -al, -ical
11. -ar
12. -ary
13. -ory
14. -ic

EXERCISE 2-4

1. patellae (*pa-TEL-ē*)
2. phenomena (*fe-NOM-e-na*)
3. omenta (*ō-MEN-ta*)
4. prognoses (*prog-NŌ-sēz*)
5. apices (*AP-i-sēz*)
6. ova (*Ō-va*)
7. spermatozoa (*sper-ma-tō-ZŌ-a*)
8. meninges (*me-NIN-jēz*)
9. emboli (*EM-bō-lī*)
10. protozoon (*prō-tō-ZŌ-on*)
11. appendix (*a-PEN-diks*)
12. adenoma (*ad-e-NŌ-ma*)
13. fungus (*FUN-gus*)
14. pelvis (*PEL-vis*)
15. foramen (*fō-RĀ-men*)
16. curriculum (*kur-RIK-ū-lum*)
17. index (*IN-deks*)
18. alveolus (*al-VĒ-ō-lus*)

Chapter Review

1. -ism
2. -ia
3. -sis, -osis
4. -y
5. -sis, -osis
6. -ia
7. -iatry
8. -ics
9. -ist
10. -ian
11. -ist
12. -ian
13. pediatrician
14. dermatologist
15. physiologist
16. gynecologist
17. -ic
18. -al
19. -ous

20. -oid
21. -al
22. -ic
23. -ary
24. -al
25. -oid
26. -ile
27. -al, -ical
28. -ar
29. -ory
30. gingivae (*JIN-ji-vē*)
31. diagnoses (*di-ag-NŌ-sēz*)
32. ganglia (*GANG-lē-a*)
33. lumina (*LŪ-mi-na*)
34. foci (*FŌ-sī*)
35. criteria (*krī-TIR-ē-a*)
36. larynges (*la-RIN-jēz*)
37. vertebrae (*VER-te-brē*)
38. nuclei (*NŪ-klē-ī*)
39. locus (*LŌ-kus*)
40. alveolus (*al-VĒ-ō-lus*)
41. bacterium (*bak-TĒ-rē-um*)
42. apex (*Ā-peks*)
43. foramen (*fō-RĀ-men*)
44. testis (*TES-tis*)
45. carcinoma (*kar-si-NŌ-ma*)

WORD BUILDING

46. parasitic
47. parasitologist
48. parasitism
49. parasitology

WORD ANALYSIS

50. specialist in care of the aged
    a. old, old age
    b. physician
    c. pertaining to
    d. specialist
51. uneven, not symmetrical
    a. not
    b. together
    c. measure
    d. pertaining to
52. lack of sensation
    a. not
    b. sensation
    c. condition of

Case Study Questions

1. c
2. d
3. a
4. -sis, -osis
5. -y
6. -ia
7. -ile
8. -ical
9. -ic
10. patella
11. ovum
12. protozoon

13. viral
14. necrosis
15. archeologist
16. internist
17. abdominal

Chapter 3

Pretest

1. d
2. a
3. c
4. a
5. b
6. d
7. b
8. c

Chapter Exercises

EXERCISE 3-1

1. b. uni-;   a. tri-;
   d. bi-;   c. tetra-
2. two
3. four
4. one
5. half
6. two
7. four
8. three
9. one
10. bi-
11. multi-
12. semi-
13. uni-

EXERCISE 3-2

1. d
2. c
3. a
4. b
5. e

EXERCISE 3-3

1. a-; not, without, lack of, absence
2. anti-; against
3. a-; not, without (root *mnem/o* means "memory")
4. dis-; absence, removal, separation
5. contra-; against, opposite
6. in-; not
7. de-; down, without, removal, loss
8. non-; not
9. unconscious
10. insignificant
11. disinfect
12. unusual
13. nonspecific
14. decongestant
15. incompatible

EXERCISE 3-4

1. dia-; through
2. per-; through
3. ad-; toward, near
4. ab-; away from
5. dia-; through
6. trans-; through

EXERCISE 3-5

1. c
2. e
3. d
4. b
5. a

EXERCISE 3-6

1. d
2. e
3. c
4. b
5. a
6. homeo-; same, unchanging
7. equi-; equal, same
8. ortho-; straight, correct, upright
9. re-; again, back
10. eu-; true, good, easy, normal
11. neo-; new
12. mega-; large, abnormally large
13. iso-; equal, same
14. normo-; normal
15. heterogeneous (*het-er-ō-JĒ-nē-us*)
16. microscopic (*mī-krō-SKOP-ik*)

EXERCISE 3-7

1. e
2. a
3. b
4. c
5. d
6. pre-; before, in front of
7. post-; after, behind
8. pro-; before, in front of
9. pre-; before, in front of
10. ante-; before

EXERCISE 3-8

1. e
2. c
3. a
4. b
5. d
6. sym-; together
7. ex-; away from, outside
8. ecto-; out, outside
9. syn-; together
10. endo-; in, within
11. endogenous (*en-DOJ-e-nus*)
12. sinistromanual (*sin-is-trō-MAN-ū-al*)
13. endoderm (*EN-dō-derm*)

Chapter Review

1. e
2. c

3. d
4. b
5. a
6. d
7. c
8. a
9. b
10. e
11. e
12. d
13. a
14. b
15. c
16. e
17. a
18. b
19. c
20. d
21. one
22. three
23. left
24. two
25. opposite
26. four
27. hyper-; over, excess, abnormally high, increased
28. trans-; through
29. dis-; absence, removal, separation
30. post-; after
31. re-; again, back
32. ex-; away from, outside
33. ad-; toward, near
34. un-; not
35. ecto-; out, outside
36. de-; removal, without
37. semi-; half, partial
38. pre-; before, in front of
39. per-; through
40. dia-; through
41. anti-; against
42. micro-; small
43. dis-; absence, removal, separation
44. endo-; in, within
45. sym-; together
46. pro-; before, in front of
47. in-; not
48. T
49. F; one
50. T
51. F; four
52. F; right
53. F; three
54. T
55. T
56. dehumidify
57. adduct
58. impermeable
59. homogeneous
60. endotoxin
61. macroscopic
62. hypoventilation
63. presynaptic

64. aseptic
65. hypersensitivity
66. macrocyte
67. prenatal
68. equilateral

WORD BUILDING
69. microcytic
70. ectocardia
71. monocytic
72. dextrocardia
73. endocardial
74. macrocytic
75. microcardia
76. of equal dimensions
    a. equal, same
    b. measure
    c. pertaining to
77. association of two or more organisms
    a. together
    b. life
    c. condition of
78. pertaining to a single colony (clone) of cells
    a. one
    b. colony, clone
    c. pertaining to

Case Study Questions

1. pre-; before, in front of
2. an-; not, without, lack of, absence
3. dis-; absence, removal, separation
4. re-; again, back
5. bi-; two, twice
6. hemi-; half, one side
7. de-; down, without, removal, loss
8. hyper-; over, excess, abnormally high, increased
9. a-; not, without, lack, absence
10. poly-; many, much
11. syn-; together
12. condition of
13. pertaining to, like, resembling
14. preoperative
15. postoperative
16. abduction
17. melanoma

Chapter 4

Pretest

1. b
2. a
3. d
4. c
5. c
6. a
7. a
8. c

Chapter Exercises

EXERCISE 4-1
1. cells
2. fiber
3. tissues
4. forms
5. nucleus
6. nucleus
7. gland
8. nipple
9. mucus
10. network
11. mucus
12. body
13. morphology (*mor-FOL-ō-jē*)
14. cytology (*sī-TOL-ō-jē*)
15. histology (*his-TOL-ō-jē*)

EXERCISE 4-2
1. d
2. c
3. e
4. b
5. a
6. d
7. c
8. e
9. b
10. a
11. gen; origin, formation
12. phag/o; eat, ingest
13. blast; immature cell, productive cell, embryonic cell
14. plas; formation, molding, development
15. troph; feeding, growth, nourishment

EXERCISE 4-3
1. sugars
2. sugar
3. water
4. starch
5. lipid, fat
6. glucose
7. fat, lipid
8. steat/o; fatty
9. lip/o; lipid, fat
10. glyc/o; sugar, glucose
11. gluc/o; glucose

Chapter Review

LABELING EXERCISE
Generalized Animal Cell
1. plasma membrane
2. nucleus
3. nuclear membrane
4. nucleolus
5. cytosol
6. smooth endoplasmic reticulum (ER)
7. rough endoplasmic reticulum (ER)

8. ribosomes
9. mitochondrion
10. Golgi apparatus
11. lysosome
12. vesicle
13. peroxisome
14. centriole
15. microvilli
16. cilia

TERMINOLOGY

1. b
2. d
3. e
4. a
5. c
6. e
7. c
8. b
9. a
10. d
11. d
12. a
13. b
14. c
15. e
16. e
17. a
18. c
19. b
20. d
21. d
22. c
23. a
24. e
25. b
26. b
27. e
28. a
29. d
30. c
31. b
32. c
33. d
34. a
35. e
36. metabolism
37. epithelial, connective, muscle, and nervous
38. histology
39. glucose
40. nucleus
41. enzyme
42. cells
43. water
44. morphology
45. mucus
46. F; lipid, fat
47. F; water
48. T
49. T
50. T
51. adenoid

52. leukoblast
53. lipase
54. mucoid
55. histioblast
56. amylase
57. amyloid
58. having a stimulating effect on the body
    a. body
    b. act on, affect
    c. pertaining to
59. destruction and disposal of damaged organelles in the cell
    a. self
    b. to eat
    c. condition of
60. reduced secretion of fatty material by the skin's sebaceous glands
    a. not, without, lack of, absence
    b. fatty
    c. condition of

Case Study Questions

1. c
2. d
3. d
4. a
5. mono-; one
6. pro-; before, in front of
7. neo-; new
8. a-; not, without, lack of, absence
9. leuk/o-; white, colorless
10. neutrophils, eosinophils, basophils
11. thromboplastin, neoplasm, dysplasia
12. lymphocytes, monocytes, cytology, leukocyte

Chapter 5

Pretest

1. d
2. b
3. b
4. a
5. b
6. d
7. b
8. a

Chapter Exercises

EXERCISE 5-1

1. abdominal (*ab-DOM-i-nal*)
2. cephalic (*se-FAL-ik*)
3. cervical (*SER-vi-kal*)
4. thoracic (*thō-RAS-ik*)
5. lumbar (*LUM-bar*)
6. peritoneum
7. abdomen
8. head
9. abdominal wall

EXERCISE 5-2

1. extremities (hands and feet)
2. arms
3. finger or toe
4. arm and head
5. foot

EXERCISE 5-3

1. circumoral
2. infrascapular
3. circumvascular
4. subcostal
5. periorbital
6. suprapatellar
7. extracellular
8. suprascapular
9. intrathoracic
10. near the nose
11. behind the peritoneum
12. above the abdomen
13. within the uterus
14. around the navel (umbilicus)
15. between the buttocks
16. above the ankle
17. within the eye
18. near the sacrum

Chapter Review

LABELING EXERCISE
Directional Terms

1. superior (cranial)
2. inferior (caudal)
3. anterior (ventral)
4. posterior (dorsal)
5. medial
6. lateral
7. proximal
8. distal

Planes of Division

1. frontal (coronal) plane
2. sagittal plane
3. transverse (horizontal) plane

Body Cavities, Lateral View

1. dorsal cavity
2. cranial cavity
3. spinal cavity (canal)
4. ventral cavity
5. thoracic cavity
6. diaphragm
7. abdominopelvic cavity
8. abdominal cavity
9. pelvic cavity

The Nine Regions of the Abdomen

1. epigastric (*ep-i-GAS-trik*) region
2. umbilical (*um-BIL-i-kal*) region
3. hypogastric (*hī-pō-GAS-trik*) region
4. right hypochondriac (*hī-pō-KON-drē-ak*) region
5. left hypochondriac region
6. right lumbar (*LUM-bar*) region

7. left lumbar region
8. right iliac (*IL-ē-ak*) region; also inguinal (*ING-gwi-nal*) region
9. left iliac region; also, inguinal region

Chapter Review

TERMINOLOGY

1. e
2. b
3. d
4. c
5. a
6. d
7. e
8. b
9. c
10. a
11. c
12. e
13. a
14. b
15. d
16. F; dorsal
17. T
18. T
19. F; frontal, coronal
20. T
21. F; inferior
22. F; prone
23. T
24. small of back
25. wrist
26. back of knee
27. base of skull
28. finger or toe
29. neck
30. abdomen
31. arm
32. around the mouth
33. above the pubis
34. below the umbilicus (navel)
35. between the ribs
36. under the tongue
37. behind the peritoneum
38. having two feet
39. dorsal
40. periocular
41. inframammary
42. anterior
43. microcephaly
44. superficial
45. distal
46. suprascapular
47. intracellular
48. inferior
49. spinal cavity; The *spinal cavity* is a dorsal cavity; the others are ventral cavities.
50. cervical region; *Cervical* refers to the neck; the others are abdominal regions.

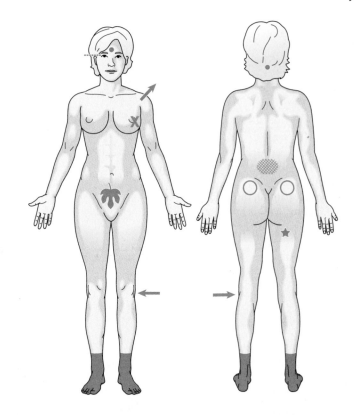

51. sagittal; *Sagittal* refers to a plane of division; the others are body positions.
52. lumb/o; The root *lumb/o* refers to the small of the back; the others refer to the extremities.
53. intracephalic
54. infrathoracic
55. extrathoracic
56. polydactyly
57. syndactyly
58. cephalothoracic
59. adactyly
60. dactylospasm
61. acephaly
62. condition in which the head is larger than average
    a. large, abnormally large
    b. head
    c. condition of
63. bluish discoloration of the hands or feet
    a. extremity
    b. blue
    c. condition of
64. pertaining to the forearm
    a. before
    b. arm
    c. pertaining to
65. pertaining to the epigastrium, the uppermost region of the abdomen
    a. on, over
    b. stomach
    c. pertaining to

Case Study Questions

1. b
2. c
3. e
4. d
5. b
6–15. See diagram.

Chapter 6

Pretest

1. d
2. c
3. b
4. a
5. c
6. c
7. a
8. d

Chapter Exercises

EXERCISE 6-1

1. pyr/o; fever
2. path/o; disease
3. py/o; pus
4. tox/o; poison
5. cancer, carcinoma
6. pus
7. fever
8. disease
9. calculus, stone

10. toxin, poison
11. hardening
12. pain
13. tumor

EXERCISE 6-2

1. b
2. a
3. d
4. e
5. c
6. xero-; dry
7. dys-; abnormal, painful, difficult
8. mal-; bad, poor

EXERCISE 6-3

1. d
2. a
3. b
4. e
5. c
6. c
7. a
8. d
9. b
10. e
11. pain in a muscle
12. any disease of muscle
13. rupture of a muscle
14. pain in a muscle
15. tumor of muscle

EXERCISE 6-4

1. e
2. d
3. b
4. a
5. c
6. softening of the spleen
7. dropping or prolapse of the spleen
8. substance poisonous or harmful to the spleen

EXERCISE 6-5

1. bacteria
2. fungus
3. bacilli
4. grapelike cluster
5. twisted chain
6. mycology (*mī-KOL-ō-jē*)
7. virology (*vī-ROL-ō-jē*)
8. bacteriology (*bak-tēr-ē-OL-ō-jē*)

Chapter Review

1. b
2. c
3. d
4. e
5. a
6. e
7. c
8. d
9. b
10. a
11. a
12. e
13. b
14. d
15. c
16. e
17. b
18. d
19. a
20. c
21. d
22. e
23. b
24. c
25. a
26. d
27. e
28. a
29. c
30. b
31. b
32. d
33. e
34. c
35. a
36. inflammation
37. neoplasm
38. metastasis
39. hernia
40. toxins; poisons
41. necrosis
42. tumor
43. carcinogenesis (*kar-sin-ō-JEN-e-sis*)
44. pyogenesis (*pī-ō-JEN-e-sis*)
45. pathogenesis (*path-ō-JEN-e-sis*)
46. oncogenesis (*ong-kō-JEN-e-sis*)
47. bronchospasm (*BRONG-kō-spazm*)
48. bronchitis (*brong-KĪ-tis*)
49. bronchostenosis (*brong-kō-sten-ō-sis*)
50. bronchorrhea (*brong-kō-RĒ-a*)
51. osteonecrosis (*os-tē-ō-ne-KRŌ-sis*)
52. osteomalacia (*os-tē-ō-ma-LĀ-shē-a*)
53. osteoclasis (*os-tē-OK-la-sis*)
54. osteoma (*os-tē-Ō-ma*)
55. osteolysis (*os-tē-OL-i-sis*)
56. T
57. F; streptococci
58. F; acute
59. T
60. F; bradycardia
61. T
62. helminths; *Helminths* are worms, the others are types of bacteria.
63. pathogen; A *pathogen* is a disease-causing microorganism, the others are terms related to neoplasia.
64. metastatic; *Metastatic* refers to the spread of cancer; the others are terms describing infections.
65. nephrotoxic (*nef-rō-TOKS-ik*)
66. pyogenic (*pī-ō-JEN-ik*)
67. nephroma (*nef-RŌ-ma*)
68. pathology (*pa-THOL-ō-jē*)
69. pyrogenic (*pī-rō-JEN-ik*)
70. nephrology (*nef-ROL-ō-jē*)
71. pathogenic (*path-ō-JEN-ik*)
72. nephropathy (*nef-ROP-a-thē*)
73. nephrogenic (*nef-rō-JEN-ik*)
74. counteracting fever
    a. against
    b. fever
    c. pertaining to
75. hardening of the arteries
    a. artery
    b. hard
    c. condition of
76. state of internal stability
    a. same
    b. stoppage, stability

Case Study Questions

1. c
2. b
3. c
4. d
5. a
6. d
7. c
8. b
9. a
10. e
11. hernia
12. gland
13. bacillus
14. sarcoma
15. malignant hyperpyrexia (also, hyperthermia)
16. human immunodeficiency virus
17. purified protein derivative
18. electrocardiogram
19. acid-fast bacillus

Chapter 7

Pretest

1. b
2. c
3. d
4. d
5. a
6. b
7. b
8. d
9. a

Chapter Exercises

EXERCISE 7-1

1. e
2. a
3. d
4. b

5. c
6. son/o; sound
7. aer/o; air (oxygen)
8. erg/o; work
9. therm/o; heat, temperature
10. chron/o; time
11. chrom/o; color
12. pressure
13. cold
14. light
15. electricity
16. sound

EXERCISE 7-2

1. a
2. d
3. b
4. e
5. c
6. d
7. a
8. c
9. e
10. b

EXERCISE 7-3

1. b
2. e
3. d
4. a
5. c
6. cystotomy (sis-TOT-ō-mē)
7. cystorrhaphy (sis-TOR-a-fē)
8. cystostomy (sis-TOS-tō-mē)
9. cystopexy (SIS-tō-pek-sē)
10. cystoplasty (SIS-tō-plas-tē)
11. arthrocentesis (ar-thrō-sen-TĒ-sis)
12. arthrotome (AR-thrō-tōm)
13. arthrodesis (ar-THROD-e-sis)
14. arthroplasty (AR-thrō-plas-tē)
15. arthrotomy (ar-THROT-ō-mē)
16. tracheotomy (trā-kē-OT-ō-mē)
17. gastropexy (GAS-trō-pek-sē)
18. colostomy (kō-LOS-tō-mē)

Chapter Review

1. c
2. b
3. a
4. e
5. d
6. c
7. d
8. b
9. e
10. a
11. c
12. a
13. e
14. d
15. b
16. b

17. c
18. a
19. e
20. d
21. a
22. c
23. e
24. b
25. d
26. chrom/o; color
27. son/o; sound
28. radi/o; radiation, x-ray
29. therm/o; heat, temperature
30. erg/o; work
31. chron/o; time
32. aer/o; air, gas, oxygen
33. light
34. cystoplasty (SIS-tō-plas-tē)
35. arthrodesis (ar-THROD-e-sis)
36. tracheostomy (trā-kē-OS-tō-mē)
37. therapy (THER-a-pē)
38. hepatotomy (hep-a-TOT-ō-mē)
39. hepatectomy (hep-a-TEK-tō-mē)
40. hepatopexy (HEP-a-tō-pek-sē)
41. hepatorrhaphy (hep-a-TOR-a-fē)
42. T
43. F; radiograph
44. T
45. F; pressure
46. T
47. T
48. remission; *Remission* is the lessening of disease symptoms; the others are examining methods.
49. syncope; *Syncope* is fainting; the others are examination instruments.
50. speculum; A *speculum* is an instrument for examining a canal; the others are surgical instruments.
51. TNM; *TNM* is an abbreviation for a system of staging cancer; the others are abbreviations for imaging techniques.
52. neurotome
53. cystoscopy
54. cystolith
55. neurorrhaphy
56. lithotripsy
57. cystopexy
58. cystorrhaphy
59. neurotripsy
60. cystotome
61. describing cells or tissues that have equal attraction for the same dyes
    a. equal, same
    b. color
    c. attracting, absorbing
    d. pertaining to
62. occurring at the same time
    a. together
    b. time
    c. pertaining to

63. test that records the heart's sounds
    a. sound
    b. heart
    c. act of recording
64. formation of color or pigment
    a. color
    b. origin, formation
    c. condition of

Case Study Questions

1. sequelae
2. palpation
3. mesocephalic
4. paracentesis
5. biopsy
6. diagnostic laparoscopy
7. hyperabduction
8. c
9. d
10. b
11. a
12. d
13. c
14. a
15. history of present illness
16. cancer
17. temperature, pulse, respiration
18. activities of daily living
19. beats per minute
20. within normal limits
21. discontinue
22. normal saline solution

Chapter 8

Pretest

1. a
2. d
3. c
4. b
5. a
6. d
7. a
8. b
9. c
10. a

Chapter Exercises

EXERCISE 8-1

1. -lytic; dissolving, reducing, loosening
2. -tropic; acting on
3. -mimetic; mimicking, simulating
4. antiinflammatory (an-tē-in-FLAM-a-tō-rē)
5. contraindicated (kon-tra-IN-di-kā-ted)
6. antiseptic (an-ti-SEP-tik)
7. counteract (COWN-ter-act)
8. antitoxin (an-tē-TOK-sin)
9. antipyretic (an-tē-pī-RET-ik)
10. hypn/o; sleep

11. toxic/o; poison
12. algesi/o; pain
13. chem/o; chemical
14. narc/o; stupor
15. narrowing of a vessel
16. study of drugs
17. dissolving mucus
18. acting on the gonads (sex glands)

Chapter Review

1. d
2. c
3. b
4. e
5. a
6. d
7. a
8. e
9. b
10. c
11. c
12. b
13. e
14. a
15. d
16. d
17. c
18. e
19. a
20. b
21. e
22. c
23. e
24. d
25. a
26. d
27. a
28. e
29. pain
30. vein
31. tolerance
32. plants, herbs
33. skin
34. toxins, poisons
35. pharmacology
36. fever
37. histamine H₂ antagonist;
    A *histamine H₂ antagonist* reduces
    stomach acid secretion; the others
    are respiratory drugs.
38. tablet; A *tablet* is a solid dosage
    form, a pill; the others are forms of
    liquid solutions.
39. antineoplastics; An *antineoplastic*
    kills cancer cells; the others are
    cardiac drugs.
40. adrenergic; An *adrenergic* is a
    sympathomimetic, which mimics the
    effects of the sympathetic nervous
    system; the others are drugs to
    eliminate sensation and relieve pain.
41. widening of the bronchi
42. under the tongue

43. reducing anxiety
44. acting on the mind
45. anticonvulsant
46. vasodilation
47. counterbalance, also imbalance
48. antitoxin
49. contraindicated
50. anticoagulant
51. as needed
52. *United States Pharmacopeia*
53. international unit
54. prescription
55. milligram
56. nonsteroidal antiinflammatory drugs
57. Food and Drug Administration
58. discontinue, also discharge
59. hypnosis
60. anxiolytic
61. toxicosis
62. thrombolytic
63. thrombosis
64. narcosis
65. mucolytic
66. administration of a solution by
    subcutaneous infusion
    a. under
    b. skin
    c. washing out
67. activated by or secreting adrenaline
    (epinephrine)
    a. adrenaline
    b. work
    c. pertaining to
68. movement of drugs within the body
    as affected by biologic function
    a. drug
    b. movement
    c. pertaining to

Case Study Questions

1. a
2. c
3. d
4. d
5. e
6. c
7. b
8. d
9. a
10. d
11. b
12. a
13. e
14. e
15. b
16. c

Chapter 9

Pretest

1. b
2. c

3. a
4. d
5. d
6. a
7. a
8. c
9. b
10. b

Chapter Exercises

EXERCISE 9-1

1. heart
2. atria
3. ventricle
4. valve
5. cardiac (*KAR-dē-ak*)
6. myocardial (*mī-ō-KAR-dē-al*)
7. atrial (*Ā-trē-al*)
8. valvular (*VAL-vū-lar*); also valvar
   (*VAL-var*)
9. ventricular (*ven-TRIK-ū-lar*)
10. pericardial (*per-i-KAR-dē-al*)
11. endocarditis (*en-dō-kar-DĪ-tis*)
12. myocarditis (*mī-ō-kar-DĪ-tis*)
13. pericarditis (*per-i-kar-DĪ-tis*)
14. atrioventricular
    (*ā-trē-ō-ven-TRIK-ū-lar*)
15. interventricular
    (*in-ter-ven-TRIK-ū-lar*)
16. cardiology (*kar-dē-OL-ō-jē*)
17. valvotomy (*val-VOT-ō-mē*);
    also, valvulotomy
    (*val-vū-LOT-ō-mē*)
18. cardiomegaly (*kar-dē-ō-MEG-a-lē*)

EXERCISE 9-2

1. vessel
2. artery
3. arteriole
4. vessels
5. aorta
6. vein
7. vessels
8. pertaining to the heart and vessels
9. within the aorta
10. inflammation of a vessel or vessels
11. rupture of an artery
12. inflammation of a vein
13. angiogram
14. aortogram
15. phlebogram; venogram
16. angiogenesis (*an-jē-ō-JEN-e-sis*)
17. angiectasis (*an-jē-EK-ta-sis*);
    also, hemangiectasis
    (*hē-man-jē-EK-ta-sis*)
18. angiopathy (*an-jē-OP-a-thē*)
19. angioplasty (*AN-jē-ō-plas-tē*)
20. intravenous (*in-tra-VĒ-nus*)
21. arteriotomy (*ar-tēr-ē-OT-ō-mē*)
22. phlebectomy (*fle-BEK-tō-mē*);
    venectomy (*vē-NEK-tō-mē*)
23. aortosclerosis
    (*ā-or-tō-skle-RŌ-sis*)

EXERCISE 9-3

1. lymph
2. lymph node
3. lymphatic vessels
4. spleen
5. thymus gland
6. tonsils
7. lymphangi/o; lymphatic vessel
8. splen/o; spleen
9. lymphaden/o; lymph node
10. tonsill/o; tonsil
11. thym/o; thymus gland
12. lymphangitis (*lim-fan-JĪ-tis*); also, lymphangiitis (*lim-fan-jē-Ī-tis*)
13. lymphoma (*lim-FŌ-ma*)
14. lymphadenopathy (*lim-fad-e-NOP-a-thē*)
15. splenomegaly (*splē-nō-MEG-a-lē*)
16. thymic (*THĪ-mik*)
17. tonsillitis (*ton-si-LĪ-tis*)

Chapter Review

LABELING EXERCISE

The Cardiovascular System

1. right atrium
2. right ventricle
3. left pulmonary artery
4. left lung
5. right lung
6. left pulmonary vein
7. left atrium
8. left ventricle
9. aorta
10. head and arms
11. superior vena cava
12. internal organs
13. legs
14. inferior vena cava

The Heart and Great Vessels

1. superior vena cava
2. inferior vena cava
3. right atrium
4. right AV (tricuspid) valve
5. right ventricle
6. pulmonary valve
7. pulmonary artery
8. right pulmonary artery (branches)
9. left pulmonary artery (branches)
10. left pulmonary veins
11. right pulmonary veins
12. left atrium
13. left AV (mitral) valve
14. left ventricle
15. aortic valve
16. ascending aorta
17. aortic arch
18. brachiocephalic artery
19. left common carotid artery
20. left subclavian artery
21. apex
22. interventricular septum
23. endocardium

24. myocardium
25. epicardium

Location of Lymphoid Tissue

1. nodes
2. tonsils
3. thymus gland
4. spleen
5. appendix
6. Peyer patches (in intestine)

TERMINOLOGY

1. c
2. a
3. e
4. b
5. d
6. b
7. c
8. e
9. a
10. d
11. e
12. a
13. b
14. c
15. d
16. c
17. a
18. d
19. b
20. e
21. b
22. e
23. d
24. a
25. c
26. atrium
27. capillaries
28. myocardium
29. aorta
30. sinoatrial (SA) node
31. right atrium
32. varicose vein, varix
33. thymus gland
34. vein
35. common iliac (*IL-ē-ak*) arteries
36. common carotid (*ka-ROT-id*) artery
37. inferior vena cava
38. subclavian veins
39. T
40. F; pulmonary circuit
41. F; vein
42. T
43. F; left ventricle
44. T
45. F; arm
46. T
47. T
48. apex; The *apex* is the pointed lower region of the heart; the others are part of the heart's conduction system.

49. murmur; A *murmur* is an abnormal heart sound; the others are terms associated with blood pressure.
50. S$_1$; S$_1$ symbolizes the first heart sound; the others are waves of the ECG.
51. cusp; A *cusp* is a flap of a heart valve; the others are lymphoid tissue.
52. without vessels
53. incision of an atrium
54. surgical removal of the spleen
55. above a ventricle
56. dilatation of a vein
57. cardiologist
58. arteriorrhaphy (*ar-tēr-ē-OR-a-fē*)
59. splenopexy (*SPLĒ-nō-pek-sē*)
60. valvotome; valvulotome (*VAL-vō-tōm; VAL-vū-lō-tōm*)
61. lymphostasis (*lim-FOS-ta-sis*)
62. lymphadenectomy (*lim-fad-e-NEK-tō-mē*)
63. aortoptosis (*ā-or-top-TŌ-sis*)
64. aortostenosis (*ā-or-tō-ste-NŌ-sis*)
65. aortogram (*ā-OR-tō-gram*)
66. preaortic (*prē-ā-OR-tik*)
67. atrial
68. thymic
69. venous
70. septal
71. sclerotic
72. splenic; splenetic
73. thrombi
74. varices
75. stenoses
76. septa
77. automated external defibrillator
78. left ventricular assist device
79. deep vein thrombosis
80. ventricular fibrillation
81. bundle branch block
82. percutaneous transluminal coronary angioplasty
83. angiitis; angitis
84. lymphadenopathy
85. lymphoma
86. angioplasty
87. lymphangiitis; lymphangitis
88. angiopathy
89. lymphadenitis
90. lymphadenoma
91. angioma
92. excision of the inner layer of an artery thickened by atherosclerosis
   a. within
   b. artery
   c. out
   d. to cut
93. permanent dilation of small blood vessels causing small, local red lesions
   a. end
   b. vessel
   c. dilation

94. inflammation of lymphatic vessels
    and veins
    a. lymphatic system
    b. vessel
    c. vein
    d. inflammation

Case Study Questions

1. diaphoresis
2. sublingual
3. stress test
4. cardiovascular
5. endarterectomies
6. murmur
7. cyanosis
8. stenosis
9. interatrial
10. substernal
11. d
12. b
13. c
14. e
15. a
16. e
17. a
18. coronary/cardiac care unit
19. acute myocardial infarction
20. coronary artery disease
21. left anterior descending
22. congestive heart failure
23. transesophageal echocardiogram
24. mitral valve replacement

Chapter 10

Pretest

1. c
2. c
3. d
4. b
5. a
6. c
7. b

Chapter Exercises

EXERCISE 10-1

1. excess albumin in the blood
2. decreased protein in the blood
3. deficiency of leukocytes (white blood cells)
4. production of erythrocytes (red blood cells)
5. presence of toxins (poisons) in the blood
6. presence of bacteria in the blood
7. deficiency of platelets (thrombocytes)
8. pyemia (*pī-Ē-mē-a*)
9. viremia (*vī-RĒ-mē-a*)
10. leukemia (*lū-KĒ-mē-a*)

EXERCISE 10-2

1. hemat/o; blood
2. myel/o; bone marrow
3. thromb/o; blood clot
4. immun/o; immunity
5. hem/o; blood
6. blood
7. bone marrow
8. erythrocytes; red blood cells
9. immunity
10. platelets; thrombocytes
11. leukocytes; white blood cells
12. blood cells
13. lymphocytes
14. blood
15. lymphoblast (*LIM-fō-blast*)
16. myeloma (*mī-e-LŌ-ma*)
17. erythropenia (*e-rith-rō-PĒ-nē-a*); also, erythrocytopenia
18. thrombolysis (*throm-BOL-i-sis*)
19. myelopoiesis (*mī-e-lō-poy-Ē-sis*)
20. granulocytosis (*gran-ū-lō-sī-TŌ-sis*)
21. lymphocytosis (*lim-fō-sī-TŌ-sis*)
22. erythrocytosis (*e-rith-rō-sī-TŌ-sis*)
23. monocytosis (*mon-ō-sī-TŌ-sis*)
24. thrombocytosis (*throm-bō-sī-TŌ-sis*)

EXERCISE 10-3

1. iron
2. potassium
3. nitrogenous compounds
4. oxygen
5. iron
6. calcium
7. kalemia (*ka-LĒ-mē-a*)
8. azotemia (*az-ō-TĒ-mē-a*)
9. natremia (*nā-TRĒ-mē-a*)
10. calcemia (*kal-SĒ-mē-a*)

Chapter Review

LABELING EXERCISE
Blood Cells

1. platelet
2. leukocyte
3. erythrocyte

Leukocytes (White Blood Cells)

1. neutrophil
2. eosinophil
3. basophil
4. lymphocyte
5. monocyte

TERMINOLOGY

1. c
2. a
3. e
4. b
5. d
6. b
7. c
8. a
9. e
10. d
11. b
12. e
13. a
14. d
15. c
16. b
17. e
18. d
19. a
20. c
21. d
22. c
23. a
24. e
25. b
26. phagocytosis
27. hemoglobin
28. electrolyte
29. platelets (thrombocytes)
30. blood cells
31. oxygen
32. blood
33. anemia
34. bone marrow
35. F; thrombocyte
36. T
37. T
38. T
39. F; neutrophil
40. T
41. increase in leukocytes (white blood cells) in the blood
42. increase in eosinophils in the blood
43. increase in erythrocytes (red blood cells) in the blood
44. increase in thrombocytes (platelets) in the blood
45. increase in neutrophils in the blood
46. increase in monocytes in the blood
47. erythroblast; erythrocytoblast
48. thrombocytopenia; thrombopenia
49. pyemia
50. immunologist
51. hemorrhage
52. septicemic (*sep-ti-SĒ-mik*)
53. lymphocytic (*lim-fō-SIT-ik*)
54. basophilic (*bā-sō-FIL-ik*)
55. hemolytic (*hē-mō-LIT-ik*)
56. thrombotic (*throm-BOT-ik*)
57. leukemic (*lū-KĒ-mik*)
58. presence of viruses in the blood
59. deficiency of neutrophils
60. substance that is toxic (poisonous) to bone marrow
61. immunity to one's own tissue
62. deficiency of oxygen in the blood
63. thrombolysis; *Thrombolysis* is destruction of a blood clot; the others pertain to formation of a blood clot.

64. EPO; *EPO* is erythropoietin, a hormone that stimulates red cell production in the bone marrow; the others are abbreviations for blood tests.
65. reticulocyte; A *reticulocyte* is an immature red blood cell; the others are types of leukocytes.
66. gamma globulin; *Gamma globulin* is the fraction of the blood plasma that contains antibodies; the others are terms associated with exaggerated immune responses.
67. leukocytic
68. leukoblast
69. myeloid
70. myelogenic
71. myeloblast
72. leukemia
73. leukopenia; leukocytopenia
74. myeloma
75. leukopoiesis; leukocytopoiesis
76. myelocytic
77. overall decrease in blood cells
    a. all
    b. cell
    c. deficiency
78. increase in the number of red cells in the blood; erythremia, erythrocythemia
    a. many
    b. cell
    c. blood
    d. condition of
79. unequal distribution of hemoglobin in red cells
    a. without
    b. same, equal
    c. color
    d. condition of
80. pertaining to dysfunctional bone marrow
    a. bone marrow
    b. abnormal
    c. formation
    d. condition of

Case Study Questions

1. b
2. c
3. d
4. b
5. b
6. e
7. d
8. d
9. c
10. a
11. c
12. e
13. b

14. b
15. c
16. d
17. e
18. b
19. a
20. immunoglobulin
21. hemoglobin
22. hematocrit
23. fresh frozen plasma
24. prothrombin time
25. partial thromboplastin time
26. disseminated intravascular coagulation

Chapter 11

Pretest

1. a
2. b
3. b
4. a
5. d
6. b
7. c
8. a

Chapter Exercises

EXERCISE 11-1

1. apnea (*AP-nē-a*)
2. dyspnea (*disp-NĒ-a*)
3. eupnea (*ūp-NĒ-a*)
4. bradypnea (*brad-ip-NĒ-a*)
5. apneic (*ap-NĒ-ik*)
6. dyspneic (*disp-NĒ-ik*)
7. eupneic (*ūp-NE-ik*)
8. bradypneic (*brad-ip-NĒ-ik*)
9. aphonia (*a-FŌ-nē-a*)
10. hypocapnia (*hī-pō-KAP-nē-a*)
11. anoxia (*an-OK-sē-a*)
12. eucapnia (*ū-KAP-nē-a*)

EXERCISE 11-2

1. rhinorrhea (*rī-nō-RĒ-a*)
2. pharyngeal (*fa-RIN-jē-al*)
3. laryngoscopy (*lar-ing-GŌS-kō-pē*)
4. pharyngitis (*far-in-JĪ-tis*)
5. laryngoplasty (*la-RING-gō-plas-tē*)
6. tracheotomy (*trā-kē-OT-ō-mē*)
7. bronchostenosis (*brong-kō-ste-NŌ-sis*); bronchoconstriction (*brong-kō-kon-STRIK-shun*)
8. bronchiolitis (*brong-kē-ō-LĪ-tis*)
9. pertaining to the nose and pharynx
10. within the trachea
11. around a bronchus
12. near the nose
13. pertaining to the bronchioles
14. dilatation of a bronchus

EXERCISE 11-3

1. pain in the pleura
2. within the lungs
3. surgical removal of a lung or lung tissue
4. plastic repair of a lung
5. study of the lungs
6. absence of a lung
7. surgical incision of the phrenic nerve
8. intrapleural (*in-tra-PLŪ-ral*)
9. supraphrenic (*sū-pra-FREN-ik*)
10. pleurocentesis (*plū-rō-sen-TĒ-sis*)
11. pneumonopathy (*nū-mō-NOP-a-thē*)
12. phrenicotripsy (*fren-i-kō-TRIP-sē*)
13. spirogram (*SPĪ-rō-gram*)

Chapter Review

LABELING EXERCISE
Respiratory System

1. frontal sinus
2. sphenoidal sinus
3. nasal cavity
4. nasopharynx
5. oropharynx
6. laryngeal pharynx
7. larynx and vocal cords
8. epiglottis
9. esophagus
10. trachea
11. right lung
12. left lung
13. mediastinum
14. right bronchus
15. terminal bronchiole
16. alveolar duct
17. alveoli
18. capillaries
19. diaphragm

TERMINOLOGY

1. d
2. c
3. e
4. a
5. b
6. e
7. a
8. b
9. c
10. d
11. c
12. a
13. d
14. e
15. b
16. d
17. c
18. a
19. b
20. e
21. c

22. a
23. e
24. b
25. d
26. smell
27. carbon dioxide
28. diaphragm
29. pleura
30. alveoli
31. bronchi
32. lungs
33. tuberculosis
34. mucus
35. coughing
36. septum
37. tidal volume
38. apnea
39. residual volume
40. T
41. T
42. F; larynx
43. F; three
44. T
45. T
46. phrenicotomy (fren-i-KOT-ō-mē)
47. pleurocele (PLŪ-rō-sēl)
48. pharyngitis (far-in-JĪ-tis)
49. bronchiolitis (brong-kē-ō-LĪ-tis)
50. tracheostomy (tra-kē-OS-tō-mē)
51. accumulation of air or gas in the pleural space
52. accumulation of blood in the pleural space
53. accumulation of pus in the pleural space
54. accumulation of fluid in the pleural space
55. narrowing of a bronchus
56. pain in the pleura
57. deficiency of oxygen in the tissues
58. any disease of the lungs
59. rapid rate of respiration
60. dilatation of the bronchi
61. plastic repair of the nose
62. dryness of the throat
63. spir/o; breathing
64. pulmon/o; lung
65. py/o; pus
66. phren/o; diaphragm
67. pneum/o; pertaining to air or gas
68. extrapulmonary
69. hypercapnia
70. expiration
71. bradypnea
72. intubation
73. pharyngeal
74. alveolar
75. nasal
76. tracheal
77. pleural
78. bronchial
79. nares

80. pleurae
81. alveoli
82. conchae
83. bronchi
84. tonsil; A *tonsil* is lymphatic tissue in the pharynx; the others are parts of the nose.
85. sinus; A *sinus* is a cavity or channel; the others are parts of the larynx.
86. asthma; *Asthma* is a chronic breathing problem caused by allergy and other factors; the others are infectious diseases.
87. URI; *URI* is an abbreviation for "upper respiratory infection"; the others are abbreviations for lobes of the lung.
88. oximetry
89. eupnea
90. hypophonia
91. hyperpnea
92. eucapnia
93. dyspnea
94. hypoxia
95. dysphonia
96. hypercapnia
97. hyperphonia
98. device for measuring air flow
    a. air
    b. rapid, swift
    c. measure
99. incomplete expansion of the alveoli
    a. incomplete
    b. expansion, dilation
100. presence of air or gas in a blood vessel of the heart
    a. air, gas
    b. heart
    c. condition of
101. respiratory disease caused by inhalation of dust particles
    a. lung
    b. dust
    c. condition of

Case Study Questions

1. b
2. c
3. d
4. b
5. d
6. e
7. wheezing
8. bronchodilator
9. lobectomy
10. diaphoresis
11. thoracotomy
12. thoracoscopy
13. hemithorax
14. mediastinoscopy

15. ventilation
16. chronic obstructive pulmonary disease
17. forced vital capacity
18. arterial blood gas
19. acute respiratory distress syndrome
20. do not resuscitate

Chapter 12

Pretest

1. d
2. c
3. a
4. c
5. a
6. b
7. c
8. c
9. a

Chapter Exercises

EXERCISE 12-1

1. oral (OR-al); stomal (STŌ-mal)
2. labial (LĀ-bē-al)
3. buccal (BUK-al)
4. dental (DEN-tal)
5. gingival (JIN-ji-val)
6. lingual (LING-gwal); glossal (GLOS-sal)
7. mouth
8. teeth
9. teeth
10. jaw
11. mouth
12. tongue
13. salivary
14. outside the cheek
15. under the tongue
16. pertaining to the lip and teeth
17. inflammation of the gums
18. dropping of the uvula
19. under the tongue
20. suture of the palate

EXERCISE 12-2

1. gastric (GAS-trik)
2. enteric (en-TER-ik)
3. pyloric (pī-LOR-ik)
4. colic (KOL-ik); also colonic (kō-LON-ik)
5. duodenal (dū-ō-DĒ-nal)
6. jejunal (je-JUN-al)
7. ileal (IL-ē-al)
8. cecal (SĒ-kal)
9. anal (Ā-nal)
10. esophagitis (ē-sof-a-JĪ-tis)
11. gastropexy (GAS-trō-pek-sē)
12. gastroenterology (gas-trō-en-ter-OL-ō-jē)

13. duodenoscopy (*dū-ō-de-NOS-kō-pē*)
14. pyloroptosis (*pī-lor-ō-TŌ-sis*)
15. jejunostomy (*je-jū-NOS-tō-mē*)
16. ileectomy (*il-ē-EK-tō-mē*)
17. anorectal (*ā-nō-REK-tal*)
18. colitis (*kō-LĪ-tis*)
19. colostomy (*kō-LOS-tō-mē*)
20. colopexy (*KŌ-lō-pek-sē*)
21. colocentesis (*kō-lō-sen-TĒ-sis*)
22. colonopathy (*kō-lō-NOP-a-thē*)
23. colonoscopy (*kō-lon-OS-kō-pē*)
24. esophagogastrostomy
    (*ē-sof-a-gō-gas-TROS-tō-mē*)
25. gastroenterostomy
    (*gas-trō-en-ter-OS-tō-mē*)
26. gastrojejunostomy
    (*gas-trō-je-jū-NOS-tō-mē*)
27. duodenoileostomy
    (*dū-ō-dē-nō-il-ē-OS-tō-mē*)
28. sigmoidoproctostomy
    (*sig-moy-dō-prok-TOS-tō-mē*)

EXERCISE 12-3

1. hepatic (*he-PAT-ik*)
2. cholecystic (*kō-lē-SIS-tik*)
3. pancreatic (*pan-krē-AT-ik*)
4. pancreatography
    (*pan-krē-a-TOG-ra-fē*)
5. cholangiography
    (*kō-lan-jē-OG-ra-fē*)
6. cholecystography
    (*kō-lē-sis-TOG-ra-fē*)
7. hepatography (*hep-a-TOG-ra-fē*)
8. choledocholithiasis
    (*kō-led-o-kō-li-THĪ-a-sis*)
9. pancreatolithiasis
    (*pan-krē-a-tō-li-THĪ-a-sis*)
10. hepatitis (*hep-a-TĪ-tis*)
11. bile
12. gallstone; biliary calculus
13. common bile duct
14. gallbladder
15. liver
16. bile duct
17. pancreas

Chapter Review

LABELING EXERCISE

The Digestive System

1. mouth
2. pharynx
3. esophagus
4. stomach
5. duodenum (of small intestine)
6. small intestine
7. cecum
8. ascending colon
9. transverse colon
10. descending colon
11. sigmoid colon
12. rectum
13. anus

14. parotid salivary gland
15. sublingual salivary gland
16. submandibular salivary gland
17. liver (cut)
18. gallbladder
19. pancreas

Accessory Organs of Digestion

1. liver
2. common hepatic duct
3. gallbladder
4. cystic duct
5. common bile duct
6. pancreas
7. pancreatic duct
8. duodenum
9. spleen
10. diaphragm

TERMINOLOGY

1. d
2. c
3. b
4. e
5. a
6. e
7. d
8. a
9. b
10. c
11. e
12. a
13. d
14. b
15. c
16. c
17. a
18. d
19. e
20. b
21. d
22. e
23. a
24. c
25. b
26. liver
27. gallbladder
28. cecum
29. tongue
30. palate
31. tooth
32. cheek
33. intestine
34. liver
35. bile
36. periodontist
37. gastrectomy
38. palatorrhaphy
39. pylorostenosis
40. pancreatitis
41. gastroenterologist
42. colostomy

43. gastroduodenostomy
44. intrahepatic
45. diverticula
46. gingivae
47. calculi
48. anastomoses
49. F; above
50. F; jejunum
51. F; saliva
52. T
53. T
54. T
55. villus; A *villus* is a tiny projection
    in the lining of the small intestine
    that aids in absorption of nutrients;
    the others are parts of the mouth.
56. spleen; The *spleen* is a lymphatic
    organ; the others are parts of the
    large intestine.
57. pylorus; The *pylorus* is the distal
    portion of the stomach; the others
    are accessory digestive organs.
58. amylase; *Amylase* is a starch-
    digesting enzyme; the others are
    disorders of the digestive tract.
59. total parenteral nutrition
60. gastroesophageal reflux disease
61. gastrointestinal
62. hydrochloric acid
63. percutaneous endoscopic
    gastrostomy (tube)
64. hepatitis A virus
65. cecitis
66. proctorrhaphy
67. ileopexy
68. proctocele
69. ileocecal
70. cecopexy
71. proctitis
72. ileorrhaphy
73. ileitis
74. pertaining to the muscular coat of
    the intestine
    a. muscle
    b. intestine
    c. pertaining to
75. radiography of the biliary tract and
    gallbladder using radionuclides
    a. bile
    b. spark (radiation)
    c. act of recording data
76. referring to any route other than
    the alimentary canal
    a. beside
    b. intestine
    c. pertaining to

Case Study Questions

1. c
2. d
3. a
4. e

5. d
6. a
7. c
8. b
9. c
10. d
11. b
12. e
13. b
14. endoscopic retrograde cholangiopancreatography
15. right upper quadrant
16. nasogastric
17. inflammatory bowel disease
18. duodenal
19. mesenteric
20. focal
21. exudate
22. occult blood
23. icterus
24. antiemetic
25. cholelithiasis
26. laparoscopic cholecystectomy
27. cholecystitis
28. cholangiogram
29. sphincter
30. biopsy

Chapter 13

Pretest

1. d
2. c
3. a
4. a
5. b
6. d
7. d
8. b

Chapter Exercises

EXERCISE 13-1

1. postrenal (*pōst-RĒ-nal*)
2. prerenal (*prē-RĒ-nal*)
3. interrenal (*in-ter-RĒ-nal*)
4. perirenal (*per-i-RĒ-nal*); circumrenal (*sir-kum-RĒ-nal*)
5. nephrology (*ne-FROL-ō-jē*)
6. nephropathy (*ne-FROP-a-thē*)
7. nephrotoxic (*nef-rō-TOK-sik*)
8. nephromalacia (*nef-rō-ma-LĀ-shē-a*)
9. nephrectomy (*ne-FREK-tō-mē*)
10. glomerulitis (*glō-mer-ū-LĪ-tis*)
11. caliectasis (*kā-lē-EK-ta-sis*); calicectasis (*kal-i-SEK-ta-sis*)
12. pyeloplasty (*pī-e-lō-PLAS-tē*)
13. pyelogram (*PĪ-e-lō-gram*)
14. renography (*rē-NOG-ra-fē*); nephrography (*ne-FROG-ra-fē*)

15. calicotomy (*kal-i-KOT-ō-mē*); caliotomy (*kā-lē-OT-ō-mē*)
16. glomerulosclerosis (*glo-mer-ū-lō-skle-RŌ-sis*)
17. pyelonephritis (*pi-e-lō-nef-RĪ-tis*)

EXERCISE 13-2

1. urology (*ū-ROL-ō-jē*)
2. urography (*ū-ROG-ra-fē*)
3. urolith (*Ū-rō-lith*)
4. uremia (*ū-RĒ-mē-a*)
5. anuria (*an-Ū-rē-a*)
6. dysuria (*dis-Ū-rē-a*)
7. polyuria (*pol-ē-Ū-rē-a*)
8. cyturia (*sī-TŪ-rē-a*)
9. hematuria (*hē-ma-TŪ-rē-a*)
10. diuresis (*dī-ū-RĒ-sis*)
11. anuresis (*an-ū-RĒ-sis*)
12. natriuresis (*nā-trē-ū-RĒ-sis*)
13. kaliuresis (*kā-lē-ū-RĒ-sis*)
14. urethropexy (*ū-RĒ-thrō-pek-sē*)
15. ureterostomy (*ū-rē-ter-OS-tō-mē*)
16. ureterolith (*ū-RĒ-ter-ō-lith*)
17. urethroscopy (*ū-rē-THROS-kō-pē*)
18. cystitis (*sis-TĪ-tis*)
19. cystopexy (*SIS-tō-pek-sē*)
20. cystoscope (*SIS-tō-skōp*)
21. cystotomy (*sis-TOT-ō-mē*)
22. supravesical (*sū-pra-VES-i-kal*)
23. urethrovesical (*ū-rē-thrō-VES-i-kal*)
24. pain in the urinary bladder
25. surgical incision of the ureter
26. through the urethra
27. formation of urine

Chapter Review

LABELING EXERCISE

Urinary System

1. right kidney
2. adrenal gland
3. abdominal aorta
4. renal artery
5. common iliac artery
6. common iliac vein
7. renal vein
8. inferior vena cava
9. right ureter
10. urinary bladder
11. urethra
12. prostate gland

The Kidney

1. renal capsule
2. renal cortex
3. renal medulla
4. pyramids of medulla
5. nephrons
6. calyx
7. hilum
8. renal pelvis
9. ureter

The Urinary Bladder

1. ureter
2. smooth muscle
3. openings of ureters
4. trigone
5. urethra
6. internal urethral sphincter
7. external urethral sphincter
8. prostate

TERMINOLOGY

1. d
2. c
3. a
4. e
5. b
6. d
7. e
8. b
9. a
10. c
11. d
12. b
13. e
14. a
15. c
16. e
17. d
18. a
19. b
20. c
21. nephron
22. glomerulus
23. renin
24. urination; voiding of urine
25. urinalysis
26. urea
27. F; kidney
28. T
29. T
30. F; cortex
31. F; urethra
32. T
33. T
34. F; potassium
35. near the kidney
36. painful or difficult urination
37. toxic or poisonous to the kidney
38. near the glomerulus
39. surgical removal of a calyx
40. narrowing of a urethra
41. pyelocaliectasis; pyelocalicectasis
42. nephromalacia
43. cystectomy
44. nephropathy
45. cystourethrogram
46. ureteropyeloplasty
47. pyelonephritis
48. ureterosigmoidostomy
49. cast; A *cast* is a solid mold of a renal nephron; the others are parts of the kidney.

50. calyx; A *calyx* is a collecting region for urine in the kidney; the others are parts of a nephron.
51. specific gravity; *Specific gravity* is a measure of density; the others are treatment procedures for the urinary system.
52. dehydration
53. hypovolemia
54. antidiuretic
55. hypernatremia
56. anuresis
57. caliceal; calyceal
58. urologic
59. uremic
60. diuretic
61. nephrotic
62. ureteral
63. urethral
64. pelves
65. calyces
66. glomeruli
67. urography
68. renal
69. intrarenal
70. renography
71. intravesical
72. suprarenal
73. urology
74. interrenal
75. vesical
76. urolith
77. intravenous pyelography
78. antidiuretic hormone
79. erythropoietin
80. intravenous urography
81. sodium
82. glomerular filtration rate
83. urinalysis
84. removal of substances from the blood by passage through a semipermeable membrane
    a. blood
    b. through
    c. separation
85. test that measures and records bladder function
    a. urinary bladder
    b. measure
    c. act of recording data
86. surgical creation of a new passage between a ureter and the bladder
    a. ureter
    b. new
    c. bladder
    d. surgical creation of an opening

Case Study Questions

1. c
2. d
3. a
4. a

5. d
6. IV urogram
7. oliguria
8. nocturia
9. ureteral laser lithotripsy
10. kidney transplant
11. lithotomy
12. urinary tract infection
13. continuous ambulatory peritoneal dialysis
14. blood urea nitrogen
15. end-stage renal disease
16. human immunodeficiency virus
17. cystometrogram
18. physiologic saline solution
19. extracorporeal shock-wave lithotripsy

Chapter 14

Pretest

1. c
2. a
3. d
4. b
5. d
6. a
7. d

Chapter Exercises

EXERCISE 14-1

1. pertaining to semen
2. pain in the testis
3. plastic repair of the scrotum
4. excision of the epididymis
5. pain in the prostate
6. any disease of a testis
7. inflammation of the testis and epididymis
8. orchiopexy (*or-kē-ō-PEK-sē*); also, orchidopexy (*or-ki-dō-PEK-sē*)
9. orchioplasty (*OR-kē-ō-plas-tē*); also, orchidoplasty (*OR-ki-dō-plas-tē*)
10. orchiotomy (*or-kē-OT-ō-mē*); also, orchidotomy (*or-ki-DOT-ō-mē*)
11. spermatocyte (*sper-MA-tō-sīt*)
12. spermatolysis (*sper-ma-TOL-i-sis*)
13. spermatorrhea (*sper-ma-to-RĒ-a*)
14. spermatogenesis (*sper-ma-tō-JEN-e-sis*)
15. spermaturia (*sper-ma-TŪ-rē-a*)
16. aspermia (*a-SPER-mē-a*)
17. hemospermia (*hē-mō-SPER-mē-a*); also, hematospermia (*hem-at-ō-SPER-mē-a*)
18. oligospermia (*ol-i-gō-SPER-mē-a*)
19. pyospermia (*pī-ō-SPER-mē-a*)
20. vasectomy (*va-SEK-tō-mē*)
21. oscheoma (*os-kē-Ō-ma*)
22. vasorrhaphy (*vas-OR-a-fē*)

23. prostatectomy (*pros-ta-TEK-tō-mē*)
24. vesiculography (*ve-sik-ū-LOG-ra-fē*)
25. vesiculitis (*ve-sik-ū-LĪ-tis*)
26. epididymotomy (*ep-i-did-i-MOT-ō-mē*)

Chapter Review

LABELING EXERCISE

Male Reproductive System

1. testis
2. epididymis
3. scrotum
4. ductus (vas) deferens
5. ejaculatory duct
6. urethra
7. penis
8. glans penis
9. prepuce (foreskin)
10. seminal vesicle
11. prostate
12. bulbourethral (Cowper) gland
13. kidney
14. ureter
15. urinary bladder
16. peritoneal cavity
17. rectum
18. anus

TERMINOLOGY

1. e
2. d
3. a
4. b
5. c
6. d
7. e
8. b
9. a
10. c
11. b
12. e
13. a
14. d
15. c
16. e
17. a
18. d
19. c
20. b
21. testis
22. scrotum
23. semen
24. testosterone
25. inguinal canal
26. epididymis
27. suture of the vas (ductus) deferens
28. absence of a testis
29. tumor of the scrotum
30. incision of the seminal vesicle
31. instrument for measuring the prostate
32. presence of blood in the semen

33. prostatotomy
34. oscheolith
35. orchiopexy; orchidopexy
36. oscheoplasty
37. vasovasostomy
38. T
39. F; scrotum
40. T
41. T
42. F; urethra
43. T
44. T
45. spermatic cord; The *spermatic cord* suspends the testis in the scrotum and contains the ductus deferens, nerves, and vessels; the others are the glands that contribute to semen.
46. semen; *Semen* is the secretion that transports spermatozoa; the others are hormones active in reproduction.
47. hernia; A *hernia* is a protrusion of tissue through an abnormal body opening; the others are sexually transmitted infections.
48. seminal
49. prostatic
50. penile
51. urethral
52. scrotal
53. hepatitis B virus
54. sexually transmitted infection
55. testicular self-examination
56. gonococcus
57. prostate-specific antigen
58. genitourinary
59. vasoplasty
60. spermatolysis
61. vesicular
62. vasography
63. vesiculitis
64. spermatic
65. spermatocyte
66. vasotomy
67. spermatogenesis
68. vesiculography
69. removal of a hydrocele by fluid drainage or partial excision
    a. fluid, water
    b. hernia, localized dilatation
    c. out
    d. cut
    e. condition of
70. destructive to sperm cells
    a. sperm
    b. agent that kills
    c. pertaining to
71. undescended testis
    a. hidden
    b. testis
    c. condition of

72. inflammation of the ductus deferens and seminal vesicle
    a. vas (ductus) deferens
    b. seminal vesicle
    c. inflammation

Case Study Questions

1. d
2. a
3. c
4. d
5. c
6. a
7. c
8. bilateral inguinal herniorrhaphy
9. strangulated hernia
10. prostatitis
11. intravesical
12. balanitis
13. phimosis
14. benign prostatic hyperplasia
15. transurethral resection of the prostate
16. bladder neck obstruction
17. urinary tract infection

Chapter 15

Pretest

1. c
2. b
3. d
4. a
5. b
6. c
7. d
8. a
9. c

Chapter Exercises

EXERCISE 15-1

1. any disease of women
2. between menstruation periods
3. formation of an ovum
4. release of an ovum from the ovary
5. pertaining to an ovary
6. inflammation of an ovary
7. gynecologist (*gī-ne-KOL-ō-jist*)
8. ovulatory (*OV-ū-la-tō-rē*)
9. menorrhagia (*men-ō-RĀ-jē-a*)
10. dysmenorrhea (*DIS-men-ō-rē-a*)
11. amenorrhea (*a-men-ō-RĒ-a*)
12. oligomenorrhea (*ol-i-gō-men-ō-RĒ-a*)
13. ovariorrhexis (*ō-var-ē-ō-REK-sis*)
14. ovariocentesis (*ō-var-ē-ō-sen-TĒ-sis*)
15. ovariocele (*o-VAR-ē-ō-sēl*)
16. oophorotomy (*ō-of-ō-ROT-ō-mē*)
17. oophoroma (*ō-of-ō-RŌ-ma*)

EXERCISE 15-2

1. within the cervix
2. pertaining to the uterus and urinary bladder
3. excision of an oviduct
4. pain in the vagina
5. plastic repair of the vagina
6. softening of the uterus
7. endoscopic examination of the uterus
8. salpingopexy (*sal-PING-gō-pek-sē*)
9. salpingography (*sal-ping-GOG-ra-fē*)
10. hydrosalpinx (*hī-drō-SAL-pinx*)
11. pyosalpinx (*pī-ō-SAL-pinx*)
12. salpingo-oophorectomy (*sal-ping-gō-ō-of-ō-REK-tō-mē*); also, salpingo-ovariectomy (*sal-ping-gō-ō-var-ē-EK-tō-me*)
13. hysteropexy (*his-ter-ō-PEK-sē*)
14. metroptosis (*mē-trō-TŌ-sis*)
15. transcervical (*trans-SER-vi-kal*)
16. metrostenosis (*mē-trō-ste-NŌ-sis*)
17. hysterosalpingogram (*his-ter-ō-sal-PING-gō-gram*)
18. uterine (*Ū-ter-in*)
19. colpocele (*KOL-pō-sēl*)
20. vaginitis (*vaj-i-NĪ-tis*)

EXERCISE 15-3

1. vulvopathy (*vul-VOP-a-thē*)
2. episiorrhaphy (*e-piz-ē-OR-a-fē*)
3. vaginoperineal (*vaj-i-nō-per-i-NĒ-al*)
4. clitoritis (*klit-o-RĪ-tis*)
5. mammogram (*MAM-ō-gram*)
6. mastitis (*mas-TĪ-tis*)
7. mastectomy (*mas-TEK-tō-mē*); also, mammectomy (*ma-MEK-tō-mē*)

EXERCISE 15-4

1. before birth
2. formation of an embryo
3. pertaining to a newborn
4. endoscopic examination of the fetus
5. developing in one amniotic sac
6. lack of milk production
7. excess secretion of milk
8. embryology (*em-brē-OL-ō-jē*)
9. neonatology (*nē-ō-nā-TOL-ō-jē*)
10. embryopathy (*em-brē-OP-a-thē*)
11. amniocyte (*AM-nē-ō-sīt*)
12. amniotomy (*am-nē-OT-ō-mē*)
13. fetoscope (*FĒ-tō-skōp*)
14. amniorrhexis (*am-nē-ō-REK-sis*)
15. postnatal (*pōst-NĀ-tal*)
16. primigravida (*pri-mi-GRAV-i-da*)
17. multigravida (*mul-ti-GRAV-i-da*)
18. nullipara (*nul-IP-a-ra*)
19. primipara (*pri-MIP-a-ra*)
20. xerotocia (*zē-rō-TŌ-sē-a*)

21. bradytocia (*brad-ē-TŌ-sē-a*)
22. galactorrhea (*ga-lak-tō-RE-a*); also, lactorrhea (*lak-tō-RE-a*)
23. galactocele (*ga-LAK-to-sēl*); also, lactocele (*LAK-tō-sēl*)

Chapter Review

LABELING EXERCISE
Female Reproductive System
1. ovary
2. fimbriae
3. oviduct (fallopian tube)
4. uterus
5. cervix
6. posterior fornix
7. vagina
8. clitoris
9. labium minus
10. labium majus
11. urinary bladder
12. urethra
13. rectum
14. anus
15. peritoneal cavity
16. cul-de-sac

Ovulation and Fertilization
1. ovary
2. fimbriae
3. ovum
4. sperm cells (spermatozoa)
5. oviduct (fallopian tube)
6. implanted embryo
7. body of uterus
8. cervix
9. vagina
10. greater vestibular (Bartholin) gland

TERMINOLOGY
1. b
2. d
3. e
4. a
5. c
6. d
7. c
8. e
9. a
10. b
11. c
12. a
13. b
14. e
15. d
16. b
17. d
18. c
19. e
20. a
21. b
22. c
23. e
24. a
25. d
26. ovary
27. ovum (egg cell)
28. placenta
29. lactation
30. abortion
31. uterus
32. breasts (mammary glands)
33. T
34. T
35. F; endometrium
36. F; corpus luteum
37. F; oviduct
38. T
39. T
40. F; embryo
41. behind the uterus
42. any disease of the uterus
43. softening of the uterus
44. pus in the oviduct
45. narrowing of the vagina
46. after birth
47. below the mammary gland (breast)
48. outside the embryo
49. woman who has never been pregnant
50. woman who has given birth three times
51. causing fetal abnormalities
52. salpingocele
53. episiorrhaphy
54. metrostenosis
55. hysterosalpingectomy
56. mammogram
57. dystocia
58. amniorrhexis
59. embryology
60. fetometry
61. newborn
62. primipara
63. nulligravida
64. postpartum
65. prenatal
66. eutocia
67. anovulatory
68. cervical
69. uterine
70. perineal
71. vaginal
72. embryonic
73. amniotic
74. ova
75. cervices
76. fimbriae
77. labia
78. labia majora; The *labia majora* are part of the vulva; the others are associated with pregnancy.
79. colostrum; *Colostrum* is the breast fluid released before milk is produced; the others are hormones involved in reproduction.
80. measles; *Measles* is an infectious disease; the others are hereditary disorders.
81. candidiasis; *Candidiasis* is a fungal infection; the others are procedures used to diagnose fetal abnormalities.
82. spina bifida; *Spina bifida* is a congenital spinal defect; the others are disorders of pregnancy.
83. episioplasty
84. cervicitis
85. mammography
86. mammoplasty
87. cervicography
88. episiotomy
89. intracervical
90. cervicoplasty
91. cervicotomy
92. transcervical
93. human chorionic gonadotropin
94. toxic shock syndrome
95. intrauterine device
96. dysfunctional uterine bleeding
97. last menstrual period
98. zygote intrafallopian transfer
99. gestational age
100. fetal heart rate
101. vaginal birth after cesarean section
102. prevention of blood vessel formation
   a. against
   b. vessel
   c. origin, formation
   d. condition of
103. excessive development of the mammary glands in the male, even to the secretion of milk
   a. woman
   b. breast
   c. condition of
104. extreme rapidity of labor
   a. sharp, acute
   b. labor
   c. condition of
105. a deficiency of amniotic fluid
   a. few, scanty
   b. fluid
   c. amnion

Case Study Questions
1. b
2. d
3. b
4. a
5. e
6. d
7. c
8. e
9. prolapsed
10. zygote

11. pelvimetry
12. fundus
13. Apgar score
14. placenta
15. dilatation and curettage
16. bilateral salpingo-oophorectomy
17. pelvic inflammatory disease
18. hormone replacement therapy
19. in vitro fertilization
20. cephalopelvic disproportion
21. obstetrics
22. gynecology
23. genitourinary

Chapter 16

Pretest

1. d
2. a
3. c
4. a
5. d
6. d

Chapter Exercises

EXERCISE 16-1

1. study of the endocrine glands or hormones
2. excision of the pituitary gland (hypophysis)
3. acting on the thyroid gland
4. condition of underactivity of the adrenal gland
5. inflammation of the pancreatic islets
6. hypothyroidism (hī-pō-THĪ-royd-izm)
7. hypoparathyroidism (hī-pō-par-a-THĪ-royd-izm)
8. hyperadrenalism (hī-per-a-DRĒ-nal-izm)
9. hyperadrenocorticism (hī-per-a-drē-nō-KOR-ti-sizm)
10. hypopituitarism (hī-pō-pi-TŪ-i-ta-rizm)
11. endocrinologist (en-dō-kri-NOL-ō-jist)
12. thyrotomy (thī-ROT-ō-mē); also, thyroidotomy (thī-roy-DOT-ō-mē)
13. adrenalopathy (a-drē-na-LOP-a-thē); also, adrenopathy (a-drē-NOP-a-thē)
14. adrenalitis (a-drē-nal-Ī-tis); also, adrenitis (a-dre-NĪ-tis)
15. insuloma (in-sū-LŌ-ma)

Chapter Review

LABELING EXERCISE

The Endocrine Glands

1. pineal
2. pituitary (hypophysis)

3. thyroid
4. parathyroids
5. thymus
6. adrenals
7. pancreatic islets
8. ovaries
9. testes

TERMINOLOGY

1. d
2. e
3. c
4. b
5. a
6. b
7. d
8. e
9. a
10. c
11. b
12. d
13. e
14. c
15. a
16. c
17. e
18. d
19. a
20. b
21. d
22. c
23. e
24. a
25. b
26. pituitary (hypophysis)
27. thyroid
28. adrenals
29. diabetes mellitus
30. hyperglycemia
31. enlargement of the adrenal gland
32. condition caused by underactivity of the pituitary gland
33. pertaining to the hypophysis (pituitary)
34. any disease of the adrenal gland
35. excision of the thyroid gland
36. physician who specializes in the study and treatment of endocrine disorders
37. insuloma
38. hypophysitis
39. adrenocortical
40. parathyroidectomy
41. hemithyroidectomy
42. thyroiditis
43. hyperadrenalism
44. thyrotropic
45. thyrolytic
46. thyropathy
47. F; ADH, antidiuretic hormone
48. T
49. F; medulla

50. F; calcium
51. F; thyroid
52. T
53. T
54. T
55. PTH; *PTH* is parathyroid hormone from the parathyroid gland; the others are hormones produced by the anterior pituitary.
56. dwarfism; *Dwarfism* is caused by hyposecretion of growth hormone: the others are caused by hypersecretion of hormones.
57. TBG; *TBG* is a test of thyroid function; the others are abbreviations associated with diabetes mellitus.
58. spleen; The *spleen* is part of the immune system; the others are endocrine glands.
59. insular
60. thyrotropic
61. adrenopathy
62. thyrolytic
63. insuloma
64. adrenomegaly
65. adrenal
66. thyromegaly
67. adrenotropic
68. thyropathy
69. benign tumor of the pituitary gland
    a. cranium
    b. pharynx (the tumor arises from tissue that forms the roof of the mouth)
    c. tumor, neoplasm
70. condition of complete underactivity of the pituitary gland
    a. all
    b. under, abnormally low
    c. pituitary gland
    d. condition of
71. usually benign tumor of the adrenal medulla or any cells that stain with chromium salts (chromaffin cells)
    a. dark, dusky
    b. color
    c. cell
    d. tumor, neoplasm
72. a toxic condition caused by hyperactivity of the thyroid gland
    a. thyroid
    b. poisonous
    c. condition of

Case Study Questions

1. b
2. a
3. d
4. a
5. c

6. d
7. a
8. b
9. c
10. e
11. jaundice
12. lipase
13. nephrectomy
14. adenoma
15. ampule
16. hyperglycemia
17. nothing by mouth/non per os
18. nasogastric
19. blood urea nitrogen
20. within normal limits
21. neutral protamine Hagedorn
22. continuous subcutaneous insulin infusion

Chapter 17

Pretest

1. b
2. c
3. a
4. c
5. a
6. c
7. b
8. c

Chapter Exercises

EXERCISE 17-1

1. pertaining to a nerve or the nervous system
2. pertaining to neuroglia, glial cells
3. pertaining to a spinal nerve root
4. pertaining to the meninges
5. pertaining to a ganglion
6. spinal cord
7. nervous system, nervous tissue
8. meninges
9. spinal nerve root
10. surgical removal of a ganglion
11. inflammation of many spinal nerve roots
12. destruction of a nerve or nervous tissue
13. tumor of the meninges
14. radiographic study of the spinal cord
15. glioma (glī-Ō-ma)
16. neuropathy (nū-ROP-a-thē)
17. myelitis (mī-e-LĪ-tis)
18. neuralgia (nū-RAL-jē-a)
19. myelogram (MĪ-e-lō-gram)

EXERCISE 17-2

1. brain
2. cerebrum, brain

3. thalamus
4. mind
5. stupor, unconsciousness
6. sleep
7. brain, cerebrum
8. cerebral (SER-e-bral)
9. cortical (KOR-ti-kal)
10. thalamic (tha-LAM-ik)
11. cerebellar (ser-e-BEL-ar)
12. ventricular (ven-TRIK-ū-lar)
13. study of the mind
14. pertaining to the brain and spinal cord
15. any disease of the brain
16. lack of sleep, inability to sleep
17. outside the medulla
18. incision of a ventricle
19. supracerebral (sū-pra-SER-e-bral)
20. encephalitis (en-sef-a-LĪ-tis)
21. intracerebellar (in-tra-ser-e-BEL-ar)
22. corticothalamic (kor-ti-kō-tha-LAM-ik)
23. ventriculogram (ven-TRIK-ū-lō-gram)

EXERCISE 17-3

1. tetraplegia (tet-ra-PLĒ-jē-a)
2. speech
3. read
4. seizures
5. partial paralysis, weakness
6. paralysis of the heart
7. lack of speech communication
8. difficulty in reading
9. obsession with fire
10. fear of women
11. partial paralysis or weakness of all four limbs
12. bradylalia (brad-ē-LĀ-lē-a)
13. hemiplegia (hem-i-PLĒ-jē-a)
14. noctiphobia (nok-ti-FŌ-bē-a); also, nyctophobia (nik-tō-FŌ-bē-a)
15. photophobia (fō-tō-FŌ-bē-a)

Chapter Review

LABELING EXERCISE
Anatomic Divisions of the Nervous System

1. brain
2. spinal cord
3. central nervous system
4. cranial nerves
5. spinal nerves
6. peripheral nervous system

Motor Neuron

1. cell body
2. nucleus
3. dendrites
4. axon covered with myelin sheath
5. axon branch
6. myelin
7. muscle

External Surface of the Brain

1. sulci
2. gyri
3. frontal lobe
4. parietal lobe
5. occipital lobe
6. temporal lobe
7. pons
8. medulla oblongata
9. cerebellum
10. spinal cord

Spinal Cord, Lateral View

1. brain
2. brainstem
3. spinal cord
4. cervical enlargement
5. lumbar enlargement
6. cervical nerves
7. thoracic nerves
8. lumbar nerves
9. sacral nerves
10. coccygeal nerve

Spinal Cord, Cross Section

1. white matter
2. gray matter
3. dorsal horn
4. ventral horn
5. central canal
6. dorsal root of spinal nerve
7. dorsal root ganglion
8. ventral root of spinal nerve
9. spinal nerve

Reflex Pathway

1. receptor
2. sensory neuron
3. spinal cord (CNS)
4. motor neuron
5. effector

TERMINOLOGY

1. c
2. b
3. e
4. a
5. d
6. c
7. e
8. a
9. d
10. b
11. d
12. c
13. e
14. a
15. b
16. a
17. d
18. b
19. c
20. e

21. b
22. d
23. a
24. e
25. c
26. c
27. a
28. e
29. b
30. d
31. cerebrum
32. neuron
33. synapse
34. neuroglia, glial cells
35. cerebrospinal fluid (CSF)
36. meninges
37. reflex
38. autonomic nervous system (ANS)
39. neurotransmitter
40. cerebellum
41. pertaining to a spinal nerve root
42. partial paralysis of half the body
43. absence of a brain
44. inflammation of many nerves
45. pertaining to the cerebral cortex and thalamus
46. treatment of mental disorders
47. total paralysis
48. softening of the brain
49. sleep disorder
50. neurology
51. myelomeningitis
52. ganglionectomy; gangliectomy
53. neuropathy
54. ventriculostomy
55. hemiplegia
56. intracerebellar
57. dyslexia
58. hydrophobia
59. monoplegia
60. T
61. T
62. T
63. F; white
64. F; peripheral
65. F; dendrite
66. T
67. F; dura
68. intramedullary
69. contralateral
70. preganglionic
71. bradylalia
72. sensory
73. ventral
74. efferent
75. ganglionic
76. cortical
77. dural
78. meningeal
79. psychotic
80. ganglia
81. ventricles

82. meninges
83. gyri
84. lumbar puncture; *Lumbar puncture* is a diagnostic procedure for sampling CSF; the others are vascular disorders.
85. hematoma; *Hematoma* is a local collection of clotted blood; the others are neoplasms.
86. mania; *Mania* is a state of elation; the others are parts of the brain.
87. CNS; *CNS* is the central nervous system; the others are behavioral disorders.
88. myeloplegia
89. aphasia
90. hemiparesis
91. myoparesis
92. dysphasia
93. ganglioplegia
94. tetraplegia
95. myelitis
96. bradyphasia
97. hemiplegia
98. gangliitis
99. hemorrhage into the spinal cord
    a. blood
    b. spinal cord
    c. condition of
100. abnormal development of the spinal cord
    a. spinal cord
    b. abnormal
    c. development
    d. condition of
101. inflammation of many nerves and nerve roots
    a. many
    b. nerve
    c. spinal nerve root
    d. inflammation of
102. disturbance of muscle coordination
    a. abnormal, difficult
    b. together
    c. work
    d. condition of

Case Study Questions

1. e
2. b
3. a
4. b
5. c
6. e
7. b
8. e
9. astrocytoma
10. craniotomy
11. seizure
12. hemiparesis
13. aphasia

14. meningitis
15. subdural hematoma
16. paranoia
17. antispasmodic
18. neuroleptics
19. psychiatrist
20. computed tomography
21. lumbar puncture
22. neurological intensive care unit (also means neonatal intensive care unit)
23. intracranial pressure
24. cerebrospinal fluid
25. cerebrovascular accident
26. transient ischemic attack
27. level of consciousness

Chapter 18

Pretest

1. c
2. b
3. a
4. c
5. c
6. a
7. c

Chapter Exercises

EXERCISE 18-1

1. abnormal sensation
2. abnormal sense of smell
3. lack of taste sensation
4. anesthesia (*an-es-THĒ-zē-a*)
5. pseudogeusia (*sū-dō-GŪ-zē-a*)
6. thermesthesia (*ther-mes-THĒ-zē-a*)
7. hyperalgesia (*hī-per-al-JĒ-zē-a*)
8. dysgeusia (*dis-GŪ-zē-a*)
9. myesthesia (*MĪ-es-thē-zē-a*)

EXERCISE 18-2

1. hearing
2. sound
3. ear
4. pertaining to hearing
5. pertaining to the ear
6. pertaining to the labyrinth (inner ear)
7. pertaining to the stapes
8. pertaining to the vestibule or vestibular apparatus
9. pertaining to the cochlea
10. otalgia (*ō-TAL-jē-a*)
11. audiometry (*aw-dē-OM-e-trē*)
12. tympanoplasty (*tim-PAN-ō-plas-tē*)
13. myringotomy (*mir-in-GOT-ō-mē*); also, tympanotomy (*tim-pan-OT-ō-mē*)
14. endocochlear (*en-dō-KOK-lē-ar*); intracochlear (*in-tra-KOK-lē-ar*)

15. vestibulocochlear
    (*ves-tib-ū-lō-KOK-lē-ar*)
16. labyrinthotomy
    (*lab-i-rin-THOT-ō-mē*)
17. salpingoscope (*sal-PING-go-skōp*)
18. stapedectomy (*stā-pē-DEK-ō-mē*)
19. inflammation of the ear
20. instrument used to measure hearing
21. any disease of the vestibule or
    vestibular apparatus
22. pertaining to the eustachian
    (auditory) tube and pharynx
23. instrument used to examine the
    tympanic membrane (eardrum)

EXERCISE 18-3

1. pertaining to the nose and lacrimal
   apparatus
2. between the eyelids
3. paralysis of the eyelid
4. excision of a lacrimal sac
5. blepharospasm (*BLEF-a-rō-spasm*)
6. dacryolith (*DAK-rē-ō-lith*)
7. dacryocystitis (*dak-rē-ō-sis-TĪ-tis*)

EXERCISE 18-4

1. eye
2. vision
3. lens
4. cornea
5. lens
6. opt/o; eye, vision
7. ophthalm/o; eye
8. pupill/o; pupil
9. phac/o; lens
10. uve/o; uvea
11. irid/o; iris
12. lent/i; lens
13. uveoscleritis (*ū-vē-ō-skle-RĪ-tis*)
14. phacomalacia (*fak-ō-ma-LĀ-shē-a*)
15. pupillary (*PU-pi-ler-ē*)
16. retinopexy (*ret-i-nō-PEK-sē*)
17. cyclitis (*sī-KLĪ-tis*)
18. ophthalmoscope
    (*of-THAL-mō-skōp*)
19. ophthalmology (*of-thal-MOL-ō-jē*)
20. iridectomy (*ir-i-DEK-tō-mē*)
21. iridoplegia (*ir-id-ō-PLĒ-jē-a*)
22. pertaining to the right eye
23. splitting of the retina
24. instrument used to incise the sclera
25. pertaining to the eye or vision
26. inflammation of the sclera
27. incision of the ciliary muscle
28. inflammation of the iris and ciliary
    body
29. pertaining to the choroid and retina
30. pertaining to the lens

EXERCISE 18-5

1. macropsia (*ma-KROP-sē-a*)
2. achromatopsia (*a-krō-ma-TOP-sē-a*)
3. diplopia (*dip-LŌ-pē-a*)

4. presbyopia (*pres-bē-Ō-pē-a*)
5. ametropia (*am-e-TRŌ-pē-a*)
6. heterometropia (*het-er-ō-me-TRŌ-pē-a*); also, anisometropia (*an-ī-sō-me-TRŌ-pē-a*)

Chapter Review

LABELING EXERCISE

The Ear

1. outer ear
2. pinna
3. external auditory canal
4. tympanic membrane
5. ossicles of middle ear
6. malleus
7. incus
8. stapes
9. eustachian (auditory) tube
10. inner ear
11. vestibule
12. semicircular canals
13. cochlea

The Eye

1. sclera
2. cornea
3. conjunctival sac
4. choroid
5. ciliary muscle
6. iris
7. pupil
8. lens
9. aqueous humor
10. vitreous body
11. retina
12. fovea
13. optic disk (blind spot)
14. optic nerve

TERMINOLOGY

1. b
2. a
3. e
4. d
5. c
6. d
7. e
8. a
9. c
10. b
11. d
12. c
13. e
14. b
15. a
16. e
17. c
18. b
19. a
20. d
21. b
22. a

23. d
24. e
25. c
26. d
27. b
28. a
29. c
30. e
31. tympanic membrane
32. ear wax
33. stapes
34. sclera
35. refraction
36. retina
37. cornea
38. proprioception
39. specialist in the study and
    treatment of hearing disorders
40. instrument for measuring the eye
41. absence of a lens
42. below the sclera
43. incision of the iris
44. incision of the tympanic membrane
    (eardrum)
45. around the lens
46. excess flow of tears
47. pertaining to the choroid and
    retina
48. inflammation of the cornea and iris
49. retinopathy
50. analgesia
51. stapedectomy
52. blepharoptosis
53. otoplasty
54. vestibulocochlear
55. tympanosclerosis; myringosclerosis
56. pupillometry
57. lacrimal
58. cyclectomy
59. salpingoscopy
60. cochlear
61. palpebral
62. vestibular
63. uveal
64. corneal
65. scleral
66. papillary
67. miosis
68. exotropia
69. sc
70. hyperopia
71. hypoesthesia, hypesthesia
72. OS
73. hyperalgesia
74. pseudosmia
75. myringoplasty
76. retinoscopy
77. salpingoscopy
78. anosmia
79. retinoschisis
80. myringoscopy
81. subretinal

82. retinopexy
83. keratoscopy
84. F; constrict
85. T
86. T
87. F; smell, olfaction
88. F; taste
89. T
90. T
91. F; tympanic membrane
92. F; tears
93. smell; *Smell* is a special sense; the others are general senses.
94. pinna; The *pinna* is part of the outer ear; the others are parts of the inner ear.
95. malleus; The *malleus* is an ossicle of the ear; the others are structures that protect the eye.
96. presbycusis; *Presbycusis* is loss of hearing due to age; the others are disorders of the eye.
97. weakness or tiring of the eyes
   a. lack of
   b. strength
   c. eye
   d. condition of
98. condition in which a cataractous lens has been removed and replaced with a plastic lens implant
   a. false
   b. lens
   c. condition of
99. a cystlike mass containing cholesterol
   a. bile (here, cholesterol, found in bile)
   b. fat
   c. tumor, neoplasm
100. a type of strabismus (squint) in which the eye deviates outward
   a. out
   b. turning
   c. condition of
101. unequal refractive power in the two eyes, heterometropia
   a. not, without
   b. equal, same
   c. measure
   d. eye
   e. condition of

Case Study Questions

1. a
2. a
3. d
4. c
5. e
6. d
7. b
8. d

9. e
10. b
11. tympanogram
12. aural
13. otitis media
14. otitis externa
15. ophthalmologist
16. intraocular
17. miosis
18. midazolam
19. hertz
20. brainstem auditory evoked potentials
21. right eye
22. intraocular lens

Chapter 19

Pretest

1. c
2. a
3. d
4. b
5. c
6. d
7. a
8. c

Chapter Exercises

EXERCISE 19-1

1. bone, bone tissue
2. bone marrow
3. joint
4. cartilage
5. bursa
6. pertaining to or resembling bone
7. formation of bone marrow
8. softening of cartilage
9. surgical puncture of a joint
10. inflammation of a bursa
11. pertaining to synovial fluid, joint or membrane
12. osteomyelitis (*os-tē-ō-mī-e-LĪ-tis*)
13. osteoblast (*OS-tē-ō-blast*)
14. myeloma (*mī-e-LŌ-ma*)
15. bursotomy (*bur-SOT-ō-mē*)
16. synovitis (*si-nō-VĪ-tis*)
17. arthroplasty (*AR-thrō-plas-tē*)
18. arthropathy (*ar-THROP-a-thē*)
19. chondroid (*KON-droyd*), also chondral, cartilaginous
20. arthroscope (*AR-thrō-skōp*)
21. hyperostosis (*hī-per-os-TŌ-sis*)
22. dysostosis (*dis-os-TŌ-sis*)

EXERCISE 19-2

1. cranial
2. costal
3. pelvic
4. iliac
5. vertebral

6. sacral
7. incision of the cranium (skull)
8. before or in front of the spinal column or vertebra
9. pain in a vertebra
10. above the pelvis
11. cranioschisis (*krā-nē-OS-ki-sis*)
12. spondylitis (*spon-di-LĪ-tis*)
13. vertebroplasty (*ver-te-brō-PLAS-tē*)
14. costectomy (*kos-TEK-tō-mē*)
15. rachiocentesis (*rā-kē-ō-sen-TĒ-sis*); also, rachicentesis (*rā-kē-sen-TĒ-sis*)
16. sacroiliac (*sā-krō-IL-ē-ak*)
17. craniosacral (*krā-nē-ō-SĀ-kral*)
18. pelvimetry (*pel-VIM-e-trē*)
19. perisacral (*per-i-SĀ-kral*)
20. coccygectomy (*kok-si-JEK-tō-mē*)
21. iliococcygeal (*il-ē-ō-kok-SIJ-ē-al*)
22. infracostal (*in-fra-KOS-tal*); subcostal (*sub-KOS-tal*)

Chapter Review

LABELING EXERCISE

The Skeleton

1. cranium
2. facial bones
3. mandible
4. vertebral column
5. sacrum
6. sternum
7. ribs
8. clavicle
9. scapula
10. humerus
11. radius
12. ulna
13. carpals
14. metacarpals
15. phalanges
16. pelvis
17. ilium
18. femur
19. patella
20. fibula
21. tibia
22. tarsals
23. calcaneus
24. metatarsals
25. phalanges

Skull from the Left

1. frontal
2. parietal
3. occipital
4. temporal
5. sphenoid
6. lacrimal
7. nasal
8. zygomatic
9. maxilla
10. mandible
11. hyoid

Vertebral Column

1. cervical vertebrae
2. thoracic vertebrae
3. lumbar vertebrae
4. sacrum
5. coccyx
6. intervertebral disk
7. body of vertebra

The Pelvic Bones

1. ilium
2. ischium
3. pubis
4. pubic symphysis
5. acetabulum
6. sacrum

Structure of a Long Bone

1. proximal epiphysis (*e-PIF-i-sis*)
2. diaphysis (*dī-AF-i-sis*)
3. distal epiphysis
4. cartilage
5. epiphyseal line (growth line)
6. spongy bone (containing red marrow)
7. compact bone
8. medullary (marrow) cavity
9. artery and vein
10. yellow marrow
11. periosteum (*per-ē-OS-tē-um*)

TERMINOLOGY

1. d
2. a
3. e
4. c
5. b
6. d
7. a
8. e
9. c
10. b
11. c
12. d
13. e
14. a
15. b
16. d
17. c
18. e
19. b
20. a
21. orthopedics
22. cartilage
23. ligament
24. sacrum
25. bursa
26. synovial fluid; synovia
27. cartilage
28. bone marrow
29. joint, joint cavity
30. vertebrae
31. spine

32. inflammation of the bone marrow
33. formation of bone
34. fusion of a joint
35. excision of a synovial membrane
36. cartilage cell
37. within bone
38. around a bursa
39. inflammation of a vertebra
40. pertaining to many joints
41. below a rib
42. pain in the coccyx
43. chondrogenesis
44. osteonecrosis
45. craniotomy
46. osteochondroma
47. arthrostenosis
48. chondrectomy
49. bursolith
50. pelvimetry
51. arthroscopy
52. sacroiliac
53. coccygectomy
54. parasacral
55. cranial
56. iliac
57. coccygeal
58. pelvic
59. vertebral
60. T
61. F; ankle
62. T
63. F; appendicular
64. T
65. T
66. F; red
67. T
68. T
69. hyoid; The *hyoid* is the bone below the mandible (lower jaw); the others are bone markings.
70. lambdoid; *Lambdoid* refers to a skull suture; the others are bones of the skull.
71. cost/o; *Cost/o* refers to a rib; the others are roots pertaining to the spine.
72. sciatic; *Sciatic* refers to the sciatic nerve that travels through the leg; the others are types of bone fractures.
73. OA; *OA* is an abbreviation for osteoarthritis; the others are abbreviations for spinal regions.
74. osteolysis
75. arthrotome
76. spondylodynia
77. arthrolysis
78. osteotome
79. arthroplasty
80. osteodynia
81. spondylolysis
82. arthrodynia

83. osteoplasty
84. disease of the (cartilaginous) growth center in children
   a. bone
   b. cartilage
   c. condition of
85. surgical fusion (ankylosis) between vertebrae
   a. vertebra
   b. together
   c. fusion, binding
86. bony outgrowth from a bone
   a. out
   b. bone
   c. condition of
87. decreased growth of cartilage in the growth plate of long bones resulting in dwarfism
   a. lack of
   b. cartilage
   c. formation, molding
   d. condition of

Case Study Questions

1. c
2. b
3. c
4. e
5. c
6. a
7. d
8. b
9. zygomatic
10. periosteum
11. meniscus
12. bilateral
13. arthroplasty
14. idiopathic
15. scapulectomy
16. fracture
17. osteotomies
18. degenerative joint disease
19. magnetic resonance imaging
20. nonsteroidal antiinflammatory drugs
21. computed tomography
22. normal saline solution
23. temporomandibular joint
24. osteogenesis imperfecta
25. open reduction internal fixation
26. posterior spinal fusion
27. estimated blood loss

Chapter 20

Pretest

1. b
2. d
3. c
4. d
5. a

6. c
7. b
8. a

Chapter Exercises

EXERCISE 20-1

1. pertaining to muscle
2. pertaining to fascia
3. pertaining to a tendon
4. pertaining to tone
5. pertaining to movement
6. muscle
7. fibers
8. fascia
9. tone
10. work
11. movement, motion
12. muscle
13. muscle; smooth muscle
14. excess muscle tone
15. suture of fascia
16. inflammation of a tendon
17. pertaining to muscle and tendon
18. binding or fusion of a tendon
19. pain in a muscle
20. treatment using movement
21. inflammation of a muscle and a tendon
22. pertaining to muscle and fascia
23. producing or generating work
24. lack of muscle tone
25. abnormality of movement
26. myopathy (mī-OP-a-thē)
27. fasciectomy (fash-ē-EK-tō-mē)
28. tenotomy (ten-OT-ō-mē)
29. polymyositis (pol-ē-mī-ō-SĪ-tis)
30. musculoskeletal (mus-kū-lō-SKEL-e-tal)
31. kinesiology (ki-nē-sē-OL-ō-jē)
32. tenomyoplasty (ten-ō-MĪ-ō-plas-tē)

Chapter Review

LABELING EXERCISE
Superficial Muscles, Anterior View

1. temporalis
2. orbicularis oculi
3. orbicularis oris
4. masseter
5. sternocleidomastoid
6. trapezius
7. deltoid
8. pectoralis major
9. serratus anterior
10. biceps brachii
11. brachioradialis
12. flexor carpi
13. extensor carpi
14. external oblique
15. internal oblique
16. rectus abdominis
17. intercostals
18. sartorius
19. adductors of thigh
20. quadriceps femoris
21. gastrocnemius
22. soleus
23. peroneus longus
24. tibialis anterior

Superficial Muscles, Posterior View

1. sternocleidomastoid
2. trapezius
3. deltoid
4. teres minor
5. teres major
6. latissimus dorsi
7. triceps brachii
8. gluteus medius
9. gluteus maximus
10. hamstring group
11. gastrocnemius
12. peroneus longus

TERMINOLOGY

1. c
2. e
3. d
4. a
5. b
6. e
7. a
8. d
9. b
10. c
11. d
12. c
13. b
14. a
15. e
16. e
17. b
18. a
19. d
20. c
21. c
22. e
23. d
24. b
25. a
26. acetylcholine
27. fascia
28. three
29. extensor
30. tendon
31. Achilles tendon
32. abduction
33. muscle, muscle tissue
34. study of muscles
35. pertaining to muscle and fascia
36. plastic repair of a tendon
37. inflammation of fibers (fibrous tissue)
38. decreased muscle tone
39. abnormally increased movement
40. myositis
41. myonecrosis
42. fasciorrhaphy
43. atony
44. fasciectomy
45. kinesiology
46. tenotomy
47. tendinous
48. antagonist
49. insertion
50. adduction
51. supination
52. flexion
53. ataxic
54. athetotic
55. spastic, spasmodic
56. clonic
57. T
58. T
59. F; insertion
60. F; posterior
61. T
62. T
63. F; four
64. T
65. osteoblast; An *osteoblast* is a bone cell; the others are related to muscle structure.
66. soleus; The *soleus* is a calf muscle; the others are muscles of the arm.
67. intercostals; The *intercostals* are between the ribs; the others are quadriceps muscles in the anterior thigh.
68. actin; *Actin* is a type of muscle filament involved in contraction; the others are types of movement.
69. EMG; *EMG* is electromyography, a method for studying the electrical energy in muscles; the others are diseases that involve muscles.
70. carpal tunnel syndrome
71. acetylcholine
72. rotator cuff
73. neuromuscular junction
74. creatine kinase
75. myoblast
76. fasciodesis
77. tenalgia
78. myolysis
79. tenodesis
80. fasciitis
81. tenolysis
82. fascial
83. myalgia

84. disorder involving muscular
    inflammation and weakness with
    skin inflammation and rash
    a. skin
    b. muscle
    c. inflammation
85. muscular weakness
    a. muscle
    b. lack of
    c. strength
    d. condition of
86. lack of smooth or accurate muscle
    movement because coordination
    between muscle components is
    lacking
    a. abnormal
    b. together
    c. work
    d. condition of
87. pertaining to muscle wasting,
    atrophy
    a. lack of
    b. muscle
    c. nourishment
    d. pertaining to

Case Study Questions

1. b
2. d
3. e
4. a
5. b
6. d
7. c
8. a
9. c
10. d
11. b
12. c
13. c
14. e
15. brachial
16. orthopedic
17. flexion
18. plantar flexion
19. physical therapy
20. range of motion
21. rule out
22. electromyogram
23. somatosensory evoked potentials
24. postanesthesia care unit

Chapter 21

Pretest

1. c
2. a
3. b
4. a

5. b
6. d
7. b

Chapter Exercises

EXERCISE 21-1

1. derm/o; skin
2. seb/o; sebum
3. melan/o; melanin
4. kerat/o; keratin, horny layer of the
   skin
5. hidr/o; sweat
6. trich/o; hair
7. onych/o; nail
8. skin
9. horny (keratinous) layer
10. melanin
11. hair
12. nail
13. sweat, perspiration
14. skin
15. dermatolysis (*der-ma-TOL-i-sis*);
    dermolysis (*der-MOL-i-sis*)
16. melanoma (*mel-a-NŌ-ma*)
17. keratogenesis (*ker-a-tō-JEN-e-sis*)
18. dermatome (*DER-ma-tōm*)
19. trichology (*trik-OL-ō-jē*)
20. hyperhidrosis (*hī-per-hī-DRŌ-sis*)
21. onychomalacia
    (*on-i-kō-ma-LĀ-shē-a*)
22. dermatology (*der-ma-TOL-ō-jē*)
23. scleroderma (*sklēr-ō-DER-ma*)
24. pyoderma (*pī-ō-DER-ma*)

Chapter Review

LABELING EXERCISE

Cross Section of the Skin

1. epidermis
2. stratum basale (growing layer)
3. stratum corneum
4. dermis (corium)
5. subcutaneous layer
6. adipose tissue
7. hair follicle
8. hair
9. arrector pili muscle
10. artery
11. vein
12. nerve
13. nerve endings
14. sudoriferous (sweat) gland
15. pore (opening of sweat gland)
16. sebaceous (oil) gland
17. touch receptor
18. pressure receptor

TERMINOLOGY

1. d
2. a
3. e

4. c
5. b
6. c
7. d
8. b
9. e
10. a
11. a
12. c
13. b
14. e
15. d
16. e
17. d
18. a
19. c
20. b
21. skin
22. sweat, perspiration
23. melanin
24. sebaceous glands
25. keratin
26. excess melanin production
27. through the skin
28. producing keratin
29. excess flow of sebum
30. thickening of the skin
31. infection of a nail and nail bed
32. dryness of the skin
33. abnormal keratin production
34. seborrheic
35. melanocyte
36. scleroderma; dermatosclerosis
37. melanoma
38. hyperkeratosis
39. dermatome
40. anhidrosis
41. hyperhidrosis
42. chromhidrosis
43. T
44. F; stratum corneum
45. T
46. T
47. F; stratum basale
48. F; hair
49. trichoid
50. onychomycosis
51. dermatolysis
52. trichology
53. onycholysis
54. dermatoid
55. onychopathy
56. trichomycosis
57. dermatopathy
58. dermatology
59. keloid; A *keloid* is a raised,
    thickened scar; the others are types
    of skin lesions.
60. escharotomy; *Escharotomy* is
    removal of scab tissue; the others
    are types of skin diseases.

61. BSA; *BSA* is an abbreviation for body surface area; the others are abbreviations for skin diseases.
62. fungal infection of the skin
    a. skin
    b. plant
    c. condition of
63. benign tumor of a sweat gland
    a. sweat
    b. gland
    c. tumor
64. ingrown toenail
    a. nail
    b. hidden
    c. condition of
65. lack of color or graying of the hair
    a. lack of
    b. color
    c. hair
    d. condition of

Case Study Questions

1. b
2. c
3. d
4. e
5. a
6. c
7. b
8. d
9. a
10. e
11. e
12. d
13. dermabrasion
14. nodule
15. dermatologist
16. subcutaneous tissue
17. erythema/erythroderma
18. hyperkeratosis
19. débridement
20. ischemia
21. full-thickness skin graft
22. split-thickness skin graft
23. sun protection factor
24. at bedtime
25. twice per day

Figure Credits

FIGURE 1-3 Cohen B. Memmler's *The Human Body in Health and Disease*. 11th ed. Baltimore: Lippincott Williams & Wilkins, 2009.

FIGURE 2-2 Smeltzer SC, Bare B. *Medical-Surgical Nursing*. 11th ed. Philadelphia: Lippincott Williams & Wilkins, 2009.

FIGURE 2-3 Taylor C, Lillis C, LeMone P. *Fundamentals of Nursing*. 6th ed. Philadelphia: Lippincott Williams & Wilkins, 2006.

FIGURE 2-4 Taylor C, Lillis C, LeMone P. *Fundamentals of Nursing*. 6th ed. Philadelphia: Lippincott Williams & Wilkins, 2006.

FIGURE 2-5 Taylor C, Lillis C, LeMone P. *Fundamentals of Nursing*. 6th ed. Philadelphia: Lippincott Williams & Wilkins, 2006.

FIGURE 2-6 Cormack DH. *Essential Histology*. 2nd ed. Philadelphia: Lippincott Williams & Wilkins, 2001.

FIGURE 2-7 Cohen B. Memmler's *The Human Body in Health and Disease*. 10th ed. Baltimore: Lippincott Williams & Wilkins, 2005.

FIGURE 2-8 Cohen B. Memmler's *The Human Body in Health and Disease*. 10th ed. Baltimore: Lippincott Williams & Wilkins, 2005.

FIGURE 2-9 Cormack DH. *Essential Histology*. 2nd ed. Philadelphia: Lippincott Williams & Wilkins, 2001.

FIGURE 2-10 Cohen B. Memmler's *The Human Body in Health and Disease*. 10th ed. Baltimore: Lippincott Williams & Wilkins, 2005.

FIGURE 3-1 Cohen B. Memmler's *The Human Body in Health and Disease*. 10th ed. Baltimore: Lippincott Williams & Wilkins, 2005.

FIGURE 3-2 Cohen B. Memmler's *The Human Body in Health and Disease*. 10th ed. Baltimore: Lippincott Williams & Wilkins, 2005.

FIGURE 3-3 Koneman EW, et al. *Diagnostic Microbiology*. 6th ed. Philadelphia: Lippincott Williams & Wilkins, 2005.

FIGURE 3-4 Bickley LS. Bates' *Guide to Physical Examination and History Taking*. 10th ed. Philadelphia: Lippincott Williams & Wilkins, 2008.

FIGURE 3-5 Cohen B. Memmler's *The Human Body in Health and Disease*. 10th ed. Baltimore: Lippincott Williams & Wilkins, 2005.

FIGURE 3-6 Taylor C, Lillis C, LeMone P. *Fundamentals of Nursing*. 6th ed. Philadelphia: Lippincott Williams & Wilkins, 2006.

FIGURE 3-7 Cohen B. Memmler's *The Human Body in Health and Disease*. 10th ed. Baltimore: Lippincott Williams & Wilkins, 2005.

FIGURE 3-8 Cohen B. Memmler's *The Human Body in Health and Disease*. 10th ed. Baltimore: Lippincott Williams & Wilkins, 2005.

FIGURE 4-1 Cohen B. Memmler's *The Human Body in Health and Disease*. 10th ed. Baltimore: Lippincott Williams & Wilkins, 2005.

FIGURE 4-2 Cohen B. Memmler's *The Human Body in Health and Disease*. 10th ed. Baltimore: Lippincott Williams & Wilkins, 2005.

FIGURE 4-3 Cohen B. Memmler's *The Human Body in Health and Disease*. 11th ed. Baltimore: Lippincott Williams & Wilkins, 2009.

FIGURE 4-5 Cohen B. Memmler's *The Human Body in Health and Disease*. 11th ed. Baltimore: Lippincott Williams & Wilkins, 2009.

FIGURE 4-6 Parts A and B: Mills SE. *Histology for Pathologists*. 3rd ed. Philadelphia: Lippincott Williams & Wilkins, 2006; Part C: Gartner LP, Hiatt JL. *Color Atlas of Histology*. 5th ed. Baltimore: Lippincott Williams & Wilkins, 2009.

FIGURE 4-7 Part A: Cormack DH: *Essential Histology*. 2nd ed. Baltimore: Lippincott Williams & Wilkins, 2001. Part B: Gartner LP, Hiatt JL. *Color Atlas of Histology*. 5th ed. Baltimore: Lippincott Williams & Wilkins, 2009.

FIGURE 4-8 Cohen B. Memmler's *The Human Body in Health and Disease*. 10th ed. Baltimore: Lippincott Williams & Wilkins, 2005.

FIGURE 4-9 Cohen B. Memmler's *The Human Body in Health and Disease*. 10th ed. Baltimore: Lippincott Williams & Wilkins, 2005.

FIGURE 4-10 Cohen B. Memmler's *The Human Body in Health and Disease*. 10th ed. Baltimore: Lippincott Williams & Wilkins, 2005.

FIGURE 5-1 Cohen B. Memmler's *The Human Body in Health and Disease*. 10th ed. Baltimore: Lippincott Williams & Wilkins, 2005.

FIGURE 5-2 Cohen B. Memmler's *The Human Body in Health and Disease*. 10th ed. Baltimore: Lippincott Williams & Wilkins, 2005.

FIGURE 5-3 Cohen B. Memmler's *The Human Body in Health and Disease*. 10th ed. Baltimore: Lippincott Williams & Wilkins, 2005.

FIGURE 5-4 Cohen B. Memmler's *The Human Body in Health and Disease*. 10th ed. Baltimore: Lippincott Williams & Wilkins, 2005.

FIGURE 5-5 Cohen B. Memmler's *The Human Body in Health and Disease*. 10th ed. Baltimore: Lippincott Williams & Wilkins, 2005.

FIGURE 6-1 Cohen B. Memmler's *The Human Body in Health and Disease*. 10th ed. Baltimore: Lippincott Williams & Wilkins, 2005.

FIGURE 6-2 Cohen B. Memmler's *The Human Body in Health and Disease*. 10th ed. Baltimore: Lippincott Williams & Wilkins, 2005.

FIGURE 6-3 Cohen B. Memmler's *The Human Body in Health and Disease*. 10th ed. Baltimore: Lippincott Williams & Wilkins, 2005.

FIGURE 6-4 Bickley LS. Bates' *Guide to Physical Examination and History Taking*. 10th ed. Philadelphia: Lippincott Williams & Wilkins, 2008.

FIGURE 6-5 Cohen B. Memmler's *The Human Body in Health and Disease*. 10th ed. Baltimore: Lippincott Williams & Wilkins, 2005.

FIGURE 7-1 Taylor C, Lillis C, LeMone P. *Fundamentals of Nursing*. 6th ed. Philadelphia: Lippincott Williams & Wilkins, 2006.

FIGURE 7-2 Taylor C, Lillis C, LeMone P. *Fundamentals of Nursing*. 6th ed. Philadelphia: Lippincott Williams & Wilkins, 2006.

FIGURE 7-3 Taylor C, Lillis C, LeMone P. *Fundamentals of Nursing*. 6th ed. Philadelphia: Lippincott Williams & Wilkins, 2006.

FIGURE 7-4 Taylor C, Lillis C, LeMone P. *Fundamentals of Nursing*. 6th ed. Philadelphia: Lippincott Williams & Wilkins, 2006.

FIGURE 7-5 Taylor C, Lillis C, LeMone P. *Fundamentals of Nursing*. 6th ed. Philadelphia: Lippincott Williams & Wilkins, 2006.

FIGURE 7-6 Taylor C, Lillis C, LeMone P. *Fundamentals of Nursing*. 6th ed. Philadelphia: Lippincott Williams & Wilkins, 2006.

FIGURE 7-8 Erkonen WE. *Radiology 101*. 2nd ed. Philadelphia: Lippincott Williams & Wilkins, 2004.

FIGURE 7-9 Erkonen WE. *Radiology 101*. 2nd ed. Philadelphia: Lippincott Williams & Wilkins, 2004.

FIGURE 7-10 Pilletteri A. *Maternal and Child Health Nursing*. 6th ed. Philadelphia: Lippincott Williams & Wilkins, 2009.

FIGURE 7-12 Taylor C, Lillis C, LeMone P. *Fundamentals of Nursing*. 6th ed. Philadelphia: Lippincott Williams & Wilkins, 2006.

FIGURE 7-13 Smeltzer SC, Bare B. *Medical-Surgical Nursing*. 11th ed. Philadelphia: Lippincott Williams & Wilkins, 2009.

FIGURE 7-14 Taylor C, Lillis C, LeMone P. *Fundamentals of Nursing*. 6th ed. Philadelphia: Lippincott Williams & Wilkins, 2006.

FIGURE 8-1 Rosedahl CB, Kowalski MT. *Textbook of Basic Nursing*. 9th ed. Philadelphia: Lippincott Williams & Wilkins, 2007.

FIGURE 8-4 Taylor C, Lillis C, LeMone P. *Fundamentals of Nursing*. 6th ed. Philadelphia: Lippincott Williams & Wilkins, 2006.

FIGURE 9-1 Cohen B. Memmler's *The Human Body in Health and Disease*. 10th ed. Baltimore: Lippincott Williams & Wilkins, 2005.

FIGURE 9-2 Cohen B. Memmler's *The Human Body in Health and Disease*. 10th ed. Baltimore: Lippincott Williams & Wilkins, 2005.

FIGURE 9-3 Cohen B. Memmler's *The Human Body in Health and Disease*. 10th ed. Baltimore: Lippincott Williams & Wilkins, 2005.

FIGURE 9-4 Smeltzer SC, Bare B. *Medical-Surgical Nursing*. 11th ed. Philadelphia: Lippincott Williams & Wilkins, 2009.

FIGURE 9-7 Bickley LS. Bates' *Guide to Physical Examination and History Taking*. 10th ed. Philadelphia: Lippincott Williams & Wilkins, 2008.

FIGURE 9-8 Cohen B. Memmler's *The Human Body in Health and Disease*. 10th ed. Baltimore: Lippincott Williams & Wilkins, 2005.

FIGURE 9-11 Smeltzer SC, Bare B. *Medical-Surgical Nursing*. 11th ed. Philadelphia: Lippincott Williams & Wilkins, 2009.

FIGURE 9-16A Cohen B. Memmler's *The Human Body in Health and Disease*. 10th ed. Baltimore: Lippincott Williams & Wilkins, 2005.

FIGURE 9-16B Porth CM. *Pathophysiology*. 8th ed. Philadelphia: Lippincott Williams & Wilkins, 2008.

FIGURE 9-17 Bickley LS. Bates' *Guide to Physical Examination and History Taking*. 10th ed. Philadelphia: Lippincott Williams & Wilkins, 2008.

FIGURE 9-18 Cohen B. Memmler's *The Human Body in Health and Disease*. 10th ed. Baltimore: Lippincott Williams & Wilkins, 2005.

FIGURE 9-19 Cohen B. Memmler's *The Human Body in Health and Disease*. 10th ed. Baltimore: Lippincott Williams & Wilkins, 2005.

FIGURE 9-20 Cohen B. Memmler's *The Human Body in Health and Disease*. 10th ed. Baltimore: Lippincott Williams & Wilkins, 2005.

FIGURE 9-21 Bickley LS. Bates' *Guide to Physical Examination and History Taking*. 10th ed. Philadelphia: Lippincott Williams & Wilkins, 2008.

FIGURE 10-1 Cohen B. Memmler's *The Human Body in Health and Disease*. 10th ed. Baltimore: Lippincott Williams & Wilkins, 2005.

FIGURE 10-2 Cohen B. Memmler's *The Human Body in Health and Disease*. 10th ed. Baltimore: Lippincott Williams & Wilkins, 2005.

FIGURE 10-3 Cohen B. Memmler's *The Human Body in Health and Disease*. 10th ed. Baltimore: Lippincott Williams & Wilkins, 2005.

FIGURE 10-4 Cohen B. Memmler's *The Human Body in Health and Disease*. 10th ed. Baltimore: Lippincott Williams & Wilkins, 2005.

FIGURE 10-5 Gartner LP, Hiatt JL. *Color Atlas of Histology*. 5th ed. Philadelphia: Lippincott Williams & Wilkins, 2009.

FIGURE 10-6 Gartner LP, Hiatt JL. *Color Atlas of Histology*. 5th ed. Philadelphia: Lippincott Williams & Wilkins, 2009.

FIGURE 10-7 Cohen B. Memmler's *The Human Body in Health and Disease*. 10th ed. Baltimore: Lippincott Williams & Wilkins, 2005.

FIGURE 10-8 Cohen B. Memmler's *The Human Body in Health and Disease*. 10th ed. Baltimore: Lippincott Williams & Wilkins, 2005.

FIGURE 10-12 Rubin E, Farber JL. *Pathology*. 5th ed. Philadelphia: Lippincott Williams & Wilkins, 2007.

FIGURE 10-13 Rubin R, Strayes DS. *Rubin's Pathology: Clinicopathologic Foundations of Medicine*. 5th ed. Baltimore: Lippincott Williams & Wilkins, 2007.

FIGURE 10-14 Rubin E, Farber JL. *Pathology*. 5th ed. Philadelphia: Lippincott Williams & Wilkins, 2007.

FIGURE 10-15 Rubin E, Farber JL. *Pathology*. 5th ed. Philadelphia: Lippincott Williams & Wilkins, 2007.

FIGURE 10-16 Rubin E, Farber JL. *Pathology*. 5th ed. Philadelphia: Lippincott Williams & Wilkins, 2007.

Box 10-6 Cormack DH. *Essential Histology*. 2nd ed. Philadelphia: Lippincott Williams & Wilkins, 2001.

FIGURE 11-1 Cohen B. Memmler's *The Human Body in Health and Disease*. 10th ed. Baltimore: Lippincott Williams & Wilkins, 2005.

FIGURE 11-2 Cohen B. Memmler's *The Human Body in Health and Disease*. 10th ed. Baltimore: Lippincott Williams & Wilkins, 2005.

FIGURE 11-3 Cohen B. Memmler's *The Human Body in Health and Disease*. 10th ed. Baltimore: Lippincott Williams & Wilkins, 2005.

FIGURE 11-4 Cohen B. Memmler's *The Human Body in Health and Disease*. 10th ed. Baltimore: Lippincott Williams & Wilkins, 2005.

FIGURE 11-5 Cohen B. Memmler's *The Human Body in Health and Disease*. 10th ed. Baltimore: Lippincott Williams & Wilkins, 2005.

FIGURE 11-6 Cohen B. Memmler's *The Human Body in Health and Disease*. 10th ed. Baltimore: Lippincott Williams & Wilkins, 2005.

FIGURE 11-7 Cohen B. Memmler's *The Human Body in Health and Disease*. 11th ed. Baltimore: Lippincott Williams & Wilkins, 2009.

FIGURE 11-9 Rubin E, Farber JL. *Pathology*. 5th ed. Philadelphia: Lippincott Williams & Wilkins, 2007.

FIGURE 11-13 Taylor C, Lillis C, LeMone P. *Fundamentals of Nursing*. 5th ed. Philadelphia: Lippincott Williams & Wilkins, 2005.

FIGURE 11-14 Cohen B. Memmler's *The Human Body in Health and Disease*. 10th ed. Baltimore: Lippincott Williams & Wilkins, 2005.

FIGURE 11-15 Taylor C, Lillis C, LeMone P. *Fundamentals of Nursing*. 5th ed. Philadelphia: Lippincott Williams & Wilkins, 2005.

FIGURE 12-1 Cohen B. Memmler's *The Human Body in Health and Disease*. 10th ed. Baltimore: Lippincott Williams & Wilkins, 2005.

FIGURE 12-2 Cohen B. Memmler's *The Human Body in Health and Disease*. 10th ed. Baltimore: Lippincott Williams & Wilkins, 2005.

FIGURE 12-3 Cohen B. Memmler's *The Human Body in Health and Disease*. 10th ed. Baltimore: Lippincott Williams & Wilkins, 2005.

FIGURE 12-4 Cohen B. Memmler's *The Human Body in Health and Disease*. 10th ed. Baltimore: Lippincott Williams & Wilkins, 2005.

FIGURE 12-5 Cohen B. Memmler's *The Human Body in Health and Disease*. 10th ed. Baltimore: Lippincott Williams & Wilkins, 2005.

FIGURE 12-10 Rubin E, Farber JL. *Pathology*. 5th ed. Philadelphia: Lippincott Williams & Wilkins, 2007.

FIGURE 12-11 Erkonen WE. *Radiology 101*. 2nd ed. Philadelphia: Lippincott Williams & Wilkins, 2004.

FIGURE 12-12 Bickley LS. Bates' *Guide to Physical Examination and History Taking*. 10th ed. Philadelphia: Lippincott Williams & Wilkins, 2008.

FIGURE 12-13 Erkonen WE. *Radiology 101*. 2nd ed. Philadelphia: Lippincott Williams & Wilkins, 2004.

FIGURE 12-16 Stedman's *Medical Dictionary for the Health Professions and Nursing*. 6th ed. Baltimore: Lippincott Williams & Wilkins, 2008.

FIGURE 12-17B Erkonen WE. *Radiology 101*. 2nd ed. Philadelphia: Lippincott Williams & Wilkins, 2004.

FIGURE 13-1 Cohen B. Memmler's *The Human Body in Health and Disease*. 10th ed. Baltimore: Lippincott Williams & Wilkins, 2005.

FIGURE 13-2 Cohen B. Memmler's *The Human Body in Health and Disease*. 10th ed. Baltimore: Lippincott Williams & Wilkins, 2005.

FIGURE 13-3 Cohen B. Memmler's *The Human Body in Health and Disease*. 10th ed. Baltimore: Lippincott Williams & Wilkins, 2005.

FIGURE 13-4 Cohen B. Memmler's *The Human Body in Health and Disease*. 10th ed. Baltimore: Lippincott Williams & Wilkins, 2005.

FIGURE 13-6 Porth CM. *Pathophysiology*. 8th ed. Philadelphia: Lippincott Williams & Wilkins, 2005.

FIGURE 13-9 Rubin E, Farber JL. *Pathology*. 5th ed. Philadelphia: Lippincott Williams & Wilkins, 2007.

FIGURE 13-12 Erkonen WE. *Radiology 101*. 2nd ed. Philadelphia: Lippincott Williams & Wilkins, 2004.

FIGURE 13-13 Rubin E, Farber JL. *Pathology*. 5th ed. Philadelphia: Lippincott Williams & Wilkins, 2007.

FIGURE 13-15 Rubin E, Farber JL. *Pathology*. 5th ed. Philadelphia: Lippincott Williams & Wilkins, 2007.

FIGURE 13-16 Rubin E, Farber JL. *Pathology*. 5th ed. Philadelphia: Lippincott Williams & Wilkins, 2007.

FIGURE 14-1 Cohen B. Memmler's *The Human Body in Health and Disease*. 10th ed. Baltimore: Lippincott Williams & Wilkins, 2005.

FIGURE 14-3 Cohen B. Memmler's *The Human Body in Health and Disease*. 10th ed. Baltimore: Lippincott Williams & Wilkins, 2005.

FIGURE 14-4 Cohen B. Memmler's *The Human Body in Health and Disease*. 10th ed. Baltimore: Lippincott Williams & Wilkins, 2005.

FIGURE 14-6 Rubin E, Farber JL. *Pathology*. 5th ed. Philadelphia: Lippincott Williams & Wilkins, 2007.

FIGURE 15-1 Cohen B. Memmler's *The Human Body in Health and Disease*. 10th ed. Baltimore: Lippincott Williams & Wilkins, 2005.

FIGURE 15-2 Cohen B. Memmler's *The Human Body in Health and Disease*. 10th ed. Baltimore: Lippincott Williams & Wilkins, 2005.

FIGURE 15-3 Cohen B. Memmler's *The Human Body in Health and Disease*. 11th ed. Baltimore: Lippincott Williams & Wilkins, 2005.

FIGURE 15-4 Cohen B. Memmler's *The Human Body in Health and Disease*. 10th ed. Baltimore: Lippincott Williams & Wilkins, 2005.

FIGURE 15-7 Rubin E, Farber JL. *Pathology*. 5th ed. Philadelphia: Lippincott Williams & Wilkins, 2007.

FIGURE 15-10 Erkonen WE. *Radiology 101*. 2nd ed. Philadelphia: Lippincott Williams & Wilkins, 2004.

FIGURE 15-12 Cohen B. Memmler's *The Human Body in Health and Disease*. 10th ed. Baltimore: Lippincott Williams & Wilkins, 2005.

FIGURE 15-13 Pilletteri A. *Maternal and Child Health Nursing*. 6th ed. Philadelphia: Lippincott Williams & Wilkins, 2009.

FIGURE 15-14 Cohen B. Memmler's *The Human Body in Health and Disease*. 10th ed. Baltimore: Lippincott Williams & Wilkins, 2005.

FIGURE 15-15 Cohen B. Memmler's *The Human Body in Health and Disease*. 10th ed. Baltimore: Lippincott Williams & Wilkins, 2005.

FIGURE 15-17 Pilletteri A. *Maternal and Child Health Nursing*. 6th ed. Philadelphia: Lippincott Williams & Wilkins, 2009.

FIGURE 15-18 Pilletteri A. *Maternal and Child Health Nursing*. 6th ed. Philadelphia: Lippincott Williams & Wilkins, 2009.

FIGURE 15-19 Pilletteri A. *Maternal and Child Health Nursing*. 6th ed. Philadelphia: Lippincott Williams & Wilkins, 2009.

FIGURE 15-20 Erkonen WE. *Radiology 101*. 2nd ed. Philadelphia: Lippincott Williams & Wilkins, 2004.

FIGURE 16-1 Cohen B. *Memmler's The Human Body in Health and Disease*. 10th ed. Baltimore: Lippincott Williams & Wilkins, 2005.

FIGURE 16-2 Cohen B. *Memmler's The Human Body in Health and Disease*. 10th ed. Baltimore: Lippincott Williams & Wilkins, 2005.

FIGURE 16-3 Cohen B. *Memmler's The Human Body in Health and Disease.* 10th ed. Baltimore: Lippincott Williams & Wilkins, 2005.

FIGURE 16-5 Cohen B. *Memmler's The Human Body in Health and Disease.* 10th ed. Baltimore: Lippincott Williams & Wilkins, 2005.

FIGURE 16-6 Courtesy of Sandoz Pharmaceutical Corporation, Princeton, NJ.

FIGURE 16-7 Rubin E, Farber JL. *Pathology.* 5th ed. Philadelphia: Lippincott Williams & Wilkins, 2007.

FIGURE 17-1 Cohen B. Memmler's *The Human Body in Health and Disease.* 10th ed. Baltimore: Lippincott Williams & Wilkins, 2005.

FIGURE 17-2 Cohen B. Memmler's *The Human Body in Health and Disease.* 10th ed. Baltimore: Lippincott Williams & Wilkins, 2005.

FIGURE 17-3 Cohen B. Memmler's *The Human Body in Health and Disease.* 10th ed. Baltimore: Lippincott Williams & Wilkins, 2005.

FIGURE 17-4 Cohen B. Memmler's *The Human Body in Health and Disease.* 10th ed. Baltimore: Lippincott Williams & Wilkins, 2005.

FIGURE 17-5 Cohen B. Memmler's *The Human Body in Health and Disease.* 10th ed. Baltimore: Lippincott Williams & Wilkins, 2005.

FIGURE 17-6 Cohen B. Memmler's *The Human Body in Health and Disease.* 10th ed. Baltimore: Lippincott Williams & Wilkins, 2005.

FIGURE 17-7 Cohen B. Memmler's *The Human Body in Health and Disease.* 10th ed. Baltimore: Lippincott Williams & Wilkins, 2005.

FIGURE 17-8 Cohen B. Memmler's *The Human Body in Health and Disease.* 10th ed. Baltimore: Lippincott Williams & Wilkins, 2005.

FIGURE 17-9 Cohen B. Memmler's *The Human Body in Health and Disease.* 10th ed. Baltimore: Lippincott Williams & Wilkins, 2005.

FIGURE 17-10 Cohen B. Memmler's *The Human Body in Health and Disease.* 11th ed. Baltimore: Lippincott Williams & Wilkins, 2005.

FIGURE 17-11 Rubin E, Farber JL. *Pathology.* 4th ed. Philadelphia: Lippincott Williams & Wilkins, 2005.

FIGURE 17-13 Smeltzer SC, Bare B. *Medical-Surgical Nursing.* 11th ed. Philadelphia: Lippincott Williams & Wilkins, 2009.

FIGURE 17-14 Erkonen WE. *Radiology 101.* 2nd ed. Philadelphia: Lippincott Williams & Wilkins, 2004.

FIGURE 17-15 Rubin E, Farber JL. *Pathology.* 5th ed. Philadelphia: Lippincott Williams & Wilkins, 2007.

FIGURE 17-16 Rubin E, Farber JL. *Pathology.* 3rd ed. Philadelphia: Lippincott Williams & Wilkins, 1999.

FIGURE 17-17 Erkonen WE. *Radiology 101. 2nd ed.* Philadelphia: Lippincott Williams & Wilkins, 2004.

FIGURE 18-1 Cohen B. *Memmler's The Human Body in Health and Disease.* 10th ed. Baltimore: Lippincott Williams & Wilkins, 2005.

FIGURE 18-2 Cohen B. *Memmler's The Human Body in Health and Disease.* 10th ed. Baltimore: Lippincott Williams & Wilkins, 2005.

FIGURE 18-3 Image provided by Anatomical Chart Co.

FIGURE 18-4 Cohen B. *Memmler's The Human Body in Health and Disease.* 10th ed. Baltimore: Lippincott Williams & Wilkins, 2005.

FIGURE 18-5 Smeltzer SC, Bare B. *Medical-Surgical Nursing.* 11th ed. Philadelphia: Lippincott Williams & Wilkins, 2009.

FIGURE 18-6 Smeltzer SC, Bare B. *Medical-Surgical Nursing.* 11th ed. Philadelphia: Lippincott Williams & Wilkins, 2009.

FIGURE 18-7 Bickley LS. Bates' *Guide to Physical Examination and History Taking.* 10th ed. Philadelphia: Lippincott Williams & Wilkins, 2008.

FIGURE 18-9 Cohen B. Memmler's *The Human Body in Health and Disease.* 11th ed. Baltimore: Lippincott Williams & Wilkins, 2005.

FIGURE 18-10 Cohen B. Memmler's *The Human Body in Health and Disease.* 10th ed. Baltimore: Lippincott Williams & Wilkins, 2005.

FIGURE 18-11 Cohen B. Memmler's *The Human Body in Health and Disease.* 10th ed. Baltimore: Lippincott Williams & Wilkins, 2005.

FIGURE 18-12 Moore KL, Dalley AF. *Clinically Oriented Anatomy.* 6th ed. Philadelphia: Lippincott Williams & Wilkins, 2009.

FIGURE 18-13 Cohen B. Memmler's *The Human Body in Health and Disease.* 10th ed. Baltimore: Lippincott Williams & Wilkins, 2005.

FIGURE 18-14 Smeltzer SC, Bare B. *Medical-Surgical Nursing.* 11th ed. Philadelphia: Lippincott Williams & Wilkins, 2009.

FIGURE 18-15 Smeltzer SC, Bare B. *Medical-Surgical Nursing.* 11th ed. Philadelphia: Lippincott Williams & Wilkins, 2009.

FIGURE 18-16 Rubin E, Farber JL. *Pathology.* 5th ed. Philadelphia: Lippincott Williams & Wilkins, 2007.

FIGURE 19-1 Cohen B. Memmler's *The Human Body in Health and Disease.* 10th ed. Baltimore: Lippincott Williams & Wilkins, 2005.

FIGURE 19-2 Cohen B. Memmler's *The Human Body in Health and Disease.* 10th ed. Baltimore: Lippincott Williams & Wilkins, 2005.

FIGURE 19-3 Cohen B. Memmler's *The Human Body in Health and Disease.* 10th ed. Baltimore: Lippincott Williams & Wilkins, 2005.

FIGURE 19-4 Cohen B. Memmler's *The Human Body in Health and Disease.* 10th ed. Baltimore: Lippincott Williams & Wilkins, 2005.

FIGURE 19-5 Cohen B. Memmler's *The Human Body in Health and Disease.* 10th ed. Baltimore: Lippincott Williams & Wilkins, 2005.

FIGURE 19-6 Rubin R, Strayer DS. *Rubin's Pathology: Clinicopathologic Foundations of Medicine.* 5th ed. Baltimore: Lippincott Williams & Wilkins, 2007.

FIGURE 19-7 Cohen B. Memmler's *The Human Body in Health and Disease.* 10th ed. Baltimore: Lippincott Williams & Wilkins, 2005.

FIGURE 19-8 Erkonen WE. *Radiology 101.* 2nd ed. Philadelphia: Lippincott Williams & Wilkins, 2004.

FIGURE 19-10 Rubin E, Farber JL. *Pathology.* 5th ed. Philadelphia: Lippincott Williams & Wilkins, 2007.

FIGURE 19-11 Erkonen WE. *Radiology 101.* 2nd ed. Philadelphia: Lippincott Williams & Wilkins, 2004.

FIGURE 19-13 Rubin E, Farber JL. *Pathology.* 5th ed. Philadelphia: Lippincott Williams & Wilkins, 2007.

FIGURE 19-15 Rubin E, Farber JL. *Pathology.* 5th ed. Philadelphia: Lippincott Williams & Wilkins, 2007.

FIGURE 19-16 Erkonen WE. *Radiology 101*. 2nd ed. Philadelphia: Lippincott Williams & Wilkins, 2004.

FIGURE 19-17B Erkonen WE. *Radiology 101*. 2nd ed. Philadelphia: Lippincott Williams & Wilkins, 2004.

FIGURE 20-2 Cohen B. Memmler's *The Human Body in Health and Disease*. 10th ed. Baltimore: Lippincott Williams & Wilkins, 2005.

FIGURE 20-3 Cohen B. Memmler's *The Human Body in Health and Disease*. 10th ed. Baltimore: Lippincott Williams & Wilkins, 2005.

FIGURE 20-4 Cohen B. Memmler's *The Human Body in Health and Disease*. 10th ed. Baltimore: Lippincott Williams & Wilkins, 2005.

FIGURE 20-5 Cohen B. Memmler's *The Human Body in Health and Disease*. 10th ed. Baltimore: Lippincott Williams & Wilkins, 2005.

FIGURE 20-6 Cohen B. Memmler's *The Human Body in Health and Disease*. 10th ed. Baltimore: Lippincott Williams & Wilkins, 2005.

FIGURE 20-7 Cohen B. Memmler's *The Human Body in Health and Disease*. 10th ed. Baltimore: Lippincott Williams & Wilkins, 2005.

FIGURE 20-8 Adapted from Frontera WR, Silver JS. *Essentials of Physical Medicine and Rehabilitation*. 2nd ed. Philadelphia: Hanley and Belfus, 2008.

FIGURE 20-9 Stedman's *Medical Dictionary*. 28th ed. Baltimore: Lippincott Williams & Wilkins, 2006.

FIGURE 21-1 Cohen B. Memmler's *The Human Body in Health and Disease*. 10th ed. Baltimore: Lippincott Williams & Wilkins, 2005.

FIGURE 21-2A Bickley LS. Bates' *Guide to Physical Examination and History Taking*. 10th ed. Philadelphia: Lippincott Williams & Wilkins, 2008.

FIGURE 21-2B Cohen B. Memmler's *The Human Body in Health and Disease*. 10th ed. Baltimore: Lippincott Williams & Wilkins, 2005.

FIGURE 21-3 Rubin E, Farber JL. *Pathology*. 5th ed. Philadelphia: Lippincott Williams & Wilkins, 2007.

FIGURE 21-4 Cohen B. Memmler's *The Human Body in Health and Disease*. 10th ed. Baltimore: Lippincott Williams & Wilkins, 2005.

FIGURE 21-5 Hall JC. Sauer's *Manual of Skin Diseases*. 9th ed. Philadelphia: Lippincott Williams & Wilkins, 2006.

FIGURE 21-6 Bickley LS. Bates' *Guide to Physical Examination and History Taking*. 10th ed. Philadelphia: Lippincott Williams & Wilkins, 2008.

FIGURE 21-7 Bickley LS. Bates' *Guide to Physical Examination and History Taking*. 10th ed. Philadelphia: Lippincott Williams & Wilkins, 2008.

FIGURE 21-8 Hall JC. Sauer's *Manual of Skin Diseases*. 9th ed. Baltimore: Lippincott Williams & Wilkins, 2006.

FIGURE 21-9 Bickley LS. Bates' *Guide to Physical Examination and History Taking*. 10th ed. Philadelphia: Lippincott Williams & Wilkins, 2008.

FIGURE 21-10 Bickley LS. Bates' *Guide to Physical Examination and History Taking*. 10th ed. Philadelphia: Lippincott Williams & Wilkins, 2008.

FIGURE 21-11 The American Cancer Society, American Academy of Dermatology.

FIGURE 21-12 Bickley LS. Bates' *Guide to Physical Examination and History Taking*. 10th ed. Philadelphia: Lippincott Williams & Wilkins, 2008.

FIGURE 21-13 Bickley LS. Bates' *Guide to Physical Examination and History Taking*. 10th ed. Philadelphia: Lippincott Williams & Wilkins, 2008.

FIGURE 21-14 Smeltzer SC, Bare B. *Medical-Surgical Nursing*. 11th ed. Philadelphia: Lippincott Williams & Wilkins, 2009.

FIGURE 21-15 Bickley LS. Bates' *Guide to Physical Examination and History Taking*. 10th ed. Philadelphia: Lippincott Williams & Wilkins, 2008.

FIGURE 21-16 Smeltzer SC, Bare B. *Medical-Surgical Nursing*. 11th ed. Philadelphia: Lippincott Williams & Wilkins, 2009.

FIGURE 21-17 Bickley LS. Bates' *Guide to Physical Examination and History Taking*. 10th ed. Philadelphia: Lippincott Williams & Wilkins, 2008.

FIGURE 21-18 Smeltzer SC, Bare B. *Medical-Surgical Nursing*. 11th ed. Philadelphia: Lippincott Williams & Wilkins, 2004.

FIGURE 21-19 Bickley LS. Bates' *Guide to Physical Examination and History Taking*. 10th ed. Philadelphia: Lippincott Williams & Wilkins, 2008.

Index of Boxes

Health Professions

Index